MEDICAL
THERAPEUTICS

MEDICAL
THERAPEUTICS

THIRD EDITION

Eric B. Larson, MD, MPH

Medical Director
University of Washington Medical Center
Seattle, Washington
Associate Dean for Clinical Affairs and Professor of Medicine
University of Washington School of Medicine

Paul G. Ramsey, MD

Vice President for Medical Affairs and
Dean of the School of Medicine
University of Washington
Seattle, Washington

W.B. SAUNDERS COMPANY
A Division of Harcourt Brace & Company
Philadelphia   London   Toronto   Montreal   Sydney   Tokyo

W.B. SAUNDERS COMPANY

A Division of Harcourt Brace & Company

The Curtis Center
Independence Square West
Philadelphia, Pennsylvania 19106

Library of Congress Cataloging-in-Publication Data

Medical therapeutics / [edited by] Eric B. Larson, Paul G. Ramsey. —
  3rd ed.
     p.   cm.
    Includes bibliographical references and index.
    ISBN 0-7216-5126-7
    1. Internal medicine.   2. Therapeutics.   I. Larson, Eric B.
II. Ramsey, Paul.
    [DNLM: 1. Therapeutics—handbooks.   WB 39 M488 1998]
    RC46.M4754   1998
    616—dc21
    DNLM/DLC

                              97-7148

MEDICAL THERAPEUTICS   ISBN 0-7216-5126-7

Printed in the United States of America

Last digit is the print number: 9   8   7   6   5   4   3   2   1

CONTRIBUTORS
CONTRIBUTORS
CONTRIBUTORS

KENNETH A. ARNDT, MD
Professor of Dermatology, Harvard Medical School; Dermatologist-in-Chief, Beth Israel Deaconess Medical Center, Boston, Massachusetts
Dermatologic Diseases

JEFFREY P. BAKER, MD
Clinical Professor, Stanford University School of Medicine, Stanford, California; Chief, Division of Gastroenterology, Santa Clara Valley Medical Center, San Jose, California
Nutritional Therapeutics

MARK BERNHARDT, MD
Consultant in Dermatology, Broward General Medical Center and Holy Cross Hospital, Fort Lauderdale, Florida
Dermatologic Diseases

ROBERT L. CARITHERS, JR., MD
Professor of Medicine, University of Washington School of Medicine; Director, Section of Hepatology, Division of Gastroenterology, University of Washington Medical Center, Seattle, Washington
Liver Diseases

WILLIAM L. DALEY, MD, MPH
Clinical Instructor of Medicine, Harvard Medical School, Boston, Massachusetts; Co-Director, Cardiac Catheterization Laboratory and Interventional Cardiology, West Roxbury Veterans Administration Medical Center, West Roxbury, Massachusetts; Physician Scientist, Brigham and Women's Hospital, Boston, Massachusetts
Cardiovascular Diseases

ALLAN S. DETSKY, MD, PhD
Professor, University of Toronto; Director, Division of General Internal Medicine and Clinical Epidemiology, The Toronto Hospital, Toronto, Ontario, Canada
Nutritional Therapeutics

DAVID C. DUGDALE, MD
Associate Professor, Department of Medicine, University of Washington School of Medicine, Seattle, Washington
General Medical Care; Fluid and Electrolyte Therapy; Hypertension

LESLIE S. T. FANG, MD, PhD
Assistant Professor of Medicine, Harvard Medical School; Chief, Walter Bauer Firm, Medical Service, Massachusetts General Hospital, Boston, Massachusetts
Renal Diseases

GREGORY C. GARDNER, MD
Associate Professor, Division of Rheumatology, University of Washington School of Medicine, Seattle, Washington
Rheumatic Disorders

BRUCE C. GILLILAND, MD
Professor of Medicine and Laboratory Medicine, Division of Rheumatology, University of Washington School of Medicine, Seattle, Washington
Rheumatic Disorders

JULIE R. GRALOW, MD
Acting Instructor, University of Washington School of Medicine; Affiliate Investigator, Fred Hutchinson Cancer Research Center, Seattle, Washington
Oncologic Therapeutics

KAREN J. HUNT, MD
Acting Assistant Professor, University of Washington School of Medicine, University of Washington Medical Center, Seattle, Washington
Oncologic Therapeutics

W. CONRAD LILES, MD, PhD
Assistant Professor of Medicine, University of Washington School of Medicine; Chairman, Infection Control Committee, and Co-Director, Infectious Diseases and Tropical Medicine Clinic, University of Washington Medical Center, Seattle, Washington
Infectious Diseases

AJIT LIMAYE, MD
Senior Fellow in Infectious Diseases and Laboratory Medicine, University of Washington School of Medicine, Seattle, Washington
Infectious Diseases

ROBERT B. LIVINGSTON, MD
Professor of Medicine and Head of the Division of Oncology, University of Washington School of Medicine; Attending Physician, University of Washington Medical Center, Seattle, Washington
Oncologic Therapeutics

TERRY J. MENGERT, MD
Associate Professor of Medicine, University of Washington School of Medicine; Attending Physician, Department of Medicine, Emergency Medicine Service, University of Washington Medical Center, Seattle, Washington
Pulmonary Conditions

STEPHEN H. PETERSDORF, MD
Assistant Professor, University of Washington School of Medicine; Acting Clinical Director, High Dose Chemotherapy Unit, University of Washington Medical Center, Seattle, Washington
Oncologic Therapeutics

THOMAS H. PRICE, MD
Professor of Medicine, University of Washington School of Medicine; Medical Director, Puget Sound Blood Center, Seattle, Washington
Hematology and Transfusion Medicine

PAUL G. RAMSEY, MD
Vice President for Medical Affairs and Dean of the School of Medicine, University of Washington, Seattle, Washington
Infectious Diseases

DOMINIC F. REILLY, MD
Assistant Professor, University of Washington School of Medicine; Director, Medicine Consult Service, University of Washington Medical Center, Seattle, Washington
General Medical Care

NORMAN R. ROSENTHAL, MD
Clinical Associate Professor of Medicine, University of Washington School of Medicine; Staff Physician, Endocrinology Section, Virginia Mason Medical Center, Seattle, Washington
Endocrinologic and Related Metabolic Disorders

RICHARD P. SHANNON, MD
Associate Professor of Medicine, Harvard Medical School, Boston, Massachusetts; Chief, Cardiovascular Division, Brockton, West Roxbury Veterans Administration Medical Center, West Roxbury, Massachusetts; Cardiovascular Division, Brigham and Women's Hospital, Boston, Massachusetts
Cardiovascular Diseases

LAWRENCE R. SOLOMON, MD
Associate Clinical Professor of Medicine, Yale University School of Medicine; Medical Director, Intermediate Care Facility, Yale University Health Services, New Haven, Connecticut
Hematology and Transfusion Medicine

A. HILLARY STEINHART, MD
Assistant Professor, University of Toronto; Staff Physician, Division of Gastroenterology, Mount Sinai Hospital, Toronto, Ontario, Canada
Nutritional Therapeutics

PHILLIP D. SWANSON, MD, PhD
Professor of Neurology, University of Washington School of Medicine; Attending Physician, University of Washington Affiliated Hospitals, Seattle, Washington
Neurologic Diseases

THOMAS R. VIGGIANO, MD
Assistant Professor of Medicine, Mayo Medical School; Staff Consultant, Mayo Clinic, St. Mary's Hospital, Rochester Methodist Hospital, Rochester, Minnesota
Gastrointestinal Diseases

KENNETH K. WANG, MD
Assistant Professor, Mayo Medical School; Consultant, Mayo Clinic and Foundation, Rochester, Minnesota
Gastrointestinal Diseases

PREFACE
PREFACE

PREFACE

Medical Therapeutics is designed to guide both seasoned and apprentice clinicians as they apply available therapies to a broad range of medical disorders. The material is presented in outline format to enable you to identify quickly specific recommendations for treatments. Descriptions of disease manifestations and pathophysiology are relatively brief. *Medical Therapeutics* is intended to help the health professional in everyday patient care, whether in the hospital or in the outpatient setting. The information presented in this manual should be used as a practical supplement to a comprehensive textbook of medicine, such as *The Cecil Textbook of Medicine* or *Harrison*.

The first edition of the *Cecil Textbook of Medicine* was published in 1927. In the subsequent seven decades, biomedical research has revolutionized the practice of medicine, and scientific advances have led to dramatic improvements in therapeutic skills. Paul Beeson, a former editor of *Cecil*, described this revolution in medical therapeutics in his paper "Changes in Medical Therapy During the Past Half Century." This paper documents the vastly expanded range of effective therapies available in all areas of medicine. Treatments recommended for 60% of diseases covered in the first edition of *Cecil* were classified as "harmful," "useless," "of questionable value," or merely "symptomatic." In 1927, only 6% of diseases had treatments considered to be "effective," "helpful," or "highly effective." In striking contrast, these ratings for effective therapy could be applied to more than 50% of diseases a half century later. The therapeutic revolution analyzed by Dr. Beeson continues, as documented in this manual devoted to therapeutics.

As editors, we have endeavored to emphasize *effective* treatments and to provide guidelines to administer and monitor treatments. The third edition contains significant new information reflecting advances and changes in therapeutics since the previous editions. Virtually all the changes are based on randomized trials or on the most rigorous published material. Most reflect improved precision in the management of acute and chronic diseases. A few changes, like eradication of *Helicobacter pylori* as a cure for peptic ulcer disease, represent dramatic changes in medical therapeutics.

Continued advances will occur, however, and we urge the user of *Medical Therapeutics* to stay current by using information in journals, especially those that emphasize therapeutics like *ACP Journal Club* and *Evidence Based Medi-*

cine, and information in drug handbooks, such as *Physicians' Desk Reference* and the *Medical Letter,* and by participation in continuing medical education programs.

ERIC B. LARSON, MD
PAUL G. RAMSEY, MD

References

Beeson PB. Changes in medical therapy during the past half century. Medicine 1980;59:79–99.
Larson EB, Sheffield JVL. Evolution of clinically important advances in general internal medicine. ACP J Club Sept/Oct 1996;A14–16.

CONTENTS

CONTENTS
CONTENTS

DOMINIC F. REILLY

CARDIAC ARRHYTHMIAS
1. **Ventricular fibrillation or pulseless ventricular tachycardia**
    a. Cardioversion 200 J, 200–300 J, up to 360 J.
    b. Start CPR; intubate; establish IV access.
    c. Epinephrine 1 mg IV; repeat every 3 to 5 minutes.
    d. Defibrillate 360 J.
    e. Lidocaine 1–1.5 mg/kg IV.
    f. Defribrillate 360 J.
    g. Repeat lidocaine 1–1.5 mg/kg to maximum of 3 mg/kg.
    h. Alternate defibrillatory shocks with additional antiarrhythmics:
       • Bretylium 5 mg/kg IV; repeat in 5 minutes at 10 mg/kg.
       • Procainamide 30 mg/min up to 17 mg/kg (1.2 g for 70 kg patient).
       • Magnesium sulfate 1–2 g IV for torsades de pointes or refractory ventricular fibrillation.
    i. Consider sodium bicarbonate 1 mEq/kg IV.
2. **Ventricular tachycardia (stable, with pulse)**
    a. Obtain control of airway; administer oxygen; establish IV access.
    b. Lidocaine 1–1.5 mg/kg IV bolus; repeat 0.5–0.75 mg/kg IV every 5 to 10 minutes up to 3 mg/kg. If successful, start IV lidocaine infusion at 1–4 mg/min.
    c. Procainamide 20–30 mg/min IV up to 17 mg/kg (1.2 g for 70 kg patient), followed by a continuous infusion of 1–4 mg/min if successful.
    d. Bretylium 5–10 mg/kg IV over 8 to 10 minutes; repeat, if needed, up to 30 mg/kg. Follow with infusion of 1–2 mg/min if successful.
    e. If no response, consider adenosine for potentially aberrant supraventricular tachycardia: adenosine 6 mg rapid IV push followed by 20 mL saline flush. If no response, repeat with 12 mg rapid IV push.
    f. Synchronous cardioversion starting at 100 J.
3. **Asystole**
    a. Initiate CPR; intubate; obtain IV access.
    b. Confirm asystole in more than one lead and check "gain" on monitor.
    c. Consider and treat possible causes (hypoxia, hyperkalemia, hypokalemia, acidosis, drug overdose, hypothermia).
    d. Consider immediate transcutaneous pacing.
    e. Epinephrine 1 mg IV; repeat every 3 to 5 minutes.
    f. Atropine 1 mg IV; repeat every 3 to 5 minutes up to 0.04 mg/kg.
    g. Consider sodium bicarbonate 1 mEq/kg IV.
4. **Pulseless electrical activity (formerly electromechanical dissociation)**
    a. Initiate CPR; intubate; obtain IV access.
    b. Consider and treat possible causes (hypoxemia, hypovolemia, cardiac

tamponade, severe acidosis, tension pneumothorax, hyperkalemia, hypothermia, pulmonary embolism, drug overdose).

   c. Epinephrine 1 mg IV; repeat every 3 to 5 minutes.

   d. Consider atropine 1 mg IV if bradycardia; repeat every 3 to 5 minutes up to 0.04 mg/kg.

   e. Consider sodium bicarbonate 1 mEq/kg IV.

5. Bradycardia

   a. Obtain control of airway; administer oxygen; establish IV access.

   b. Atropine 0.5–1 mg IV; repeat every 3 to 5 minutes up to 0.04 mg/kg.

   c. Transcutaneous pacing.

   d. Dopamine 5–20 µg/kg/min IV.

   e. Epinephrine 2–10 µg/kg/min IV.

   f. Transvenous pacemaker.

6. Paroxysmal supraventricular tachycardia

   a. Obtain control of airway; administer oxygen; establish IV access.

     Unstable

   b. Consider sedation.

   c. Synchronous cardioversion 50 J, 100 J, 200 J, 300 J, and 360 J.

     Stable

   b. Consider vagal maneuvers.

   c. Adenosine 6 mg IV rapid push, followed by 20 mL saline flush. If no response, repeat with 12 mg IV.

   d. Verapamil 2.5–5 mg IV over 2 to 3 minutes; repeat in 15 to 30 minutes with 5–10 mg IV.

   e. Consider the *cautious* use of beta blockers (esmolol, propranolol) or synchronous cardioversion starting at 50 J.

7. Premature ventricular contractions (PVCs)

   a. Correct hypoxemia and electrolyte abnormalities. In general, pharmacologic therapy is not required unless there is evidence of ongoing myocardial ischemia.

   b. Lidocaine 1 mg/kg IV load, with 1–4 mg/min IV infusion.

   c. Consider magnesium sulfate 8–16 mEq IV over 5 to 60 minutes, followed by 4–8 mEq/h infusion.

SHOCK

1. Cardiogenic

   a. Dobutamine (250 mg in 500 mL D_5W = 500 µg/mL). Start at low dose and increase according to hemodynamic response (2–20 µg/kg/min).

   b. Dopamine (200 mg in 250 mL D_5W = 800 µg/mL). Start at low dose and increase according to hemodynamic response (2–5 µg/kg/min initially; may increase to 50 µg/kg/min).

   c. Consider nitroprusside (50 mg in 250 mL D_5W = 200 µg/mL); start at 0.1–5 µg/kg/min and titrate according to hemodynamic response to a maximum dose of 10 µg/kg/min.

2. **Septic**
   a. Support blood pressure with fluid (crystalloid or colloid).
   b. Dopamine as above; *or*
   c. Norepinephrine (Levophed) (4 mg in 500 mL D_5W = 8 µg/mL); start at low dose and increase according to hemodynamic response (2–32 µg/min).

3. **Anaphylactic**
   a. Epinephrine 0.3–0.5 mg (0.3–0.5 mL of a 1:1000 dilution) given SC or IM or 0.1–0.25 mg (1–2.5 mL of a 1:10,000 dilution) given IV if hypotension present.
   b. Support blood pressure with fluids, and vasopressors if necessary.
   c. Consider corticosteroids.

STATUS ASTHMATICUS
   a. Albuterol or metoproterenol inhaled via nebulizer; repeat as necessary.
   b. Methylprednisolone 125 mg IV.
   c. Epinephrine 0.3–0.5 mg (0.3 mL of 1:1000 dilution) SC or IM or terbutaline 0.25 mg SC; may repeat once in 15 to 30 minutes.
   d. Aminophylline 5–6 mg/kg IV over 20 to 30 minutes, followed by infusion at 0.2–0.5 mg/kg/h.

PULMONARY EDEMA
   a. Furosemide (Lasix) 0.5–1 mg/kg IV.
   b. Morphine sulfate 1–3 mg IV.
   c. Nitroglycerin 5–25 µg/min IV or 1–2 inches of paste.

HYPERKALEMIA
   a. Calcium gluconate 10 mL or 1 ampule IV over 2 to 5 minutes (use if K^+ > 8 mmol/L or ECG changes are present).
   b. Sodium bicarbonate 50 mEq or 1 ampule IV over 2 to 5 minutes.
   c. Glucose (250 mL of 20% glucose) IV *and* regular insulin 10 units IV.
   d. Sodium polystyrene sulfonate (Kayexalate) 15–30 g in 50–100 mL of water given orally *or* 50 g of Kayexalate *plus* 50 g sorbitol in 250 mL of water rectally (retain for 30 to 45 minutes).
   e. Consider hemodialysis.

HYPERTENSIVE ENCEPHALOPATHY
   a. Nitroprusside 50 mg in 250 mL D_5W = 200 µg/mL. Start at 0.25–2.5 µg/kg/min and titrate according to hemodynamic response. Invasive arterial monitoring recommended; *or*
   b. Labetalol 20 mg IV initially; then 40–80 mg IV every 10 minutes. May also be given as continuous infusion of 2 mg/min IV. Do not exceed a total cumulative dose of 300 mg IV; *or*

    c. Esmolol 5 g diluted in 480 mL D_5W. Loading dose of 500 µg/kg over 1 minute followed by maintenance infusion dose of 50 µg/kg/min for 4 minutes. May increase infusion by increments of 50 µg/kg/min every 4 minutes up to a maximum rate of 200 µg/kg/min; each preceded by a loading dose of 500 µg/kg/min for 1 minute.

STATUS EPILEPTICUS

    a. Benzodiazepines for immediate control: diazepam 5–10 mg IV or lorazepam 1–2 mg IV.

    b. Phenobarbital or phenytoin for prolonged control: phenobarbital 150–400 mg IV; may repeat in 20 minutes with 150–250 mg IV; or phenytoin 1000 mg IV loading dose. (Do not exceed 50 mg/min; monitor blood pressure closely for hypotension and do not mix phenytoin with solution other than sodium chloride.)

NOTICE

Medicine is an ever-changing field. Standard safety precautions must be followed, but as new research and clinical experience broaden our knowledge, changes in treatment and drug therapy become necessary or appropriate. Readers are advised to check the product information currently provided by the manufacturer of each drug to be administered to verify the recommended dose, the method and duration of administration, and contraindications. It is the responsibility of the treating physician relying on experience and knowledge of the patient to determine dosages and the best treatment for the patient. Neither the publisher nor the editors assume any responsibility for any injury and/or damage to persons or property.

The Publisher

1

GENERAL MEDICAL CARE

DAVID C. DUGDALE
DOMINIC F. REILLY

Therapeutic plans must be individually tailored for patients, taking into consideration such factors as age, underlying diseases, and psychosocial issues.

Evaluation of therapeutic efficacy, compliance, potential drug interactions, adverse effects, and cost should be routine as part of the planning and monitoring of medical care. Unexpected or new adverse effects of a medication should be reported to the Food and Drug Administration.

I. MEDICAL ORDER WRITING

Medical orders communicate essential patient information and therapeutic plans. If you use a systematic approach to order writing and if you write legibly and avoid ambiguity and confusing abbreviations, you will minimize errors. The mnemonic ADCA VAN DIMLS stands for the essential order categories.

Admitting order: noting physician(s) responsible for the patient
Diagnosis
Condition
Allergies
Vital signs: frequency of monitoring and conditions for which the physician(s) should be notified
Activity level
Nursing: instructions for general care
Diet
Intravenous (IV) orders
Medication orders
Laboratory studies
Special orders: miscellaneous instructions

Personal discussion of medical orders with the individual who will carry them out improves patient care. Regular review of orders—especially medications—helps ensure appropriate care.

II. DRUG INTERACTIONS AND EFFECTS

A. Calculation of Drug Doses

Many adverse effects occur when dosages inappropriate for a patient's size or physiologic status are ordered. Others are mediated by interactions between medications. Constant attention to detail is required to maintain therapeutic effect while minimizing adverse effects. The following information may be useful in calculating drug doses.

1. CREATININE CLEARANCE = $[(140 - \text{age})/\text{serum creatinine (mg/dL)}] \times \text{weight (kg)}/72$ (multiply by 0.85 for women)
   (A good estimate if serum creatinine less than 5 mg/dL)

2. IDEAL BODY MASS
    a. **Women:** 45 kg for first 152 cm (60 in.) + 0.9 kg/cm over 152 *or* 2.3 kg/in. over 60
    b. **Men:** 48 kg for first 152 cm (60 in.) + 1.1 kg/cm over 152 *or* 2.8 kg/in. over 60
3. BODY SURFACE AREA (BSA)
    a. **Nomogram:** See Figure 1–1.
    b. **Formula:** BSA (m^2) = square root of {[height (cm) × weight (kg)]/3600}
4. ALTERATION OF DRUG DOSE IN RENAL DYSFUNCTION. See page 247.

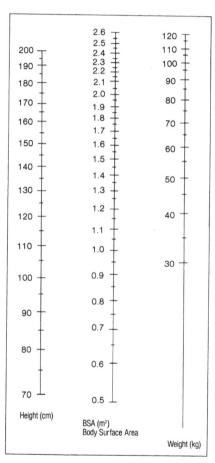

FIGURE 1–1. Body surface area (BSA) nomogram. The BSA is indicated where a straight line connecting the height and weight levels intesects the surface area column. (Adapted from Behrman RE, Vaughan VC. Nelson's Textbook of Pediatrics, 12th ed. Philadelphia: W.B. Saunders Company; 1983, p 1814.)

B. Pharmacokinetics and Pharmacodynamics

Morbidity from drug interactions may be avoided by using only essential drugs, monitoring compliance and adverse effects, and measuring drug levels and effects when appropriate. Drug interactions may be pharmacodynamic, in which one drug changes a patient's response to another drug without affecting its serum level (e.g., the induction of digoxin toxicity by diuretic-induced hypokalemia or added sedation using both narcotics and benzodiazepines), or pharmacokinetic, in which the object drug's pharmacokinetics and, therefore, serum level are changed. **Mechanisms of pharmacokinetic interactions** include:

1. ABSORPTIVE EFFECTS (enteral route) may be mediated by binding (e.g., cholestyramine and digoxin) or pH (e.g., antacids and tetracycline) effects.

2. DISTRIBUTION EFFECTS, such as by altered protein binding, may occur with medications that are greater than 90% protein bound. Drug effects generally correlate with free drug levels, which may be altered by competition for protein binding. For example, sodium valproate may increase free serum phenytoin levels. Onset of such an interaction may be delayed, depending on the level of the second drug that is required to produce it.

3. CLEARANCE EFFECTS may occur with medications that induce (barbiturates and rifampin) or inhibit (cimetidine, isoniazid) the hepatic microsomal enzyme system, altering the clearance of other medications (Table 1–1). Cessation of a microsomal inducer may allow toxic accumulation of another medication (e.g., rifampin and theophylline).

4. METABOLIC EFFECTS may cause an increased risk of toxicity (e.g., induction of hypothyroidism by a medication may alter the clearance of many drugs).

Hansten PD, Horn JR. Drug Interactions and Updates Quarterly. Vancouver, WA: Applied Therapeutics Inc.; 1996.

III. MANAGEMENT OF PAIN

Pain, the most common presenting symptom, suggests anatomic or physiologic derangement. Symptomatic treatment should not be offered until diagnostic possibilities have been considered and, if necessary, evaluated. Treatment with narcotics is contraindicated in undiagnosed acute abdominal pain and head injuries. It may complicate assessment and management. The salicylates and the other nonsteroidal anti-inflammatory drugs (NSAIDs) (Table 1–2) are widely used to control pain and inflammation. Although the medications are used interchangeably, not all are approved by the Food and Drug Administration for both indications. The proper treatment of pain depends on the underlying disease, chronicity of pain, and psychosocial factors. Nonpharmacologic treatment may be useful.

A. Acetaminophen

Acetaminophen (Table 1–2) is widely used for mild to moderate pain. Phenacetin is a related compound that is metabolized to acetaminophen but

TABLE 1-1. **Drugs That May Induce or Inhibit the Hepatic Oxygenase System**

INDUCERS	INHIBITORS
Barbiturates	Allopurinol
Carbamazepine	Amiodarone
Cigarette smoking*	Chloramphenicol
Ethanol (chronic)	Cimetidine
Griseofulvin	Diltiazem
Phenytoin	Disulfiram
Rifabutin	Ethanol (acute)
Rifampin	Erythromycin
	Fluconazole
	Fluoxetine
	Haloperidol
	Isoniazid
	Itraconazole
	Ketoconazole
	Monoamine oxidase inhibitors
	Oral contraceptives
	Paroxetine
	Phenothiazines
	Quinidine
	Quinolone antibiotics
	Tricyclic antidepressants
	Verapamil

*Reference: Schein JR. Cigarette smoking and clinically significant drug interactions. Ann Pharmacother 1995;29:1139–1148.

is rarely employed as a single analgesic agent. The mechanism of action of acetaminophen is not clearly defined, and its anti-inflammatory effect is weak. Acetaminophen is especially useful in the presence of aspirin allergy, warfarin treatment, upper GI sensitivity to anti-inflammatory agents, and bleeding disorders.

Acetaminophen is absorbed rapidly from the GI tract, and 90% is excreted in the urine after conjugation by the liver. Its primary toxic effect, hepatic necrosis, is seen in acute overdosage. Hepatic damage may occur with chronic therapeutic use in those with prior liver disease (Ann Intern Med 1986;104:399–404).

Although acetaminophen can induce synthesis of hepatic microsomal enzymes, this does not occur with standard doses, and significant drug interactions are unusual.

B. Salicylates

Salicylates are the most commonly used analgesics. Some formulations include caffeine, sedatives, or antihistamines, but there is no evidence of enhanced analgesic effect when these agents are added.

The most common route of administration is oral. Rectal (absorption is erratic) and parenteral (as sodium thiosalicylate) formulations are available.

TABLE 1-2. Nonnarcotic Analgesics

DRUG NAME	TRADE NAME	USUAL ADULT ORAL DOSE (mg)	MAXIMUM ADULT DAILY DOSE (mg)	CHEMICAL CLASS	COMMENT
Acetaminophen	Tylenol	325–650 q4–6h	4000	Aminophenol	Hepatotoxicity if overdosed and in persons with cirrhosis
SALICYLATES					
Acetylsalicylic acid	Aspirin	325–975 q4h	6000	Salicylate	Antagonizes effect of probenecid; increases effect of sulfonylureas; reduces renal clearance of methotrexate
Choline magnesium trisalicylate	Trilisate	500–1000 q12h	3000	Salicylate	Antagonizes effect of probenecid; increases effect of sulfonylureas; reduces renal clearance of methotrexate
Salsalate	Disalcid	500–1000 q8h; 750–1500 q12h	3000	Salicylate	Antagonizes effect of probenecid; increases effect of sulfonylureas; reduces renal clearance of methotrexate
SHORT-ACTING NSAIDs					
Diclofenac potassium	Cataflam	50 tid	200	Acetic acid	Formulation is immediate release
Diclofenac sodium	Voltaren	25–75 bid-tid	200	Acetic acid	Formulation is delayed release
Fenoprofen calcium	Nalfon	300–600 q6h	3200	Propionic acid	Highly protein bound (to albumin)
Ibuprofen	Motrin, Rufen	400–600 q6h	3200	Propionic acid	Also approved for primary dysmenorrhea; available in nonprescription strength (200 mg)
Indomethacin	Indocin, Indocin SR	25–50 q8h or 75 q12h (sustained release)	200	Acetic acid	Available in suppository, suspension, and sustained-release forms

Table continued on following page

7

TABLE 1–2. Nonnarcotic Analgesics *(Continued)*

DRUG NAME	TRADE NAME	USUAL ADULT ORAL DOSE (mg)	MAXIMUM ADULT DAILY DOSE (mg)	CHEMICAL CLASS	COMMENT
SHORT-ACTING NSAIDs *(Continued)*					
Ketoprofen	Orudis, Oruvail	50–75 q6–8h	300	Propionic acid	High rate of dyspepsia (11%); available in sustained-release form and nonprescription strength (12.5 mg)
Ketorolac	Toradol	10 q4–6h	40	Acetic acid	100% bioavailable; indicated only as continuation of parenteral ketorolac
Meclofenamate sodium	Meclomen	50–100 q6h	400	Anthranilic acid	High rate of diarrhea (10–33%)
Mefenamic acid	Ponstel	500, then 250 q6h	1000	Anthranilic acid	Also approved for primary dysmenorrhea
Tolmetin sodium	Tolectin	400 q6–8h	2000	Acetic acid	High rate of nausea (11%)
INTERMEDIATE-ACTING NSAIDs					
Diflunisal	Dolobid	500 q12h	1500	Salicylate derivative	Not metabolized to salicylate; increases acetaminophen level by 50% when coadministered
Etodolac	Lodine	200–400 bid–qid	1200	Acetic acid	Antacids reduce peak concentration by 20%
Flurbiprofen	Ansaid	50–100 bid–tid	300	Propionic acid	May cause CNS stimulation
Naproxen	Naprosyn	250–500 q8–12h	1250	Propionic acid	Approved for acute gout; may increase effect of protein-bound drugs, such as phenytoin, sulfonylureas, and warfarin; available in nonprescription strength (220 mg)
Naproxen sodium	Anaprox	275–550 q8–12h	1375	Propionic acid	Approved for acute gout; may increase effect of protein-bound drugs, such as phenytoin, sulfonylureas, and warfarin
Sulindac	Clinoril	150–200 q12h	400	Acetic acid	Approved for acute gout

LONG-ACTING NSAIDs				
Nabumetone	Relafen	500–750 bid; 1000–1500 qd		High rate of diarrhea (14%)
Oxaprozin	Daypro	600–1200 qd	Propionic acid	Highly protein bound
Piroxicam	Feldene	10–20 qd	Oxicam	High rate of dyspepsia (20%); may increase effect of protein-bound drugs, such as phenytoin, sulfonylureas, and warfarin
		1500	Nonacidic	
		1800		
		20		
PARENTERAL NSAID				
Ketorolac	Toradol	30 or 60 initially, then 15–30 q6h (all IM)	Acetic acid	Total duration of treatment should not exceed 5 days; 30 mg equal to 6–12 mg morphine sulfate but 10 times as expensive
		150 1st day, then 120 qd		

1. ADVERSE EFFECTS OF ASPIRIN
    a. **Gastric intolerance.** The most common adverse effect is gastric intolerance. **Gastritis** and **peptic ulcer disease** may occur. Enteric-coated preparations (e.g., Ecotrin) and combinations with antacids (e.g., Ascriptin) are available but may achieve lower salicylate blood levels.
    b. **Aspirin sensitivity** (bronchospasm, rhinosinusitis, urticaria, and anaphylaxis) is part of a triad including asthma and nasal polyps. Some degree of aspirin sensitivity may occur in 10% to 20% of asthmatics. Some NSAIDs may also cause the same reactions. Normal sinus x-rays indicate a low risk of sensitivity and predict less severe reactions if they occur. Desensitization protocols are available (J Allergy Clin Immunol 1984;74:617–622).
    c. **Other adverse effects** are (1) an **antiplatelet effect** that lasts for the lifetime of the platelet (approximately 2 weeks). Nonacetylated salicylates have less antiplatelet effect, similar to NSAIDs. (2) **Tinnitus** at high doses. (3) Aspirin treatment is associated with the development of **Reye's syndrome** in children and teenagers with viral infections, such as influenza and varicella.
    d. **Significant drug interactions with salicylates** include (1) increase of prothrombin time in warfarin-treated patients, (2) decrease of the uricosuric effect of probenecid and sulfinpyrazone, and (3) increase in methotrexate plasma levels due to decreased renal clearance.

C. NSAIDs

The NSAIDs (Table 1–2), although more convenient than salicylates, are more expensive, and their clear superiority over aspirin as analgesic or anti-inflammatory agents has not been established. In general, the shorter-acting agents are preferred as analgesics; longer-acting agents are easier for chronic use as anti-inflammatories. Parenteral forms are available. NSAIDs are metabolized in the liver and excreted in urine. In some cases there is a fecal component of excretion.

1. ADVERSE EFFECTS OF NSAIDs
    a. **Reversible platelet inhibition.**
    b. **Gastric intolerance** that may be associated with gastritis and peptic ulcer disease. The risk of NSAID-induced ulcer disease is reduced by misoprostol and omeprazole but not by histamine H_2 blockers or sucralfate.
    c. **Acute renal failure** (especially in the elderly and in patients with prerenal conditions) due to a decrease in glomerular filtration rate caused by alteration in renal prostaglandins. Nephrotoxicity may be less common with sulindac (Arch Intern Med 1990;150:268–270).
    d. **Hyperkalemia** due to a hyporeninemic-hypoaldosteronemic state.
    e. **Central nervous system effects,** including confusion, delirium, and dizziness, are especially more common in the elderly.
    f. **Impaired antihypertensive effects** of diuretics (due to sodium retention) and beta blockers.

D. Narcotics

Narcotic use for analgesia (Table 1–3) should be carefully controlled. However, less than 1% of cases of narcotic addiction begin with physician prescriptions. In general, narcotics are underused for acute pain and overused for chronic pain.

Narcotic orders often specify as needed, or prn, use. A more effective technique for inpatients is to give the medication unless refused by the patient or somnolence or respiratory depression occurs. A trough in analgesic effect is avoided, and the pain behavior that is central to the addictive process is minimized.

1. ADVERSE EFFECTS OF NARCOTICS
   a. **Respiratory depression** is unlikely to occur in a patient still in pain. It can be reversed with intravenous naloxone injected over 10 to 15 seconds; bolus dosing should be avoided in patients using narcotics chronically.
   b. **Postoperative confusion** is commonly due to narcotics.
   c. Histamine release and a non-IgE-mediated **anaphylactoid response** (e.g., appearance of perivenous erythema after IV narcotic injection).
   d. **Nausea,** more common in ambulatory patients, can usually be managed by choosing an alternative narcotic. Narcotics have a direct central effect that is antagonized by antidopaminergic agents such as prochlorperazine. A vestibular component, if present, may respond to meclizine or dimenhydrinate. Gastric stasis responsive to metoclopramide may occur, especially in patients receiving narcotics long term.
   e. **Smooth muscle spasm** may lead to abdominal cramps, urinary retention, or worsening of biliary colic. Meperidine and codeine have less pharmacologic effect on biliary tract pressure than morphine has.
   f. **Constipation** may result because of decreased propulsive contraction.

2. ADJUNCTIVE AGENTS
   a. The combination of 650 mg of aspirin or acetaminophen and 30 mg of codeine has an analgesic effect equal to that of 60 mg of codeine.
   b. Hydroxyzine 25 to 100 mg IM is also used to potentiate narcotic effect but appears to act primarily as a sedative.

3. ADMINISTRATION. The standard initial dose of morphine sulfate in a 70 kg adult is 10 mg IM. Peak analgesia occurs at 1 hour, with onset in 30 minutes.

   When immediate effect is required, morphine sulfate may be given intravenously. Peak analgesia occurs at 20 minutes, and peak respiratory depression occurs at 10 minutes. The usual starting dose is 2–8 mg (higher for pain).

   Patient-controlled analgesia may allow better pain control in postoperative patients at risk for respiratory complications (Arch Intern Med 1990;150:1897–1903).

TABLE 1–3. Narcotic Analgesics

DRUG NAME	TRADE NAME	COMMON ADULT DOSES (mg) AND ROUTES	PARENTERAL DOSE (mg) EQUAL TO 10 mg MORPHINE SULFATE IM	ORAL DOSE (mg) EQUAL TO LISTED PARENTERAL DOSE	COMMENT
NARCOTICS					
Fentanyl	Sublimaze, Duragesic (transdermal)	0.05–0.1 q1–2h IM or IV; 0.025–0.1/h transdermal (base dose on total morphine dose); 0.2–0.4 as lozenge	0.125	NA	Primary use is IV or epidurally for perioperative analgesia; transdermal form available but costly; lozenge effective for analgesia or conscious sedation
Oxymorphone	Numorphan	1–1.5 q4–6h IM; 5 q4–6h PR	1	NA	Major use is perioperative
Hydromorphone	Dilaudid	2 q4–6h PO; 1–2 q4–6h IM; 3 q6–8h PR	1.5	7.5	High abuse potential
Levorphanol	Levo-Dromoran	2 q6–8h PO	2	4	Long acting
Methadone	Dolophine	5–10 q4–6h PO or PR	8	20	Different $t_{1/2}$ for analgesia and prevention of opiate withdrawal
Morphine sulfate	Roxanol	5–20 q4h IM; 5–20 q6h PR; 10–30 q4h Sl; 10–30 q4h PO or PR	10	60 (single dose)	Oral bioavailability poor; sublingual or suppository form useful for breakthrough pain
Morphine, sustained release	MS Contin	15–100 q6–12h PO	10	30 (repeated doses)	Not appropriate for prn use

Drug	Trade names	Dose			Comments
Oxycodone	Percocet, Percodan, Tylox, Oxycodone, Oxycontin CII	5–10 q4–6h PO; 10–40 q12h PO	15	25	Often combined with aspirin (Percodan) or acetaminophen (Percocet, Tylox); slow-release form available for q12h dosing
Hydrocodone	Vicodin, Lortab	5–10 q4–6h PO	NA	30	Only available combined with acetaminophen or aspirin
Pentazocine	Talwin	30–60 q3–4h IM; 50–100 q4h PO	45	135	Mixed agonist-antagonist
Meperidine	Demerol	50–125 q3–4h IM or IV; 50–100 q4h PO	75	250	Metabolite normeperidine may accumulate with prolonged use, causing excitation or seizures
Codeine	Codeine	15–60 q4h PO	130	200	Schedule II unless combined with acetaminophen or aspirin; used as cough suppressant
Propoxyphene	Darvon	32–100 q4h PO	180	360	Less abuse potential than codeine at usual doses
NARCOTIC-LIKE AGENTS					
Buprenorphine	Buprenex	0.3 q6h IM	0.3	NA	Mixed agonist-antagonist; schedule V controlled substance
Butorphanol	Stadol	1–4 q3–4h IM	2–3	NA	Mixed agonist-antagonist; not a controlled substance
Nalbuphine	Nubain	10 q6h IM, IV, or SC	10	NA	Mixed agonist-antagonist; not a controlled substance
Tramadol	Ultram	50–100 q4–6h PO	NA	NA	100 mg equianalgesic to 60 mg codeine; seizure risk in high doses

E. Narcotic-like Agents

Tramadol is a centrally acting analgesic that binds **mu-opioid receptors** and inhibits the reuptake of serotonin and norepinephrine. Although it originally was thought to have narcotic-like potency without the potential for dependence syndromes, postmarketing experience has refuted this. Additionally, it appears to lower the seizure threshold in some patients. In spite of its current popularity, tramadol's advantages over narcotics are minimal.

F. Chronic Pain

Chronic pain management differs in many ways from acute pain management. Psychosocial issues are often paramount. However, they may be concealed by the patient or may be otherwise inapparent clinically. Somatic pathology is often less apparent. Regional (i.e., nerve blocks) and nonpharmacologic approaches are helpful in the management of selected chronic pain syndromes.

Narcotics should be avoided in chronic pain management. The major exception is patients with **terminal malignant disease,** in whom narcotic dependence may be expected and required doses may be very high. Patient surveys indicate that undertreatment of pain is common (N Engl J Med 1994;330:592–596).

When narcotics are used long term, longer-acting agents (e.g., methadone, sustained-release morphine, or sustained-release oxycodone orally or fentanyl transdermally) should be given on a fixed schedule. One method is the "pain cocktail," which usually contains methadone, acetaminophen, and hydroxyzine. With this technique, the patient is unaware of minor dosage adjustments, which is useful in some circumstances. Continuous subcutaneous infusion of high concentration narcotics is feasible when chronic parenteral narcotics are required.

G. Nontraditional Analgesics

Various medications that are not traditional analgesics are useful in chronic pain management:

1. TRICYCLIC ANTIDEPRESSANTS, most commonly amitriptyline, desipramine, and nortriptyline, have been used, especially if neuropathic pain is suspected. The typical dose is 25 to 100 mg at bedtime. Fluphenazine (a neuroleptic) 2 mg qd or bid may also be effective.

2. PHENYTOIN AND CARBAMAZEPINE (usual doses 300 mg qd and 200–400 mg bid, respectively) are useful for neuropathic pain, sometimes as the sole agent. They may be effective in doses that yield serum levels below quoted therapeutic levels.

3. ETIDRONATE DISODIUM (5 mg/kg/d) and other bisphosphonates (pamidronate, alendronate) may help the bone pain associated with cancer and Paget's disease.

4. BETA BLOCKERS, notably propranolol and nadolol, are used for headache disorders, either therapeutically or prophylactically, solely or adjunctively.

5. DEXTROAMPHETAMINE (5–20 mg bid) may reverse sedation in cancer patients using narcotics chronically.

6. **BELLADONNA AND OPIUM SUPPOSITORIES** (30 mg of opium PR, qd or bid) may help the pain associated with rectal or bladder tenesmus (e.g., after prostatectomy and rectal or bladder cancer).

Carr DB, Jacox AK, Chapman CR, et al. Acute pain management: operative or medical procedures and trauma. Clinical practice guideline No. 1. Rockville, MD: Agency for Health Care Policy and Research, 1992 (AHCPR publication No. 92-0020).

Jacox A, Carr DB, Payne R. New clinical practice guidelines for the management of pain in patients with cancer. N Engl J Med 1994;330:651–655.

Jacox AK, Carr DB, Payne R, et al. Management of cancer pain. Clinical practice guideline No. 9. Rockville, MD: Agency for Health Care Policy and Research, 1994 (AHCPR publication No. 94-0592).

McQuay H, Carroll D, Jadad AR, Wiffen P, Moore A. Anticonvulsant drugs for management of pain: a systematic review. Br Med J 1995;311:1047–1052.

Watson CPN. Antidepressant drugs as adjuvant analgesics. J Pain Symptom Manage 1994; 9:392–405.

IV. FEVER

A. Definition and Manifestations

Fever, a body temperature (measured orally) above 38°C, often requires diagnostic testing before symptomatic treatment. Although fever may be part of the host defense system, some patients benefit from antipyresis.

If fever is not controlled, elderly patients may become confused, children and epileptic patients may have seizures, and the increased metabolic rate may aggravate heart disease. Furthermore, patients with fever are often uncomfortable.

B. Management

1. **ASPIRIN AND ACETAMINOPHEN** are both effective in lowering body temperature in doses of 325–650 mg PO or PR. Acetaminophen is the drug of choice in children and teenagers when viral illnesses are suspected.

   In patients with prolonged or recurrent fever, the drugs may be given every 3 to 4 hours until the underlying illness resolves (unless temperature must be monitored as a measure of therapeutic efficacy). When antipyretics are used irregularly only for a specified temperature elevation, the patient may be subjected needlessly to the discomforts of recurrent sweating and chilling.

2. **IBUPROFEN, INDOMETHACIN, KETOROLAC, AND CORTICOSTEROIDS** are potent antipyretics useful in selected circumstances.

3. **PHYSICAL MEASURES** for treatment of fever (sponge baths and cooling blankets) are usually reserved for treatment of heat stroke.

Styrt B, Sugarman B. Antipyresis and fever. Arch Intern Med 1990;150:1589–1597.

V. CONSTIPATION

A. Causes

Constipation is common among inpatients because of inactivity, dietary change, or medication side effects. Commonly implicated medications include narcotics, aluminum- or calcium-containing antacids, tricyclic antidepressants, phenothiazines, calcium channel blockers, and iron salts.

B. Management

Constipation should not be treated without consideration of possible underlying causes, such as metabolic and bowel abnormalities. There are few contraindications to transient laxative use in inpatients, but chronic use in outpatients should be discouraged. Classes of laxatives (Table 1–4) include:

1. BULKING AGENTS, usually the drugs of choice for outpatients, may be less useful for inpatients because of delayed onset of effect. Increased bulk causes increased peristaltic activity and decreased transit time. Bulk laxatives may affect medication absorption.

2. EMOLLIENT LAXATIVES are also safe, with the exception of mineral oil, which may lead to fat-soluble vitamin deficiency and lipid pneumonitis. They are the drugs of choice for hard, dry stools.

3. CATHARTIC LAXATIVES induce hyperosmolarity in the intestinal lumen and decrease water absorption. They are contraindicated in patients with abdominal pain of uncertain cause. Injudicious use can induce fluid and electrolyte abnormalities.

4. STIMULANT LAXATIVES promote fluid accumulation in the gut lumen and enhance intestinal motility. All stimulant laxatives are contraindicated in patients with abdominal pain of uncertain cause. They are habit forming, and chronic use may cause neurologic damage with colonic atony, dilation, and hypomotility.

5. SUPPOSITORIES AND ENEMAS are useful in bowel preparation for radiographic procedures but should not be used in other circumstances if oral agents are effective.

   Bisacodyl, an effective stimulant available as a suppository, acts in 15 to 30 minutes and is usually better tolerated than enemas.

   Enemas increase rectal peristalsis by distention. Some preparations (e.g., potassium bitartrate) produce carbon dioxide to enhance this effect. Other substances used as enemas include glycerin, sorbitol, and tap water. The main criterion for selection is ease of administration.

Romero Y, Evans JM, Fleming KC, Phillips SF. Constipation and fecal incontinence in the elderly population. Mayo Clin Proc 1996;71:81–92.

VI. DIARRHEA

A. Causes

Diarrhea is a common symptom of disease, but it also can be a medication side effect. Common offenders include magnesium-containing antacids, antibiotics (with and without *Clostridium difficile* infection), laxatives, quinidine, and colchicine. Diarrhea should not be treated symptomatically before other possible causes are ruled out. Drugs that inhibit motility often should be withheld if acute mucosal inflammation is suspected.

B. Management

Adequate fluid intake should be ensured (oral or IV) while avoiding excessive osmotic loads. Acute diarrheal illnesses may decrease intestinal

TABLE 1–4. Laxatives

AGENT	USUAL ADULT DOSE AND ROUTE	TIME TO EFFECT	COMMENT
BULK AGENTS			
Methylcellulose (Citrucel)	4–6 g tid PO	Onset 12–24 h; full effect 2–3 d	May reduce absorption of digoxin, salicylates, and nitrofurantoin if given simultaneously
Psyllium (Metamucil, Perdiem Plus)	3–6 g qd–tid PO	Same as above	Same as above; may also reduce absorption of warfarin; some preparations contain sugar
Bran	6 g qd PO	Same as above	Cheap; no drug interactions
EMOLLIENT AGENTS			
Dioctyl sodium sulfosuccinate (DSS, Colace)	50–360 mg qd PO	1–3 d	Available as capsule, solution, and tablet
Dioctyl potassium sulfosuccinate (Dialose)	100–240 mg qd PO	Same as above	Available as capsule
Dioctyl calcium sulfosuccinate (Surfak)	50–240 mg qd PO	Same as above	Available as capsule
CATHARTIC AGENTS			
Magnesium hydroxide (Milk of Magnesia)	30–60 mL qd PO (82–164 mEq Mg)	3–6 h; low dose: 6–8 h	Avoid in renal failure; commonly used at HS in low dose; double-strength formulations available; may decrease tetracycline absorption
Lactulose (Chronulac)	10–20 g qd PO (15–30 mL)	24 h	Poorly absorbed disaccharide also used in hepatic encephalopathy; often used in elderly patients
Sorbitol	15–30 mL of 70% solution qd PO	3–6 h	Nonabsorbable; less expensive than lactulose but as effective; also given rectally to treat hyperkalemia
Magnesium citrate	100–200 mL qd PO (77–154 mEq Mg)	3–6 h	Avoid in renal failure; induces watery stool
Sodium sulfate (Golytely)	2–4 L PO	1–3 h	Induces watery stool; commonly used in bowel preparation

Table continued on following page

TABLE 1-4. **Laxatives** *(Continued)*

AGENT	USUAL ADULT DOSE AND ROUTE	TIME TO EFFECT	COMMENT
STIMULANT AGENTS			
Senna (Senokot)	5–15 mL qd PO	Onset 6 h; 12–24 h to full effect	May induce melanosis coli; available as powder or liquid
Cascara sagrada	5 mL qd PO	Onset 8 h	May induce melanosis coli
Bisacodyl (Dulcolax)	5–15 mg qd PO; 10 mg qd PR	6–12 h PO; 15–30 min PR	Tablets contain tartrazine dye; do not give orally within 1 h of antacids; suppository may cause mild proctitis
Castor oil	15–60 mL PO	1–6 h	Induces semifluid stool; active in small intestine; cramping common; should be reserved for bowel preparation

lactase activity, and lactose restriction for 3 to 5 days is often helpful. Oral glucose-electrolyte solutions are useful in some circumstances, especially in pediatrics.

1. BULKING AGENTS (Table 1–5) lead to formed stools by absorption of water but may increase electrolyte losses. Bulking agents are more useful in the management of chronic diarrhea associated with irritable bowel syndrome, colostomy, and ileostomy.

2. KAOLIN (hydrated aluminum silicate) AND PECTIN (polygalacturonic acid) are combined for their supposed adsorbent and mucosal-protective properties. Stool fluidity decreases, but overall stool weight or frequency does not. Adverse effects, with the exception of drug interactions, are usually minimal.

3. BISMUTH SUBSALICYLATE (Pepto-Bismol) decreases intestinal fluid secretion by affecting the intestinal prostaglandins. It effectively prevents and treats traveler's diarrhea (usually due to enterotoxigenic *Escherichia coli*) (N Engl J Med 1993;328:1821–1827). It is contraindicated in patients with a coagulopathy or a history of aspirin hypersensitivity or when Reye's syndrome is possible. Significant salicylate absorption may occur. In one study, the use of 8 ounces of Pepto-Bismol over 3.5 hours caused absorption of salicylate equivalent to 2600 mg of aspirin (J Pediatr 1981;99:654–656).

4. NATURAL ANTIMUSCARINICS. Preparations that contain natural antimuscarinics (e.g., atropine, scopolamine) or **synthetic anticholinergics** inhibit intestinal motility and cramping. However, they involve anticholinergic risks (acute glaucoma, urinary retention, CNS side effects). At dosages low enough to be free of adverse effects, these agents are not effective in severe diarrhea and should not be used if acute mucosal inflammation is suspected.

5. NARCOTICS exert an antidiarrheal effect by decreasing intestinal motility and reducing secretory activity mediated by opioid receptors. At standard doses, the antidiarrheal narcotics do not cause analgesia, but doses above recommended levels can cause euphoria and physical dependence. This risk is highest with camphorated tincture of opium, less with diphenoxylate, and even less with loperamide.

    Diphenoxylate and loperamide are equally effective for acute diarrhea. However, loperamide is more effective in chronic diarrhea due to inflammatory bowel disease. These agents should be avoided if acute mucosal inflammation is suspected (JAMA 1973;226:1525–1528). In acute ulcerative colitis, opiates may increase the risk of toxic megacolon.

6. CHOLESTYRAMINE, a bile acid binder, should be considered for diarrhea due to excessive intraluminal bile acids (e.g., ileal resection) and in patients with pseudomembranous colitis.

Brownlee HJ, ed. Management of acute nonspecific diarrhea. Am J Med 1990;88(Suppl 6A): 1S–37S.
Mercadante S. Diarrhea in terminally ill patients: pathophysiology and treatment. J Pain Symptom Manage 1995;10:298–309.

TABLE 1–5. **Antidiarrheals**

AGENT	USUAL ADULT DOSE	DRUG INTERACTIONS	COMMENT
BULK OR ADSORBENT AGENTS			
Psyllium (Metamucil, Perdiem Plus)	3 g qd–tid	*See Table 1–4*	Must be given with water
Methylcellulose (Citrucel)	4–6 g bid–tid	*See Table 1–4*	Must be given with water
Kaolin-pectin (Kaopectate)	60–120 mL after each bowel movement	May reduce absorption of digoxin and tetracyclines	Kaopectate tablets contain a different absorbent
PROSTAGLANDIN SYNTHESIS INHIBITOR			
Bismuth subsalicylate (Pepto-Bismol)	524 mg (2 pills or 30 mL) every 30 min; maximum 8 doses qd	Increased risk of bleeding in those taking warfarin	Changes stool color to black
ANTIMUSCARINIC AGENTS			
Kaolin, pectin, hyoscyamine, atropine, scopolamine (Donnagel)	30 mL, then 15 mL every 3 h, up to 60 mL qd	Decreased absorption of digoxin and chloroquine	Anticholinergic side effects; available with paregoric
OPIOID AGENTS			
Tincture of opium (Paregoric)	5–10 mL up to qid	Increased depression with CNS depressants	5 mL equivalent to 2 mg morphine
Diphenoxylate, 2.5 mg and atropine 0.025 mg (Lomotil)	2 tablets up to qid	Increased depression with CNS depressants	Contraindicated in invasive infectious diarrhea and acute ulcerative colitis
Loperamide (Imodium)	4 mg, then 2 mg after each stool; maximum 16 mg qd	Increased depression with CNS depressants	Same as above; more potent than diphenoxylate; available without prescription
BILE ACID BINDER			
Cholestyramine (Questran)	4 g tid–qid	Decreased absorption of many drugs, e.g., chlorothiazide, digoxin, thyroxine, warfarin, and phenobarbital	Must be given with water; give other drugs 1 h before or 4 h after dose

VII. NAUSEA AND VOMITING

A. Causes

Nausea is the most common adverse drug effect. Nausea and vomiting are mediated by a medullary center that receives afferents from the GI tract, the cortical centers, the vestibular system, and the dopaminergic chemoreceptor trigger zone (CTZ), a medullary center.

After possible diagnoses have been considered, symptomatic treatment should be used to reduce patient discomfort, to avoid electrolyte disturbances, to reduce risk of aspiration of gastric contents, and to avoid gastroesophageal injury.

B. Management

1. **AIRWAY PROTECTION** is important in the management of nausea and vomiting; a stuporous patient may require an endotracheal tube. Placement of a nasogastric tube and positioning the patient with the head elevated by 15 to 30 degrees may help.

2. **ANTIEMETICS** (Table 1–6).

   a. **Emetrol** is a mixture of dextrose, levulose, and phosphoric acid that may be effective in mild nausea or motion sickness. It is the only antiemetic judged safe during pregnancy.

   b. **Antacids** may help when there is a peptic component, as in reflux esophagitis.

   c. **Some antihistamines with H₁ specificity** are effective for nausea associated with motion sickness or vestibular disorders. They are less effective than the neuroleptics in nausea due to other causes. The antihistamines depress labyrinthine excitability and vestibulo-cerebellar pathways. They may cause sedation and anticholinergic symptoms, such as dry mouth and urinary retention.

   d. **Meclizine** and **dimenhydrinate** are used primarily for nausea of motion sickness or vestibular dysfunction. The latter is more effective for motion sickness, and prophylactic use is superior. Parenteral preparations of **hydroxyzine** and **diphenhydramine** are available. The IV route (diphenhydramine and dimenhydrinate only) is preferred in patients receiving cancer chemotherapy. Drug interactions, aside from additive sedative effects, are unusual for this class of medications. Transdermal **scopolamine** is no longer available in the United States.

   e. **Metoclopramide** has central antidopaminergic and peripheral cholinergic activities. It stimulates gastric emptying and decreases gastroesophageal reflux. The usual starting dose is 10 mg qid. For chemotherapy-induced nausea, the dosage may be up to 2 mg/kg q2h for two doses, then 1 mg/kg q3h for three doses. Doses should be halved if the creatinine clearance is less than 40 mL/min.

   Sedation is a common effect (10% for 10 mg qid, 70% for 1–2 mg/kg). Other common adverse effects include dystonic reactions and pseudoparkinsonism. Metoclopramide potentiates the risk of dystonic reactions to phenothiazines and may precipitate a hyper-

TABLE 1–6. Antiemetics

AGENT	CLASS	USUAL ADULT DOSE AND ROUTE	ANTICHOLINERGIC EFFECT	POTENTIAL FOR DYSTONIA	COMMENT
Dextrose, levulose, phosphoric acid (Emetrol)		15–30 mL PO q15min	0	0	Available without prescription; safe in pregnancy
Dimenhydrinate (Dramamine)	Histamine (H_1) blocker	50–100 mg PO, IM, or IV q4h	1–2+	0	Available without prescription
Diphenhydramine (Benadryl)	H_1 blocker	25–100 mg PO, IM q6h; 25–75 mg IV q4h	3+	0	Most sedating of the H_1 blockers; available as elixir
Hydroxyzine (Vistaril, Atarax)	H_1 blocker	25–100 mg PO, IM q6h	2+	0	Mild anxiolytic; not for IV use; available as elixir
Meclizine (Antivert)	H_1 blocker	12.5–37.5 mg PO tid	1–2+	0	Single daily dose useful as motion sickness prophylaxis
Trimethobenzamide (Tigan)	Chemoreceptor trigger zone (CTZ) effect	250 mg PO tid-qid; 200 mg PR, IM tid-qid	1+	1+	Suppository contains benzocaine; pregnancy category B
Metoclopramide (Reglan)	CTZ effect	10–20 mg PO qid; 1–2 mg/kg IV q2h; see text	0	2–4+	Risk of dystonia is dose dependent: 0.2% for low dose, 25% for very high dose
Droperidol (Inapsine)	CTZ effect	1.25–2.50 mg IV or IM q4h	1+	2+	High rate of sedation; onset in 3–10 min
Chlorpromazine (Thorazine)	Phenothiazine	10–25 mg PO q4–6h; 25–50 mg IM q3–4h; 25–100 mg PR q8h	3+	2–3+	Also useful for hiccups; more sedating and higher frequency of hypotension than with prochlorperazine

Drug	Class	Dose			Comments
Prochlorperazine (Compazine)	Phenothiazine	5–10 mg PO, IM or IV q6h; 25 mg PR q12h	2+	3+	Available as elixir
Promethazine (Phenergan)	Phenothiazine	12.5–25 mg PO, PR, or IM q4–6h	3+	2+	More sedating than prochlorperazine; also useful for motion sickness and as an antihistamine; available as elixir
Granisetron (Kytril)	Serotonin$_3$ receptor antagonist	1 mg PO 60 min before chemotherapy and 12 h later; 0.01/kg IV 60 min before chemotherapy, then 12 h and 24 h later	0	0	Should be used on a scheduled basis rather than prn; headache a common side effect; effect may be reduced by SSRIs
Ondansetron (Zofran)	Serotonin$_3$ receptor antagonist	8 mg PO 30 min before chemotherapy and q8h for up to 48 h; 8–12 mg IV 30 min before chemotherapy and q4h for 2 doses or 32 mg IV 30 min before chemotherapy as single dose	0	0	Should be used on a scheduled basis rather than prn; headache a common side effect; effect may be reduced by SSRIs
Dexamethasone (Decadron)	Steroid	10–20 mg IV q12h; 8 mg PO q6h	0	0	Used as 2–3 d course of adjunctive treatment for nausea or chemotherapy
Methylprednisolone (Solu-Medrol)	Steroid	250–500 mg IV q6h	0	0	Used similarly to dexamethasone
Dronabinol (Marinol)	Cannabinoid	5–10 mg/m^2 PO q4–6h	0	0	Schedule II

tensive crisis in patients taking MAO inhibitors. It may decrease absorption of drugs absorbed from the stomach (e.g., digoxin).

f. **Neuroleptic drugs** act at the CTZ, where they have antidopaminergic effects. All neuroleptics except thioridazine have some antiemetic effect, usually at doses substantially below their neuroleptic dosage. These drugs are less useful in nausea due to local action on the GI tract or vestibular dysfunction. They have sedative, alpha-adrenergic blocking, and anticholinergic actions.

Acute dystonic reactions, which may occur with any of these agents, can be treated with diphenhydramine 25–50 mg or benztropine mesylate 1–2 mg IM or IV, followed by a course of oral therapy. The neuroleptics are metabolized in the liver; their effect may be diminished by microsomal inducers.

g. **Antagonists of the serotonin type 3 receptor** are agents proven effective against chemotherapy-induced nausea. The prototype agent, **ondansetron,** is available in intravenous and oral forms. Side effects, including headache, lightheadedness, and transaminase elevations, are seldom serious. A major advantage is the lack of antidopaminergic side effects. All agents from this class are relatively high in cost, but single-dose regimens of a longer-acting agent, **granisetron,** often are effective. The role of this class in treatment of nausea due to causes other than cancer chemotherapy is not well defined.

h. **Cannabinoids,** such as dronabinol or nabilone, are as effective as prochlorperazine or metoclopramide. The main adverse effects of tetrahydrocannabinol are depersonalization, dysphoria, and somnolence. The risk of dysphoria is markedly reduced by combination treatment with prochlorperazine.

3. PROPHYLACTIC COMBINATION TREATMENT of nausea should be given to patients receiving emetogenic chemotherapy. Severe nausea is an important and potentially avoidable cause of poor compliance with chemotherapy regimens. High doses of metoclopramide, droperidol, prochlorperazine, and promethazine are effective prophylactically. Intravenous diphenhydramine is also used commonly, although not as a single agent. It prevents dystonic reactions. Brief courses of **dexamethasone** or **methylprednisolone** are proven adjuncts. Low doses of **lorazepam** may be helpful in decreasing the discomfort of nausea as well as anticipatory nausea associated with chemotherapy.

Grunberg SM, Hesketh PJ. Control of chemotherapy-induced emesis. N Engl J Med 1993; 329:1790–1796.

VIII. PSYCHOSIS AND DELIRIUM

A. Neuroleptics

Drugs used to treat psychosis (Table 1–7) are collectively called neuroleptics. The largest class is the phenothiazines; there are several other chemical classes. All are equally effective antipsychotics at equipotent doses. All have greater or lesser antidopaminergic, anticholinergic, and alpha-adrenergic blocking properties. Newer agents, such as risperidone and clozapine, have

TABLE 1-7. Neuroleptics

AGENT	EQUIVALENT DOSE (mg)	USUAL* ADULT TOTAL DAILY ORAL DOSE (mg) AND SCHEDULE	SINGLE* IM DOSE (mg)	SEDATION	RELATIVE MAGNITUDE OF EXTRAPYRAMIDAL EFFECT	RELATIVE MAGNITUDE OF HYPOTENSIVE EFFECT	COMMENT
PHENOTHIAZINES							
Chlorpromazine (Thorazine)	100	200–800; qd–qid	25–100	3+	2+	3+	Increases valproic acid level; used for hiccups
Fluphenazine (Prolixin)	2	2–40; tid–qid	1.25–2.50	1+	3+	1+	Available as decanoate for long-acting injection therapy
Mesoridazine (Serentil)	50	75–400; tid	25	3+	1+	2+	Increased toxicity when used with propranolol
Perphenazine (Trilafon)	10	8–64; bid–qid	5–10	2+	2+	1+	—
Thioridazine (Mellaril)	100	150–800; bid–qid	NA	3+	1+	2+	Increased toxicity when used with propranolol
Trifluoperazine (Stelazine)	5	2–40; bid	1–2	1+	3+	1+	Decreases effect of warfarin; increased toxicity when used with propranolol
NONPHENOTHIAZINE NEUROLEPTICS							
Clozapine (Clozaril)	50	50–900; qd–bid	NA	3+	1+	3+	Used only after failure of several other agents; causes agranulocytosis (1% risk), most often during wk 4–8 of therapy

Table continued on following page

TABLE 1-7. **Neuroleptics** *(Continued)*

AGENT	EQUIVALENT DOSE (mg)	USUAL* ADULT TOTAL DAILY ORAL DOSE (mg) AND SCHEDULE	SINGLE* IM DOSE (mg)	SEDATION	RELATIVE MAGNITUDE OF EXTRAPYRAMIDAL EFFECT	RELATIVE MAGNITUDE OF HYPOTENSIVE EFFECT	COMMENT
Haloperidol (Haldol)	2	2–40; bid–tid	2–5	1+	3+	1+	Available as decanoate for long-acting injection therapy
Loxapine (Loxitane)	10	20–100; bid–qid	12.5–50	1+	2+	1+	Increased toxicity when used with guanabenz
Risperidone (Risperdal)	1	2–8; bid	NA	1+	1+	1–2+	Clearance of risperidone increased by carbamazepine
Thiothixene (Navane)	5	6–60; tid	2–4	2+	2+	2+	—

*Lower doses are recommended for frail elderly persons. Doses listed are "antipsychotic doses," usually used in conjunction with a psychiatrist.

significant antiserotonergic properties. The agent should be chosen on the basis of possible side effects and history of efficacy. In general, the less potent neuroleptics are more sedating, cause more postural symptoms, have more anticholinergic effects, and have fewer associated movement disorders (with the exception of tardive dyskinesia).

B. Treatment

1. TREATMENT OF ACUTE MAJOR PSYCHOSIS consists of frequent doses of parenteral drugs. Haloperidol 5 mg IM or chlorpromazine 50–100 mg IM may be used hourly until control is achieved, followed by additional doses every 4 to 8 hours for the first 24 to 72 hours.

   In most cases, lower doses or a parenteral benzodiazepine should be used initially in frail elderly persons. Patients must be monitored for development of hypotension or acute dystonia.

2. CONFUSION OR DELIRIUM should not be treated symptomatically with neuroleptics until underlying conditions, such as medication toxicity, electrolyte imbalance, infection, hypoxia, hepatic insufficiency, and cardiovascular disease, have been ruled out or treated primarily. General supportive measures are also important in the management of psychosis, delirium, and confusion.

   Disturbance of the patient should be minimized, and the room lights should be dimmed at night. Attendants may be required and are preferred to restraints.

   Family members may help reassure the patient. They need to know that the patient's bizarre behavior is not willful and that it will in most cases resolve without sequelae.

   After complicating medical illnesses have been ruled out, symptomatic treatment with low doses (0.5–2 mg hs) of haloperidol may be helpful. In agitated, critically ill patients, higher doses or a parenteral benzodiazepine may be necessary. All neuroleptics have the potential to cause several extrapyramidal syndromes. **Acute dystonia** is more common in young patients. It may be treated with diphenhydramine 25–50 mg IM or benztropine mesylate 1–2 mg IM; subsequent oral therapy may be required for days to several weeks. A syndrome identical to **Parkinson's disease** may occur, especially in the elderly. Usually, the offending drug must be discontinued. **Tardive dyskinesia** is a late complication of neuroleptic use and has no effective treatment.

3. NEUROLEPTIC MALIGNANT SYNDROME is a potentially fatal emergency characterized by fever, stupor, catatonia, hemodynamic instability, and myoglobinemia (Med Clin North Am 1993;77:477–492). Recognition with immediate discontinuation of the neuroleptic and prompt treatment are essential.

Kane JM. Drug therapy: schizophrenia. N Engl J Med 1996;334:34–41.

IX. INSOMNIA

Possible underlying disorders, ranging from metabolic diseases to sleep apnea, should be considered before symptomatic treatment of insomnia.

Short-term treatment of insomnia is safe if side effects of hypnotic drugs are carefully monitored. Chronic use of hypnotics for insomnia is not recommended because of difficulty with habituation, side effects, and questionable efficacy. Objective improvement in daytime functioning as a result of hypnotic use has never been demonstrated.

A. Benzodiazepines

Benzodiazepines (Table 1–8) are usually the drugs of choice for insomnia and anxiety. They have a favorable therapeutic index, with minimal effects on respiration at commonly used dosages.

Addiction and withdrawal syndromes may occur. Dangerous withdrawal syndromes are rare for daily doses of less than 20 mg diazepam. Moderate symptoms, such as dysphoria, irritability, and insomnia, may occur in up to one third of patients.

The shorter-acting agents are more likely to produce withdrawal symptoms as well as rebound insomnia after only short-term use. **The benzodiazepines should be avoided during pregnancy** because of the risk of fetal abnormalities.

The selection of one benzodiazepine agent over another is based on pharmacokinetic differences. All are well absorbed orally, but only lorazepam and midazolam are consistently and rapidly absorbed when given IM.

All are metabolized by the liver. Lorazepam and oxazepam are cleared solely by glucuronidation, which is less affected by age and comorbidity, and are preferred for patients with underlying liver disease. Some have long-lived active metabolites that are responsible for part of their effect. Estazolam, clonazepam, lorazepam, midazolam, oxazepam, and temazepam have no active metabolites; alprazolam and triazolam have only short-lived ones.

Diazepam has the most rapid onset of action of all benzodiazepines used orally, reaching peak concentration within 30 to 60 minutes of an oral dose. It is generally not used as a hypnotic because of long-lived active metabolites.

Agents marketed as **hypnotics** include estazolam, flurazepam, quazepam, temazepam, and triazolam. Triazolam and flurazepam reach peak effect in 1 to 2 hours, whereas estazolam, quazepam, and temazepam have peak effect in 2 to 3 hours. Flurazepam and quazepam have long-lived active metabolites. They are widely used for insomnia and are more effective after the first night. Their effects persist for 1 to 2 days after discontinuation. Quazepam is more expensive than flurazepam and has no definite therapeutic advantage. Triazolam has the shortest duration of action but is more often associated with rebound insomnia; temazepam and estazolam have intermediate durations of action. Of these three agents, temazepam is the least expensive.

B. Zolpidem

Zolpidem has high-affinity binding at a benzodiazepine-receptor subtype located in the cerebellum and cerebral cortex. It decreases sleep latency and increases sleep time as well as flurazepam and triazolam. It does not appear to cause tolerance or withdrawal symptoms after prolonged use, and daytime sedation is unusual. The usual dose is 10 mg, or 5 mg for elderly

TABLE 1-8. Sedatives and Hypnotics

AGENT	HALF-LIFE OF EFFECT INCLUDING ACTIVE METABOLITES (h)	ADULT DOSE, mg* (ORAL UNLESS STATED) FOR HYPNOTIC USE	COMMENT
ANTIHISTAMINES			
Diphenhydramine (Benadryl)	4-6	25-50	Highest rate of anticholinergic effects; most sedating of the antihistamines
Hydroxyzine (Vistaril, Atarax)	6-24	25-50	Used as an anxiolytic at higher dose, up to 100 mg
Pyrilamine (Rynatan)	4-6	25-50	Relatively little anticholinergic effect
BARBITURATES			
Pentobarbital (Nembutal)	15-48	100 PO or 120-200 PR	Barbiturates should not be used as hypnotics for more than 2 consecutive weeks; all have been linked to fetal abnormalities, although they are safer in pregnancy than benzodiazepines; drug interactions common due to induction of hepatic microsomal system (e.g., warfarin, corticosteroids, phenytoin, estrogens)
Secobarbital (Seconal)	15-40	100 PO or 200 PR	
Amobarbital (Amytal)	8-42	65-200	
BENZODIAZEPINES			
Short-Acting			
Midazolam (Versed)	1-3	See comment	Primary use is IM or IV for conscious sedation; usual initial dose is 1-2 mg, repeat as needed q3-5min; usual total dose 2.5-5 mg
Oxazepam (Serax)	5-10	15-30	Commonly used for alcohol withdrawal
Triazolam (Halcion)	1.5-3	0.125-0.25	Not used as an anxiolytic

*Lower doses recommended for frail elderly persons.

Table continued on following page

TABLE 1–8. Sedatives and Hypnotics *(Continued)*

AGENT	HALF-LIFE OF EFFECT INCLUDING ACTIVE METABOLITES (h)	ADULT DOSE, mg* (ORAL UNLESS STATED) FOR HYPNOTIC USE	COMMENT
Intermediate-Acting			
Alprazolam (Xanax)	11–19	0.5–1	Not commonly used as a hypnotic; used for panic disorder (2–6 mg/d)
Estazolam (ProSom)	10–24	1–2	Not used as an anxiolytic
Lorazepam (Ativan)	10–20	1–2	Can be used IM; use 1–2 mg q1h for acute agitation (fewer side effects than haloperidol)
Temazepam (Restoril)	10–17	15–30	Most used as an anxiolytic; $t_{1/2}$ in elderly women greater than in elderly men
Long-Acting			
Chlordiazepoxide (Librium)	30–90	25–50	Commonly used for alcohol withdrawal
Clonazepam (Klonopin)	18–50	0.5–1	FDA approved as adjunctive anticonvulsant
Clorazepate (Tranxene)	50–80	15–30	Also used for alcohol withdrawal
Diazepam (Valium)	30–90	5–10	Commonly used for alcohol withdrawal; used IV for seizures, maximal rate of administration is 5 mg/min due to risk of cardiovascular collapse
Flurazepam (Dalmane)	50–100	15–30	Not used as an anxiolytic; 15 mg as effective as 30 mg for most patients
Prazepam (Centrax)	50–100	10–20	Primarily used as an anxiolytic
Quazepam (Doral)	28–114	7.5–15	Not used as an anxiolytic

		See text for further comments
MISCELLANEOUS DRUGS		
Chloral hydrate (Noctec)	4–10	500–1000	Many patients require up to 2000 mg; may increase warfarin effect; do not use if renal or hepatic function is impaired
Glutethimide (Doriden)	5–22	250–500	Decreases effect of warfarin; seriously consider alternative drugs to glutethimide
Meprobamate (Miltown)	6–17	800	FDA approved only for anxiety; seriously consider alternative drugs to meprobamate
Zolpidem (Ambien)	6–8	5–10	Controlled substance (schedule IV) in spite of lack of tolerance or withdrawal symptoms; use lower dose in elderly or in patients with hepatic impairment (pharmacologic $t_{1/2}$ quadrupled to 10 h in cirrhotics)
PURE ANXIOLYTIC		
Buspirone (Buspar)	—	5–20 mg tid	May be a selective anxiolytic; minimal sedative activity; may displace digoxin from plasma proteins

*Lower doses recommended for frail elderly persons.

patients. Its cost is significantly greater than all benzodiazepines used to treat insomnia.

C. Barbiturates

The only major indications for barbiturates are as adjuncts to anesthesia and as anticonvulsants. When these drugs are used as hypnotics, tolerance begins to develop within a few days. The effect on total sleep time is halved after 2 weeks. Their therapeutic index is low.

D. Chloral Hydrate

Chloral hydrate is a hypnotic that, in commonly used doses (500–1000 mg), shortens time to sleep but does not change total time asleep. It is useful for sleep induction before electroencephalographic (EEG) recording because of its relatively slight effect on EEG patterns. Its therapeutic index is between that of the benzodiazepines and that of the barbiturates.

E. Glutethimide and Meprobamate

Glutethimide is a sedative that has significant anticholinergic action as well as long-lived active metabolites. Meprobamate is also used as a hypnotic. The use of both drugs should be abandoned because of the potential for dependence and abstinence syndromes and lack of advantages over the benzodiazepines.

X. ANXIETY

Anxiety may be a symptom of depression, psychosis, substance abuse, or panic disorder. Any of the agents discussed for insomnia may be used to treat anxiety symptomatically, but only hydroxyzine, buspirone, and the benzodiazepines are widely employed.

A. Hydroxyzine

Hydroxyzine has the advantage of lack of dependence or abstinence syndromes, although high doses (50–100 mg qid), may be required to treat anxiety.

B. Benzodiazepines

The benzodiazepines are effective as anxiolytics and are commonly used at one third to one half of the hypnotic dose administered bid to qid. The agents with active long-lived metabolites have the advantage of less frequent dosing once effect has been established. Benefit for 4 months of continuous use has been documented. The effectiveness of longer-term use is unproved, and dependence can occur.

C. Buspirone

A new class of drugs, represented by buspirone, is available to treat anxiety with minimal sedation and liability for dependence. The anxiolytic effect may have a latency of onset of 1 to 2 weeks. Its role in the treatment of anxiety disorders is not clearly defined.

XI. SEDATION DURING MEDICAL PROCEDURES

For sedation during diagnostic and therapeutic procedures, diazepam (2–10 mg IV), lorazepam (1–2 mg IV), and midazolam (0.5–2 mg IV) are preferred because of their ease of use. The rapid redistribution of diazepam gives it the shortest duration of action (10 to 30 minutes). Lorazepam and midazolam may also be given IM, but the onset of action is slower than by the IV route.

Bone RC, Levine RL, Barkin RL, et al. Recognition, assessment, and treatment of anxiety in the critical care patient. Disease-a-Month 1995;41:296–359.
Farney RJ, Walker JM. Office management of common sleep-wake disorders. Med Clin North Am 1995;79:391–414.
Gillin JC, Byerley WF. The diagnosis and management of insomnia. N Engl J Med 1990;322: 239–248.

XII. DEPRESSION

Depression, with a prevalence of 3% to 9%, may be a manifestation of a major affective disorder or a bipolar illness. Metabolic disorders or drugs may cause depression. Commonly implicated drugs include alcohol, sedatives, cimetidine, alpha-methyldopa, reserpine, beta blockers, and corticosteroids.

A. Suicide

Assessment of the risk of suicide is a critical part of managing depression. Features that suggest a high risk include detailed thought to a suicide plan, coexistence of alcoholism, social isolation, male gender, and advanced age. A high risk of suicide usually mandates hospital admission.

B. Antidepressant Medications

Antidepressants (Table 1–9) are effective in all types of depression. A medication is usually selected to address the most bothersome symptom(s) with a minimum of side effects. Which drug will be the most effective is not predictable.

All antidepressants have a latency of antidepressant effect of up to 4 weeks. Because the average duration of an untreated depressive event is 9 months, antidepressants are usually given for 8 to 12 months and then tapered.

1. **TCAs.** There are several important side effects of tricyclic antidepressants (TCAs). Anticholinergic effects, sedation, a fine tremor, and postural hypotension are the most common. **Cardiotoxicity** includes heart block, bundle branch block, and bradyarrhythmias or tachyarrhythmias. Atrial arrhythmias and premature ventricular contractions are not contraindications to therapy, but concomitant therapy with type I antiarrhythmics should be cautious because of similarity of effect. TCAs are contraindicated in acute MI.

   Significant additive effects may occur with other CNS sedatives. Cimetidine, fluoxetine, and paroxetine increase the pharmacologic effects of most TCAs. The TCAs are well absorbed orally and have half-lives long enough to allow once-daily administration if side effects permit.

TABLE 1-9. Drugs Used in the Affective Disorders

AGENT	USUAL ADULT DOSE RANGE (mg) (LOWER DOSES RECOMMENDED FOR ELDERLY PERSONS)	RELATIVE SEDATION	RELATIVE ANTICHOLINERGIC EFFECT	RELATIVE DELAY OF CARDIAC CONDUCTION	RELATIVE POSTURAL HYPOTENSION	COMMENT
TRICYCLIC ANTIDEPRESSANTS						
Amitriptyline (Elavil, Endep, Enovil)	75–300	3	2	3	3	Used for chronic pain
Clomipramine (Anafranil)	25–250	2	2	2	2	Primary use is for obsessive-compulsive disorder; may lower seizure threshold; may increase plasma concentration of protein-bound drugs (e.g., digoxin, warfarin)
Desipramine (Norpramin, Pertofrane)	75–300	1	1	3	1	Used for chronic pain; metabolite of imipramine
Doxepin (Adapin, Sinequan)	75–300	3	3	1	3	Potent antihistamine (receptor subtypes 1 and 2)
Imipramine (Janimine, Tofranil)	50–300	2	2	3	2	Used for chronic pain, panic disorder, and headache
Nortriptyline (Aventyl, Pamelor)	50–150	1	1	2	2	Used for chronic pain, panic disorder, and headache; metabolite of amitriptyline
Protriptyline (Vivactil)	15–60	0	2	2	1	Used in central sleep apnea
Trimipramine (Surmontil)	50–300	2	2	3	2	—
TETRACYCLIC ANTIDEPRESSANTS						
Amoxapine (Asendin)	200–600	2	1	1	1	Metabolite has neuroleptic side effect
Maprotiline (Ludiomil)	75–300	2	1	1	1	May lower seizure threshold

	Dosage Range (mg/day)					Comments
HETEROCYCLIC ANTIDEPRESSANTS						
Nefazodone (Serzone)	200–600	2	1	0	1	Give in divided doses on bid schedule; do not administer with terfenadine or astemizole; risk of priapism in males and similar phenomenon in females; may increase plasma concentration of protein-bound drugs (e.g., digoxin, warfarin)
Trazodone (Desyrel)	150–600	3	1	0	2	Risk of priapism in males and similar phenomenon in females; may increase plasma concentration of protein-bound drugs (e.g., digoxin, warfarin); should be given as divided doses
MISCELLANEOUS AGENTS						
Bupropion (Wellbutrin)	300–450	0	0	1	0	Single dose should not exceed 150 mg; inhibits dopamine reuptake; given bid or tid
Venlafaxine (Effexor)	75–375	1	1	1	0	Inhibits serotonin and norepinephrine reuptake; given bid or tid
MONOAMINE OXIDASE INHIBITORS (MAOIs)						
Isocarboxazid (Marplan)	10–30	2	1	0	3	—
Phenelzine (Nardil)	15–90	2	1	0	3	Also used in panic disorder
Tranylcypromine (Parnate)	20–60	1	1	0	3	—

Table continued on following page

TABLE 1-9. Drugs Used in the Affective Disorders *(Continued)*

AGENT	USUAL ADULT DOSE RANGE (mg) (LOWER DOSES RECOMMENDED FOR ELDERLY PERSONS)	RELATIVE SEDATION	RELATIVE ANTICHOLINERGIC EFFECT	RELATIVE DELAY OF CARDIAC CONDUCTION	RELATIVE POSTURAL HYPOTENSION	COMMENT
SELECTIVE SEROTONIN REUPTAKE INHIBITORS (SSRIs)						
Fluoxetine (Prozac)	20–40 (starting dose 10 in the elderly)	0	0	0	0	Up to 60 mg/d for obsessive-compulsive disorder; $t\frac{1}{2}$ of fluoxetine 24–72 h; $t\frac{1}{2}$ of active metabolite (norfluoxetine) 96–144 h
Paroxetine (Paxil)	20–50 (starting dose 10 in the elderly)	1	1	0	1	No active metabolite; $t\frac{1}{2}$ of paroxetine 21 h
Sertraline (Zoloft)	50–200 (starting dose 12.5–25 in the elderly)	0	0	0	0	$t\frac{1}{2}$ of sertraline 26 h; $t\frac{1}{2}$ of active metabolite (desmethylsertraline) 62–104 h

There is a roughly linear correlation between therapeutic effect and serum levels for most agents, and routine drug level monitoring is not necessary. Lower doses (Table 1–9) are recommended in frail, elderly persons.

2. **SSRIs.** Selective serotonin-reuptake inhibitors (SSRIs) are widely used antidepressants that are generally better tolerated than the TCAs. They are as effective as TCAs in the management of depressed outpatients and do not have the significant anticholinergic, hypotensive, sedative, and cardiotoxic effects that frequently limit treatment with TCAs. The SSRIs are also effective in panic disorder, usually at doses lower than that used for depression. Common side effects include anorexia, anxiety, insomnia, diarrhea, and sexual dysfunction. Paroxetine and fluoxetine are known to inhibit some of the isoenzymes of the cytochrome P450 system and they reduce the clearance of diazepam, metoprolol, encainide, flecainide, and many TCAs.

3. **MAOIs.** Monoamine oxidase inhibitors (MAOIs) are rarely used as first-line antidepressant agents and appear to be more effective in atypical depression, panic disorder, and depression with psychomotor retardation. Because of inhibition of MAO in the GI tract, foods rich in tyramine or tryptophan are contraindicated. Implicated foods include cheese, wine, beer, yogurt, chicken liver, chocolate, bananas, avocados, and sour cream (Arch Intern Med 1991;151:873–884).

Many medications, such as alpha-methyldopa, amphetamines, caffeine, L-dopa, meperidine, phenothiazines, SSRIs, sympathomimetics, and TCAs should not be administered simultaneously with the MAOIs. Consumption of such foods or medications may cause severe hypertension. Orthostatic hypotension, tremor, and insomnia may occur with all of the MAOIs.

4. **LITHIUM.** Lithium, usually in the form of lithium carbonate, is the mainstay of chronic treatment for mania. Acute treatment may also require sedatives or neuroleptics. Lithium carbonate is well absorbed orally and is usually administered two or three times per day. Lithium has a half-life of 20 to 24 hours in patients with normal renal function. Sodium depletion, NSAIDs, and thiazides decrease lithium clearance. Urinary alkalinizers, such as potassium citrate, increase lithium clearance.

The average daily dose of lithium carbonate is 900–1500 mg, and an increment of 300 mg corresponds to a change in serum level of 0.2 mEq/L. **Monitoring of serum levels is essential** because of a narrow therapeutic range, and 0.8 to 1.2 mEq/L (10 hours after the previous dose) is considered optimal.

With therapeutic lithium concentrations, thyroxine synthesis may be impaired, although most patients remain euthyroid. Nephrogenic diabetes insipidus, leukocytosis, electrocardiographic abnormalities, and neurologic symptoms may also result from lithium use.

Preskorn SH, Baker BS. Outpatient management of the depressed patient. Disease-a-Month 1995;41:75–140.

XIII. PRESSURE SORES

The pressure sore (decubitus ulcer) has a prevalence among hospital inpatients of 3% to 11%. Patients with hypoalbuminemia, fecal incontinence, and fractures are at greatest risk of developing pressure sores. Pathophysiologic factors include external pressure sufficient to close the cutaneous capillaries exerted for more than 2 hours, shear forces on the skin producing damage to dermal structures, and external friction causing damage to the stratum corneum. The presence of moisture accelerates epidermal breakdown by interfering with natural reparative processes.

A. Preventive Measures

Preventive measures should be used for all patients at risk of pressure sores. Frequent turning of a patient (every 1 to 2 hours) normally permits adequate blood supply, although underlying microvascular disease may further impair capillary function.

Although cushioning systems may help, none have consistently lowered pressures below capillary closing pressure. Air-fluidized bed and mattress systems are effective but not practical for general use.

Cutaneous shear forces may be decreased by the use of sheepskin and clothing that is free of particulate matter. Proper positioning—whether lying or sitting—also helps minimize shear forces. Skin care to maintain appropriate levels of moisture may require intervention to dry the skin as well as judicious use of emollients to minimize fragility. Early pressure lesions may be confused with cellulitis (Table 1–10). If such lesions progress to ulceration and tissue necrosis, surgical debridement is usually necessary.

B. Management

Management of established pressure sores is similar to the management of ulcerative lesions in general, with debridement of necrotic tissue by mechanical means (instruments, Water-Pik, whirlpool) or by topical means (wet to dry dressing with gauze soaked in normal saline or hydrogen peroxide or biochemical agents, such as collagenase, fibrinolysin-deoxyribonuclease, or papain). Studies of alternatives to wet to dry dressings have been poorly controlled, and no convincing advantages have been demonstrated.

Once the wound is free of necrotic debris, it should be kept moist with

TABLE 1–10. **Staging of Pressure Sores**

STAGE	DESCRIPTION
I	Nonblanchable erythema of intact skin
II	Partial-thickness skin loss involving epidermis or dermis or both
III	Full-thickness skin loss involving damage or necrosis of subcutaneous tissue that may extend down to, but not through, underlying fascia
IV	Full-thickness skin loss with extensive destruction, tissue necrosis, or damage to muscle, bone, or supporting structures

minimal trauma. Topical antibiotics (e.g., silver sulfadiazine) or vapor-permeable occlusive dressings should be used.

Patients should receive nutritional support if needed, and measures should be taken to avoid new pressure sores.

Allman RM. Pressure ulcers among the elderly. N Engl J Med 1989;320:850–853.
Bergstrom N, Bennett MA, Carlson CE, et al. Treatment of pressure ulcers. Clinical practice guideline No. 15. Rockville, MD: Agency for Health Care Policy and Research, 1995 (AHCPR publication No. 95-0653) 1 (800) 358-9295.
Smith DM. Pressure ulcers in the nursing home. Ann Intern Med 1995;123:433–442.

XIV. URINARY INCONTINENCE

Urinary incontinence occurs in 20% of hospitalized elderly patients and 50% of nursing home residents. Many events, including hospitalization, may cause transient urinary incontinence.

New medications may promote urinary retention and overflow incontinence (anticholinergics, analgesics, sedatives) or increased flow (diuretics). Alpha-adrenergic agonists and antagonists, theophylline, and calcium channel blockers may also contribute to the development of incontinence.

A. Evaluation of the Incontinent Patient

A history, physical examination, and record of the timing of micturition and incontinence may suggest drug reactions or functional incontinence.

Urinalysis may provide evidence of a tumor, stone, or infection, leading to specific evaluation and treatment. **Measurement** of the postvoid residual urine volume (in and out bladder catheterization or with a portable ultrasound device) is important to evaluate for bladder outlet obstruction. A postvoid residual volume over 150 to 200 mL is abnormal and requires further evaluation.

B. Incontinence Due to an Acute Illness

Patients with incontinence due to an acute medical illness have a good prognosis for recovery of urinary function when their medical problem resolves. Judicious use of **absorptive undergarments** may be very helpful, although care must be taken to avoid skin breakdown.

For men, **condom catheters** may help but may cause skin breakdown, contribute to bladder infections, and aggravate confusion. The use of indwelling bladder catheters is generally not an appropriate long-term solution, although they may be required in selected cases. Intermittent bladder catheterization is preferred.

C. Detrusor Hyperactivity

Detrusor hyperactivity is the most common cause of chronic incontinence in the elderly. It results from insufficient inhibition of the detrusor muscle by the CNS (e.g., cerebrovascular disease, Alzheimer's disease, normal pressure hydrocephalus) or hyperexcitability of the afferent pathways (e.g., bladder or pelvic infection, tumor, fecal impaction, uterine prolapse, or prostatic hypertrophy).

The pattern of micturition is erratic, but usually with voided volumes over 150 mL. There is usually a warning period before micturition. Bladder training, in which the patient voids voluntarily every 1 to 2 hours, may keep the bladder volume within the detrusor capacity.

Drug therapy of detrusor hyperactivity uses **anticholinergic agents,** such as propantheline bromide (Pro-Banthine) 15–120 mg qd administered bid to qid, imipramine (Tofranil) 25–150 mg qd administered bid to qid, and oxybutynin (Ditropan) 5–20 mg qd administered bid to qid.

Detrusor-sphincter dyssynergia may also be present. **Alpha-adrenergic blockers** that may help relax the smooth muscle internal sphincter include prazosin (Minipress) 2–20 mg qd administered bid to tid, terazosin (Hytrin) 1–10 mg at bedtime, doxazosin (Cardura) 1–8 mg at bedtime and phenoxybenzamine (Dibenzyline) 10–60 mg qd given bid to tid.

D. Overflow Incontinence

Overflow incontinence usually causes frequent, small amounts of urinary leakage from a distended bladder, particularly with physical exertion, coughing, sneezing, or Valsalva maneuver.

It may result from bladder outlet obstruction, detrusor-sphincter dyssynergia, or detrusor weakness, usually due to a drug effect or a neurologic lesion, such as radiculopathy or neuropathy. After an episode of acute overdistention (600 to 800 mL or more), the bladder may be hypotonic but recover its tone after 7 to 14 days of catheter decompression.

Mechanical obstruction should be treated surgically or with catheter drainage. Maneuvers, such as Valsalva maneuver or suprapubic compression, may also help.

Drug therapy for overflow incontinence uses alpha-adrenergic blockers to allow internal sphincter relaxation (see above). Detrusor tone may be augmented by bethanechol (Urecholine, Duvoid) 30–150 mg qd administered tid.

E. Sphincter Insufficiency

Sphincter insufficiency most commonly appears as stress incontinence. It is common in parous postmenopausal women but may occur in men with surgically damaged internal sphincters. Initial management of women is with pelvic floor exercises and, in postmenopausal patients, topical estrogens [conjugated estrogen (Premarin) cream 1–2 g intravaginally at bedtime]. Alpha-adrenergic drugs, such as phenylpropanolamine 50–150 mg qd administered bid to qid, imipramine (see Detrusor Hyperactivity above), and surgical correction are other potential treatments.

Fantl JA, Newman DK, Colling J, et al. Managing acute and chronic urinary incontinence. Clinical practice guideline No. 2. Rockville, MD: Agency for Health Care Policy and Research, 1992 (AHCPR publication No. 92-0686) 1 (800) 358-9295.

Ouslander JG, Schnelle JF. Incontinence in the nursing home. Ann Intern Med 1995;122:438–449.

Wein AJ. Pharmacology of incontinence. Urol Clin North Am 1995;22:557–577.

XV. DRUG OVERDOSES

A. Incidence

1. It is estimated that 4.3 million poisonings occurred in the United States in 1993.

2. Toxic sequelae to drugs may be intentional, accidental, or iatrogenic

and should be considered in any patient with an altered mental status, seizures, or cardiac arrhythmias. A thorough history, physical examination, and appropriate laboratory testing are required to direct therapy.

3. The local poison control center should be contacted for specific assistance.

B. Immediate Assessment and Treatment

1. Ensure safety of treatment staff. Patients suffering toxic effects from environmental chemicals, such as tear gas or insecticides, may pose a hazard to staff (usually because of contaminated clothes). Until decontamination can be completed, staff should wear gowns, gloves, and airway protection (as needed).

2. Ensure adequate airway, breathing, and circulation. The cervical spine should be immobilized in cases of trauma, neck pain, or altered mental status. Usually, a large-bore IV catheter should be placed while blood samples are obtained for analysis. Vital signs, cardiac rhythm, neurologic status, and oxygen saturation should be monitored continuously.

3. Laboratory studies that should be routine include:
   a. **Serum electrolytes, glucose, BUN, creatinine, osmolarity, and pregnancy test.** An elevated anion gap suggests ingestion of alcohol, toluene, methanol, paraldehyde, iron, isoniazid, ethylene glycol, salicylates, or strychnine. Serum drug levels and general toxicology screens may be helpful, and some blood should be retained for future use.
   b. **Arterial blood gases** should be determined, including the carboxyhemoglobin level, if applicable.
   c. **A 12-lead ECG** should be done.

4. In the patient with an altered level of consciousness, immediate treatment should include thiamine 100 mg IV, glucose 25 g IV, naloxone 0.8–2 mg IV (two to five ampules). Use a higher dose if opiate excess is strongly suspected. The dosage for children is 0.01 mg/kg.

5. Seizures should be treated by protecting the airway and administering diazepam (5–10 mg IV) or lorazepam (2–4 mg IV or IM). Phenytoin 15–18 mg/kg may be given IV at 50 mg/min if these are not effective.

6. Cardiac arrhythmias
   a. **Supraventricular tachycardia** occurs in many overdoses, especially if anticholinergic drugs are involved. Appropriate advanced cardiac life support (ACLS) protocols should be followed for their management.
      (1) ***Adenosine*** 6 mg (1 ampule) IV push followed by a 20 mL saline flush. If no response, repeat with 12 mg, *or*
      (2) ***Propranolol*** 1–3 mg IV over 3 to 4 minutes. Repeat in 5 to 10 minutes as needed to control rate to a maximum of 0.1 mg/kg. Propranolol is relatively contraindicated in cases of digoxin overdose.
      (3) In cases of anticholinergic poisoning, ***Physostigmine*** 0.5–1 mg

given over 2 minutes, repeated q15min, up to a total of 6 mg may be required for refractory arrhythmias. **Atropine** 0.5 mg for each 1 mg of physostigmine may be required to treat adverse effects. Physostigmine is contraindicated in patients with suspected TCA overdose, conduction disturbance, widening of the QRS complex, or CHF.

  b. **Ventricular ectopy or tachycardia** should be treated with the proper ACLS protocols: **lidocaine** 1 mg/kg IV loading dose, with 2–4 mg/min infusion. Phenytoin and propranolol may also be effective. Procainamide and quinidine should be avoided.

7. MEASURES TO DECREASE ABSORPTION of any ingested toxin should be initiated (see below).

8. OTHER ADDITIONAL TREATMENTS should be given based on the initial clinical impression, supplemented by laboratory tests. Comorbid conditions (e.g., bronchospasm, infections) should be treated appropriately.

9. A PATIENT WITH DRUG TOXICITY should be considered suicidal until proved otherwise. No patient should be discharged from the emergency room without a psychiatric assessment. When doubt exists, hospital admission is appropriate.

C. Measures to Stop Absorption

1. IN PATIENTS TOXIC FROM TOPICAL ABSORPTION, contaminated clothes and equipment should be removed, and the skin should be cleansed with copious irrigation.

2. IN PATIENTS WHO HAVE INGESTED A TOXIN, decontamination of the GI tract may be appropriate. Consultation with a poison control center is advised.

  a. **In an awake patient,** give syrup of ipecac (15 mL for children, 30 mL for adults) and water (15 mL/kg for children, 1000 mL for adults). Repeat this in 20 minutes; if no emesis occurs, perform **gastric lavage.** Use caution when giving ipecac to patients who have ingested sedatives, as their level of consciousness may decline rapidly.

  b. **Gastric lavage** (36 French tube through mouth or nose) may be done in an awake patient (head down, left lateral decubitus position). Lavage with at least 5 L of warmed water. Use 300 mL aliquots in adults, 10 mL/kg aliquots in children.

  c. There are important **contraindications to emesis or lavage.**

  (1) Patients with impaired mental status or gag reflex should be lavaged only after intubation with a cuffed endotracheal tube.

  (2) Patients who have ingested antiemetics, amphetamines, camphor, chlordane, cocaine, cyclic antidepressants, hydrocarbons, isoniazid, lindane, nicotine, or strychnine should not be given ipecac to induce emesis.

  (3) Patients who have ingested a caustic substance (acid, alkali) should not be lavaged or receive ipecac.

(4) Patients who have ingested a long-chain hydrocarbon (gasoline, mineral spirits, turpentine, kerosene) should not be lavaged because of the risk of aspiration pneumonitis. Patients who have ingested aromatic or halogenated hydrocarbons (benzene, toluene), camphor, phenol, heavy metals, or insecticides should be lavaged after intubation with a cuffed endotracheal tube.

3. ACTIVATED CHARCOAL should be given (50–100 g) after the stomach is cleared of pill fragments unless acetaminophen toxicity is suspected (it binds *N*-acetylcysteine, the antidote for acetaminophen toxicity). Repeated doses (every 4 to 6 hours) may be useful in drugs with enterohepatic circulation (e.g., TCAs).

D. Measures to Enhance Drug Excretion

Measures to enhance drug excretion should be used for some situations.

1. FORCED DIURESIS (3–6 mL/kg/h) may be helpful for some agents. This is accomplished by volume loading, followed by furosemide or mannitol, with careful observation of fluid and electrolyte status (especially serum potassium).

   a. **Neutral diuresis** may aid excretion of isoniazid and bromides.

   b. **Acid diuresis** (urine pH less than 5.5) may be induced with ascorbic acid (500–2000 mg PO or IV) or ammonium chloride (100 mEq in 1000 mL of 0.9% sodium chloride infused at a rate of <5 mL/min in adults). It may help excretion of phencyclidine (PCP), strychnine, amphetamines, quinine, and quinidine. It should be avoided in patients who may have myoglobinuria (e.g., drug-induced, prolonged coma, or crush injury).

   c. **Alkaline diuresis** (urine pH greater than 7.5) may be induced with 1–2 mEq/kg of IV sodium bicarbonate over 60 to 120 minutes. This increases the excretion of salicylates, phenobarbital, TCAs, and the herbicide 2,4-dichlorophenoxyacetic acid (2,4-D).

2. CHARCOAL HEMOPERFUSION may be indicated with toxicity due to the insecticide paraquat or theophylline. Patients with overdoses of chloral hydrate, chlorophenothane, digoxin, digitoxin, ethchlorvynol, glutethimide, methaqualone, methotrexate, methophenobarbital, phenobarbital, phenytoin, and TCAs also may benefit, depending on their clinical status.

3. HEMODIALYSIS. Poisoning with the following agents is usually an indication for hemodialysis: ethylene glycol, lithium, methanol, salicylic acid, and *Amanita phalloides* mushrooms.

   Many other chemicals are dialyzable. Depending on their clinical status, some patients may benefit from hemodialysis after ingestion of acetaminophen, arsenic, bromide, carbamazepine, chloral hydrate, ethanol, and isopropyl alcohol.

E. Specific Antidotes

Some toxins have specific antidotes (Table 1–11). They may affect the metabolism of toxins to produce less toxic substances (e.g., ethanol for methanol), protect specific organs from damage (e.g., *N*-acetylcysteine for

TABLE 1–11. Specific Toxin Antidotes

TOXIN	ANTIDOTE	ANTIDOTE ADMINISTRATION
Acetaminophen	N-Acetylcystine	140 mg/kg PO loading dose, then 70 mg/kg PO q4h for 17 doses; repeat a dose if patient vomits within 1 h of its administration
Anticholinergic agents (examples include antihistamines, antiparkinsonian drugs, antipsychotic agents, atropine)	Physostigmine	Use only if necessary to manage coma, convulsions, dysrhythmias, or delirium; dose is 1–2 mg IV over 5 min; effect lasts 20–60 min; may repeat dose; do not exceed 6 mg over time
Benzodiazepines	Flumazenil	0.2 mg IV over 30 s; if no response in 30 s give 0.3 mg IV over 30 s; subsequent doses of 0.5 mg IV may be given, each over 30 s and 1 min between doses, to a total of 3–5 mg
Beta blockers	Glucagon	50–150 µg/kg IV over 1 min, followed by continuous infusion of 1–5 mg/h titrated to vital signs
Calcium channel blockers, hydrofluoric acid, fluorides	Calcium (calcium chloride for calcium channel blocker overdose; calcium gluconate for hydrofluoric acid or fluoride exposure)	*For calcium-channel-blocker overdose:* give 1 g calcium chloride IV over 5 min; continuously monitor cardiac rhythm *For hydrofluoric acid burns:* infiltrate each cm² of dermis and SC tissue with 0.5 mL of 10% calcium gluconate as needed for pain control; a calcium gel may also be applied to the burn surface *For PO fluoride ingestion:* give 10 g calcium gluconate in 250 mL water PO; maximum dose 30 g/d
Cyanide	Amyl nitrite, sodium nitrite, and sodium thiosulfate	Inhale amyl nitrite ampule for 30 s of every min; give 100% O_2 between amyl nitrite inhalations; use a new ampule q3min and continue until sodium nitrite can be given IV; sodium nitrite dose is 300 mg IV (10 mL of a 3% solution) at a rate of 2.5–5 mL/min; then administer 12.5 g of sodium thiosulfate IV
Cyclic antidepressants	Sodium bicarbonate	1–3 mEq/kg IV as necessary to maintain blood pH at 7.5; alkalinization results in increased protein binding of cyclic antidepressant and minimizes the amount of free drug available; useful in management of cyclic antidepressant-induced cardiac arrhythmias or hypotension

Digitalis glycosides	Digoxin-specific antibody fragments	Milligrams of digoxin ingested divided by 0.6 = number of vials required; if amount ingested is unknown but life-threatening dysrhythmias are present give 20 vials; if 6 h postingestion dig level is available, the number of vials to administer is = (dig level in ng/mL × 5.6 × wt in kg) divided by 600
Iron	Deferoxamine mesylate	15 mg/kg/h IV; or 90 mg/kg IM (maximum of 1 g per injection) q8h; maximum dose is 6 g in 24 h; use only IV route for life-threatening exposures; during therapy, monitor urine output, urine color, and iron levels
Methanol, ethylene glycol	Ethanol	Loading dose is 10 mL/kg of 10% ETOH in D_5W solution IV over 30 min; also begin a maintenance dose of 0.66–1.3 mL/kg/h IV of 10% solution; maintain blood ethanol concentration at 100–150 mg/dL; watch glucose and sodium levels closely; if patient is being dialyzed, add 91 mL/h to maintenance dose
Isoniazid, hydrazine, monomethyl-hydrazine mushrooms	Pyridoxine	*Unknown amount ingested:* give 5 g IV over 5 min *Known amount ingested:* give 1 g pyridoxine IV q5min for every gram ingested; an overdose of pyridoxine may cause neuropathy
Organophosphate or carbamate insecticides	Atropine	Begin with 2 mg IV test dose; then administer 2–4 mg IV q10–15min as needed until cessation of secretions occurs; for organophosphate insecticide poisoning, pralidoxime chloride 1–2 g IV q6h should be administered after initial treatment with atropine

From Mengert TJ, et al. Emergency medical therapeutics, 4th ed. Philadelphia: W.B. Saunders; 1996, p 875.

acetaminophen), or enhance excretion (e.g., chelating agents for heavy metals). In most cases of drug toxicity, removal of exposure and supportive therapy are the mainstays of treatment.

Kulig K. Initial management of ingestions of toxic substances. N Engl J Med 1992;326:1677–1681.
Mengert TJ. Standard therapy of the poisoned/overdose patient. In: Mengert TJ, Eisenberg MS, Copass MK, eds. Emergency Medical Therapy, 4th ed. Philadelphia: W.B. Saunders; 1996.

XVI. MEDICATIONS AND PREGNANCY

Approximately 3% of neonates have recognized congenital malformations, but only 10% of these are linked to specific agents. The time of greatest risk of major morphologic abnormalities is between 18 and 60 days of gestation. Only a few medications have been shown to be teratogenic in humans; likewise, only a small number are known to be safe. A larger number are known animal teratogens in doses exceeding common clinical use, and the majority carry an unknown risk (Table 1–12).

The Food and Drug Administration has established **five categories of risk** of medication use.

- **A:** Controlled studies in humans failed to demonstrate a risk to the fetus.
- **B:** No evidence of risk in humans: either animal findings show risk but human findings do not, or, if no adequate human studies have been done, animal findings are negative.
- **C:** Human studies have not been done; animal studies may be positive or not done.
- **D:** Available data show risk to the fetus, but potential benefits may outweigh the potential risks.
- **X:** Contraindicated during pregnancy.

This classification is helpful at the extreme ranges of risk. Unfortunately, most drugs fall in categories B and C.

Some medications given after the first trimester may cause fetal harm without leading to major malformations. When administered after the fourth month of pregnancy, the tetracycline antibiotics may cause staining of the teeth. The deciduous teeth are most frequently involved, but the permanent teeth may be affected if tetracyclines are used close to term. Heparin, the anticoagulant of choice during pregnancy, is not associated with congenital defects but carries an increased risk of fetal loss. Narcotics and barbiturates used late in pregnancy may cause dependence and withdrawal syndromes in the neonate.

As few medications are 100% safe during pregnancy, the best strategy is to use a **minimum number of medications** for as short a time as possible. Combination products, both prescription and nonprescription, should be avoided. Use of a reference text or consultation with an individual with special interest in teratology may help when choosing medications.

Folic acid supplementation before conception can reduce the risk of congenital neural tube defects. The U.S. Public Health Service recommends that women planning conception consume a minimum of 0.4 mg/d of folic acid.

Briggs GG, Freeman RK, Yaffe SJ. Drugs in Pregnancy and Lactation, 4th ed. Baltimore: Williams & Wilkins; 1994.

Text continued on page 51

TABLE 1–12. Medication Use During Pregnancy

CLASS OF DRUG	GENERALLY CONSIDERED SAFE[1]	PROBABLY SAFE BUT WITH FEWER DATA AVAILABLE	SOME RISK DOCUMENTED OR SUSPECTED[2]	CONTRAINDICATED[3]
Analgesics	Acetaminophen	Aspirin[4] Methadone[5] Morphine[5] Meperidine[5]	Ibuprofen and NSAIDs[4] Colchicine Codeine[5]	Dihydroergotamine
Antiasthmatics	—	Cromolyn sodium Ipratropium Terbutaline	Albuterol Isoetharine Metaproterenol Salmeterol Theophylline	—
Anti-infectives	Ampicillin Cephradine[6] Erythromycin[7] Penicillin	Azithromycin Amphotericin B Clindamycin Clotrimazole Dicloxacillin Ethambutol Nafcillin Nitrofurantoin[8] Sulfonamides[5]	Acyclovir Chloroquine Fluconazole Gentamicin[9] Isoniazid Ketoconazole Metronidazole[10] Rifampin Trimethoprim[11] Vancomycin	Chloramphenicol Ciprofloxacin Clarithromycin Griseofulvin Norfloxacin Ofloxacin Streptomycin Tetracyclines Tobramycin[10]
Anticoagulants	—	—	Dipyridamole Heparin[12] Low molecular weight heparin	Warfarin
Anticonvulsants	—	—	Carbamazepine[13] Phenobarbital[13] Phenytoin[13]	Paramethadione[13] Trimethadione[13] Valproic acid[13]

Table continued on following page

47

TABLE 1–12. Medication Use During Pregnancy (*Continued*)

CLASS OF DRUG	GENERALLY CONSIDERED SAFE[1]	PROBABLY SAFE BUT WITH FEWER DATA AVAILABLE	SOME RISK DOCUMENTED OR SUSPECTED[2]	CONTRAINDICATED[3]
Antidepressants	—	Fluoxetine Paroxetine Sertraline	Amitriptyline Desipramine Doxepin Nortriptyline Venlafaxine	—
Antiemetics	Emetrol	Metoclopramide Ondansetron Promethazine	Cisapride Prochlorperazine	—
Antihistamines	—	Chlorpheniramine Loratadine Meclizine	Astemizole Diphenhydramine Hydroxyzine Terfenadine	—
Antihypertensives	Hydralazine Methyldopa Metoprolol[14]	Atenolol[14] Bumetanide[15] Clonidine Furosemide[15] Nadolol[14] Propranolol[14]	Chlorothiazide[15] Nifedipine Nitroprusside Phenoxybenzamine Prazosin Spironolactone[15] Triamterene[15]	ACE inhibitors
Cardiac drugs	—	Adenosine Atropine Digoxin Lidocaine Quinidine	Amiodarone Disopyramide Nifedipine Nitroglycerin Procainamide Verapamil	HMG-CoA reductase inhibitors
Decongestants	—	—	Phenylpropanolamine Pseudoephedrine	—

Endocrine	Levothyroxine	Prednisone[16]	Cortisone Dexamethasone Glyburide[17] Propylthiouracil[18]	Bromocriptine Danazol Estrogens Methimazole
Gastrointestinal	Kaolin-pectin[19] Loperamide Milk of Magnesia Psyllium	Cimetidine Docusate Famotidine Ranitidine Sucralfate	Cholestyramine Cisapride Omeprazole Sulfasalazine[4]	Chenodiol Misoprostol
Psychotropics	—	—	Chlorpromazine Haloperidol Perphenazine	Lithium
Sedatives	Chloral hydrate	—	Alprazolam Chlordiazepoxide Diazepam	Estazolam Quazepam Temazepam Triazolam
Vaccinations	—	—	Inactivated *Haemophilus influenzae* type b Hepatitis A Hepatitis B Influenza Oral polio Tetanus/diphtheria toxoid	Live virus Measles Mumps Rubella Varicella

Table continued on following page

49

TABLE 1–12. Medication Use During Pregnancy *(Continued)*

CLASS OF DRUG	GENERALLY CONSIDERED SAFE[1]	PROBABLY SAFE BUT WITH FEWER DATA AVAILABLE	SOME RISK DOCUMENTED OR SUSPECTED[2]	CONTRAINDICATED[3]
Miscellaneous	—	Guaifenesin Purified Protein Derivative for skin testing	—	Alendronate Antineoplastic agents Auranofin Etretinate Iodine Isotretinoin Thalidomide Tretinoin

[1]No drug can be considered unequivocally safe during pregnancy. The risks and benefits must be weighed in each case.
[2]Degree of risk is quite variable in this class; these drugs may be useful if potential benefit outweighs potential risk.
[3]Use should be avoided in all but exceptional circumstances.
[4]Avoid use during last trimester.
[5]May cause neonatal toxicity when used at term.
[6]First-generation cephalosporins are probably safe. Many second-generation and third-generation cephalosporins contain an *N*-methylthiotetrazole side chain that may cause fetal testicular toxicity.
[7]Avoid erythromycin estolate owing to risk of neonatal hepatic toxicity.
[8]Avoid use at term owing to risk of hemolysis in neonates deficient in glucose-6-phosphate dehydrogenase.
[9]Not clearly teratogenic, but there is risk of fetal ototoxicity.
[10]Avoid use in first trimester.
[11]Generally should not be used owing to its activity as a folate antagonist.
[12]Not teratogenic, but increased rate of fetal loss may occur; however, this is the anticoagulant of choice during pregnancy.
[13]The use of anticonvulsants during pregnancy may involve increased risk to the fetus. The risks and benefits must be carefully weighed. The simultaneous administration of folate may be beneficial.
[14]Beta blocker use at term may result in neonatal bradycardia and hypoglycemia.
[15]Use of diuretics is usually considered inappropriate during pregnancy.
[16]Little risk has been documented with low doses of prednisone. However, higher doses or more potent steroids may increase the risk of fetal malformations.
[17]Use of oral hypoglycemic agents is considered inappropriate during pregnancy; insulin should be used.
[18]Considered the drug of choice for treating hyperthyroidism during pregnancy.
[19]Long-term use may reduce iron absorption and result in anemia.

Gilstrap LC, Little BB. Drugs and Pregnancy. New York: Elsevier; 1992.
Kuller JM. Effects on the fetus and newborn of medications commonly used in pregnancy. J Perinat Neonatal Nurs 1990;3:73–87.

XVII. PERIOPERATIVE MEDICAL CARE

The goals of the **preoperative medical evaluations** are to identify the patient's medical problems, assess the risk for surgery, and create a plan for perioperative management of the medical problems. Effective preoperative consultation requires **concise and explicit communication** between the consultant and the surgical-anesthesia team. Recommendations for medications should include the dosage, route, frequency, and duration of therapy.

Important components of the preoperative assessment include the past medical and surgical history (including complications), allergies, medications, habits, family and social history, a review of systems, and a summary of available laboratory studies. The preoperative consultation should include an **assessment of the patient's surgical risk,** suggestions for **managing the medical problems** perioperatively, and recommendations for appropriate **prophylactic therapy.**

Risk assessment addresses the general risk of surgery as well as specific surgical risks (e.g., cardiac complications). General risk factors for perioperative complications include increasing age (>65 years), the number and severity of medical problems, exercise tolerance, the type and duration of surgery and anesthesia, and a history of previous perioperative complications. The American Society of Anesthesiologists (ASA) classification assesses a patient's general risk of surgery (Table 1–13). The risk of complications is highest for vascular, orthopedic, thoracic and abdominal procedures.

A. Cardiovascular Disease

The most familiar **index for cardiac risk assessment** is a point scale based on the presence of specific risk factors (Table 1–14). Another popular risk assessment tool modifies Goldman's original index to include more detailed information about prior MIs, the presence of angina, and a history of pulmonary edema (Detsky AS, et al).

1. **APPROPRIATE PATIENT SELECTION.** Reduction of perioperative cardiac complications is best accomplished by appropriate patient selection

TABLE 1–13. **American Society of Anesthesiologists Classification**

ASA CLASS	DISEASE STATE	SURGICAL MORTALITY
1	Healthy	Very low (0.01%)
2	Mild/moderate systemic illness	Low (0.1%)
3	Severe systemic illness	Moderate (0.66%)
4	Severe, life-threatening illness	High (4.6%)
5	Moribund	Very high (9.2%)

From Dripps RD, Lamont A, Eckenhoff JE. The role of anesthesia in surgical mortality. JAMA 1961;178:261. Copyright 1961, American Medical Association.

TABLE 1–14. **Goldman Cardiac Risk Index**

FACTOR	POINTS
Myocardial infarction within 6 mo	10
Age > 70 y	5
S3 gallop or jugular venous distention	11
Significant aortic stenosis	3
Rhythm other than NSR with PACs	7
More than 5 PVC/min	7
Poor medical condition	3
K^+ <3 mEq/L, HCO_3^- <20 mEq/L	
BUN >50 mg/dL, creatinine >3 mg/dL	
Po_2 <60 mm Hg, Pco_2 >50 mm Hg	
Liver disease, bedridden	
Abdominal, thoracic, or aortic surgery	3
Emergency operation	4
Total	53

CLASS	POINTS	RISK OF CARDIAC COMPLICATION	RISK OF DEATH
I	0–5	0%	0.2%
II	6–12	5%	2%
III	13–25	11%	2%
IV	>25	22%	56%

and attentive perioperative care. Patients with uncontrolled cardiovascular illness, such as unstable angina, uncompensated CHF, significant valvular heart disease, and uncontrolled hypertension, should, if possible, have their surgery delayed until their medical problems are corrected. Stable angina with an exercise tolerance of greater than four blocks of walking and two flights of stairs does not increase perioperative cardiac risk.

2. ANESTHESIA. A thorough assessment of the patient's medical problems and risk assessment will help the anesthesiologist and patient decide on the best anesthetic choice. Some types of **anesthesia may worsen underlying cardiac problems.** For example, spinal anesthetics frequently cause venodilatation, which decreases cardiac preload. This could have potentially devastating effects on a patient with critical aortic stenosis. For that reason, the choice of anesthetic agents and techniques is best left to the anesthesiology team after discussion of the patient's medical problems and risks.

3. HEMODYNAMIC MONITORING. Invasive hemodynamic monitoring (arterial, central venous, or pulmonary artery catheterization) may be helpful in managing patients with CHF, valvular heart disease, or significant coronary artery disease, particularly if substantial fluid shifts may be expected. Since postoperative fluid mobilization may require 48 hours, monitoring is usually continued for that period.

4. **MEDICAL PROBLEMS.** Close attention to the patient's medical problems perioperatively is vital to minimizing complications. The serum **electrolytes** should be checked frequently and kept well within the normal range. Patients with significant coronary disease may benefit from maintaining the **hematocrit** near or above 30%. **Tachycardia** should be avoided by maintaining adequate intravascular volume and by controlling pain, anxiety, and fever. Close attention to the patient's **pulmonary status** is important in decreasing the risk of perioperative cardiac complications, particularly arrhythmias.

5. **MEDICATION MANAGEMENT.** Proper perioperative medication management can help reduce complications. Patients receiving **antihypertensive and antianginal therapy** should generally receive these medications on the day of surgery and postoperatively if possible. Many patients are transiently hypotensive postoperatively as a result of fluid shifts and narcotic analgesia. It is best to use **short-acting agents** and to include parameters for which the medication should be held (e.g., diltiazem 60 mg PO q6h, hold for systolic blood pressure <100 mm Hg). **Diuretics** are usually held perioperatively and used only prn for the first few days after surgery. Many authors recommend stopping the antihypertensive **guanethidine** (Ismelin) 2 weeks before surgery to avoid potential drug interactions.

6. **SPECIFIC MEDICATIONS**
   a. **Beta adrenergic blockers.** Patients who take beta blockers are at risk for a withdrawal syndrome, including hypertension and tachycardia, which begins 24 hours after the last dose. The medication should be taken on the morning of surgery (with a small sip of water) and continued postoperatively, if at all possible. Short-acting beta blockers (metoprolol 25–50 mg bid PO or per nasogastric tube) may be absorbed even in patients with a postoperative ileus. Alternatively, IV beta blockers (propranolol 0.5–3 mg IV every 4 to 6 hours or a continuous infusion of esmolol) may be substituted, with appropriate monitoring. Beta blockers should be discontinued in patients who develop hypotension, pulmonary edema, heart block, or bronchospasm.
   b. **Digoxin.** When digoxin is used in the management of CHF, the indications for perioperative use are the same as for chronic use. It may be helpful in patients at high risk for perioperative supraventricular tachycardia (SVT), such as elderly patients undergoing thoracic surgery, patients with valvular heart disease, or patients with a history of SVT.
   c. **Antiarrhythmics** should generally be continued perioperatively if possible (PO or IV). Close monitoring of therapeutic levels and serum electrolytes is essential. Patients with life-threatening arrhythmias may benefit from cardiology consultation, the placement of defibrillator pads before starting surgery, and having antiarrhythmic agents readily available in the operating room.
   d. **Anticoagulants.** For patients considered at **low risk** for complications from discontinuing their anticoagulation (stroke prophylaxis in nonvalvular atrial fibrillation, prosthetic aortic valve, bioprosthetic

heart valve, remote deep venous thrombosis), anticoagulation can usually be discontinued 3 days before surgery and resumed postoperatively when the patient is taking medications orally.

For patients at **high risk** from discontinuing their anticoagulation (prosthetic mitral valve, atrial fibrillation with mitral stenosis, known intravascular thrombus, previous dialysis shunt thrombosis, hypercoagulable state), the following protocol should be considered:

*(1) **Discontinue warfarin*** 2 days before the procedure.

(2) Admit the patient 1 day before the procedure. Check the **prothrombin time** on admission. Begin IV **heparin** and titrate into the therapeutic range.

(3) If the admission prothrombin time is elevated, give **vitamin K** 1–5 mg SC. **Discontinue** the **heparin** 6 to 8 hours before the procedure. Check the **coagulation studies** immediately before the procedure.

*(4) **Resume the heparin*** postoperatively when possible from a surgical standpoint (generally within 24 to 48 hours). Resume warfarin when patient is able to take it orally.

B. Pulmonary Disease

The primary perioperative pulmonary complications are pneumonia, atelectasis, and respiratory failure. **Risk factors** for pulmonary complications include the surgical site (highest for thoracic and upper abdominal procedures), age >60 years, a history of chronic obstructive pulmonary disease (COPD) with dyspnea or productive cough, surgery longer than 3 hours, smoking (especially if currently smoking), obesity, forced expiratory volume in 1 second (FEV_1) less than 2 L, baseline P_{CO_2} greater than 45 mm Hg, ASA classification >2, and low serum albumin.

The use of intensive bronchodilators, adequate hydration, incentive spirometry (with preoperative teaching), early mobilization, and avoidance of sedatives minimizes pulmonary complications. Preoperative corticosteroids (prednisone 20–40 mg PO qd for 7 days) may be beneficial in patients with severe **COPD or asthma.** Postoperatively, the steroids should be tapered by 50% per day back to preoperative doses, as tolerated. Chest physiotherapy may be helpful for patients with localized pulmonary infiltrates but is of minimal benefit in others. Patients with chronically infected sputum benefit from **preoperative antibiotic treatment.** Smokers should **discontinue smoking before surgery** (although benefits may not be fully realized unless the patient discontinues smoking at least 8 weeks before surgery).

C. Prophylactic Therapy

Prophylactic therapy should be recommended for all patients undergoing significant procedures.

1. PULMONARY. INCENTIVE SPIROMETRY AND EARLY POSTOPERATIVE MOBILIZATION should be recommended in almost all cases.

2. DEEP VENOUS THROMBOSIS (Table 1–15). Although several prophylactic regimens exist, the optimal duration of DVT prophylaxis in unclear. At

TABLE 1–15. Risk Factors for Deep Venous Thrombosis

Prior thromboembolism	Obesity
Age >40 y	Multiple trauma
Leg or hip fracture	Malignancy
Myocardial infarction	Prolonged immobilization
Hip or knee arthroplasty	Coronary artery bypass surgery
Abdominal surgery	Gynecologic malignancy
Major urologic procedures	Neurosurgical procedures
Congestive heart failure	

a minimum, prophylaxis should continue until the patient is fully ambulatory. Estrogen-containing **oral contraceptives** should be discontinued 3 weeks before elective surgery. Postmenopausal estrogen replacement therapy need not be discontinued.

  a. Heparin 5000 units SC q12h is reasonable for most low-risk to moderate-risk patients. Although the risk of serious hemorrhagic complications is minimal with SC heparin, it should be avoided in patients with recent neurosurgical or ophthalmologic procedures.

  b. Sequential compression devices are an alternative particularly well suited for patients who have contraindications to anticoagulant usage. Their use may be initiated in the operating room.

  c. Warfarin may be used perioperatively in high-risk patients, but with a greater risk of hemorrhagic complications. Warfarin 5–10 mg may be given the night before surgery and continued postoperatively to maintain an international normalized ratio (INR) between 2 and 3. Close laboratory monitoring is essential.

  d. Several **low molecular weight heparins** are used for DVT prophylaxis and may be particularly well suited for high-risk patients. Their cost is high. Regimens include **enoxaparin** 30 mg SC bid or **dalteparin** 2500 IU SC qd beginning 1 to 2 hours before surgery.

  3. ENDOCARDITIS PROPHYLAXIS. Patients with prosthetic heart valves, congenital heart disease, rheumatic or other valvular heart disease, mitral valve prolapse with regurgitation, idiopathic hypertrophic subaortic stenosis, or prior endocarditis should have antibiotic prophylaxis before nonsterile procedures (Table 1–16). Patients with left-sided lesions, prior endocarditis, and prosthetic valves are at the highest risk. Prophylaxis is recommended for dental procedures or procedures in the upper respiratory tract that may result in bleeding. It is also recommended for procedures involving instrumentation of the GI-GU tract or incision and drainage of infected areas.

D. Management of Specific Problems

  1. PAIN AND NAUSEA. Control of postoperative pain and nausea requires careful attention to avoid toxic effects, most commonly excess sedation and confusion. The phenothiazines or other dopaminergic antagonists are the drugs of choice.

  2. FEVER. Fever is common in the first 24 to 48 hours after surgery. It frequently resolves with improvement in pulmonary toilet (incentive

TABLE 1–16. **Endocarditis Prophylaxis for Adults**

PROCEDURE	DRUG
RESPIRATORY OR ORAL PROCEDURES	
Low Risk	
No penicillin allergy	Amoxicillin 3 g PO 1 h before, then 1.5 g PO 6 h after procedure
Penicillin allergy	Erythromycin 1 g PO 2 h before, then 500 mg PO 6 h after procedure
High Risk (Previous Endocarditis, Prosthetic Valves, and Left-Sided Lesions)	
No penicillin allergy	Ampicillin 2 g IM/IV with gentamicin 1.5 mg/kg (not to exceed 80 mg) 30 min before procedure, then amoxicillin 1.5 g PO 6 h after procedure
Penicillin allergy	Vancomycin 1 g IV start 1 h before procedure
GASTROINTESTINAL OR GENITOURINARY PROCEDURES	
No penicillin allergy	Ampicillin 2 g IM/IV with gentamicin 1.5 mg/kg (not to exceed 80 mg) 30 min before procedure, then amoxicillin 1.5 g PO 6 h after procedure
Penicillin allergy	Vancomycin 1 g IV with gentamicin 1.5 mg/kg (not to exceed 80 mg) start 1 h before procedure; may be repeated 8 h later

spirometry and mobilization) and time. Regardless, patients with postoperative fevers should be evaluated. However, in the absence of localized physical findings or evidence of toxicity (e.g., hypotension), an extensive laboratory evaluation is not needed. If the patient has had a bladder catheter, a urinalysis should be performed.

3. DIABETES. Patients with **type I diabetes** should receive insulin perioperatively either SC or IV. Patients with **type II diabetes** treated with **oral agents** should have their agent discontinued preoperatively and resumed postoperatively when the patient resumes oral intake. The oral hypoglycemic agent metformin (Glucophage) should be discontinued 48 hours before surgery to minimize the risk of lactic acidosis. A variable-dose **regular insulin** regimen or low doses of **long-acting insulin** provided on a scheduled basis (before meals and at bedtime) may be used until the patient is able to resume the preoperative regimen. Patients with **type II diabetes who use insulin** should receive half of their usual morning dose of intermediate-acting insulin on the morning of surgery and a variable-dose regular insulin regimen, with a dextrose-containing IV solution. All patients with diabetes should have close monitoring of their glucose perioperatively (e.g., capillary glucose at before mealtimes and at bedtime).

4. STEROID DEPENDENCE. Patients who have received physiologic doses of corticosteroids for more than 2 weeks in the 6 months before surgery should receive stress dose steroids perioperatively, hydrocortisone 50–100 mg IV on call to the operating room and q8h postoperatively. Taper the steroids by 50% per day, back to preoperative doses as

tolerated. Patients who remain under significant physiologic stress postoperatively (e.g., ventilator dependent, sepsis) should receive stress doses of steroids until they improve.

Clagett GP, Anderson FA, Levine MN, et al. Prevention of venous thromboembolism. Chest 1992;102:391S–407S.

Detsky AS, Abrams HB, McLaughlin JR, et al. Predicting cardiac complications in patients undergoing non-cardiac surgery. J Gen Intern Med 1986;1:211–219.

Durack DT. Prevention of infective endocarditis. N Engl J Med 1995;332:38–44.

Eagle KA, Brundage BH, Chaitman BR, et al. Guidelines for perioperative cardiovascular evaluation for noncardiac surgery. Report of the American College of Cardiology/American Heart Association Task Force on Practice Guidelines. J Am Coll Cardiol 1996;27:910–948.

Goldman L, Caldera DL, Nussbaum SR, et al. Multifactorial index of cardiac risk in noncardiac surgical procedures. N Engl J Med 1977;297:845–850.

Hall JC, Tarala RA, Hall JL, Mander J. A multivariate analysis of the risk of pulmonary complications after laparotomy. Chest 1991;99:923–927.

2 2 2 2 2 2 2 2

FLUID AND ELECTROLYTE THERAPY

DAVID C. DUGDALE

I. NORMAL FLUID AND ELECTROLYTE PHYSIOLOGY

In healthy individuals, the renal, pulmonary, and endocrine systems maintain the body water and electrolytes within the physiologic range. When regulatory mechanisms fail, the physician must supplement or alter natural fluid and electrolyte inputs.

A. Total Body Water (TBW)

TBW accounts for approximately 50% of body weight in females and 60% of body weight in males. Approximately two thirds of TBW is intracellular.

The **extracellular fluid** comprises intravascular fluid (one fourth of extracellular fluid, or one twelfth of TBW) and extravascular fluid composed primarily of interstitial fluid, with small amounts in the bone and dense connective tissues.

Fluids administered IV distribute between the intravascular and extravascular spaces in fractions determined by the fluids' protein and sodium content.

B. Normal Fluid and Electrolyte Balance (Table 2–1)

As the maximal concentrating ability of the renal tubule is 1200 milliosmoles (mOsm)/L, excretion of the daily average production of 600 mOsm requires a minimum urine output of 500 mL. **Insensible losses** (skin, respiratory tract) increase by 100 to 300 mL/day for each degree C of fever. When oral intake is decreased, maintenance fluid and electrolytes must be provided. If feasible, the enteral route is preferred because of its lower rate of complications.

If parenteral supplements are required, IV **dextrose** solutions are used. A dose of 100–200 g/d (3.4 kcal/g) avoids ketosis and lessens body protein catabolism.

Although the renal conservation of **sodium** (Na) is very effective, maintenance Na is usually given, 80–120 mEq/d. Obligatory renal and fecal **potassium** losses must be replaced (60–100 mEq/d).

Total **maintenance** fluid and electrolyte needs for adults are typically met with 2–3 L (or 35 mL/kg of body weight) of 5% dextrose containing either 0.2% or 0.45% NaCl and 20 to 30 mEq of KCl/L. For maintenance longer than

TABLE 2–1. Fluid Fluxes in a Healthy Man (mL/d)

INTAKE	QUANTITY	OUTPUT	QUANTITY
Ingested fluid	1400	Urine	1500
Fluid in food	850	Skin	500
Water of oxidation	350	Respiratory tract	400
		Stool	200

TABLE 2–2. **Information for Calculation of Fluid and Electrolyte Replacement**

COMMON CONVERSIONS
1 mEq Na = 23 mg Na = 58.5 mg NaCl
1 g Na = 2.54 g NaCl = 43 mEq Na
1 g NaCl = 0.39 g Na = 17 mEq Na
1 mEq K = 39 mg K = 74.5 mg KCl
1 g K = 1.91 g KCl = 26 mEq K
1 g KCl = 0.52 g K = 13 mEq K
1 mEq Ca = 20 mg Ca = 0.5 mmol Ca
1 g Ca = 50 mEq Ca = 25 mmol Ca
1 mEq Mg = 0.12 g $MgSO_4 \cdot 7H_2O$
1 g Mg = 10.2 g $MgSO_4 \cdot 7H_2O$ = 82 mEq Mg
10 mmol P_i = 0.31 g P_i
1 g P_i = 32 mmol P_i

COMMON AMPULES
7.5% $NaHCO_3$ = 50 mL = 44.6 mEq Na
50% Dextrose = 50 mL = 25 g Dextrose
10% $CaCl_2 \cdot 2H_2O$ = 10 mL = 13.6 mEq Ca
10% Ca gluconate = 10 mL = 4.6 mEq Ca
50% $MgSO_4 \cdot 7H_2O$ = 2 mL = 8.1 mEq Mg
46% K phosphate = 10 mL = 30 mmol (930 mg) P_i with 44 mEq K
42% Na phosphate = 10 mL = 30 mmol (930 mg) P_i with 40 mEq Na

5 days, addition of calcium, magnesium, phosphate, and vitamins should be considered (Tables 2–2 and 2–3).

II. DISTURBANCES OF BODY FLUID VOLUME

The management of body fluid volume disturbances is based on three principles:
- Diagnosis and treatment of disorders that create or maintain imbalances
- Correction of abnormalities of volume status while providing maintenance therapy

TABLE 2–3. **Electrolyte Content of Intravenous Fluids (in mEq/L)**

IV FLUID	mOsm/L	Na	K	Ca	Cl	HCO_3^- EQUIVALENT
0.45% NaCl (half-normal saline)	154	77	-	-	77	---
0.9% NaCl (normal saline)	308	154	-	-	154	---
3% NaCl	1026	513	-	-	513	---
Ringer's lactate	272	130	4	30	109	28
5% Dextrose in water	252	50 g/L of dextrose, no electrolytes				
5% Dextrose with quarter-normal saline	320	34	-	-	34	---
5% Dextrose with half-normal saline	406	77	-	-	77	---

TABLE 2–4. **Electrolyte Content of Selected Body Fluids**

	ELECTROLYTE CONCENTRATIONS (mEq/L)				
FLUID	Na	K	Cl	HCO$_3$$^-$	H
Sweat	30–60	5	40–80	—	—
Gastric	40–80	5–20	80–120	—	10–80
Bile	130–160	5	80–120	40–50	—
Pancreatic	120–150	5	60–80	70–90	—
Ileostomy	60–120	10	60–130	30–50	—
Stool					
Normal	5	50	5	—	—
Diarrhea	50–100	20	20–60	30–50	—

- Correction of remaining electrolyte disturbances (unless life threatening at presentation)

A vast number of disease processes lead to fluid and electrolyte abnormalities. Knowledge of body fluid content (Table 2–4) allows estimation of derangements, but clinical and laboratory measurements are required for precise assessment.

The **urgency** of volume deficit correction is determined by clinical criteria. Moderate intravascular volume depletion may produce **thirst** as its only symptom. Tachycardia, decreased skin turgor and axillary sweat, decreased urine output, and modest azotemia with the blood urea nitrogen (BUN) elevated disproportionately to the serum creatinine may be seen. The estimated deficit should be corrected over 24 to 48 hours.

More severe volume depletion is associated with **postural hypotension** and **oliguria.**

Initial treatment is the rapid (up to 1000 mL/h) administration of 0.9% NaCl (normal saline) until postural hypotension has resolved. Only 25% of administered normal saline remains in the intravascular space. Hypertonic saline should not be used just for volume expansion.

Once the severe deficit is corrected, slower replacement continues (e.g., 0.45% NaCl, 75–150 mL/h), and electrolyte disturbances can be treated.

Volume loss sufficient to cause **resting hypotension** usually results from **hemorrhage** and may require infusion of blood or plasma protein products.

Clinical criteria may correlate imperfectly with volume status, especially in the face of renal, cardiac, or infectious diseases. The use of central venous (in the absence of cardiopulmonary disease) or pulmonary artery pressure monitoring may help guide therapy.

III. DISTURBANCES OF SERUM SODIUM CONCENTRATION

Abnormalities of the serum Na concentration result from free water imbalance. In some cases, treatment of an associated volume deficit is an important first step. Symptoms of hyponatremia or hypernatremia may be mild or overshadowed by volume-related symptoms.

A rapidly developed abnormality of serum Na causes more symptoms than a slowly developed one. Hyponatremia with serum Na above 125 mEq/L rarely causes symptoms. The symptoms of hypernatremia correlate better with the degree of hyperosmolality than the serum Na. Hyponatremia and hypernatremia produce neurologic symptoms ranging from lethargy and coma to irritability, muscular twitching, and seizures.

A. Hyponatremia

So-called **pseudohyponatremia** may occur with severe hyperlipidemia (lipemic serum) or hyperglobulinemia. The Na concentration per liter of plasma water is normal, and the apparent hyponatremia does not affect the clinical status.

The presence of a large amount of osmotically active solute (glucose is most common) causes true hyponatremia. For each increase by 100 mg/dL of the serum glucose above normal, the serum Na decreases by 1.6 mEq/L (e.g., a serum glucose of 600 mg/dL causes a Na reduction of 8 mEq/L).

Important **causes** of hyponatremia include:
- Fluid loss with hypotonic replacement
- Diuresis induced by drugs or osmotic loads
- Edematous states
- Endocrine diseases (hypothyroidism, deficiency of glucocorticoids or mineralocorticoids)
- Syndrome of inappropriate secretion of antidiuretic hormone (SIADH), characterized by inappropriately high urine osmolarity
- Extreme polydipsia (usually greater than 15 L/d)

Treatment of hyponatremia depends on its degree and whether symptoms are present. **Hypovolemia** should be corrected if the underlying diseases allow. If **symptoms are minimal** or hyponatremia is moderate (serum Na greater than 120 mEq/L) or chronic, water intake restriction to 1000 mL/d is appropriate initial treatment. In patients with CHF, angiotensin-converting enzyme (ACE) inhibitors help correct hyponatremia. The ADH antagonist demeclocycline 900–1200 mg/d may help in patients with SIADH. Furosemide may help by causing excretion of dilute urine but may also require volume replacement.

If symptoms are severe and acute, the amount of sodium required to raise the serum concentration to 125 mEq/L should be administered over 6 hours. The rate should not exceed 0.5 to 1.0 mEq/L/h or 12 mEq/L/d, so extreme cases may require more than 6 hours.

$$\text{Na deficit} = (125 - Na_{measured}) \times TBW$$

NaCl (3%) may be given IV with furosemide (20–80 mg IV) to prevent volume overload, if it occurs. Rapid correction to Na above 125 mEq/L is rarely necessary and may be associated with a central demyelination syndrome.

B. Hypernatremia

This may result from:
- Hypotonic fluid loss (sweat)
- Osmotic diuresis (glucose)
- Adrenal hyperfunction

- Diabetes insipidus
- Inappropriate IV fluid use

The **goal of treatment** is to provide half of the water deficit in 12 to 24 hours, then the rest in another 24 hours. During the first 2 days of treatment, the Na should be reduced by no more than 0.5 mEq/L/h.

$$\text{Free water deficit} = \left[\frac{(\text{serum Na})}{140} - 1 \right] \times \text{TBW}$$

Because a volume deficit is usually present, **initial treatment** is with normal saline until the patient becomes euvolemic. Overly rapid correction of the serum Na (or osmolarity) may produce cerebral edema and death.

Karp BI, Laureno R. Pontine and extrapontine myelinolysis: a neurologic disorder following rapid correction of hyponatremia. Medicine 1993;72:359.
Mulloy AL, Caruana RJ. Hyponatremic emergencies. Med Clin North Am 1995;79:155.
Palevsky PM, Bhagrath R, Greenberg A. Hypernatremia in hospitalized patients. Ann Intern Med 1996;124:197.

IV. DISTURBANCES OF SERUM POTASSIUM CONCENTRATION

A. Hypokalemia

Hypokalemia is usually asymptomatic. In patients with **chronic hypokalemia,** the level of serum K that requires treatment is controversial. In the absence of premature ventricular contractions, ischemic heart disease, and digoxin therapy, one might withhold replacement unless the serum K is less than 3.2 mEq/L. If hypokalemia is due to medications (e.g., diuretics taken for hypertension), the use of a potassium-containing salt substitute (50–70 mEq K/tsp), change in diet, or change of medication should be considered.

The **symptoms** of hypokalemia are primarily neuromuscular, ranging from weakness to cramps to paralysis. Ventricular arrhythmias, a renal concentrating defect, ileus, rhabdomyolysis, and aggravation of hepatic encephalopathy may also result from hypokalemia.

Causes of hypokalemia include:

- Gastrointestinal loss (vomiting, diarrhea)
- Renal loss (metabolic alkalosis, use of diuretics, gentamicin, carbenicillin, or amphotericin B, excess mineralocorticoid effect, renal tubular acidosis, Mg depletion)
- Extracellular to intracellular shifts (acute alkalosis, insulin therapy)

The serum K may remain normal even with a body deficit of 100 to 200 mEq, as is seen typically with acidemia. If the serum K is 2 to 4 mEq/L and renal function is normal, it increases by 1 mEq/L for each 100 to 200 mEq of K administered.

K can be replaced orally (Table 2–5) or IV. Liquid K supplements have a disagreeable taste and may cause gastric irritation. Slow-release supplements are better tolerated but may cause GI ulcers or may be only partially utilized.

IV administration of more than 10 mEq of K per hour causes phlebitis. Central IV lines allow rates up to 20 to 30 mEq/h. Such high rates of administration are usually reserved for emergent treatment of arrhythmias. ECG monitoring is mandatory. Mg-depleted patients require Mg supplements to fully correct their K deficit.

TABLE 2–5. **Oral Potassium Supplements**

FORM	STRENGTH (%)	DOSE	COMMENT
LIQUID			
Potassium chloride	5, 7.5, 10, 15, 20	15 mL of 10% liquid contains 20 mEq K	Some brands contain sugar, saccharin, alcohol, flavorings, or tartrazine
Potassium gluconate	10	45 mL of 10% liquid contains 20 mEq K	Some brands contain alcohol or saccharin
POWDER			
Potassium chloride	15, 20, 25 mEq K per package		Some brands contain alcohol or saccharin
TABLETS			
Potassium chloride	1, 3.3, 4, 6.7, 8, 10, 20 mEq K per tablet		Some brands contain sugar, saccharin, or tartrazine; some are effervescent mixtures of salts; some are chewable; wax matrix formulations have lower risk of GI complications

B. Hyperkalemia

Artifactual elevations **(pseudohyperkalemia)** may occur with thrombocytosis (usually platelet count above $1,000,000/mm^3$) or leukocytosis (more than $100,000/mm^3$). The plasma K remains normal. Sample hemolysis, usually due to the use of small needles or laboratory delay, also elevates K determinations.

Hyperkalemia can lead to **muscle weakness and cardiac arrhythmias.** Common **causes** include:

- Excessive intake (usually iatrogenic)
- Poor **renal excretion** (renal failure, obstructive uropathy, adrenal insufficiency, and many drugs: K-sparing diuretics, NSAIDs, angiotensin-converting enzyme, ACE inhibitors)
- Redistribution phenomena (acidemia, rhabdomyolysis, succinylcholine, digoxin toxicity)

The urgency of **treatment** is dictated by the presence of electrocardiographic changes (peaked T waves, prolonged P-R interval, absent P waves, widened QRS complex, ventricular arrhythmias). If ECG changes are present, cardiac monitoring and frequent serial K measurements are indicated.

IV **Ca gluconate,** 10–20 mL of a 10% solution, injected over 1 to 5 minutes blunts the effect of hyperkalemia on neuromuscular membranes within 5 minutes. The effect lasts about 30 minutes. It should be used cautiously if the patient has been receiving digoxin.

The administration of **insulin, albuterol,** or **sodium bicarbonate (NaHCO$_3$)** causes movement of extracellular K into the intracellular space. Insulin's effect occurs in 15 minutes and albuterol's in 30 minutes. The effect of bicarbonate is variable and may be delayed by 1 to 4 hours. The redistribution effects last several hours.

Insulin should be given as 5–10 U of regular insulin IV with 50 mL of 50% dextrose, followed by 10% dextrose IV at 50 mL/h to avoid late hypoglycemia.

Albuterol may be given via nebulizer [20 mg (8 times the usual dose for bronchospasm) in 4 mL of normal saline] over 10 minutes.

Individual ampules of **NaHCO₃** (44.6 mEq) may be used cautiously or mixed with 10% dextrose in water and given over 30 to 60 minutes.

K is removed from the body by the **cation exchange resin, Na polystyrene sulfonate** (Kayexalate): 1 g of resin removes 1 mEq of K in exchange for 1.5 mEq of Na. The resin's effect begins 1 to 2 hours after an oral dose. The oral dose is 15–30 g with 50–100 mL of 20% **sorbitol** or a **phenolphthalein-based laxative** (more effective than sorbitol) up to four times per day. Resin 50 g with 200 mL of 20% sorbitol may also be given as a retention enema every 4 hours; this route of administration produces a more rapid effect than the oral route.

Hemodialysis may be useful in the patient with acute renal failure and volume excess. Prior treatment with albuterol may reduce the efficiency of K removal by hemodialysis.

Allon M. Treatment and prevention of hyperkalemia in end-stage renal disease. Kidney Int 1993;43:1197.

Ponce SP, Jennings AE, Madins NE, et al. Drug-induced hyperkalemia. Medicine 1985;64:357.

V. DISTURBANCES OF SERUM CALCIUM CONCENTRATION

Calcium is a divalent cation that exists in serum as a free ion and bound to plasma proteins. Alkalemia increases the fraction that is bound to protein, lowering the ionized Ca concentration. The ionized Ca is physiologically active, and symptoms correlate with its level. The serum level of Ca is under the control of a complex regulatory system involving the parathyroid gland, kidneys, and vitamin D metabolism.

Most laboratories measure the total serum Ca. Hypoalbuminemia causes a low total serum Ca without affecting the ionized Ca or causing symptoms. For each 1 g/dL decrease in serum albumin concentration, the total Ca concentration falls by 0.8 mg/dL.

A. Hypocalcemia

The primary **sign** of acute hypocalcemia is **tetany.** It may be elicited by inflating a sphygmomanometer around the arm to cause carpal spasm (Trousseau's sign). Muscle spasm, lethargy, seizures, and Chvostek's sign (elicited by percussion over the facial nerve) may be present.

Major **causes** of hypocalcemia include:
- Hypoparathyroidism (usually after thyroid or parathyroid surgery)
- Hypomagnesemia (usually at levels below 0.8 mEq/L)
- Pancreatitis
- Tumor lysis syndrome
- Rhabdomyolysis
- Vitamin D deficiency
- Chronic renal failure

Treatment of acute hypocalcemia is 10–30 mL of 10% Ca gluconate given over 10 minutes. Since the effect of a bolus of Ca gluconate wanes after 2 hours, it must be followed by continuous infusion of 5–15 mg/kg/h of Ca gluconate (0.5–1.5 mg/kg/h of elemental Ca). Serial Ca levels must be measured.

If the serum level of inorganic phosphate (P_i) is very high, IV Ca must be used carefully. When the Ca-P_i product (with both in mg/dL units) exceeds 65, there is a risk of metastatic calcification.

If magnesium (Mg) deficiency is present, it must be treated while monitoring K balance.

Longer-term treatment uses oral Ca supplements (Table 2–6). They are usually well tolerated, although constipation may occur. Noncarbonate Ca salts are better absorbed than Ca carbonate if hypochlorhydria is present, but a carbonate is usually less expensive. Measurement of urinary Ca excretion may be indicated in some circumstances.

B. Hypercalcemia

The **symptoms** of hypercalcemia, including fatigue, confusion, nausea, vomiting, constipation, and polyuria (due to a reversible renal tubular defect), usually begin at serum levels between 11 and 12 mg/dL. A shortened Q-T interval, premature ventricular contractions, and an idioventricular rhythm may also occur. Hypercalcemia above 15 mg/dL or severe symptoms require emergency treatment.

Primary hyperparathyroidism or malignancy causes 90% of cases of hypercalcemia. Other **causes** include:

- Granulomatous diseases
- Hyperthyroidism
- Immobilization
- Milk-alkali syndrome
- Drug effects (lithium, thiazides, vitamin D)

Most hypercalcemic patients are volume depleted. Management of the underlying pathologic state is crucial to the long-term **treatment** of hypercalcemia. Treatment agents are listed in order of most to least rapid effect.

Normal saline to correct volume depletion followed by more normal saline with **furosemide**-induced diuresis is rapidly effective and should be used in all patients. Calciuresis begins immediately, and the serum Ca may fall by 4 mg/dL in 24 hours.

TABLE 2–6. **Oral Calcium Supplements**

SALT	% ELEMENTAL Ca BY WEIGHT	DOSE AVAILABLE IN mg (TOTAL)	COMMENT
Ca glubionate	6	1800	Syrup form, 5 mL dose
Ca gluconate	9	500, 650, 975, 1000	
Ca lactate	13	325, 650	
Ca citrate	21	950, 2376	
Ca acetate	25	250, 500, 667, 1000	Pill and capsule forms available
Ca phosphate	39	1565	
Ca carbonate	40	350, 420, 500, 650, 750, 850, 1250, 1500	Chewable, powder, and liquid forms available

Salmon calcitonin is effective in conditions with rapid bone turnover, most notably immobilization, vitamin D excess, and thyrotoxicosis. It is less effective in hypercalcemia due to malignancy or hyperparathyroidism. The initial dose is 4 U/kg SC or IM, which may be repeated every 6 to 12 hours. It acts in 3 to 4 hours but is not useful for long-term therapy of hypercalcemia. Giving a test dose (to exclude allergy) should be considered. Synthetic **human calcitonin** may be used as an alternative (0.5 mg/d SC).

Plicamycin (mithramycin) inhibits osteoclast activity and works in most patients. It is given as an infusion over 4 to 6 hours at a dose of 25 μg/kg. It acts in 8 to 24 hours and may be repeated every 2 to 4 days. It has potential for serious toxicity, including thrombocytopenia and renal and hepatic damage.

Bisphosphonates directly inhibit osteoclast function. Although available in oral preparations, they should be used IV for acute hypercalcemia. Their effect occurs over 1 to 3 days. Specific agents include **pamidronate** (60–90 mg IV infused over 2–3 h) and **etidronate** (7.5 mg/kg IV over 4 h each day for 3 days).

Gallium nitrate inhibits bone resorption and is useful in persons with malignancy-associated hypercalcemia. Its effect takes 1 to 3 days. The dose is 200 mg/m^2/d IV for up to 5 days. It is contraindicated if the serum creatinine is above 2.5 mg/dL and may cause nephrotoxicity.

Glucocorticoids (daily dosage equivalent to 60 mg of prednisone) are especially useful in patients with granulomatous diseases, hematologic malignancies, breast cancer, and vitamin D excess. The maximal effect is reached in 24 to 48 hours.

Oral phosphate should be used if the serum P_i is less than 3 to 4 mg/dL. The initial dose is 250 mg of elemental P_i tid or qid. Oral P_i therapy is frequently limited by diarrhea. IV P_i, although extremely effective, is risky and should be considered only in extreme emergencies.

Edelson GW, Kleerekoper M. Hypercalcemic crisis. Med Clin North Am 1995;79:79.
Reber PM, Heath H. Hypocalcemic emergencies. Med Clin North Am 1995;79:93.
Zaloga GP. Hypocalcemic crisis. Crit Care Clin 1991;7:191.

VI. DISTURBANCES OF SERUM PHOSPHORUS CONCENTRATION

Phosphorus is present in the serum in several anionic forms. The content is expressed as milligrams of elemental inorganic phosphorus (P_i) per deciliter. Normally, the P_i concentration decreases by 1 to 1.5 mg/dL after meals. Alkalemia also decreases the P_i level.

A. Hypophosphatemia

Mild to moderate hypophosphatemia (1 to 2.5 mg/dL) is common in hospitalized patients and usually has no clinical consequences. Adequate nutrition and treatment of the underlying illness usually are sufficient therapy. If needed, oral replacement is 250 mg of P_i two or three times daily and is limited primarily by diarrhea (Table 2–7).

Patients with P_i concentrations below 1 mg/dL may have severe **symptoms,** including anorexia, bone pain, muscle weakness (including respiratory muscles), CHF, hemolysis, and rhabdomyolysis.

TABLE 2–7. **Oral Phosphate Supplements**

PREPARATION	FORM	P$_i$ DOSE (mg) PER UNIT	CATIONS PER UNIT
K-Phos Neutral	Tablet	250	1.1 mEq K
			13 mEq Na
Neutra-Phos	Capsule	250	7.1 mEq K
			7.1 mEq Na
Neutra-Phos-K	Capsule	250	14.2 mEq K
Phospho-Soda	Liquid (6.7 mL)	1000	40 mEq Na

Causes include:
- Feeding of malnourished patients (e.g., chronic alcoholics)
- Treatment of diabetic ketoacidosis
- Respiratory alkalosis
- GI malabsorption (may be due to aluminum-containing antacids)
- Renal wasting (Fanconi syndrome)

Severe hypophosphatemia may be treated as follows: 2–6 mg/kg of P$_i$ should be given IV over 6 hours and repeated until the serum P$_i$ reaches 2 mg/dL. Extra caution is needed for patients with renal failure or hypercalcemia (increased risk of metastatic calcification). Hypocalcemia may result from therapy.

The initial IV fluid management of hospitalized **chronic alcoholics** should include 6–8 g of P$_i$ as the Na or K salt. Otherwise, resumption of a normal diet is usually sufficient.

B. Hyperphosphatemia

Elevated levels of serum P$_i$ occur in chronic renal failure, hypoparathyroidism, vitamin D excess, tumor lysis syndrome, and rhabdomyolysis. Usually, there are no symptoms unless hypocalcemia or metastatic calcification develops.

Dietary restriction of phosphate (and protein) and use of phosphate binders (aluminum hydroxide or carbonate suspensions, 15–30 mL tid initially or calcium carbonate 650 mg tid) with meals are helpful.

Peppers MP, Geheb M, Desai T. Hypophosphatemia and hyperphosphatemia. Crit Care Clin 1991;7:201.

VII. DISTURBANCES OF SERUM MAGNESIUM CONCENTRATION

Like Ca, Mg is a divalent cation with many actions in the neuromuscular system. Through its effect on parathyroid hormone release and action, Mg is important in Ca regulation. The normal serum concentration is 1.6 to 2.4 mEq/L (2 to 3 mg/dL).

A. Hypomagnesemia

Hypomagnesemia can produce irritability, confusion, weakness, fasciculations, nystagmus, and seizures. Serious symptoms are rare until the concentration is less than 0.8 mEq/L. Symptoms may be aggravated by coincident hypocalcemia.

Common **causes** include:
- Poor nutrition (e.g., chronic alcoholism)
- Intestinal malabsorption
- Renal wasting (diuretics, cisplatin, gentamicin, amphotericin B, pentamidine, cyclosporine, primary hyperaldosteronism, diabetic ketoacidosis)
- Acute pancreatitis
- Postoperative hypoparathyroidism

Urgent **treatment** uses IV Mg sulfate, 1–2 g (as a 50% solution) diluted to 5% concentration in D_5W and infused over 10 to 15 minutes. In patients suspected of having Mg deficiency, 1–2 mL of 50% Mg sulfate may be given IM as needed or added to maintenance IV fluids.

Oral Mg supplements may be given as Mg oxide (400 mg pill, contains 20 mEq of Mg, taken one to three times daily) or Milk of Magnesia (10 mL contains 30 mEq of Mg, taken one or two times daily), but diarrhea often limits the dose.

B. Hypermagnesemia

Symptoms and signs of hypermagnesemia include:
- Serum level of 3 to 5 mEq/L: hypotension and nausea
- Serum level of 5 to 7 mEq/L: hyporeflexia and somnolence
- Serum level above 12 mEq/L causes coma
- Prolongation of the Q-T interval and QRS duration, T wave peaking, atrioventricular block, and cardiac arrest may also occur at high serum levels

Hypermagnesemia results from excess administration or ingestion of a laxative or antacid that contains Mg by a patient with renal insufficiency (serum creatinine above 3 to 4 mg/dL).

IV Ca gluconate 10–20 mL of a 10% solution given over 5 minutes temporarily reverses the effects of Mg toxicity. Saline diuresis with **furosemide** increases urinary Mg excretion in patients with adequate renal function. In patients with advanced renal failure, dialysis is the only other modality available. In patients with residual renal function, forced diuresis may help.

Al-Ghamdi SMG, Cameron EC, Sutton RAL. Magnesium deficiency: pathophysiologic and clinical overview. Am J Kidney Dis 1994;24:737.
Van Hook JW. Hypermagnesemia. Crit Care Clin 1991;7:215.

VIII. ACID-BASE DISTURBANCES

Acid is continuously produced by normal metabolism. The blood pH is regulated by buffer systems and the excretory ability of the lungs and kidneys.

Buffer systems (bicarbonate, phosphate, proteins) rapidly absorb newly produced acid.

Carbon dioxide, produced from carbonic acid, is excreted by the lungs.

The kidney excretes **hydrogen ions** into the urine, thereby regenerating bicarbonate. Hydrogen ions in the urine are buffered by ammonia and phosphate species.

A pathologic process that causes alveolar hypoventilation or hyperventilation results in a primary increase or decrease in the partial pressure of carbon dioxide (PCO_2) and leads to **respiratory acidosis or alkalosis,** respectively.

A process that causes a primary increase or decrease in the serum bicarbonate (HCO_3^-) concentration results in a **metabolic alkalosis or acidosis,** respectively.

When the blood pH goes above or below normal, alkalemia or acidemia is present.

The kidney compensates for respiratory disturbances, and the lungs compensate for metabolic disturbances. The compensation is not complete. Thus, the primary disturbance can be identified by evaluating the arterial pH and PCO_2 and serum HCO_3^- (the measured CO_2 of the serum electrolytes).

When arterial blood gases are determined, only two of the quantities are measured directly. The third is calculated on the basis of the Henderson-Hasselbalch equation:

$$pH = 6.1 + \log[HCO_3^-/(0.03 \times PCO_2)]$$

Most acid-base disturbances have only one primary pathophysiologic process. Compensation by the lung (change in minute ventilation) occurs rapidly; renal compensation requires several hours to days. If overcompensation or undercompensation occurs, a mixed acid-base disturbance is present. Predictive rules are available to make this distinction (Tables 2–8 and 2–9).

A. Metabolic Acidosis

Generation of excess acid or loss of alkali results in metabolic acidosis. Calculation of the **anion gap** [$AG = Na - (Cl + CO_2)$] allows a simplified **diagnostic approach.** The traditional normal AG range is 8 to 16 mEq/L, but variations in laboratory techniques may lower the reference range by up to 5 mEq/L.

Causes of metabolic acidosis with **increased AG** include:
- Renal failure
- Ketoacidosis (diabetic or alcoholic)
- Lactic acidosis
- Drug intoxication (methanol, paraldehyde, salicylate, ethylene glycol)
  Causes of metabolic acidosis with a **normal AG** include:
- Gastrointestinal loss of alkali (diarrhea, ureteroileostomy)
- Renal tubular acidosis
- Acetazolamide
- Cholestyramine
- Obstructive uropathy

TABLE 2–8. **Simple Acid-Base Disturbances**

DISTURBANCE	PRIMARY CHANGE	pH	COMPENSATORY CHANGE
Metabolic acidosis	Decreased bicarbonate	Decreased	Decreased PCO_2
Metabolic alkalosis	Increased bicarbonate	Increased	Increased PCO_2
Respiratory acidosis	Increased PCO_2	Decreased	Increased bicarbonate
Respiratory alkalosis	Decreased PCO_2	Increased	Decreased bicarbonate

---

TABLE 2-9. **Expected Compensatory Changes in Acid-Base Disturbances**

Normal arterial blood pH: 7.35–7.45
Normal arterial P_{CO_2}: 35–45 mm Hg
Normal total CO_2: 24–30 mEq/L

EXPECTED COMPENSATORY CHANGE
ΔHCO_3^- = change in measured bicarbonate (mEq/L)
ΔP_{CO_2} = change in arterial P_{CO_2} (mm Hg)

DISORDER	EXPECTED CHANGE
Metabolic acidosis	$\Delta P_{CO_2} = (1-1.5) \times \Delta HCO_3^-$
Metabolic alkalosis	$\Delta P_{CO_2} = (0.25-1) \times \Delta HCO_3^-$
Respiratory acidosis	
Acute	$\Delta HCO_3^- = 0.1 \times \Delta P_{CO_2} \pm 3$
Chronic	$\Delta HCO_3^- = 0.4 \times \Delta P_{CO_2} \pm 4$
Respiratory alkalosis	
Acute	$\Delta HCO_3^- = (0.1-0.3) \times \Delta P_{CO_2}$*
Chronic	$\Delta HCO_3^- = (0.2-0.5) \times \Delta P_{CO_2}$†

*Change to below 18 mEq/L is unusual.
†Change to below 14 mEq/L is unusual.

- Administration of HCl or NH_4Cl
- Sulfur ingestion
- Hyperparathyroidism

In acute metabolic acidosis, correction of the underlying pathophysiology is crucial. If arterial pH falls below 7.15 or hemodynamic collapse occurs, $NaHCO_3$ may be given on the basis of an estimate of the **bicarbonate deficit:**

$$HCO_3^- \text{ deficit} = \text{weight} \times 0.5^* \times (\text{target } HCO_3^- - \text{actual } HCO_3^-)$$
$$^*\text{use } 0.8 \text{ if pH} < 7.1$$

To avoid **overshoot alkalemia,** the target HCO_3^- is usually 15 to 18 mEq/L. One half of the deficit is given over 3 to 4 hours, using D_5W with one to three ampules of $NaHCO_3$ added.

The end point of treatment is determined by clinical and laboratory data, as the volume of distribution of HCO_3^- is variable, and acid production may be ongoing. Bicarbonate replacement is not important in toxin ingestion (e.g., salicylates, methanol) and is rarely needed for diabetic ketoacidosis. Rapid correction may lead to hypokalemia or hypocalcemia, with their attendant morbidity.

Treating chronic metabolic acidosis often requires administration of bicarbonate or citrate.

B. Respiratory Acidosis

Respiratory acidosis is caused by **alveolar hypoventilation.** It may result from neuromuscular disease, sedative drugs, mechanical airway obstruction, or severe intrinsic lung disease. The treatment is restoration of ventilation. If acidemia is life threatening and ventilatory support must be delayed, small amounts of IV $NaHCO_3$ may be given.

C. Metabolic Alkalosis

Metabolic alkalosis can occur with **volume depletion,** when the urinary chloride concentration is usually less than 10 mEq/L. **Causes** include:
- Vomiting
- Nasogastric suction and fluid loss
- Excessive diuresis

Metabolic alkalosis may also be associated with **mineralocorticoid excess,** usually with urinary chloride levels above 20 mEq/L. Examples include:
- Cushing's syndrome
- Primary hyperaldosteronism
- Bartter's syndrome.

Treatment of the first group is aimed at the underlying disorder. Volume restoration with NaCl allows bicarbonate excretion. Potassium deficits are often present and should be treated, as they help promote and maintain metabolic alkalosis. If prolonged nasogastric suction is expected, agents that inhibit gastric acid secretion may lessen the alkalosis.

Treatment of the mineralocorticoid excess is aimed at the underlying disorder. KCl is given. Excess alkali consumption should be avoided. Sodium should be replaced with NaCl.

If alkalemia is causing cardiac arrhythmias (usually pH greater than 7.6), 0.15 molar HCl in sterile water may be given IV through a central venous catheter.

The bicarbonate excess may be calculated in the same way as in metabolic acidosis. Half of the acid may be administered over 4 hours or until signs of alkalemia abate.

Acetazolamide, 250–500 mg tid, which increases renal alkali excretion, is also useful.

D. Respiratory Alkalosis

Hyperventilation leads to an increased blood pH. **Causes** include:
- Sepsis
- Salicylate toxicity
- Hepatic disease
- Pregnancy
- Excessive mechanical ventilation
- Anxiety
- Pain
- Hypoxia
- Intrinsic pulmonary disease
- Central nervous system disease (e.g., encephalitis)

Treatment is aimed at the underlying cause. If complications appear, the respiratory drive may be blunted with sedatives, such as IV lorazepam (1–2 mg), midazolam (2–5 mg), or morphine sulfate (5–10 mg).

E. Mixed Acid-Base Disturbances

Diagnosis of mixed disorders is based on the clinical setting and results of laboratory studies. Common examples include patients with cirrhosis treated with diuretics (respiratory and metabolic alkalosis) and salicylate intoxication (respiratory alkalosis and metabolic acidosis). Once diagnosed, the disturbances are treated as described previously in this chapter, with priority determined by clinical criteria.

Gabow PA. Disorders associated with an altered anion gap. Kidney Int 1985;27:472–483.

Schelling JR, Howard RL, Winters D, Linas SL. Increased osmolal gap in alcoholic ketoacidosis and lactic acidosis. Ann Intern Med 1990;113:580–582.

Winter SD, Pearson JR, Gabow PA, Schultz AL, Lepoff RB. The fall of the serum anion gap. Arch Intern Med 1990;150:311–313.

3 33 33 33 33 33 33

INFECTIOUS DISEASES

AJIT LIMAYE
W. CONRAD LILES
PAUL G. RAMSEY

33333333333333

The clinical management of infectious disease has become increasingly complex, with new pathogens, new patterns of antimicrobial resistance, and larger numbers of immunocompromised patients. Antimicrobial therapy selection is based on many factors, including established efficacy in the clinical situation at hand, host factors, drug toxicity, pharmacokinetics, and the relative cost of a given antimicrobial agent compared with other agents.

I. SELECTION AND USE OF ANTIMICROBIAL AGENTS: GENERAL CONSIDERATIONS

Empiric antimicrobial therapy directed against the spectrum of probable infecting organisms must often be given before definitive microbiologic identification and antimicrobial susceptibility information are available. In certain instances, broad-spectrum antimicrobial therapy is warranted. If the clinical situation is acute, empiric therapy via the IV route is usually begun immediately after specimens are collected. In less serious, stable clinical circumstances, therapeutic decisions may be delayed until the results of microbiologic culture are in, and initial therapy may be oral or parenteral.

A. Host Factors

Several factors about the patient should be considered in selecting antibiotics.

1. AGE. In young children and the elderly, **gastric pH is decreased,** allowing increased absorption of agents such as penicillins and other orally administered beta-lactams. Absorption of weak acids such as ketoconazole may be decreased. Young age and inadequate glucuronyl transferase production can lead to **gray syndrome** in neonates and young children treated with chloramphenicol. When given to pregnant women or newborns, **sulfonamides** displace bilirubin and may result in **kernicterus. Tetracycline** given to children younger than age 8 years may cause **tooth discoloration.**

2. RENAL FUNCTION. Toxic levels of penicillins, aminoglycosides, tetracyclines, and quinolones may develop as renal function declines, leading possibly to **nephrotoxicity** and **ototoxicity,** particularly with **aminoglycosides. Neurotoxic reactions** may result with increased levels of **penicillins and cephalosporins.**

3. HEPATIC DYSFUNCTION. Hepatic dysfunction may lead to **impaired metabolism** of macrolides, rifamycins, imidazoles, chloramphenicol, and linconoid drugs. The risk of aminoglycoside-induced nephrotoxicity is increased in patients with underlying cirrhosis or hepatic failure.

4. METABOLIC ABNORMALITIES. Slow acetylation of isoniazid is genetically determined and is associated with **polyneuritis. Glucose-6-phosphate dehydrogenase (G-6-PD) deficiency** may predispose patients to

75

hemolysis when such antibiotics as sulfonamides, nitrofurantoin, furazolidone, chloramphenicol, and pyrimethamine are used. The action of sulfonylurea hypoglycemics may be potentiated by sulfonamides and chloramphenicol.

5. SITE OF INFECTION. The site of infection determines the route and dose of antibiotic to be given. To treat meningitis effectively, the agent must be lipid soluble to cross the **blood-brain barrier.** The vegetations of bacterial endocarditis and devitalized bone or tissue are other areas where penetration may be poor. Local conditions, such as pH or the presence of a foreign body, also alter the choice of antimicrobial therapy (e.g., aminoglycosides are ineffective at pH <7.0).

6. HISTORY OF PREVIOUS ADVERSE EFFECTS. A history of adverse effects from a particular class of antibiotics must be considered before prescribing a similar antibiotic.

7. PREGNANCY. Pregnant patients should be identified before antibiotics are prescribed. Virtually all antibiotics cross the placenta and are excreted in breast milk to some extent. Most penicillins (except ticarcillin), cephalosporins, and erythromycins can be used safely in pregnant women.

B. Drug Interactions and Dosing Recommendations

Major adverse effects and drug interactions are summarized in Table 3–1, and dosing recommendations for antimicrobial agents are found in Table 3–2.

C. Identification of the Infecting Organism

The **gram stain** is one of the simplest, quickest, and least expensive methods of identifying bacteria and fungi. In normally sterile body fluids (pleural, pericardial, peritoneal, cerebrospinal, and synovial fluids, urine, and the buffy coat component of blood), the morphologic characteristics of microorganisms provide specific information to guide therapy. For body substances that contain "normal" flora as well as potential pathogens (sputum, stool, and vaginal secretions), findings from gram stains are more difficult to interpret. Gram stains may reveal polymorphonuclear leukocytes in an infected fluid even when the etiologic agent is not apparent. Immunologic methods for antigen detection can be useful as a rapid diagnostic tool (e.g., fluorescent antibody stains for *Legionella* and selected viruses, such as herpes simplex virus and cytomegalovirus).

D. Antimicrobial Susceptibility

Antimicrobial agents listed as "preferred agents" (green shading) or "alternative agents" (gray shading) in Table 3–3 should be used when the suspected pathogen has been isolated from culture and the organism has been shown to be sensitive. As some preferred agents may not be active against all strains of a suspected pathogen, more broad-spectrum coverage provided by other antimicrobial agents (gray shading) may be considered before culture results are obtained in appropriate acute clinical situations. For example, since not all strains of *Haemophilus influenzae* are sensitive to ampicillin, another agent should be used initially in the setting of suspected

Text continued on page 88

TABLE 3-1. Adverse Effects and Drug Interactions

ANTIMICROBIAL	MAJOR ADVERSE EFFECTS	DRUG INTERACTIONS
Acyclovir	Possible bone marrow suppression	Probenecid: ↑ acyclovir toxicity
Amantadine	Central nervous system effects (e.g., disorientation)	Anticholinergics: hallucinations, confusion
Aminoglycosides	Ototoxicity, maculopapular rash, neuromuscular blockade ↑ Nephrotoxicity with amphotericin B, cephalosporins, loop diuretics	Inactivated by high levels of carbenicillin, ticarcillin ↑ Effects of neuromuscular blocking agents
Amphotericin B	Acute tubular necrosis ↑ Nephrotoxicity with aminoglycosides Hypokalemia Hypomagnesemia	↑ Digitalis toxicity ↑ Effects of neuromuscular blocking agents
Aztreonam	Phlebitis, eosinophilia	
Carbenicillin and ticarcillin	Bleeding disorders Hypokalemia	↓ Effect of aminoglycosides
Cephalosporins	Anaphylaxis, serum sickness, leukopenia, pseudomembranous colitis, maculopapular rash, erythema multiforme ↑ Bleeding, hypoprothrombinemia ↑ Nephrotoxicity with aminoglycosides, loop diuretics Interstitial nephritis Pseudomembranous colitis	Disulfiram-like reaction with alcohol and cefamandole, moxalactam, cefoperazone, cefotetan
Chloramphenicol	Aplastic anemia, hemolysis in glucose-6-phosphate dehydrogenase (G-6-PD) deficiency	Acetaminophen: ↑ chloramphenicol level Barbiturates: ↑ effects ↓ chloramphenicol effect Warfarin: ↑ anticoagulant effect Phenytoin: ↑ toxicity ↓ chloramphenicol effect Sulfonylureas: ↑ effect
Clindamycin	Pseudomembranous colitis	↑ Effects of neuromuscular blocking agents

Table continued on the following page

77

TABLE 3-1. Adverse Effects and Drug Interactions

ANTIMICROBIAL	MAJOR ADVERSE EFFECTS	DRUG INTERACTIONS
Erythromycin	Diarrhea, cholestatic jaundice	Carbamazepine, digoxin, theophylline: ↑ levels
Imipenem with cilastatin	Thrombocytopenia, encephalopathy, seizures, phlebitis, nausea, diarrhea	
Isoniazid (INH)	Anemia, peripheral neuropathy, drug-induced lupus Chronic hepatitis, cytotoxic effects ↑ INH hepatotoxicity with rifampin	Aluminum: ↓ INH absorbed Carbamazepine: ↑ toxicity of both Disulfiram: psychosis, ataxia
Ketoconazole	Possible inhibition of adrenal corticosteroid synthesis with prolonged use	Antacids, cimetidine: ↓ ketoconazole levels Cyclosporine: ↑ cyclosporine levels Alcohol: disulfiram-like reaction
Metronidazole	Peripheral neuropathy	Anticoagulants: ↑ anticoagulant effect Disulfiram: organic brain syndrome Barbiturates: ↓ metronidazole effect
Penicillins	Maculopapular rash, photosensitivity, erythema multiforme, anaphylaxis, serum sickness, anemia, leukopenia, diarrhea, pulmonary infiltrates, drug-induced lupus, encephalopathy (with high doses) Interstitial nephritis (especially with methicillin), glomerulonephritis Hepatitis with oxacillin Pseudomembranous colitis Seizures with high-dose therapy	↓ Effect of aminoglycoside in renal failure Oral contraceptives: ↓ effect with ampicillin
Pentamidine	Nephrotoxicity, hepatotoxicity Hypoglycemia, hypotension, phlebitis, bone marrow depression	

Drug	Adverse Effects	Drug Interactions
Quinolones	Dizziness, headache, nausea, leukopenia, eosinophilia, rash	↑ Effect of theophylline with ciprofloxacin, enoxacin
Rifampin	Anemia Orange coloration of body secretions	↓ Effect of anticoagulants, barbiturates, beta blockers, oral contraceptives, corticosteroids, digoxin, quinidine, sulfonylureas ↑ INH hepatotoxicity
Sulfonamides	Anaphylaxis, serum sickness, aplastic anemia, pulmonary infiltrates, maculopapular rash, photosensitivity, drug-induced lupus Glomerulonephritis	↑ Effect of warfarin, phenytoin, sulfonylureas, theophylline
Tetracyclines	Photosensitivity, discoloration of developing teeth, nausea, epigastric distress Prerenal azotemia	↑ Effect of warfarin, digoxin, lithium Antacids, iron: ↓ tetracycline absorption Barbiturates, phenytoin: ↓ doxycycline levels
Trimethoprim	Rash, bone marrow depression	
Vancomycin	Ototoxicity	Aminoglycosides: ↑ nephrotoxicity

TABLE 3–2. Dosing Recommendations for Antimicrobial Agents

	STANDARD DOSAGE (NORMAL RENAL FUNCTION)	DOSAGE INTERVAL FOR CREATININE CLEARANCE (mL/min)			SUPPLEMENT AFTER DIALYSIS*
		80–50	50–10	<10	
Aztreonam	0.5–2 g IV q6–12h	8–12 h	12–24 h	24–36 h	Yes (H)
Aminoglycosides†,‡					
Amikacin	5–7.5 mg/kg IV q8–12h	12 h	24–36 h	36–72 h	Yes (H,P)
Gentamicin	1–2 mg/kg IV q8h	8–12 h	12–24 h	24–72 h	Yes (H,P)
Tobramycin	1–2 mg/kg IV q8h	8–12 h	12–24 h	24–72 h	Yes (H,P)
Amphotericin B	Initial test dose, 1 mg IV, then 0.5–1.5 mg/kg IV q24h	24 h	24 h	24–48 h	No
Cephalosporins					
First Generation					
Cefadroxil	0.5–1 g PO q12–24h	12–24 h	24 h	36–48 h	Yes (H)
Cephradine	0.5 g PO q6h	6 h	8 h	12–24 h	Yes (H,P)
Cephalexin	0.25–0.5 g PO q6h	6 h	8–12 h	24–48 h	Yes (H)
Cephalothin	1–2 g IV q4–6h	6 h	8 h	12 h	Yes (H,P)
Cephapirin	1 g IV q4–6h	6 h	8 h	12 h	Yes (H)
Cefazolin	1–2 g IV q6–8h	8 h	12 h	24–48 h	Yes (H)
Second Generation					
Cefaclor	0.25–0.5 g PO q8h	8 h	8 h	8 h	Yes (H)
Cefonicid	1–2 g IV q24h	24 h	24 h	3–5 d	No (H,P)
Cefotetan	1–2 g IV q12h	12 h	24 h	48 h	Yes (H)
Cefoxitin	1–2 g IV q4–6h	8 h	8 h	24–48 h	Yes (H), No (P)
Cefuroxime	0.75–1.5 g IV q8h	8–12 h	24–48 h	24 h	Yes (H,P)
Third Generation					
Cefoperazone	1–2 g IV q8–12h	8–12 h	8–12 h	8–12 h	Yes (H)
Cefotaxime	1–2 g IV q4–6h	4–6 h	6–12 h	12–24 h	Yes (H)
Ceftazidime	1–2 g IV q6–8h	8–12 h	12–24 h	24–48 h	Yes (H,P)
Ceftizoxime	1–2 g IV q6–8h	8 h	12 h	12–24 h	Yes (H,P)
Ceftriaxone	1–2 g IV q12–24h	12–24 h	24 h	24 h	No
Chloramphenicol†	1 g IV q6h	6 h	6 h	6 h	Yes (H), No (P)
Clindamycin	0.15–0.45 g PO q6h; 0.15–0.9 g IV q6h	6 h	6 h	6 h	No (H,P)
Erythromycin	0.25–0.5 g PO q6h; 0.25–1 g IV q6h	6 h	6 h	6 h	No (H,P)
Imipenem	0.5–1 g IV q6–8h	6–8 h	6–12 h	12–24 h	Yes (H)
Metronidazole	0.25–0.5 g PO q8h; 0.5–0.75 g IV q8h	8 h	8–12 h	12–24 h	Yes (H), No (P)

Penicillins

Agent	Dose				Dialysis
Penicillins					
Penicillin G	1–3 MU IV q4–6h	6–8 h	8–12 h	12–24 h	Yes (H), No (P)
Penicillin V	0.25–0.5 g PO q6h	6–8 h	8–12 h	12–24 h	Yes (H), No (P)
Penicillinase-Resistant Penicillins					
Dicloxacillin	0.5 g PO q6h	6 h	6 h	6 h	No (H)
Nafcillin§	0.5–2 g IV q4–6h	4–6 h	4–6 h	4–6 h	No (H)
Methicillin	1–2 g IV q4–6h	6 h	8 h	12 h	No (H,P)
Broad-Spectrum Penicillins					
Amoxicillin	0.25–0.5 g PO q8h	8 h	12 h	12–24 h	Yes (H), No (P)
Amoxicillin-clavulanate	One tablet (250 or 500 mg amoxicillin/125 mg clavulanate) PO tid	8 h	12 h	12–24 h	N/A
Ampicillin	0.5–1 g PO q6h; 1–2 g IV q4–6h	6 h	8 h	12 h	Yes (H), No (P)
Ampicillin-sulbactam	1–2 g/0.5–1 g IV q6h	6–8 h	12 h	24 h	Yes (H), No (P)
Carbenicillin	4–5 g IV q4–6h	6–8 h	12–24 h	24–48 h	Yes (H,P)
Ticarcillin	2–3 g IV q4–6h	8–12 h	12–24 h	24–48 h	Yes (H,P)
Ticarcillin-clavulanate	One (3 g ticarcillin/0.1 g clavulanate) vial q4–6h	8–12 h	12–24 h	24–48 h	N/A
Azlocillin	2–3 g IV q4–6h	4–6 h	6–8 h	12 h	Yes (H)
Mezlocillin	2–4 g IV q4–8h	4–6 h	6–8 h	8–12 h	Yes (H)
Piperacillin	3–4 g IV q4–6h	4–6 h	6–8 h	12 h	Yes (H)
Trimethoprim-Sulfamethoxazole	160/800 mg PO q12h; 10–20 mg/kg/d IV based on trimethoprim component divided into q6h or q12h schedule	12 h	18 h	24–48 h	No (P)
Tetracyclines	0.25–0.5 g PO q6h; 0.5–1 g IV q12h	– – – – – – – Contraindicated – – – – – – –			
Doxycycline	0.1 g PO or IV q12h	12–24 h	12–24 h	12–24 h	No (H,P)
Vancomycin†	0.5–1 g IV q12–24h	1–2 d	2–4 d	4–7 d	No (H,P)
Quinolones					
Ciprofloxacin	0.25–0.75 g PO q12h; 0.4 g IV q12h	12 h	12–24 h	24 h	Yes (H,P)
Norfloxacin	0.4 g PO q12h	12 h	12–24 h	24 h	N/A

*H, hemodialysis; P, peritoneal dialysis; N/A, not applicable.

†Levels should be followed.

‡For more specific dosing information, see Hull JH, Sarubbi FA. Gentamicin serum concentrations: pharmocokinetic predictions. Ann Intern Med 1976;85:183–189. Patients with moderate-to-severe renal insufficiency should receive a loading dose of 1–2 mg/kg of all aminoglycosides (except amikacin, which is 5–7.5 g/kg).

§Dose should be reduced in combined renal and hepatic failure.

For further information, see Bennett WM, Aronoff GR, Morrison G, et al. Drug prescribing in renal failure: dosing guidelines for adults. Am J Kidney Dis 1983;3:155, and Van Scoy RE, Wilson WR. Antimicrobial agents in adult patients with renal insufficiency: initial dosage and general recommendations. Mayo Clin Proc 1987;62:1142.

TABLE 3-3. Antimicrobial Agents of Choice Against Selected Organisms

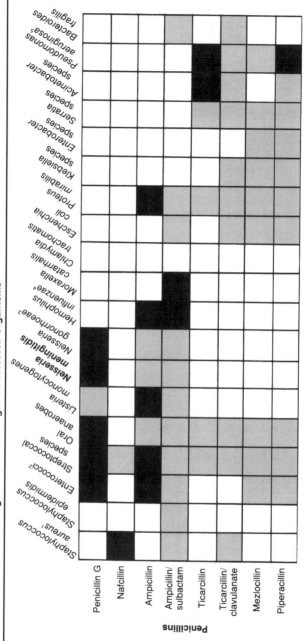

KEY: Appropriate antibiotics for treatment of clinical infections caused by various bacteria are depicted. Green-shaded squares denote "preferred agent(s)" for therapy; "alternate agents" are designated by the gray-shaded squares. These choices of antimicrobial therapy are based in part on antibiotic sensitivity data from the University of Washington Medical Center. Since these data represent solely the experience from a single hospital, information in this table may not be accurate for other hospitals. It is important to be aware of local antimicrobial sensitivity patterns when choosing antibiotic therapy.

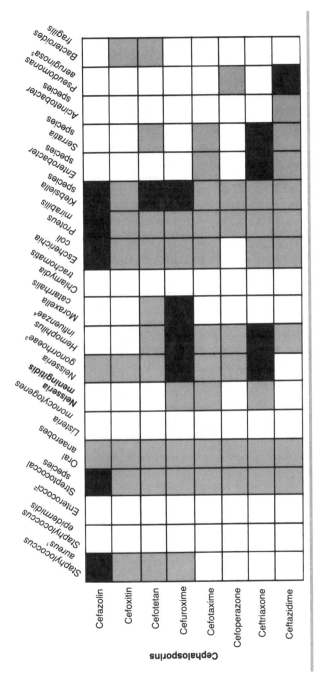

[1]"Methicillin-resistant" strains of Staphylococcus aureus (MRSA) are found in some hospitals and will be resistant to multiple beta-lactams. In general, infections due to MRSA should be treated with vancomycin.

[2]Use penicillin (or ampicillin or vancomycin) with an aminoglycoside for systemic infections.

[3]In regions where penicillinase producers are prevalent, use a cephalosporin (e.g., ceftriaxone) or ciprofloxacin.

[4]For penicillinase producers, use a second- or third-generation cephalosporin (e.g., cefuroxime or ceftriaxone), ampicillin/sulbactam, or TMP/SMX.

[5]Combination therapy is optimal: an aminoglycoside plus an extended-spectrum penicillin or a third-generation cephalosporin. TMP/SMX, trimethoprim-sulfamethoxazole.

Table continued on following page

TABLE 3–3. Antimicrobial Agents of Choice Against Selected Organisms (Continued)

	Staphylococcus aureus[1]	Staphylococcus epidermidis	Enterococci[2]	Streptococcal species	Oral anaerobes	Listeria monocytogenes	Neisseria meningitidis	Neisseria gonorrhoeae[3]	Hemophilus influenzae[4]	Moraxella catarrhalis	Chlamydia trachomatis	Escherichia coli	Proteus mirabilis	Klebsiella species	Enterobacter species	Serratia species	Acinetobacter species	Pseudomonas aeruginosa[5]	Bacteroides fragilis
Aminoglycoside																			
Gentamicin																			
Tobramycin																			
Amikacin																			
Broad-spectrum agents																			
Imipenem																			
Aztreonam																			
Ciprofloxacin																			
TMP/SMX																			

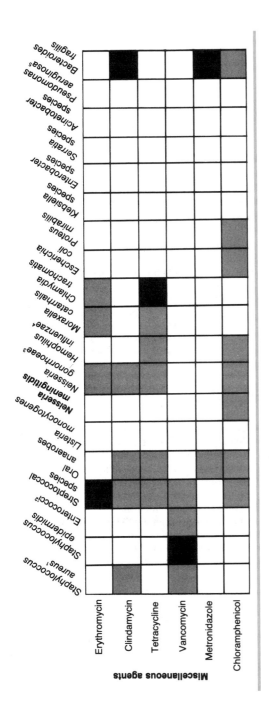

H. influenzae meningitis (e.g., ceftriaxone or chloramphenicol) until the antimicrobial sensitivity pattern is known. If the isolate is sensitive to ampicillin, the antibiotic coverage can be narrowed to the appropriate "preferred agent." A number of methods are available to determine antimicrobial susceptibility.

1. **DISK DIFFUSION.** The disk diffusion method involves placing antibiotic-permeated paper disks on a solid medium that has been inoculated with a pure culture of the patient's organism. The method is simple and inexpensive and has been standardized for most organisms. Within 24 hours, most bacteria can be rated as susceptible, intermediate, or resistant on the basis of the size of the zone of inhibition around each antibiotic disk. This technique cannot be applied to fastidious or slow-growing organisms and has not been standardized for anaerobes.

2. **AGAR OR BROTH DILUTION.** Agar or broth dilution techniques provide quantitative susceptibility information about an organism. These serial dilution methods are used to determine the lowest concentration of antibiotic that will inhibit visible bacterial growth after an 18- to 24-hour period. This level is called the **minimal inhibitory concentration (MIC).** An organism is considered sensitive to an antibiotic when the MIC of the antibiotic to that organism is no more than one fourth of the obtainable peak serum concentration. The **minimal bactericidal concentration (MBC)** may be found by subculturing the dilution tubes that do not show growth into antibiotic-free media. The subculture from the lowest antibiotic concentration that suppresses overnight growth is designated as that organism's MBC.

E. Combination Antimicrobial Therapy

Most infections can be treated with a single antimicrobial agent. The simultaneous use of two or more antimicrobial agents has effects on the host and the flora. Combination therapy is appropriate only in specific situations. In vitro, an antimicrobial combination can have one of three different effects on a microorganism: (1) **additive,** in which the activity of the drugs in combination is equal to the sum of their separate activities, (2) **synergistic,** in which the activity of the drug combination is greater than the sum of their separate activities, and (3) **antagonistic,** in which the combined activity of the agents is less than the sum of their independent effects. Although these effects can be demonstrated by several methods in the laboratory, clinical trials documenting the in vivo effects of the in vitro findings are limited.

There are several commonly cited reasons for using combination antimicrobial therapy:

1. **PREVENTION OF EMERGENCE OF RESISTANT ORGANISMS.** If the spontaneous mutation of microorganisms were the most common method of acquiring resistance, combination therapy would decrease this occurrence. However, tuberculosis and, perhaps, infections due to *Pseudomonas aeruginosa* or Enterobacteriaceae are the only diseases for which this rationale should routinely lead to the use of multiple agents.

2. **TREATMENT OF POLYMICROBIAL INFECTIONS.** Intraabdominal, pelvic, and genital tract infections, as well as abscesses in other locations, are

caused by aerobic and anaerobic flora. These infections may require combination therapy to cover the broad variety of organisms involved.

3. **THERAPY FOR INFECTIONS OF UNKNOWN ETIOLOGY IN SEVERELY ILL OR IMMUNOCOMPROMISED PATIENTS.** Broad-spectrum initial coverage may be necessary until the causative pathogen or pathogens become apparent. A commonly employed regimen is a third-generation cephalosporin or extended-spectrum penicillin combined with an aminoglycoside.

4. **DECREASED TOXICITY.** Theoretically, it may be possible to lower the dose of a potentially toxic agent when used in combination with another effective antimicrobial.

5. **SYNERGISM.** Although many synergistic antimicrobial combinations have been demonstrated in the laboratory, combination therapy has been proved more effective than a single agent in only a few clinical situations. The most widely accepted combination is penicillin plus an aminoglycoside for enterococcal endocarditis. A combination of an antipseudomonal penicillin with an aminoglycoside against *Pseudomonas aeruginosa* is also widely accepted. Fixed drug combinations, such as trimethoprim with sulfamethoxazole, work by inhibiting two steps in the folic acid cycle. Beta-lactam agents in combination with beta-lactamase inhibitors, such as amoxicillin or ticarcillin plus clavulanate (Augmentin and Timentin, respectively), act synergistically.

F. Assessment of Antimicrobial Therapy

Effective antimicrobial therapy should result in clinical improvement of the patient, as evidenced by normalization of temperature and white blood cell count, accompanied by subjective improvement and disappearance of the pathogen from the infection site. The duration of antibiotic therapy should be determined on the basis of clinical response. Not enough well-controlled studies are available to make decisions concerning length of therapy in most situations. In general, most acute bacterial infections for which antibiotics penetrate well to the site of infection should be treated for at least 3 to 5 days *after* clinical signs of infection have resolved. Some chronic infections, such as osteomyelitis, and infections involving sites that are penetrated poorly by antibiotics, such as vegetations in bacterial endocarditis, may require much longer antibiotic courses after symptoms and signs of infection have resolved.

1. **THE SERUM BACTERICIDAL TITER** has been used to monitor therapy in bacterial endocarditis. Serial dilutions of the patient's serum are incubated with a standardized inoculum of the infecting organism. The highest dilution that inhibits growth is determined. A serum bactericidal titer of 1:8 or greater correlates with successful outcome in most serious infections. In bacterial endocarditis, a titer greater than 1:64 is desirable. The lack of standardization and consistency of this test has made its use controversial.

2. **MEASUREMENTS OF ANTIMICROBIAL SERUM CONCENTRATIONS** are useful to avoid toxicity from elevated levels of agents, such as the aminoglycosides and vancomycin, especially in patients with impaired renal

function. Measurement can also be used to ensure adequate peak levels of these agents.

If a patient does not improve clinically, there are several factors to consider:

- Inadequate drug delivery resulting from poor compliance or poor absorption of the agent
- Inadequate dosage or prolonged antibiotic-free intervals between doses
- Poor antibiotic penetration to the site of infection, as, for example, in endocarditis
- Presence of abscess or abscesses that require drainage
- Presence of a foreign body
- Emergence of a resistant pathogen or superinfection with a new pathogen
- A new infection site, such as pneumonia, urinary tract infections, or phlebitis in the hospitalized patient
- Drug fever
- Altered host defenses

II. PROPHYLACTIC USE OF ANTIMICROBIAL AGENTS

A. Antimicrobial Prophylaxis for Surgery

Preoperative prophylactic antibiotics are used in some situations (Table 3–4). The antibiotic chosen should have a narrow spectrum of coverage directed against the most likely infecting pathogen or pathogens. Its cost, safety, and efficacy must be considered and the prophylaxis tailored to each situation. Prophylactic antibiotics must reach high tissue levels during the operation. For this reason, a dose should usually be given on call to the operating room and repeated only if the surgery is delayed or prolonged. A maximum of three doses should be given for most operations, except for "contaminated cases" (e.g., a perforated viscus), when a longer course is indicated. It is also common practice to give more than three doses when prosthetic joints and heart valves are to be implanted, although additional benefit has not been established clearly in these situations. Administration beyond 72 hours increases the risk of bacterial resistance and drug toxicity without decreasing the risk of infection.

Appropriate prophylactic antimicrobial use must be coupled with proper surgical technique and judgment. Factors that contribute to the development of wound infection in clean surgical procedures include prolonged hospitalization before the procedure, extended operative time, excessive use of wound drains, and razor shaving of the operative field the night before surgery. A preoperative shower with an antiseptic soap has been shown to decrease the incidence of wound infection.

Hirschman JV, Inui TS. Antimicrobial prophylaxis: a critique of recent trials. Rev Infect Dis 1980; 2:1–23.

Hull JH, Sarubbi FA. Gentamicin serum concentrations: pharmacokinetic predictions. Ann Intern Med 1976;85:183.

Medical Letter. The choice of antimicrobial drugs. Med Lett Drugs Ther 1986;28:33–40.

Sarubbi FA, Hull JH. Amikacin serum concentrations: predication of levels and dosage guidelines. Ann Intern Med 1978;89:612–618.

Symposium on antimicrobial agents. Mayo Clin Proc 1987;62:789–1031.

TABLE 3-4. Antimicrobial Prophylaxis for Surgery

TYPE OF SURGERY	LIKELY PATHOGENS	DOSAGE BEFORE SURGERY*
Cardiovascular	*Staphylococcus epidermidis, S. aureus, Corynebacterium* sp.	Cefazolin or vancomyin,† 1 g IV
Orthopedic (including prosthetic joint placement)	*S. aureus, S. epidermidis*	Cefazolin or vancomycin,† 1 g IV
Head and neck	*S. aureus,* streptococci, oral anaerobes	Cefazolin, 1 g IV
High-risk gastroduodenal or biliary tract	Enteric gram-negative bacilli, gram-positive cocci, group D streptococci, *Clostridium*	Cefazolin, 1 g IV
Colorectal	Enteric gram-negative bacilli, anaerobes	Oral: neomycin, plus erythromycin base, 1 g of each at 1 PM, 2 PM, and 11 PM the day before surgery‡ Parenteral: cefoxitin, 1 g IV
Appendectomy	Enteric gram-negative bacilli, anaerobes	Cefotetan, 1 g IV
Vaginal or abdominal hysterectomy; high-risk cesarean section	Enteric gram-negative bacilli, anaerobes, group B and D streptococci	Cefazolin, 1 g IV
Abortion	As above, but test for *Chlamydia*	Tetracycline, 500 mg PO qid, or doxycycline, 100 mg PO bid; continue for 7 days if *Chlamydia* culture positive
Ruptured viscus	Enteric gram-negative bacilli, anaerobes, group D streptococci	Clindamycin, 600 mg IV q6h, plus gentamicin or tobramycin, 1.5 mg/kg IV or IM, with or without ampicillin, 1.5 g IV q6h; *or* cefotetan alone or with gentamicin or tobramycin; *or* imipenem, 500 mg IV q6h
Traumatic wounds§	*S. aureus,* group A streptococcus, *Clostridium, Pasteurella*	Ampicillin-sulbactam, 1.5–3 g IV q4–6h, with or without gentamicin or tobramycin; *or* cefazolin, 1 g q6–8h IM or IV; *or* ticarcillin-clavulanate, 3.1 g IV q4–6h

*Parenteral prophylactic antimicrobials for clean and clean-contaminated surgery can be given as a single dose just before the operation. For prolonged operations, additional intraoperative dosages should be given q4–8h for the duration of the procedure. For dirty surgery, therapy should usually be continued for 5 to 10 days.

†For hospitals in which methicillin-resistant *S. aureus* and *S. epidermidis* frequently cause wound infection, or for patients with penicillin or cephalosporin allergy.

‡After appropriate diet and catharsis (see Nichols RL. Postoperative infections and antimicrobial prophylaxis. In: Mandell GL, Douglas RG, Bennett JE, et al., eds. Principles and Practice of Infectious Diseases, 2nd ed. New York: Wiley, 1985, p. 1641.)

§For bite wounds, in which likely pathogens may also include oral anaerobes, *Eikenella corrodens* (humans), and *Pasteurella multocida* (dogs and cats), some consultants recommend use of amoxicillin-clavulanic acid (Augmentin) or ampicillin-sulbactam (Unasyn).

Adapted from recommendations presented in Med Lett Drugs Ther 1987;29:91–94. Modifications based on local usage.

B. Antimicrobial Prophylaxis for Prevention of Endocarditis

The American Heart Association issued new recommendations for the prevention of bacterial endocarditis in dental and medical procedures in 1990.

1. PROPHYLAXIS IS RECOMMENDED for patients with:
   - Prosthetic cardiac valves, including bioprosthetic and homograft valves
   - Most congenital cardiac anomalies
   - Hypertrophic cardiomyopathy
   - Mitral valve prolapse with associated audible murmur of valvular regurgitation
   - A history of previous bacterial endocarditis, even in the absence of heart disease
   - A history of rheumatic and other acquired valvular dysfunction, even following corrective valvular surgery

2. PROPHYLAXIS IS NOT RECOMMENDED for patients with:
   - Isolated secundum atrial septal defect
   - Mitral valve prolapse without valvular regurgitation
   - Physiologic, functional, or innocent heart murmurs
   - Cardiac pacemakers and implantable defibrillators
   - A history of previous coronary artery bypass graft surgery
   - A history of previous rheumatic fever or Kawasaki's disease without valvular dysfunction
   - A history of surgical repair without residua beyond 6 months of secundum atrial septal defect, ventricular septal defect, or patent ductus arteriosus

3. Patients with increased risk of bacterial endocarditis should receive antibiotic PROPHYLAXIS WHEN UNDERGOING THE FOLLOWING PROCEDURES:
   - Dental procedures likely to result in gingival bleeding (including professional dental cleaning)
   - Tonsillectomy
   - Adenoidectomy
   - Rigid bronchoscopy
   - Surgical procedures involving manipulation of the respiratory mucosa
   - Cholecystectomy and biliary tract surgery
   - Cystoscopy
   - Urethral surgery
   - Prostatic surgery
   - Incision and drainage of infected tissue
   - Upper endoscopy
   - Vaginal hysterectomy
   - Urethral catheterization, urinary tract surgery, and vaginal delivery when infection is present

   a. **For dental, oral, or upper respiratory tract procedures** the recommended **prophylactic regimen** is **amoxicillin, 3 g PO 1 hour before the procedure, followed by 1.5 g PO 6 hours after the initial dose.** In penicillin-allergic patients, either erythromycin (1 g PO 2 hours before the procedure, followed by 500 mg PO 6 hours after the initial dose) or clindamycin (300 mg PO 1 hour before the procedure, followed by 150 mg 6 hours after the initial dose) may be employed.

b. For genitourinary or gastrointestinal procedures, the recommended regimen for prophylaxis against endocarditis is **ampicillin, 2 g IV or IM, plus gentamicin, 1.5 mg/kg (not to exceed 80 mg) 30 minutes before the procedure, followed by amoxicillin, 1.5 g PO 6 hours after the initial dose (or the parenteral regimen may be repeated once 8 hours after the initial dose).** In penicillin-allergic patients, the recommended regimen is vancomycin 1 g IV, plus gentamicin 1.5 mg/kg (not to exceed 80 mg) 1 hour before the procedure. Repeat administration of vancomycin and gentamicin can be considered 8 hours after the initial doses. An alternate regimen for low-risk patients is amoxicillin 3 g PO 1 hour before the procedure, followed by 1.5 g PO 6 hours later.

Dajani AS, et al. Prevention of bacterial endocarditis: recommendations by the American Heart Association. JAMA 1990;264:2919–2922.

III. OTITIS AND SINUSITIS

A. Otitis Externa

Otitis externa, infection of the external auditory canal, can be divided into four categories, as follows:

1. ACUTE LOCALIZED OTITIS EXTERNA usually occurs as a pustule or furuncle caused by *Staphylococcus aureus.* Erysipelas due to group A streptococcus may also be present in the canal. **Treatment** for both conditions is **local heat and systemic antibiotics** (dicloxacillin or erythromycin). Incision and drainage may be needed for some patients.

2. ACUTE DIFFUSE OTITIS EXTERNA (swimmer's ear) occurs in warm, humid environments. **Treatment** consists of local **irrigation with hypertonic saline (3%) and cleansing with mixtures of alcohol (70% to 95%) and acetic acid.** Burow's solution (50%) may reduce inflammation. Topical treatment with solutions containing antibiotics (neomycin and polymixin) and a steroid is effective also (e.g., Cortisporin Otic). Systemic antibiotics are not necessary unless invasive otitis is suspected.

3. CHRONIC OTITIS EXTERNA is secondary to irritating drainage from chronic suppurative otitis media, and **treatment is that of a middle ear infection.**

4. INVASIVE OTITIS EXTERNA (also called malignant otitis externa) occurs most frequently in the elderly diabetic patient and results from the spread of infection into the adjacent soft tissues, cartilage, and bone. **Treatment includes surgical debridement of the canal, along with topical application of antipseudomonal antibiotics and steroids. Systemic therapy** directed against *Pseudomonas aeruginosa* (**an aminoglycoside and a beta-lactam antibiotic,** such as carbenicillin or ticarcillin) for 4 to 6 weeks is also necessary. Hemorrhagic external otitis caused by *P. aeruginosa* has also been described in association with hot tub use and also may require IV antibiotic administration.

B. Otitis Media

1. ACUTE OTITIS MEDIA characterized or accompanied by symptoms of an upper respiratory tract infection, ear pain, drainage, and decreased hearing is commonly due to *Streptococcus pneumoniae* and nontypable *Haemophilus influenzae*. Less frequent pathogens include group A streptococcus, *Staphylococcus aureus,* and *Moraxella catarrhalis*. Gram-negative bacilli may have a role in chronic suppurative otitis and in infections in immunosuppressed patients. Therapy is usually initiated without knowledge of the pathogen and should be directed toward covering *Streptococcus pneumoniae* and *H. influenzae.* **Amoxicillin, 250 mg PO tid,** is the initial agent of choice for adults. **Amoxicillin-clavulanate, 250 mg PO tid,** is an option when the prevalence of ampicillin-resistant *H. influenzae* is appreciable or when *M. catarrhalis* is suspected. In the **penicillin-allergic patient, trimethoprim-sulfamethoxazole, 1 double-strength tablet 160 mg/800 mg PO bid or an oral cephalosporin (i.e., cefuroxime axetil 250 mg qid)** can be administered. Decongestants and antihistamines are of no proven benefit. The presence of bullous myringitis suggests possible infection by *Mycoplasma pneumoniae.* **Erythromycin, 250 mg qid, is the treatment of choice.**

2. CHRONIC OTITIS MEDIA following recurrent episodes of acute infection and prolonged duration of middle ear effusion has been managed by chemoprophylaxis and immunoprophylaxis. Chemoprophylaxis with once-a-day antimicrobial therapy has been successful in children. Immunoprophylaxis with pneumococcal vaccine may reduce the incidence of acute otitis media due to serotypes of *Streptococcus pneumoniae* included in the vaccine. Persistent middle ear effusion is most successfully treated by insertion of tympanostomy tubes.

3. MASTOID INFECTION may accompany otitis media, and tympanocentesis cultures are useful to guide antibiotic selection. Initial therapy should include antimicrobial coverage for *Streptococcus pneumoniae* and *H. influenzae,* with additional coverage for *Staphylococcus aureus* and gram-negative enteric bacilli if the clinical course has been prolonged.

Doroghazi RM, Nadol JB, Hyslop NE. Invasive external otitis: report of 21 cases and review of the literature. Am J Med 1981;71:603–614.

Nelson JD. Changing trends in the microbiology and management of acute otitis media and sinusitis. Pediatr Infect Dis 1986;5:749–753.

C. Maxillary Sinusitis

Over 90% of acute (<3 weeks in duration) sinusitis involves the maxillary sinuses. Treatment is usually empiric and is directed toward *Streptococcus pneumoniae,* nonencapsulated *H. influenzae,* and *M. catarrhalis.* **Amoxicillin 250–500 mg PO tid, amoxicillin-clavulanate (Augmentin) 250–500 mg PO tid, or trimethoprim-sulfamethoxazole 160 mg/800 mg, 1 tablet twice a day for a 10-day course, is recommended.** Oxymetazoline hydrochloride nasal spray 3 times a day (not to be used for more than 3 days) may reduce mucosal swelling. Follow-up with repeat transillumination and sinus radiographs or computed tomography is indicated for patients who do not respond to therapy. Consultation with an ENT specialist should be considered for patients with chronic symptoms, especially if sinus x-rays show persistent air-fluid levels or complete opacification of the airspace.

D. Nosocomial Sinusitis

Nosocomially acquired sinusitis, a common problem in ICU patients with indwelling nasal or oral tubes, is usually caused by antibiotic-resistant gram-negative rods. Effective treatment depends on the results of cultures from material obtained by direct sinus puncture. Initial treatment should cover *Pseudomonas aeruginosa* until culture results are available and indwelling tubes are removed, if possible.

E. Chronic Sinusitis

Cultures of material obtained by direct maxillary sinus puncture in patients with sinusitis of longer than 3 months' duration usually show a predominance of anaerobic flora or *Staphylococcus aureus*. Antimicrobial therapy directed at oral anaerobic flora and *Staphylococcus aureus* may be helpful in these individuals, but no well-controlled studies are available to guide antibiotic use. Surgical procedures to create better drainage should be considered if symptoms do not respond to antimicrobial therapy. Patients with chronic sinusitis and severe asthma may respond well to surgical drainage, often with considerable improvement in their response to treatment for bronchospasm.

F. Complications of Sinusitis

1. Untreated FRONTAL SINUSITIS can lead to cranial osteomyelitis, frontal subperiosteal abscess, epidural abscess, subdural abscess, and brain abscess. Initial antimicrobial therapy for mild frontal sinusitis is the same as that for maxillary sinusitis. Close observation is necessary, however, as these patients may require hospitalization for IV therapy or surgical intervention.

2. Orbital cellulitis is a complication of ETHMOID SINUSITIS. The causative bacteria that have been described include *Staphylococcus aureus, H. influenzae, Streptococcus pneumoniae,* and *Streptococcus pyogenes.* Early treatment with IV antibiotics is essential, and these patients should be followed carefully by an otolaryngologist.

3. SPHENOID SINUSITIS is rare but is associated with severe complications because of the proximity of the sphenoid sinus to several important structures. **Cavernous sinus thrombosis,** pituitary insufficiency, bitemporal hemianopsia, subdural abscess, internal carotid infection, and meningitis can result from extension of infection.

4. SEPTIC CAVERNOUS SINUS THROMBOSIS is most frequently caused by *S. aureus.* **Initial antimicrobial therapy should include IV administration of a semisynthetic penicillin or vancomycin in the penicillin-allergic patient. Broad-spectrum coverage** directed against aerobic gram-negative rods is also indicated, pending culture results. Heparin therapy is controversial.

5. **MUCORMYCOSIS AND ASPERGILLOSIS,** caused by opportunistic organisms, are types of **fungal sinusitis** seen in diabetic and immunosuppressed patients. **Surgical treatment is usually necessary, along with administration of systemic amphotericin B.** Unless these fungal infections are diagnosed very early in the clinical course, osteomyelitis is usually present in affected patients. Aggressive early surgical therapy may improve the prognosis of fungal sinusitis.

Daley CL, Sande M. The runny nose: infections of the paranasal sinuses. Infect Dis Clin North Am 1988;2:131–147.

Gualtney JM, Scheld WM, Sande MA, et al. The microbial etiology and antimicrobial therapy of adults with acute community-acquired sinusitis. J Allergy Clin Immunol 1992;90:457–462.

Hamory BH, Sande MA, Sydnor A, et al. Etiology and antimicrobial therapy of acute maxillary sinusitis. J Infect Dis 1979;139:197–202.

IV. PHARYNGEAL INFECTIONS

A. Pharyngitis

The goal in the diagnosis and treatment of acute pharyngitis is to separate pharyngitis due to group A streptococcal disease and other serious throat infections from those that are benign and self-limited. Most pharyngitis is caused by a virus. A throat culture should be done in adults who have a history of rheumatic fever, contact with a person known to have streptococcal pharyngitis, or clinical signs suggesting possible streptococcal infection, such as fever, pharyngeal exudate, and cervical adenopathy.

1. **GROUP A STREPTOCOCCAL PHARYNGITIS.** Treatment may be initiated on the basis of either a positive throat culture or high clinical suspicion and then discontinued if the culture is negative. **Penicillin V 250 mg PO qid for 10 days or benzathine penicillin G 1.2 MU in a single IM dose is recommended.** The latter treatment, while painful, eliminates the problem of the patient's compliance. **The penicillin-allergic patient can be given erythromycin, 250 mg PO qid for 10 days.** Initiation of treatment within 1 week of the onset of streptococcal pharyngitis should prevent rheumatic fever. A repeat throat culture after clinically successful treatment is not necessary. Oral therapy suffices for most patients with pharyngitis. Hospitalization and parenteral therapy are required if adequate hydration cannot be maintained or there is danger of airway compromise. Severe odynophagia suggests possible complications (e.g., epiglottitis or peritonsillar abscess). Pharyngitis due to other beta-hemolytic streptococci is rare and does not require antimicrobial therapy.

2. **GONOCOCCAL PHARYNGITIS.** Treatment is described on p. 106.

3. **VIRAL PHARYNGITIS.** Viral pharyngitis caused by type A influenza may benefit from early use of amantadine, 100 mg PO bid or 200 mg PO qd, or rimantidine, 100 mg PO bid. Herpetic oropharyngeal infection in the immunosuppressed patient can be treated with acyclovir 250 mg/m^2 every 8 hours IV for 7 days.

4. **LUDWIG'S ANGINA (ANAEROBIC PHARYNGITIS).** This type of pharyngitis can be treated with an oral penicillin or cephalosporin initially. It may,

however, spread to the soft tissues of the neck and require surgical drainage and IV antibiotics.

B. Epiglottitis

When epiglottitis is suspected on the basis of clinical findings or lateral neck radiographic abnormalities, **initial IV antibiotic therapy should be directed against** *Haemophilus influenzae.* However, *Streptococcus pneumoniae,* other streptococci, *Staphylococcus aureus,* and *H. parainfluenzae* also have been implicated in cases of epiglottitis in normal hosts, and *Pseudomonas aeruginosa* may cause epiglottitis in the immunosuppressed patient. Hospitalization for IV antimicrobial therapy and close observation is indicated for adults with epiglottitis.

C. Peritonsillar Abscess

Streptococcus pyogenes is the organism most frequently associated with peritonsillar abscess, but other pathogens, including *Staphylococcus aureus,* have been noted. Drainage, along with appropriate antimicrobial therapy, is often needed for successful treatment.

D. Odontogenic Infection

Drainage and extraction of the affected tooth are essential. Oral microflora, particularly anaerobes, are the most frequently involved organisms. **Amoxicillin 500 mg PO tid, penicillin VK 500 mg PO qid,** or **erythromycin 500 mg PO qid for 7 to 10 days** as an adjunct to drainage/extraction is appropriate. For more serious infections, **clindamycin 300 mg PO qid** or **amoxicillin-clavulanate 500 mg PO tid** may be considered.

Ramsey PG, Weymuller EA. Complications of bacterial infection of the ears, paranasal sinuses, and oropharynx in adults. Emerg Med Clin North Am 1985;3:143–159.

V. TRACHEOBRONCHITIS

A. Acute Bronchitis

Most cases of acute bronchitis are associated with viruses (rhinovirus, coronavirus, influenza A and B viruses, adenovirus, measles virus) or are caused by *Mycoplasma pneumoniae.* **Treatment** is symptomatic with cough suppressants, rest, and hydration. Antibiotics are not recommended unless infection with *M. pneumoniae* or *Bordetella pertussis* is suspected. During influenza A epidemics, treatment with amantadine or rimantidine may be considered if the illness is of less than 48 hours' duration.

B. Chronic Bronchitis: Acute Infectious Exacerbations

Respiratory viruses frequently exacerbate chronic bronchitis. Since patients with chronic bronchitis are often colonized with *Streptococcus pneumoniae,* unencapsulated *Haemophilus influenzae,* and *Moraxella catarrhalis,* a sputum gram stain will usually reveal these organisms during periods of acute exacerbation. After a sputum culture has been obtained, antimicrobial therapy may be directed against *H. influenzae* and *S. pneumoniae.* **Amoxicillin 250 mg PO tid, tetracycline 500 mg PO qid,** or **trimethoprim-**

sulfamethoxazole, 1 double-strength tablet (160 mg/800 mg) PO bid, may be chosen. If *Moraxella catarrhalis,* which often produces penicillinase, is suspected by gram stain, **amoxicillin-clavulanate 250 mg PO tid** should be employed. Prophylactic and chronic antibiotic therapy is controversial and should be considered only in selected patients with frequent exacerbations. Influenza and pneumococcal vaccines should be given to these patients.

C. Bacterial Tracheitis

Bacterial tracheitis is uncommon in adults, with the exception of patients who have had tracheal injury due to viral infection or intubation. Community-acquired organisms include *Staphylococcus aureus,* group A beta-hemolytic streptococci, and *Haemophilus influenzae* type B. Hospital-acquired infection is more likely to be caused by gram-negative pathogens. In the ICU, it is important to differentiate colonization from infection. Fever, stridor, dyspnea, or grossly purulent sputum suggests infection. Empiric therapy should be directed toward the organisms seen on the gram stain when infection is suspected.

VI. PNEUMONIA

Initial antimicrobial therapy for pneumonia is often based on limited information and may be empiric. A sputum gram stain and subsequent culture provide the most valuable information to guide therapy. The method of sputum collection (expectorated, nasotracheal, transtracheal needle aspiration, bronchoscopic, or open lung biopsy) should be tailored to the condition of the individual patient. A satisfactory sputum sample contains fewer than 10 epithelial cells and more than 25 white blood cells per low-power field with a predominating organism. When an expectorated sputum specimen is inadequate and does not enable the clinician to detect an etiologic agent, a more invasive method for obtaining sputum may be considered before beginning therapy. Alternatively, in selected patients, other information, such as age group, predisposing conditions, and where the pneumonia was acquired, can be used to guide initial antibiotic selection.

Because of difficulties in establishing a definitive bacteriologic diagnosis in community-acquired pneumonia, interest has focused on empiric treatment regimens based on the most likely pathogens for given epidemiologic groups. Guidelines for the initial management of adults with community-acquired pneumonia published by the American Thoracic Society are shown in Table 3–5.

A. Community-Acquired Pneumonia: Factors to Consider in Antibiotic Selection

1. YOUNG ADULTS. *Mycoplasma pneumoniae,* respiratory viruses, *Chlamydia pneumoniae,* and pneumococcus are the major etiologic agents. *Legionella* may cause approximately 1% of cases in this population. Empiric therapy with erythromycin is often employed if sputum is not available and the patient is not severely ill.

2. OLDER ADULTS. Bacterial pathogens are more common than in younger adults (*Streptococcus pneumoniae, Legionella pneumophila, Haemophi-*

TABLE 3-5. American Thoracic Society Guidelines for Initial Management of Adults with Community-Acquired Pneumonia

1. Outpatient pneumonia without comorbidity and 60 years of age or younger: macrolide *or* tetracycline

2. Outpatient pneumonia with comorbidity or 60 years of age or older: second-generation cephalosporin *or* TMP-SMX *or* beta-lactam/beta-lactamase inhibitor
   ±
   erythromycin or other macrolide

3. Hospitalized patients with community-acquired pneumonia: second- or third-generation cephalosporin *or* beta-lactam/beta-lactamase inhibitor
   ±
   erythromycin or other macrolide

4. Severe hospitalized community-acquired pneumonia: third-generation cephalosporin with antipseudomonal activity *or* other antipseudomonal agents, such as imipenem-cilastin or ciprofloxacin
   +
   erythromycin or other macrolide

From American Thoracic Society guidelines for the initial management of adults with community-acquired pneumonia: diagnosis, assessment of severity, and initial antimicrobial therapy. Am Rev Respir Dis 1993;148:1418–1426.

lus influenzae, and *Staphylococcus aureus*). Vigorous attempts to identify the etiologic agent are indicated.

3. NURSING HOME RESIDENTS AND THE ELDERLY. Pneumonia is more likely to be due to gram-negative organisms, including *Klebsiella pneumoniae, H. influenzae,* and *Enterobacter aerogenes.* Pneumococcal and staphylococcal pneumonias are also prevalent.

4. ALCOHOLISM. As the causative agent of pneumonia associated with alcoholism, *S. pneumoniae* is most common, followed by anaerobes, *H. influenzae, K. pneumoniae,* and *Mycobacterium tuberculosis.*

5. ASPIRATION PNEUMONIA. When consciousness is altered or normal airway protective reflexes are impaired, the resulting pneumonia reflects the flora of the oropharynx. *Bacteroides melaninogenicus, Fusobacterium* spp., and anaerobic gram-positive cocci are the most common anaerobes isolated. *Streptococcus* spp. are the most common aerobes isolated in community-acquired aspiration pneumonia, whereas gram-negative bacilli and *S. aureus* are the most common aerobic isolates in the hospital setting.

6. CHRONIC OBSTRUCTIVE PULMONARY DISEASE. *H. influenzae, S. pneumoniae,* and *Moraxella catarrhalis* predominate as the causes of pneumonia associated with chronic obstructive pulmonary disease.

7. CYSTIC FIBROSIS. In pneumonia associated with cystic fibrosis, *S. aureus* and *H. influenzae* prevail in younger patients, followed later by *Pseudomonas aeruginosa.*

8. POSTINFLUENZA BACTERIAL PNEUMONIAS. *S. pneumoniae, S. aureus,* or *H. influenzae* may cause this type of pneumonia.

B. Hospital-Acquired Pneumonia: Factors to Consider in Antibiotic Selection

The oropharynx is often colonized with gram-negative organisms. Anaerobes are also in high concentration and may be aspirated. Colonization with these organisms must be distinguished from infection and therapy directed accordingly. Mechanical ventilation markedly increases the risk of pulmonary superinfection and nosocomial pneumonia. The presence of radiographic infiltrates, fever, and purulent sputum strongly suggests pneumonia, but infection may be difficult to distinguish from bacterial colonization in the severely ill patient. Misguided, prolonged broad-spectrum antibiotic therapy may result in colonization and subsequent infection with multiply resistant organisms. Most nosocomial pneumonias occurring in the setting of mechanical ventilation are caused by enteric and nonenteric aerobic gram-negative rods.

C. Principles of Therapy

For most patients with pneumonia, hospitalization is indicated for IV antibiotics and hydration, monitoring of respiratory status, and good pulmonary toilet. Oxygen should be given, if indicated by respiratory status. Young people with mycoplasmal, mild pneumococcal, or viral pneumonia may be followed closely as outpatients and treated with oral antibiotics.

After appropriate cultures are obtained, initial antibiotic coverage should be directed at the most likely pathogen or pathogens indicated by the sputum gram stain, considering the mode of acquisition and host factors. Initial coverage should be broader in the seriously ill patient, pending results of diagnostic studies.

D. Therapy by Organism for Pneumonia

1. **GRAM-POSITIVE ORGANISMS**
   a. *Streptococcus pneumoniae.* In the young, healthy adult, erythromycin or penicillin V, given orally, may be adequate. If extrapulmonary sites are involved or the patient is seriously ill, **aqueous penicillin G, 1–2 MU IV q4h,** should be given. **Procaine penicillin G, 300,000–600,000 U q12h IM,** can be used if the patient is not hospitalized. Therapy should be continued for at least 2 to 3 days after the temperature returns to normal. Elderly individuals and patients with extrapulmonary sites should receive at least 7 days of parenteral therapy.

   Given the increasing prevalence of resistant isolates in many communities, **initial therapy for serious pneumococcal infections should include a third-generation cephalosporin (i.e., ceftriaxone or cefotaxime) or vancomycin or both** until antimicrobial susceptibilities are available. Pneumococcal isolates with intermediate resistance to penicillin (i.e., MIC ≥0.1 µg/mL, <1 µg/mL) may be treated with high-dose penicillin G (i.e., 20–24 MU/d) or a third-generation cephalosporin, but highly resistant strains (i.e., MIC ≥1 µg/mL) must be treated with vancomycin.

   b. *Staphylococcus aureus.* A beta-lactamase stable penicillin (e.g., **nafcillin)** should be used initially until the organism's susceptibilities are known. Treatment is usually continued for 3 to 4 weeks.

2. GRAM-NEGATIVE ORGANISMS. Most gram-negative pneumonias are hospital acquired and result from aspiration of oropharyngeal contents. Two antimicrobial agents should be used initially when the pathogen is unknown. Treatment is usually continued for 2 to 3 weeks, guided by the response of the patient.

   a. *Klebsiella pneumoniae.* **Mild disease may be treated with a single agent (e.g., a first-generation cephalosporin, such as cefazolin 1 g IV q8h or cephalothin 2 g IV q6h).** An **aminoglycoside** should be added for synergy in more seriously ill patients, especially for the first few days of therapy. Depending on susceptibility data, a single second-generation or third-generation cephalosporin (e.g., ceftriaxone) may be used.

   b. *Pseudomonas aeruginosa.* **Combination therapy with an anti-pseudomonal penicillin (e.g., ticarcillin) or cephalosporin (e.g., ceftazidime) plus an aminoglycoside (e.g., gentamicin) is indicated.** A third-generation cephalosporin alone is not adequate, and the role of other single agents (e.g., imipenem) remains unproved.

   c. *Haemophilus influenzae.* **Known beta-lactamase-negative strains should be treated with ampicillin, 1–2 g IV q4–6h for 10 days.** Patients with a penicillin allergy may receive **cefuroxime or ceftriaxone.** If cephalosporins cannot be given, chloramphenicol is an alternative. Ampicillin-resistant organisms can be treated with cefuroxime, a third-generation cephalosporin, ampicillin-sulbactam, or chloramphenicol.

3. ASPIRATION PNEUMONIA WITH MIXED ORGANISMS
   a. **Community-acquired infection. Penicillin G, 1–2 MU IV q4h, is usually adequate.** The patient with a penicillin allergy may receive a first-generation cephalosporin or clindamycin.

   b. **Hospital-acquired infection.** Broad-spectrum antibiotics (e.g., cephalosporin and aminoglycoside combinations or imipenem-cilastatin) are usually begun to cover gram-negative organisms until culture results are known. Newer antibiotics, such as ticarcillin-clavulanate and piperacillin-tazobactam, also provide excellent coverage.

4. OTHER INFECTIONS
   a. *Mycoplasma pneumoniae.* Infection with this organism may be treated with **erythromycin or tetracycline, 250–500 mg PO q6h** for 2 weeks.

   b. **Legionnaire's disease (*L. pneumophila* and *L. micdadei*). Erythromycin, 0.5–1 g IV or PO q6h** for 3 weeks, should be given to patients with this disease.

   c. **Q fever and psittacosis. Either tetracycline 500 mg PO qid, doxycycline 100 mg PO bid, or chloramphenicol 50 to 100 mg/kg/d PO or IV (divided into q6h doses)** given for 2 weeks is effective against these diseases.

   d. **Viral pneumonia.** Influenza is the most common cause of viral pneumonia in adults. Amantadine or rimantidine may speed improvement (Table 3–6).

TABLE 3–6. Antiviral Chemotherapy

VIRUS	DISEASE OR GOAL OF TREATMENT	TREATMENT
Nonimmunocompromised Host		
Herpes simplex virus (HSV)	Primary genital HSV	Topical: 5% acyclovir (ACV) ointment 5×/d for 7 d
		PO: ACV, 200 mg 5×/d for 10 d*
		IV: ACV, 5 mg/kg q8h for 5 d
	Recurrent	PO: ACV, 200 mg 5×/d for 5 d
	Suppression	PO: ACV, 200–400 mg bid–tid for 4–6 mo
	Encephalitis	IV: ACV 10–15 mg/kg q8h for 10 d
	Keratoconjunctivitis	Topical: 1% trifluorothymidine ophthalmic solution, 1 drop q2h while awake (9 drops/d maximum)
		After reepithelialization, 1 drop 5×/d for 7 d
		PO: ACV, 800 mg 5×/d for 10 d
		IV: ACV, 5 mg/kg q8h (rarely indicated)
Varicella zoster virus (VZV)	Prophylaxis against varicella	IM: varicella zoster immune globulin, 625 U (5 vials)
	Primary varicella (chickenpox)	PO: ACV, 800 mg 5×/d for 7 d
		IV: ACV, 10 mg/kg q8h for 7 d
	Zoster (shingles)	PO: ACV, 800 mg 5×/d for 7 d
		Famciclovir, 500 mg tid for 7 d
		Valacyclovir, 1 g tid for 7 d
Immunocompromised Host		
HSV	Prophylaxis	PO: ACV, 400 mg 5×/d
		IV: ACV, 250 mg/m² q8h
	Treatment	PO: ACV, 400 mg 5×/d for 10 d (or until 3 d after healing)
	Suppression	IV: ACV, 250 mg/m² q8h for 7 d
		PO: ACV, 200–400 mg 2–3×/d; increase if reactivation occurs

VZV	Zoster or varicella	IV: ACV, 500 mg/m² q8h for 7 d
	Prophylaxis	IM: varicella zoster immune globulin, 625 U (5 vials)
Influenza A	Prophylaxis	PO: amantadine or rimantadine, 200 mg/d for 5–7 wk† or only for 10–14 d after influenza vaccination
	Treatment	PO: amantadine or rimantadine, 200 mg/d for 3–5 d† (start within 24–48 h of disease onset)
Respiratory syncytial virus	Treatment	Aerosol: ribavirin (diluted to 20 mg/ml) given 12 h/d for 3 d

*Adjustments for renal impairment:
1. Acyclovir: for the following creatinine clearance ranges, give 1.73 mg/m² at these adjusted intervals:
>50 mL/min, dose q8h
24–50 mL/min, dose q12h
10–25 mL/min, dose q24h
<10 mL/min, halve dose q24h
2. Amantadine: daily amantadine dose (in mg) = 200 × (patient's creatinine clearance in mL/min ÷ 120).

†In elderly, use 1.4 mg/kg/d if normal renal function.

For additional information, see the following references: Dorsky DI, Crumpacker CS. Drugs five years later: acyclovir. Ann Intern Med 1987;107:859–874. Gold D, Corey L. Acyclovir prophylaxis for herpes simplex virus infection. Antimicrob Agents Chemother 1987;31:361–367. Hermans PE, Cockerill FR. Antiviral agents. Mayo Clin Proc 1987;62:1108–1115. Knight V, Gilbert BE (eds). Antiviral chemotherapy. Infect Dis Clin North Am 1987;vol 1, no 2.

e. *Pneumocystis carinii.* Infection with this organism is discusse-dunder "Acquired Immunodeficiency Syndrome (AIDS)" (see Tables 3–10 and 3–12, pp. 132 and 137).

f. *Pseudomonas pseudomallei.* This agent is endemic to Southeast Asia and the South Pacific. Therapy should be based on susceptibility data. Tetracycline 500 mg qid or trimethoprim-sulfamethoxazole, 1 double-strength tablet (160 mg/800 mg) PO bid, is often effective. Ceftazidime (1.5 g IV q8h) should be administered to the severely ill patient.

g. *Yersinia pestis* (plague) and *Francisella tularensis* (tularemia). An aminoglycoside (streptomycin or gentamicin) is the agent of choice. Tetracycline may also be effective, but relapses or treatment failures have been observed with short courses (e.g., those less than 2 weeks).

American Thoracic Society. Guidelines for the initial management of adults with community-acquired pneumonia: diagnosis, assessment of severity, and initial antimicrobial therapy. Am Rev Respir Dis 1993;148:1418–1426.

E. Lung Abscess

Lung abscesses appear radiographically as one or more large cavities with air-fluid levels or as multiple small cavities, as seen in necrotizing pneumonia. Most abscesses form after aspiration of oropharyngeal organisms. Necrotizing pneumonias are usually caused by anaerobes, *Klebsiella,* other gram-negative bacteria, or *Staphylococcus aureus.* Septic emboli to the lung may also result in abscess formation. Transtracheal aspiration, empyema fluid, blood cultures, or percutaneous transthoracic aspiration often is needed to obtain useful specimens for culture. Therapeutic options include:

1. BRONCHOSCOPY may be required therapeutically, as well as diagnostically, if the patient is not expectorating sputum and improving. Postural drainage is also helpful. Patients not responding to these methods and to antibiotics may need surgical drainage.

2. HIGH DOSE PENICILLIN (6–12 MU/d) can be successful in the mildly ill patient. Because of the increased incidence of penicillin-resistant anaerobes, **metronidazole** should be added in serious anaerobic infections, pending susceptibility data. **Clindamycin** is a good choice in the penicillin-allergic patient. Imipenem, ticarcillin-clavulanate, ampicillin-sulbactam, and chloramphenicol are also active against most anaerobes.

3. A PENICILLINASE-RESISTANT PENICILLIN is preferred for known staphylococcal abscesses. Vancomycin or a cephalosporin may be appropriate in the patient allergic to penicillin. For group A streptococcal infection, penicillin G is the agent of choice. Two agents (an aminoglycoside and a cephalosporin) should be used for infection due to *K. pneumoniae* or other facultative or aerobic gram-negative bacilli in the seriously ill patient.

Bartlett JG. Antibiotics in lung abscess. Semin Respir Infect 1991;6:103–111.

F. Tuberculosis

Pulmonary disease is the most common clinical manifestation of *Mycobacterium tuberculosis* infection. The diagnosis is suggested by chest x-ray and is confirmed by isolation of the organism from sputum. Newer culture techniques have shortened the time needed to demonstrate the organism. Acid-fast bacilli (AFB) can often be visualized on stained sputum smears. Fluorochrome smears have improved the sensitivity and specificity of sputum examination. Skin test reactivity identifies those who have been exposed to the organism but who have subclinical disease. However, there are a number of reasons that patients have false-negative skin test reactions, including overwhelming tuberculosis.

1. THERAPY. Antimicrobial therapy for active tuberculosis should always include at least two agents to which the organism is known to be susceptible. More than one active agent appears to be necessary to prevent the emergence of resistant strains. Therapy for active tuberculosis must be prolonged because of the slow growth of the organism.

   a. **6-month therapy.** A 6-month regimen consisting of isoniazid (INH), rifampin, pyrazinamide (PZA), and pyridoxine given for 2 months, followed by INH, rifampin, and pyridoxine given for 4 months is the first-line regimen for patients with fully susceptible organisms who comply with treatment. For initial empiric therapy of active tuberculosis in most patients, a four-drug regimen—**INH (300 mg), rifampin (600 mg), PZA (25 mg/kg/d),** and **ethambutol (15–25 mg/kg/d)**—with **pyridoxine (50 mg PO qd)** added to reduce INH toxicity, is appropriate, unless drug-resistant TB is suspected (in which case, individualized therapy must be designed in consultation with the local public health department). If the organism is sensitive to all agents, ethambutol may be discontinued, and a 6-month course can be completed as described above. If the organism is resistant to either INH or rifampin, consultation with the local public health department tuberculosis section is strongly advised. An alternative to daily therapy is three times weekly therapy with INH, rifampin, PZA, and ethambutol all administered for 6 months. Directly observed therapy is mandatory for all intermittent regimens and should be strongly considered for all patients. The treatment regimens for active pulmonary tuberculosis are identical in HIV-infected and HIV-noninfected individuals.

   b. **9-month therapy.** For persons who are unable to take PZA, a regimen of **INH, rifampin, and pyridoxine** may be administered for a total of 9 months. **Ethambutol** should also be included in the initial empiric regimen but may be discontinued if the organism is sensitive to both INH and rifampin.

   c. **Special treatment circumstances.** The following guidelines are useful in specific situations:

      (1) ***When INH cannot be used*** because of suspected or documented resistance or other reasons, rifampin and ethambutol may be used for 18 months.

      (2) ***When rifampin cannot be used,*** INH and ethambutol can be used for 18 months, with streptomycin for the first 6 to 8 weeks.

      (3) ***When neither INH nor rifampin is an option,*** at least three drugs to which the organism is sensitive should be used for at least 18 months.

(4) ***In patients with renal disease,*** neither ethambutol nor streptomycin is recommended. Pyrazinamide or ethionamide should be considered.

(5) ***In end-stage renal disease,*** INH and rifampin can be used in the usual doses and given after dialysis. Pyridoxine supplementation is necessary.

(6) ***Pregnancy.*** 9-month therapy can be used. INH, rifampin, and ethambutol should be given during the first 6 to 8 weeks. Streptomycin and pyrazinamide should be avoided.

2. FOLLOW-UP. Uncomplicated pulmonary tuberculosis can be managed in the outpatient setting. Contacts of the patient have usually been exposed before diagnosis. A patient's sputum is usually not infectious after 2 weeks of effective therapy. Sputum smears and cultures should be performed monthly until 3 consecutive specimens are negative. Cultures are then obtained at 2- to 3-month intervals and at 6 months after therapy is completed. Chest x-rays are often done monthly until sputum cultures yield negative findings and then at 2- to 3-month intervals. Follow-up radiographs are obtained at the completion of therapy and if reactivation is suspected. **The local public health department should be involved in the follow-up of patients and in contact tracing.** Contacts with evidence of active disease should be identified and treated.

3. ISONIAZID THERAPY FOR SUBCLINICAL INFECTION (POSITIVE TUBERCULIN SKIN TEST BUT NO EVIDENCE OF ACTIVE TUBERCULOSIS). INH may be given for subclinical infection when a positive tuberculin skin test (TST) indicates the presence of viable bacilli with potential for reactivation. The decision to use prophylactic therapy should take into consideration the relative risk of developing active disease weighed against the risk of developing INH-related hepatitis (the incidence of which increases with age). The recent increase in tuberculosis cases in the United States has led to recommendations for preventive therapy for a broad range of individuals who are at increased risk of developing active tuberculosis. The interpretation of the TST for different populations is shown in Table 3–7. **Preventive therapy** consists of INH alone in a single oral daily dose of 300 mg for at least 6 months (12 months for HIV-infected individuals). Consultation with the local public health department for preventive therapy for patients with potential INH-resistant TB strains, as well as for directly observed therapy, is strongly urged. Patients should be counseled about symptoms of hepatitis and seek prompt medical attention if these symptoms develop. Mild aminotransferase elevation occurs in 10% to 20% of patients and is not necessarily a contraindication to continuing therapy. Patients should be followed on at least a monthly basis while on preventive therapy.

Cohn DL, Catlin BJ, Peterson KL, et al. A 62-dose, 6-month therapy for pulmonary and extrapulmonary tuberculosis. Ann Intern Med 1990;112:407–415.

Combs DL, O'Brien RJ, Geiter LJ. USPHS tuberculosis short-course chemotherapy trial 21: effectiveness, toxicity, and acceptability. Ann Intern Med 1990;112:397–406.

Dutt AK, Moers D, Stead WW. Short-course chemotherapy for extrapulmonary tuberculosis. Ann Intern Med 1986;104:7–12.

Van Scoy RE, Wilkowske CJ. Antituberculous agents. Mayo Clin Proc 1987;62:1129–1136.

TABLE 3-7. **Interpretation of Positive Tuberculin Skin Test**

POSITIVE TST (mm INDURATION)	PATIENT GROUP	PREVENTIVE TREATMENT
>5	Close contacts of active TB case	All
	HIV positive	All
	Chest x-ray suggestive of old TB	All
>10	Injection drug users	All
	Diseases that increase TB risk*	All
	Foreign-born from TB endemic countries	†
	Medically underserved low-income populations, including high-risk ethnic groups	†
	Residents of facilities for long-term care (e.g., correctional institutions, nursing homes, mental institutions)	†
>15	All others	†

*Diabetes mellitus, prolonged therapy with corticosteroids (>15 mg prednisone for >2–3 weeks), immunosuppressive therapy, hematologic and reticuloendothelial malignancies, end-stage renal disease, clinical situations associated with substantial rapid weight loss or chronic undernutrition (including postgastrectomy).
†All patients with a positive TST from these groups should receive preventive therapy if they are under 35 years of age. For patients with a positive TST who are over 35 years of age, preventive therapy should be strongly considered for those who have been in close contact with a newly diagnosed active case of TB or who have had a documented recent TST conversion (within 2 years). Others should be considered for preventive therapy on a case by case basis.

VII. CELLULITIS AND ANIMAL BITES

A. Cellulitis

Cellulitis is most frequently caused by group A streptococci and *Staphylococcus aureus*. Cultures of the leading edge rarely yield the causative agent but may be useful to identify rare pathogens (e.g., gram-negative rods) in some patients. Skin biopsies more frequently yield the causative organism but are rarely used except in complicated cases. Blood cultures seldom reveal the pathogen.

Initial antimicrobial therapy should be based on clinical presentation and a patient's underlying risk factors. Therapy can be adjusted based on the clinical response or according to blood and skin culture results, if positive. Antibiotics are usually given for 7 to 10 days. When there is clinical improvement, the course can be completed with oral agents. Patients with **cellulitis of the lower extremity can usually be treated effectively with a semisynthetic penicillin,** such as nafcillin, or with a **cephalosporin.** *Haemophilus influenzae* should be suspected in children or in adults with facial cellulitis. Aerobic gram-negative organisms may occasionally cause cellulitis in patients with diabetes or in immunosuppressed individuals. More broad-spectrum therapy is indicated for these patients, especially if they are severely ill.

Hook EW, Hooton TM, Horton CA, et al. Microbiologic evaluation of cutaneous cellulitis in adults. Arch Intern Med 1986;146:295–297.

B. Animal Bites

Therapy for animal bites primarily consists of local care and tetanus prophylaxis (Table 3–8). Prophylactic antibiotics should be considered as adjunctive therapy. Local care consists of adequate wound irrigation and debridement. The risk of bacterial infection increases with delay in local care. Infections resulting from animal bites are often caused by *Pasteurella multocida,* whereas human bites are often complicated by *Staphylococcus aureus* infections. Aerobic and anaerobic cultures should be obtained from wound exudate. Gram stain may reveal the infecting organism. Penicillin is the antibiotic of choice for *Pasteurella multocida.* Patients with cirrhosis are at risk for serious infections caused by *Capnocytophagus canimorsus* following dog bites. Penicillin is the preferred antibiotic for treatment of these infections.

Goldstein EJ. Bite wounds and infection. Clin Infect Dis 1992;14:633–638.

VIII. SEXUALLY TRANSMITTED DISEASES

A. Gonorrhea

The increasing incidence of penicillin-resistant strains has made alternatives to penicillin important in the treatment of gonorrhea. Gram stains and cultures should be obtained from all sites that may be potentially infected because of the patient's sexual practices. Rectal culture should be standard procedure for all women because of the potential for inoculation of this area from infected cervicovaginal secretions. Pharyngeal and cervical gram stains are unreliable. Up to 50% of patients with gonococcal cervicitis or urethritis have concomitant *Chlamydia trachomatis* infection. Thus, each of the regimens for treatment of gonococcal infection must be combined with a regimen against *C. trachomatis.* Contact tracing, notification, and treatment are an important aspect of evaluation of patients with sexually transmitted diseases and is often best accomplished by the local public health department.

1. **UNCOMPLICATED GONOCOCCAL ANOGENITAL OR PHARYNGEAL INFECTION**
   - Ceftriaxone 125 mg IM × 1, *or*
   - Spectinomycin*† 2 g IM × 1, *or*
   - Cefixime 400 mg PO × 1, *or*
   - Ciprofloxacin* 500 mg PO × 1, *or*
   - Ofloxacin* 400 mg PO × 1

     Each of these regimens must be combined with presumptive treatment for *C. trachomatis* infection (see section on treatment of nongonococcal urethritis).

2. **PERSISTENT GONOCOCCAL INFECTION AFTER PREVIOUS TREATMENT; OR KNOWN CASES OF PENICILLIN RESISTANCE.** Ceftriaxone 250 mg IM may be used. As an alternative, spectinomycin 2 g IM may be administered but is not effective for pharyngeal infection.

---

*May be used even in patients with a history of anaphylaxis or immediate urticaria to penicillin.
†Spectinomycin is not effective for pharyngeal infection.

TABLE 3–8. Immunizations

DISEASE	VACCINE TYPE*	SCHEDULE
ROUTINE IMMUNIZATIONS		
Measles	LV†	Routine childhood
Mumps	LV†	Routine childhood
Rubella	LV†	Routine childhood; if not, before pregnancy
Poliomyelitis (oral poliovaccine, or OPV)	LV†	Routine childhood
Poliomyelitis (inactivated polio vaccine, or IPV)	KV	Nonimmunized adults
Pertussis	KB	Routine childhood
Diphtheria	BT	Routine childhood, booster every 10 y
Tetanus	BT	Routine childhood, booster every 10 y, and if tetanus-prone wound occurs, *with* tetanus immune globulin
Haemophilus influenzae type b	BP	Routine childhood
TRAVEL IMMUNIZATIONS		
Yellow fever	LV†	Single shot every 10 y
Rabies, human diploid cell vaccine (HCDV)	KV	Preexposure: 3 doses; booster every 2 y
		Postexposure: 5 doses with rabies immune globulin
Japanese encephalitis	KV	Limited availability: 3 shots, booster every 4 y
Cholera	KB	2 shots, booster every 6 mo (single dose fulfills most travel requirements)
Typhoid	KB	2 shots (Note: oral vaccine now available)
Plague	KB	3 shots, booster every 6–12 mo
Meningococcus infection	BP	Single shot, no boosters (rarely needed)
Hepatitis A	KV	Single shot, booster at 6–12 mo

*LV, live virus; KV, killed virus; KB, killed bacteria; BT, bacterial toxoid; BP, bacterial polysaccharide; IG, immune globulin.
†Live virus vaccines are generally contraindicated in pregnancy and immunocompromised patients.

Table continued on following page

TABLE 3–8. Immunizations (Continued)

DISEASE	VACCINE TYPE*	SCHEDULE
SPECIAL IMMUNIZATIONS		
Influenza A and B	KV	Single shot annually, for elderly, those with chronic diseases, and those with high exposure risk
Hepatitis B	KV	3 shots (at 0, 1, and 6 mo); need for boosters unknown; indicated for those at risk of exposure; postexposure in unimmunized person, give with HBIG
Pneumococcus infection	BP	Single shot, booster not needed for at least 5 y; indicated for elderly and chronically ill
Hepatitis B immune globulin (HBIG)	IG	Give within 24–48 h of exposure to blood containing high titer of HB_sAg or within 14 d of sexual contact; give with hepatitis B vaccine (additional HBIG needed 1 mo later if given without vaccine)
Immune globulin	IG	Give within 14 d of exposure to hepatitis A
Rabies immune globulin (RIG)	IG	Give postexposure in those unimmunized with rabies vaccine
Tetanus immune globulin	IG	Give postexposure with tetanus toxoid
Varicella vaccine	LV†	Consider for nonimmune health care workers
Varicella zoster immune globulin	IG	Give postexposure in immunocompromised patients

3. PENICILLIN-ALLERGIC PATIENTS
   a. **History of late onset, atypical, or undocumented penicillin allergy.** Cefixime 400 mg PO or ceftriaxone 125–250 mg IM, plus doxycycline 100 mg PO bid for 7 days, can be used; the patient should be observed for 30 minutes after being given cephalosporin. Alternatively, ciprofloxacin 500 mg PO followed by doxycycline may be employed.
   b. **History of anaphylaxis or immediate urticaria.** Spectinomycin 2 g IM or ciprofloxacin 500 mg PO, plus doxycycline (100 mg bid) for 7 days, may be selected.

4. MANAGEMENT OF CONTACTS. All partners at risk should be examined, cultured, and treated. Although there is no time period that will encompass all circumstances, in most cases the following should be considered **minimal** criteria.
   a. **Symptomatic patients.** All partners within **2 weeks before onset** of symptoms should be examined.
   b. **Asymptomatic patients.** All partners within **4 weeks before diagnosis** should be examined.

B. Syphilis

Penicillin remains the drug of choice for syphilis, and there are no resistant strains. *Treponema pallidum* cannot be cultured. Diagnosis is made by darkfield examination of any lesions and by serology.

For all stages of syphilis, penicillin is the treatment of choice; if tetracycline is given, it is extremely important to counsel the patient firmly about adherence to the regimen, as deletion of only a few doses or slight shortening of therapy significantly increases the failure rate.

1. EARLY SYPHILIS (PRIMARY, SECONDARY, AND EARLY LATENT SYPHILIS UP TO 1 YEAR IN DURATION). Benzathine penicillin G 2.4 MU IM in a single dose should be given, *or* tetracycline 500 mg qid for 15 days (if there is well-documented allergy to penicillin) may be used. In addition, patients should be counseled about the possibility of a Jarisch-Herxheimer reaction.

2. LATE SYPHILIS (MORE THAN 1 YEAR IN DURATION), EXCLUDING NEUROSYPHILIS. Benzathine penicillin G 2.4 MU IM weekly for three doses (total 7.2 MU) is the treatment of choice. Tetracycline 500 mg qid for 30 days (if there is well-documented allergy to penicillin) is an alternative.

3. NEUROSYPHILIS IN PATIENTS INFECTED 1 YEAR OR MORE, BOTH SYMPTOMATIC AND ASYMPTOMATIC
   a. **Treatment of choice.** Hospitalization is required for administration of penicillin G, 2–3 MU IV q4h for 10 days, followed by benzathine penicillin G, 2.4 MU IM weekly for three doses.
   b. **Outpatient alternative.** The following is effective: procaine penicillin G 2.4 MU IM once daily, plus probenecid 500 mg qid, both for 10 days, followed by benzathine penicillin G 2.4 MU IM weekly for three doses.
   c. **Patients with history of penicillin allergy.** The patient should be referred for penicillin skin testing. If skin testing confirms an allergy,

penicillin desensitization should be considered. A 10-day course of ceftriaxone may be an effective alternative, but data are incomplete. The efficacy of erythromycin and tetracycline is not established for neurosyphilis.

4. FOLLOW-UP
   a. **Syphilis in pregnancy.** The follow-up of pregnant patients with syphilis is individualized, but most patients should be seen on the following schedules.
   b. **Early syphilis (primary, secondary, and early latent).** A clinical examination should be performed 1 week after treatment; the serology (quantitative Venereal Disease Research Laboratory [VDRL]) should be repeated 1, 3, 6, and 12 months after treatment.
   c. **Neurosyphilis.** The serology should be repeated as for late syphilis, and follow-up lumbar punctures should be given at 3- to 4-month intervals until results are normal (includes patients having early syphilis with abnormal cerebrospinal fluid).

5. MANAGEMENT OF CONTACTS
   a. **Contacts of patients with early syphilis** should receive routine history, examination, and syphilis serology, including rapid plasma reagin (RPR). Treatment should be administered for all contacts within the preceding 3 months.
   b. In **contacts of patients with late syphilis,** serologic studies should be performed (including fluorescent treponemal antibody absorption [FTA-ABS] even if the VDRL is negative) in all long-term (e.g., marital) contacts and in the children of infected women.

C. Nongonococcal and Postgonococcal Urethritis

The major causes of nongonococcal urethritis (NGU) and postgonococcal urethritis (PGU) are *Chlamydia trachomatis* and, less often, *Ureaplasma urealyticum.* A gram stain should be performed, along with culture for *Neisseria gonorrhoeae* and *C. trachomatis.*

1. INITIAL OR ISOLATED EPISODE (NO EPISODE WITHIN THE PREVIOUS 6 WEEKS). Doxycycline 100 mg bid (or tetracycline 500 mg qid) may be given for 7 days, *or* erythromycin stearate or base 500 mg qid (or enteric-coated erythromycin base 666 mg tid), can be used for 7 days when a tetracycline is contraindicated or not tolerated.

   Trimethoprim-sulfamethoxazole (Bactrim, Septra), one double-strength tablet bid for 7 days, can be administered if neither tetracycline nor erythromycin is tolerated. Other options include ofloxacin 300 mg PO bid for 7 days or azithromycin 1 g PO in a single dose for patients unlikely to comply with multiple-dose therapy.

   Sexual abstention should be advised until symptoms have resolved and treatment of both patient and partner is complete.

2. IMMEDIATE TREATMENT FAILURE (PERSISTENT URETHRITIS WHILE ON THERAPY OR RECRUDESCENCE IMMEDIATELY AFTER TREATMENT COMPLETION). Urethritis must be confirmed by examination and laboratory studies. A urethral wet mount and culture for *Trichomonas* should be obtained; if the wet mount is negative, the patient should be retreated with erythromycin,

as above (or with tetracycline, as above, if erythromycin was used initially), pending the results of the *Trichomonas* culture.

3. **RECURRENCE OF URETHRITIS WITHIN 6 WEEKS FOLLOWING APPARENT RESOLUTION.** It should be confirmed that the treatment regimen was followed and that sexual contact limitations were followed (or that the partner was examined and treated). The patient should be treated with erythromycin 500 mg qid for 2 to 4 weeks or with doxycycline 100 mg bid for 2 to 4 weeks (if the original treatment was erythromycin).

4. **MANAGEMENT OF CONTACTS.** Regular partners and source contacts should be examined and treated with doxycycline, tetracycline, or erythromycin. In contacts of men with recurrent NGU, the need and value of treatment are unknown.

D. Mucopurulent Cervicitis

The leading cause of nongonococcal mucopurulent cervicitis (MPC) is *Chlamydia trachomatis.* However, other considerations include herpetic cervicitis, trichomoniasis, candidiasis, vaginitis due to foreign bodies or chemical irritation, and IUDs, all of which may be associated with polymorphonuclear neutrophils (PMNs) in endocervical smears and occasionally with other signs suggestive of MPC. The diagnosis of MPC should be made with caution when any of these conditions is present.

1. **TREATMENT OF NONGONOCOCCAL MUCOPURULENT CERVICITIS.** Doxycycline 100 mg bid may be administered for 7 days, or erythromycin base or stearate 500 mg qid (or enteric-coated erythromycin base 666 mg tid) may be given for 7 days. In the case of severe gastrointestinal intolerance, erythromycin should be given with food, the dose should be halved, and therapy should be extended to 14 days.

Persistent or recurrent MPC should be **retreated** if therapeutic compliance appears to have been suboptimal. If the patient has a new or untreated partner, or if the initial antibiotic was erythromycin, a switch to tetracycline or doxycycline is in order.

2. **MANAGEMENT OF CONTACTS.** When NGU or gonorrhea is present, the condition should be treated accordingly. In those with no urethritis, regular and source contacts should be treated as for NGU. Treatment of other contacts should be deferred, pending culture results.

E. Pelvic Inflammatory Disease

Neisseria gonorrhoeae and *Chlamydia trachomatis* are the most common causes of pelvic inflammatory disease (PID). A cervical gram stain, plus cultures for *N. gonorrhoeae* and *C. trachomatis* should be performed. Culturing the cervix for other bacteria is not necessary. When PID is suspected, IUDs should be removed if present. Hospitalization is recommended when patients are unable or unwilling to follow outpatient regimens, as well as when pregnancy, pelvic abscess, or an unclear diagnosis is a consideration.

1. **INPATIENTS.** Doxycycline 100 mg IV bid and either cefoxitin 2 g IV q6h or cefotetan 2 g IV q12h should be given for at least 48 hours after the patient clinically improves. An alternative regimen is clindamycin 600

mg IV q6h plus gentamicin 1.5 mg/kg q8h. After discharge from the hospital, doxycycline 100 mg PO bid should be continued for a total of 10 to 14 days.

2. OUTPATIENTS. Either ceftriaxone 250 mg IM or cefoxitin 2 g IM plus probenecid 1 g PO should be combined with doxycycline 100 mg PO bid for 14 days. An alternative is ofloxacin 400 mg PO bid combined with either clindamycin 450 mg PO qid or metronidazole 500 mg PO bid for 14 days.

3. MANAGEMENT OF CONTACTS. Examination and urethral smear and culture for *Neisseria gonorrhoeae* and *Chlamydia trachomatis* are imperative for all contacts within the preceding 4 weeks, regardless of symptoms. When gonorrhea or NGU is present, the condition should be treated accordingly. Persons in whom no urethritis is present should be treated as for NGU.

F. Bacterial Vaginosis

Bacterial vaginosis (BV) is associated with an overgrowth of *Gardnerella vaginalis* and anaerobic bacteria, with a decrease in the normal *Lactobacillus* flora. Saline wet mount or gram stain of the vaginal secretions does not indicate BV, since it is frequently isolated in low numbers from normal women. Asymptomatic patients are usually not treated unless the discharge is especially profuse.

1. TREATMENT OF SYMPTOMATIC PATIENTS. Metronidazole 500 mg bid should be administered for 7 days. Alcohol consumption should be avoided for 12 hours before and 24 hours after completion of therapy. This drug is contraindicated in pregnancy. As an alternative, amoxicillin-clavulanate 500 mg tid or clindamycin 300 mg PO tid may be given for 7 days (effective in 50% of patients). These drugs may be used if the patient is pregnant or cannot tolerate metronidazole.

2. RESISTANT OR RECURRENT BV. The optimal treatment for recurrent BV is unknown. Options include retreatment with metronidazole or amoxicillin and simultaneous retreatment of the patient and her regular sexual partner. If an IUD is present, its removal should be considered.

G. Trichomonal Vaginitis

Trichomonas vaginalis can be identified by microscopic examination of a saline wet mount of vaginal secretions. Culture should also be performed. The **treatment for trichomonal vaginitis is metronidazole, 2 g PO in a single dose.** Alcohol consumption should be avoided for 12 hours before and 24 hours after completion of therapy. In addition, sexual abstention is recommended until symptoms have improved and the partner or partners have been treated.

1. TREATMENT FAILURE (PERSISTENCE OR RECURRENCE DESPITE SEXUAL ABSTENTION OR AFTER INTERCOURSE ONLY WITH A TREATED PARTNER). Metronidazole 500 mg bid may be administered for 7 days in cases of continued persistence or if there are two or more recurrences when reinfection is unlikely.

2. **PREGNANT WOMEN.** Clotrimazole vaginal tablets or 1% cream, 1 tablet, or 1 applicatorful daily can be used for 7 days. Metronidazole is contraindicated in the first trimester and is of uncertain safety in the second and third trimesters.

3. **MANAGEMENT OF CONTACTS.** Treatment should not be dispensed or prescribed for unexamined partners, nor should it be given to patients for distribution to partners. In regular partners or source contacts, a routine genitourinary examination should be performed. The contact should be treated with metronidazole, 2 g in a single dose.

H. *Candida* Vulvovaginitis

Candidiasis is usually due to *Candida albicans.* Diagnosis is by microscopic examination of a wet mount or gram stain of vaginal secretions. Culture is not routinely advised. Clotrimazole vaginal tablets or 1% cream, 1 dose daily, may be given for 7 days. Miconazole nitrate 2% vaginal cream, 1 application daily at bedtime, can be used for 7 days. Alternatively, in nonpregnant patients, fluconazole 200 mg PO may be employed.

I. Acute Epididymitis

Acute epididymitis is often due to *Neisseria gonorrhoeae* or *Chlamydia trachomatis.* A gram stain, as well as cultures of urethral swabs for these organisms, should be performed. Treatment recommendations are:

1. **CHLAMYDIAL EPIDIDYMITIS (PROVEN OR SUSPECTED).** Doxycycline 100 mg bid (or tetracycline 500 mg qid) can be administered for 10 days.

2. **GONOCOCCAL EPIDIDYMITIS.** An effective treatment is ceftriaxone 250 mg IM (single dose), plus doxycycline or tetracycline, as described above, for 10 days.

3. **NONCHLAMYDIAL, NONGONOCOCCAL EPIDIDYMITIS.** Begin therapy with 250 mg of ceftriaxone IM (single dose), followed by doxycycline 100 mg bid, while awaiting urinalysis and culture results. A case of documented bacterial epididymitis should be referred for urologic consultation.

Celum CL, Handsfield HH. Sexually Transmitted Diseases Clinical Practice Guidelines. Seattle: Seattle–King County Department of Public Health, 1993.
Drugs for sexually transmitted diseases. Med Lett 1995;37:117–122.
Handsfield HH, ed. Sexually transmitted diseases. Infect Dis Clin North Am 1987;Vol 1, No 1.
Holmes KK, Mardh P-A, Sparling PF, et al. Sexually Transmitted Diseases. New York: McGraw-Hill, 1990.

IX. URINARY TRACT INFECTIONS

The most commonly isolated pathogens infecting the urinary tract are from the Enterobacteriaceae family. Most uncomplicated urinary tract infections (UTI) are caused by *Escherichia coli.* Other frequently isolated bacteria are *Klebsiella, Enterobacter, Serratia, Proteus,* and *Providencia.* Coagulase-negative staphylococci, particularly *Staphylococcus saprophyticus,* are becoming more widely recognized as urinary tract pathogens, especially in young women. Infections with *Pseudomonas* spp., enterococci, and *Staphylococcus aureus* are associated with the use of urinary tract instrumentation.

Chlamydia trachomatis is linked with acute urethral syndrome (AUS) in women.

A gram stain and culture of the urine are key in directing antimicrobial therapy. Colony counts of greater than 100,000/mL constitute "significant bacteriuria." Lower colony counts (10^2 to 10^4/mL) may be considered significant if obtained as a midstream urine specimen from a symptomatic female with pyuria. Sterile pyuria in a symptomatic woman suggests AUS. A yield of three or more types of bacteria in a culture probably is due to contamination. Blood cultures are essential for the patient with suspected pyelonephritis.

A. Acute Uncomplicated Urinary Tract Infection: Therapy

Traditional therapy for women with an acute, uncomplicated UTI has been a 7- to 10-day course of antibiotics. Three-day therapy may be as effective as 10-day therapy. Most UTIs in healthy, young, nonpregnant women without genitourinary tract abnormalities are due to *Escherichia coli* or *Staphylococcus saprophyticus.*

1. REGIMEN OF CHOICE. The therapy of choice is trimethoprim-sulfamethoxazole, one double-strength tablet PO bid for 3 days. If the patient is allergic to sulfonamides, amoxicillin 500 mg tid may be given for 3 days. If the patient is allergic to sulfonamides and penicillin, doxycycline 100 mg bid can be administered for 3 days. For more resistant organisms, the following can be considered: amoxicillin-clavulanate (250/125 mg PO tid), oral cephalosporins (cephalexin 250–500 mg PO qid), or a quinolone (ciprofloxacin 250–500 mg PO bid).

2. FOLLOW-UP. A urinalysis of a midstream specimen and culture should be performed 3 to 7 days after completion of treatment. Women who have been given 3 days of trimethoprim-sulfamethoxazole should return if symptoms persist or recur. Men with UTI should be referred for urologic evaluation.

B. Acute Urethral Syndrome (AUS)

Acute urethral syndrome, characterized by sterile pyuria, is often due to *Chlamydia trachomatis* (*Neisseria gonorrhoeae* and other causes of vaginitis must also be considered). Treatment is a 7-day course of doxycycline 100 mg PO bid or tetracycline 500 mg PO qid. An empiric trial may also be useful in patients with sterile cultures and no pyuria. Although tuberculosis should be considered in an older individual with sterile pyuria, *Mycobacterium tuberculosis* genitourinary infection is rare in young women.

C. Urinary Tract Infection in Males

A UTI in a male is considered complicated. Gonorrhea and NGU must be ruled out. In addition, a urine gram stain and culture must be performed. Many infections have a prostatic focus, and a localization test should be considered. While awaiting culture results, **empiric treatment** may be begun with **trimethoprim-sulfamethoxazole (1 double-strength tablet PO bid for 14 days)** or ciprofloxacin (250–500 mg PO bid for 14 days). Urologic evaluation is recommended.

D. Pyelonephritis

Pyelonephritis (fever, chills, flank pain, and white blood cell casts in the urine) may be treated on an outpatient or inpatient basis, depending on factors involving the patient.

1. **OUTPATIENTS.** Recommended therapy includes either trimethoprim-sulfamethoxazole (1 double-strength tablet PO bid) or ciprofloxacin (500 mg PO bid) for 14 to 21 days to ensure eradication of infection.

2. **INPATIENTS. Ampicillin (1 g IV q4-6h) with IV aminoglycoside** therapy should be initiated pending culture results. Vancomycin may be substituted for ampicillin in the case of penicillin allergy. Patients may be discharged soon after clinical improvement but should receive oral antibiotics on an outpatient basis to complete a 14- to 21-day course.

3. **FOLLOW-UP.** The urine culture should be repeated 1 to 2 weeks after completion of therapy. Ultrasound examination of the kidneys and urologic evaluation should be considered in those patients not responding to appropriate antimicrobial therapy.

E. Asymptomatic Bacteriuria

Asymptomatic bacteriuria often clears spontaneously in healthy nonpregnant females and does not require treatment. It should, however, be treated in pregnant women. Therapy for asymptomatic bacteriuria in the elderly is controversial.

Patients with bacteriuria and indwelling catheters should not be treated unless they are symptomatic. Symptomatic UTIs should be treated with antibiotics for short periods of time to sterilize the urine, but long courses should not be used to avoid selecting resistant organisms. Chronic antibiotic suppression is not effective in patients with chronic indwelling catheters.

F. Acute Bacterial Prostatitis

In acute bacterial prostatitis (fever and perineal discomfort), the urinalysis and culture generally yield positive findings. **Trimethoprim-sulfamethoxazole (1 double-strength tablet bid for at least 14 days) or ciprofloxacin (250–500 mg PO bid) is recommended.**

G. Chronic Bacterial Prostatitis

Chronic bacterial prostatitis may cause recurrent UTIs in men. Localization studies and urologic evaluation are recommended. **Prolonged treatment (6 to 12 weeks) with trimethoprim-sulfamethoxazole (1 double-strength tablet PO bid) or ciprofloxacin (500 mg PO bid)** may be effective.

Andriole VT. Urinary tract infections in the 90's: pathogenesis and management. Infection 1992;20:S251–S256.

Johnson JR, Stamm WE. Urinary tract infections in women: diagnosis and treatment. Ann Intern Med 1989;111:906–917.

Latham RH, Wong ES, Larson A, et al. Laboratory diagnosis of urinary tract infection in ambulatory women. JAMA 1987;254:3333–3337.

Lipsky BA, Ireton RC, Fihn SD, et al. Diagnosis of bacteriuria in men: specimen collection and culture interpretation. J Infect Dis 1987;155:847–854.

Stamm WE, Hooton TM. Management of urinary tract infections in adults. N Engl J Med 1993;329:1328–1334.

X. INFECTIOUS DIARRHEA

Infectious diarrhea is diagnosed largely on the basis of stool cultures. Special techniques may be necessary to isolate likely pathogens based on clinical history. Gram stains of stool are generally not useful to identify specific organisms, with the exception of patients with *Campylobacter* gastroenteritis and *Staphylococcus aureus* enterocolitis. Gram stains, however, may reveal PMNs that would raise the possibility of an infectious cause requiring specific treatment.

Therapy is supportive in most cases of infectious diarrhea. The majority of patients can be rehydrated orally. Antispasmodics may actually be harmful in some cases, and in general, such drugs as diphenoxylate hydrochloride with atropine (Lomotil) should be avoided.

Treatment of diarrhea due to the following diseases is mainly supportive and does not require antimicrobials: viral gastroenteritis; infection with *Clostridium perfringens, S. aureus, E. coli 0157:H7, Bacillus cereus, Vibrio parahaemolyticus,* and *Aeromonas hydrophila;* and Ciguatera, scombroid, and shellfish poisoning. Table 3–9 provides recommendations for treating specific infections.

XI. BONE AND JOINT INFECTIONS

A. Infectious Bursitis

Infectious bursitis usually involves the prepatellar or olecranon bursa and is characterized by pain and swelling. A gram stain of the bursa aspirate often provides an etiologic diagnosis even when the culture is negative. *Staphylococcus aureus* is the most common agent. Streptococci are the next most common bacteria involved, especially group A beta-hemolytic strains. Other organisms, such as atypical mycobacteria, are uncommon.

In most cases, the initial therapy should be parenteral with a semisynthetic penicillinase-resistant penicillin (nafcillin 1–1.5 g IV q4–6h). In patients with mild disease, oral therapy (dicloxacillin 250–500 mg PO qid) may be used. The duration of treatment should be 14 to 21 days. Adequate drainage is required in all patients.

B. Intervertebral Disc Space Infections

Most intervertebral disc space infections in adults occur postoperatively. The operative site is often healed, with no signs of infection at presentation. Blood cultures should be done, and material for culture should be obtained from the disc space by needle aspiration. Cultures from the wound rarely reflect the true pathogen. *Staphylococcus aureus* is the most common pathogen, followed by *Staphylococcus epidermidis* and enteric gram-negative organisms.

Therapy is guided by the gram stain and by culture of the material obtained by needle aspiration. If gram-positive cocci are involved, nafcillin should be given empirically. For infection with gram-negative bacteria, a cephalosporin or a penicillinase-resistant penicillin plus an aminoglycoside should be used. If cultures are negative, therapy should be directed against *S. aureus.* If no improvement is noted after 2 to 3 weeks of appropriate antimicrobial therapy, aspiration should be reattempted. Surgery to obtain

TABLE 3-9. **Treatment of Infectious Diarrhea**

ORGANISM	THERAPY
Salmonella	
S. choleraesuis	Uncomplicated gastroenteritis: supportive only
S. enteritidis	Antibiotics may prolong the carrier state
	Septicemia: treat as for enteric fever
S. typhi	Enteric fever: ciprofloxacin, 500 mg PO bid for 14–21 d
	Alternates: ampicillin, 1–2 g IV q6h, *or* trimethoprim-sulfamethoxazole (TMP-SMZ), one double-strength tablet PO q12h, ceftriaxone, 1 g IV/IM q12h
	Carriers (excreting >6 mo) with cholelithiasis: cholecystectomy, failing alternative antibiotics for 30 d
	Avoid antidiarrheal agents
Shigella	
S. sonnei	Bacillary dysentery: ampicillin (do not use amoxicillin), 500 mg
S. flexneri	IV or PO q6h for 5–7 d, *or* TMP-SMZ, one double-strength tablet PO q12h for 5 d (for ampicillin-resistant strains), *or* ciprofloxacin, 500 mg PO q12h
	Avoid antidiarrheal agents
Yersinia sp.	
Y. enterocolitica	Enterocolitis and mesenteric adenitis: supportive care only
	Septicemia: tetracycline, 500 mg PO q6h, *or* doxycycline, 100 mg PO q6h, TMP-SMZ, one double-strength tablet PO q12h
Y. pseudotuberculosis	Septicemia: ampicillin, 1–2 g IV q6h
Enteropathogenic	
Escherichia coli	Traveler's diarrhea: ciprofloxacin, 500 mg PO bid, *or* TMP-SMZ, one double-strength tablet PO bid, for 5 d, reduces duration
Campylobacter	Protracted symptoms: ciprofloxacin, 500 mg PO bid, *or* erythromycin, 500 mg PO qid for 3–4 wk
Clostridium difficile	Antibiotic-associated diarrhea: vancomycin, 125–500 mg PO qid for 7 d, *or* metronidazole, 500 mg PO tid for 10 d; oral cholestyramine may be used as adjunctive symptomatic therapy

For further information, see Gorbach SL, ed. Infectious diarrhea. Infect Dis Clin North Am 1988;vol 2, no. 3.

tissue for culture and to provide adequate drainage should be considered. The duration of therapy should be at least 6 to 8 weeks.

C. Infectious Arthritis

The most important step in the diagnosis of infectious arthritis is examination of fluid obtained by direct joint aspiration. A gram stain and aerobic and anaerobic cultures should be obtained; in addition, a total leukocyte count and differential, a glucose level determination, and examination for crystals should be done. In patients with chronic arthritis and in immunosuppressed patients, mycobacterial and fungal cultures may be useful. Synovial tissue biopsy may be required for diagnosis of chronic arthritis (e.g., tuberculous arthritis).

1. **ETIOLOGIC AGENTS.** Of **bacterial agents,** gonococcal infection is the most common cause of monoarticular arthritis in those 15 to 40 years old. In

adults with nongonococcal arthritis, *Staphylococcus aureus* is implicated in the majority of cases. *Streptococcus* spp. are the next most common causative agents. Gram-negative bacilli cause infectious arthritis in patients who are immunosuppressed or chronically debilitated and in those who are IV drug users. Anaerobic infections rarely occur. Of the **nonbacterial agents,** viral hepatitis and rubella are often complicated by arthritis. Parvovirus B19 has recently been recognized as a cause of acute arthritis. *Mycobacterium kansasii* and *M. tuberculosis* are uncommon causes of infectious arthritis. *Sporothrix schenckii* is the most common fungus that produces infectious arthritis. Arthritis is a feature of Lyme disease due to *Borrelia burgdorferi* (see under Lyme disease section).

2. **THERAPY.** Appropriate therapy includes both adequate drainage of the joint (aspiration, arthroscopic, or open) and antimicrobial administration. Repeated aspiration is important both for removal of purulent material and to assess the effectiveness of antimicrobial therapy by repeat gram stain, culture, and leukocyte count. Initial therapy should be parenteral. Oral antibiotics may be used later in the course if adequate serum levels can be obtained. The duration of therapy should be at least 3 weeks and should be longer in gram-negative infections and in those that do not respond promptly. Intraarticular installation of antibiotics is of dubious clinical value.

   a. *Staphylococcus aureus.* For arthritis produced by this organism, nafcillin 9–12 g/d may be given in divided doses every 4 hours.

   b. **Streptococci.** Penicillin G 10 MU/d may be administered in divided doses every 4 hours. In penicillin-allergic patients, vancomycin or clindamycin may be substituted.

   c. **Gonococcal arthritis.** In areas where there are no penicillin-resistant strains of *Neisseria gonorrhoeae,* the following may be given: penicillin G, 10 MU/d for 3 days, followed by amoxicillin 500 mg PO tid for a total of 7 days of antibiotic therapy. When penicillin-resistant *N. gonorrhoeae* is a possibility, ceftriaxone is the drug of choice. In the patient allergic to penicillin, spectinomycin is an alternative. Once clinical improvement has occurred, therapy can be completed with an oral quinolone such as ciprofloxacin.

   d. **Gram-negative bacilli.** Gentamicin (4.5–5 mg/kg/d in divided doses every 8 hours) and ticarcillin (15–18 g/d in divided doses every 4 hours) may be administered.

   e. **Initial treatment if Gram stain is negative.** If no organisms are seen on the initial gram stain in a young, healthy adult, therapy with penicillin should be started. In a patient with risk factors for *S. aureus* and gram-negative infections, nafcillin and gentamicin should be given, pending culture results.

   f. **Lyme arthritis.** Arthritis develops late in the disease and is treated with high-dose IV penicillin or IV ceftriaxone (see below).

   g. **Fungal arthritis.** Arthritis caused by fungi is treated with amphotericin B, with the addition of 5-flucytosine if the organism is sensitive, or with systemic azoles such as itraconazole or fluconazole.

h. **Prosthetic joint infections.** These infections are best eradicated by removal of the prosthesis, together with debridement and antibiotic therapy. If detected very early, some infections may be cured with prolonged parenteral therapy (6 weeks), followed by oral antibiotics (3 months). Therapy must be individualized.

Smith JW, Piercy EA. Infectious arthritis. Clin Infect Dis 1995;20:225–230.

D. Lyme Disease

Lyme disease, a multisystem inflammatory disorder caused by the spirochete *Borrelia burgdorferi,* is transmitted via the bite of *Ixodes* ticks. Three clinical stages of illness are described. Stage 1 disease (localized disease) consists of constitutional flu-like symptoms and a characteristic expanding skin lesion (erythema chronicum migrans). This lesion develops at the site of the tick bite and may be associated with regional lymphadenopathy. Stage 2 disease (disseminated) is characterized by additional skin lesions, migratory joint and muscle pains, regional or generalized lymphadenopathy, hepatitis, cardiac abnormalities (conduction system abnormalities, myocarditis, and pericarditis), and neurologic manifestations (meningitis, cranial neuropathies, and peripheral radiculopathy) that occur from weeks to months after the tick bite. Stage 3 disease (persistent), which may develop weeks to years after exposure to the spirochete, is associated with arthritis and, less commonly, chronic neurologic symptoms or skin disease (acrodermatitis chronicum atrophicans).

Oral antibiotic therapy generally shortens stage 1 disease and prevents development of later stages in most patients. **Doxycycline (100 mg PO bid) or tetracycline (250 mg PO qid) for 14 to 28 days is recommended for most patients with stage 1 disease,** although treatment failures have been reported. **Amoxicillin (500 mg PO qid) or erythromycin (250 mg PO qid) for 14 to 28 days** can be used also. A Jarisch-Herxheimer reaction may occur in some patients. **Mild stage 2 disease** (e.g., facial palsy alone or a cardiac abnormality limited to first-degree atrioventricular block) should be treated with a course of oral antibiotics. For **advanced stage 2 or stage 3 disease,** therapy with ceftriaxone (1–2 g IV qd) or penicillin G (3 MU IV q4h) for 21 to 28 days is recommended and appears to be effective for many patients. Chronic arthritis seen in stage 3 disease may respond to prolonged oral doxycycline (100 mg PO bid for 30 to 90 days).

Nocton JJ, Steere AC. Lyme disease. Adv Intern Med 1995;40:69–117.

E. Acute Osteomyelitis

Osteomyelitis is classified by its presumed pathogenesis as hematogenous, contiguous, or associated with peripheral vascular disease, each with its unique microbiology. In all cases of osteomyelitis, vigorous attempts should be made to determine the etiologic agent. Blood cultures are particularly important in hematogenous osteomyelitis. Needle aspiration of soft tissue or bone, joint fluid analysis, and open biopsy may be necessary to identify the organism.

1. HEMATOGENOUS OSTEOMYELITIS. *Staphylococcus aureus* is the most common pathogen. Gram-negative bacilli occur frequently in patients with sickle cell disease *(Salmonella),* in heroin addicts *(Pseudomonas),* and

in patients with debilitating diseases. Anaerobic osteomyelitis is rare but can occur after anaerobic bacteremia.

Treatment consists of parenteral bactericidal agents in high doses. Therapy is usually continued for at least 4 weeks. Oral therapy may be attempted if the causative agent has been isolated and bactericidal levels can be attained with an appropriate oral antibiotic. Initial therapy, pending culture results, should be directed against *S. aureus* with a penicillinase-resistant semisynthetic penicillin. If gram-negative organisms are suspected on the basis of the clinical situation (e.g., in an IV drug user), an aminoglycoside should be added. Most cases of hematogenous osteomyelitis will be cured without surgery, unless there is poor clinical response or the hip joint is involved. Immobilization should be dictated by local symptoms.

2. CONTIGUOUS FOCI OSTEOMYELITIS. Osteomyelitis due to a nearby focus of infection develops indolently in older adults, often postoperatively, or with the presence of adjacent soft tissue infections. Blood cultures do not frequently yield positive results in this form of osteomyelitis but are indicated. Draining wounds often yield mixed cultures, and open biopsy or needle aspiration is necessary to determine the pathogen. *S. aureus* is still the most common agent isolated, but cultures are frequently mixed. *Staphylococcus epidermidis* is considered a pathogen, especially when prosthetic devices are present. Mixed infections often involve gram-negative bacteria. *Pseudomonas aeruginosa* is associated with puncture wounds of the feet and *Pasteurella multocida* with animal bites.

Therapy should be parenteral and directed toward the suspected pathogen. The duration of therapy should be at least 4 weeks. Surgical debridement of adjacent wounds is an important component of proper management.

3. OSTEOMYELITIS ASSOCIATED WITH PERIPHERAL VASCULAR DISEASE. This type of osteomyelitis most commonly occurs in the small bones of older diabetic patients, who are predisposed to tissue ischemia and trauma. Blood cultures usually are not helpful. Bone cultures obtained by needle aspiration or open biopsy are necessary to define the pathogens. Most infections are mixed, often staphylococci and streptococci, or a combination of staphylococci, streptococci, and organisms of the Enterobacteriaceae family. Anaerobes may also be present.

Antimicrobial therapy should be directed toward the etiologic agent for 4 to 6 weeks. Often, surgical intervention is necessary, especially that involving limited amputations in diabetics.

F. Chronic Osteomyelitis

Persistent pain may be the only symptom of chronic osteomyelitis, and sinus tract or wound drainage may be the only clinical sign. Blood culture and wound sinus cultures are generally not helpful. Needle aspiration or open biopsy should be performed before antimicrobial therapy is started. Surgery is also often necessary for debridement. Staphylococcal and gram-negative infections are common. Cure often requires extensive debridement, with excision of all grossly involved bone. Patients who are not surgical candidates may be treated with chronic or intermittent suppressive therapy. The optimal length of therapy has not been well defined. Parenteral agents may be given for 4 to 6 weeks, followed by oral agents for 6 months or longer.

G. Vertebral Osteomyelitis

This disease is a form of hematogenous osteomyelitis that is usually associated with UTI or pelvic infection in older adults or IV drug use or endocarditis in younger adults. Blood cultures are frequently not positive but should be done. It is essential to obtain material for culture by needle aspiration or open biopsy. *Staphylococcus aureus* is the most common pathogen. After a UTI, gram-negative organisms may be involved. *Pseudomonas aeruginosa* is a common infecting organism in IV drug users. Parenteral antibiotics effective against the identified pathogen are recommended for 4 to 6 weeks.

H. Tuberculous Osteomyelitis

Bone is a common extrapulmonary site of tuberculosis. A chest x-ray, a tuberculin skin test, and needle or open biopsy are part of the workup. The organism implicated is usually *Mycobacterium tuberculosis,* although rare cases of "atypical" mycobacteria have been reported. The recommended treatment is isoniazid and rifampin plus possibly other antimycobacterial agents for a prolonged period of 1 to 2 years.

I. Fungal Osteomyelitis

Fungal osteomyelitis caused by *Candida, Aspergillus,* or *Rhizopus* spp. is most frequently seen in the immunosuppressed host as part of a disseminated infection. Amphotericin B is indicated, but surgical intervention is often necessary for successful therapy.

Laughlin RT, Wright DG, Moder JT, et al. Osteomyelitis. Curr Opin Rheumatol 1995;7:315–321.

XII. INFECTIVE ENDOCARDITIS

The majority of patients with infective endocarditis (IE) have a history of underlying heart disease of either rheumatic or congenital origin. Some have no detectable valvular abnormalities but experience bacteremia, which leads to infection of the normal valve. The clinical presentation of endocarditis may be nonspecific (fever, fatigue, and arthralgia) or more suggestive of the diagnosis (fever, new heart murmur, and peripheral stigmata). The disease is described as "acute" or "subacute" based on the onset of symptoms. The key to laboratory diagnosis is the blood culture. Bacteremia is usually low grade and continuous. The urgency with which blood cultures must be obtained before instituting antimicrobial therapy depends on the presentation of the patient.

A. Etiologic Agents

The majority of IE cases are caused by streptococci or staphylococci. Of the streptococci, viridans streptococci predominate, followed by nonenterococcal group D streptococci and the enterococci. Previously damaged valves are infected with more virulent organisms, such as *Staphylococcus aureus*, pneumococci, gonococci, and group A beta-hemolytic streptococci. Infections caused by enterococci and *Haemophilus* spp. are variable in presentation. Coagulase-positive staphylococci are the most common staphylococci isolated from patients with IE who had previously normal valves. Coagulase-negative staphylococci frequently cause prosthetic valve IE. Less common causes are gram-negative bacilli, anaerobic bacteria, and fungi.

B. Therapy

All patients should be hospitalized for high-dose IV antibiotics and observed carefully for arrhythmias and hemodynamic deterioration. Antimicrobial therapy is based on isolation of the etiologic agent and determination of antimicrobial susceptibility. Initial treatment of the patient with acute IE should be directed toward *S. aureus* with **nafcillin (2 g q4h) plus gentamicin (1 mg/kg q8h). Vancomycin (1 g q12h)** may be substituted for nafcillin in the penicillin-allergic patient. Presumed IE with negative blood cultures is usually treated with penicillin or ampicillin plus an aminoglycoside for 4 weeks. When an organism is isolated, the MIC and MBC of the appropriate antibiotics should be ascertained. Knowing serum bactericidal levels may be helpful when somewhat resistant organisms are involved or if a course of therapy will be completed with oral antibiotics. In vitro killing should be achieved with peak serum dilutions of at least 1:8 and preferably 1:16 or more.

C. Specific Therapy Based on Isolated Organism

1. VIRIDANS STREPTOCOCCI. Viridans streptococci sensitive to penicillin are most successfully killed with a combination of **aqueous penicillin G 2–4 MU IV q4h or procaine penicillin 1.2 MU IM q6h,** combined with **gentamicin** 1 mg/kg body weight IV q8h for the initial 1 to 2 weeks, followed by **penicillin** alone for a total antibiotic treatment duration of 4 weeks. Patients particularly susceptible to aminoglycoside toxicity may be treated with IV penicillin alone for 4 weeks. The second 2 weeks of penicillin therapy alone may be given orally if the patient is reliable and serum bactericidal levels are adequate on the usual dose of penicillin V, 1 g PO q6h, with 0.5 g of probenecid with each dose. Resistant viridans streptococci should be treated like enterococci. In the patient with a history of severe penicillin allergy or positive skin testing, cephalothin, 8–12 g/d in divided doses every 4 hours, may be given. Vancomycin 1 g q12h is another alternative. Therapy should be continued for 4 weeks.

2. GROUP D STREPTOCOCCI. These are classified as nonenterococcal or enterococcal. Infection with nonenterococcal *Streptococcus bovis* can be treated like that with susceptible viridans streptococci if the MICs are similar. For patients with enterococcal endocarditis, an aminoglycoside should be added for the full course of therapy. **Penicillin 3 MU IV q4h, along with gentamicin 1 mg/kg IV q8h (or streptomycin 0.5 g q12h IM**), is suggested for at least 4 to 6 weeks. In the patient with a history of penicillin allergy, skin testing and desensitization, if necessary, should be performed. Vancomycin, 1 g q12h, plus an aminoglycoside for

4 to 6 weeks is an alternative treatment. Recently, enterococci isolated from patients in Michigan, Massachusetts, and other locations have shown "high-level" resistance to all aminoglycosides. At present, endocarditis with these highly resistant enterococcal isolates cannot be treated effectively with antibiotics.

3. STAPHYLOCOCCI. **Nafcillin 2 g IV q4h** or a **cephalosporin** (cephalothin 2 g IV q4h) should be started initially. If the isolate is subsequently found to be penicillin sensitive, penicillin G, 3 MU IV q4h, may be substituted. The addition of gentamicin, 1 mg/kg q8h, for the first 3 to 7 days may clear the bacteremia more rapidly. Therapy should continue for 6 weeks. If the patient is allergic to penicillin or the staphylococci are resistant to methicillin, vancomycin, 1 g IV q12h, is recommended. "Tolerant" staphylococci may be more difficult to treat. Concomitant gentamicin therapy or the addition of rifampin may be indicated.

4. ENTERIC GRAM-NEGATIVE RODS. Infection with *Escherichia coli* or *Proteus mirabilis* can be treated with a combination of ampicillin (2 g IV q4h) and gentamicin (1.7 mg/kg IV q8h). *Klebsiella* spp. require a combination of a cephalosporin and an aminoglycoside. Infection with *Serratia marcescens* is often refractory to medical therapy alone, and valve replacement may be required. *Pseudomonas* endocarditis is treated with gentamicin or tobramycin (1.7 mg/kg q8h) plus piperacillin (18 g/d). Left-sided *Pseudomonas* endocarditis usually requires a combined medical-surgical approach. Medical therapy should be continued for 6 weeks.

5. OTHER AEROBIC BACTERIA. Endocarditis attributable to *Haemophilus* spp. (non–beta-lactamase producers) may be treated successfully with 2–3 g of ampicillin IV q6h for 4 weeks. Infection with *H. parainfluenzae* can be managed with 200–300 mg/kg/d of ampicillin plus 4.5–5 mg/kg/d of gentamicin, in divided doses q8h for 6 to 8 weeks. Pneumococcal, gonococcal, and meningococcal endocarditis should be treated with penicillin G, 3 MU IV q4h for 4 weeks.

6. ANAEROBIC BACTERIA. Penicillin G 3 MU IV q4h is usually the drug of choice, except for patients with infection caused by *Bacteroides fragilis*. Metronidazole is the drug of choice in these patients.

7. FUNGAL ENDOCARDITIS. A combined medical-surgical approach is warranted. Amphotericin B, 0.5 mg/kg/d, plus 5-flucytosine, 150 mg/kg/d PO, is recommended pending results of sensitivity tests.

D. Prosthetic Valve Endocarditis

Prosthetic valve endocarditis (PVE) is often divided into early PVE (within 2 months of valve replacement) and late PVE (more than 2 months postoperatively). *Staphylococcus epidermidis* is the most common cause of early PVE. Late PVE is usually produced by viridans streptococci. There may be a delayed appearance of microorganisms acquired in the perioperative period, such as *S. epidermidis, Candida* spp., diphtheroids, or gram-negative bacilli.

Antimicrobial therapy for PVE follows the same guidelines as that for native valve endocarditis. However, **initial therapy while cultures are**

pending should be directed toward _S. epidermidis,_ with vancomycin plus gentamicin. Surgery should be considered on an individual basis.

E. Endocarditis in Intravenous Drug Users

S. aureus is the most frequently isolated organism in IV drug users with endocarditis. Other organisms include streptococci, including enterococci; gram-negative bacilli, including _Pseudomonas;_ and fungi, usually _Candida._ There is some regional variation. Treatment is the same as for native valve endocarditis. **Empiric coverage, pending culture results, should be directed against _S. aureus_ and aerobic gram-negative rods (e.g., nafcillin 2 g IV q4h and gentamicin 1.7 g/kg IV q8h).** Recent evidence indicates that uncomplicated right-sided _S. aureus_ endocarditis may be effectively treated with a 2-week course of nafcillin (1.5 g IV q4h) and tobramycin (1 mg/kg IV q8h). Vancomycin may be substituted for nafcillin for patients allergic to penicillin.

Chambers HF, Miller RT, Newman MD. Right-sided _Staphylococcus aureus_ endocarditis in intravenous drug abusers: 2-week combination therapy. Ann Intern Med 1988;109:619–624.

Coleman DL, Horwitz RI, Andriole VT. Association between serum inhibitory and bactericidal concentration and therapeutic outcome in bacterial endocarditis. Am J Med 1982;73:260–267.

Kaye D. Prophylaxis for infective endocarditis: an update. Ann Intern Med 1986;104:419–423.

Sande MA, Scheld WM. Combination antibiotic therapy of bacterial endocarditis. Ann Intern Med 1980;92:390–395.

Wilson WR, Guilani ER, Danielson GK. Symposium on infective endocarditis. Mayo Clin Proc 1982;57:145–148.

Wilson WR, Karchmer AW, Adjani AS, et al. Antibiotic treatment of adults with infective endocarditis due to streptococci, enterococci, staphylococci, and HACEK microorganisms. JAMA 1995;274:1706.

XIII. PERITONITIS

A. Spontaneous Bacterial Peritonitis

The majority of cases of spontaneous bacterial peritonitis occur in patients with alcoholic cirrhosis and ascites. The most commonly isolated organisms are _Escherichia coli,_ pneumococci, other streptococci, and _Pseudomonas, Enterobacter, Klebsiella,_ and _Clostridium_ spp. Nephrotic patients are most commonly infected with pneumococci. Gram stain and culture of the peritoneal fluid are essential. Culture yield is enhanced by bedside inoculation of peritoneal fluid into blood culture bottles. Blood cultures often are positive for the same organism. Empiric therapy should be directed at the organism suggested by the gram stain, if positive. **Empiric therapy with ampicillin plus an aminoglycoside** has been traditionally recommended. However, concerns regarding aminoglycoside-associated nephrotoxicity have led to alternative empiric regimens, such as ampicillin plus aztreonam, a third-generation cephalosporin such as cefotaxime or ceftriaxone, or ampicillin-sulbactam. Following primary therapy, some authorities favor prophylactic maintenance on TMP-SMX or ciprofloxacin to reduce the risk of recurrence.

B. Secondary Peritonitis

Secondary peritonitis is usually polymicrobial and caused by organisms from the GI tract. The facultative organisms commonly isolated are

*Bacteroides fragilis, Bacteroides melaninogenicus, Peptococcus, Peptostrep-
tococcus, Fusobacterium, Eubacterium lentum,* and *Clostridium.* Peritoneal
fluid gram stain and culture, as well as blood cultures, are important in
isolating the pathogen. After the appropriate specimens for culture are
obtained, antimicrobial therapy should be started. There are several alternatives:

- **Clindamycin** (600 mg IV q6–8h) or **metronidazole** (a loading dose of 15
  mg/kg, then 7.5 mg/kg IV q6h) with **ampicillin** (1.5–2 g IV q4h) or **penicillin**
  (2 MU IV q4h) and an **aminoglycoside** (tobramycin or gentamicin 1.7
  mg/kg IV q8h)
- **Ampicillin-sulbactam** (1.5 g IV q4–6h) with or without an aminoglycoside
- **Cefotetan** (2 g IV q12h) and an aminoglycoside
- **Chloramphenicol** (50–100 mg/kg IV/d divided into doses q6h) plus an
  aminoglycoside and ampicillin
- **Imipenem-cilastatin,** 0.5–1 g IV q6h

Bhuva M, Ganger D, Jensen D. Spontaneous bacterial peritonitis: an update on evaluation,
management, and prevention. Am J Med 1994;97:169–175.
Felisart J, Rimona A, Arroyo V, et al. Cefotaxime is more effective than is ampicillin-tobramycin
in cirrhotics with severe infections. Hepatology 1985;5:457–462.

C. Peritonitis During Continuous Ambulatory Peritoneal Dialysis (CAPD)

The most frequently isolated organism is *S. epidermidis,* followed by *S.
aureus, Streptococcus* spp., and then gram-negative enteric pathogens.
Intraperitoneal administration of cephalothin may be given. Vancomycin
should be given both intraperitoneally and IV. Antimicrobials should be
given for 10 days to 3 weeks. Fungal peritonitis due to *Candida* spp. may also
be encountered and should be treated with amphotericin B 0.5 mg/kg/d IV.
A change of the catheter may be required to eradicate infection.

XIV. CNS INFECTIONS

A. Meningitis

When a patient has symptoms suggestive of meningitis (fever, headache,
altered mental states, and stiff neck), the first consideration should be
therapy, not specific diagnosis. Antimicrobial therapy based on the most
likely pathogen should be initiated within 30 minutes of presentation. In the
absence of papilledema and other signs of increased intracranial pressure, a
lumbar puncture should be obtained rapidly. The results of cerebrospinal
fluid studies can be used, along with additional clinical information, to alter
the initial therapy, if necessary.

1. LIKELY ORGANISMS BASED ON CHARACTERISTICS OF THE PATIENT
   a. **Age.** *Streptococcus pneumoniae* is the most common cause of
   bacterial meningitis in adults over the age of 40 years, and *Neisseria
   meningitidis* is the most common causative agent in individuals aged
   18 to 40. *Haemophilus influenzae,* enteric gram-negative bacilli,
   streptococci, staphylococci, and *Listeria monocytogenes* are much
   less frequently seen in normal hosts but must be considered more
   likely in specific situations.

b. **Shunt-associated meningitis.** Up to 30% of all ventricular shunts become infected. The most common organisms found are *Staphylococcus epidermidis, Staphylococcus aureus,* streptococci, diphtheroids, *Bacillus* spp., gram-negative enteric organisms, *Propionibacterium acnes,* and mixed groups. Antimicrobial therapy should be given systemically and intraventricularly in most cases. *Staphylococcus aureus* shunt infection can usually be treated with cephalothin IV and intraventricularly (0.3 mg/mL of estimated cerebrospinal fluid volume) once or twice a day. *S. epidermidis* infections will usually require both systemic and either intraventricular or intrathecal vancomycin therapy (e.g., vancomycin 20 mg intrathecally daily). Addition of systemic rifampin 600 mg PO or IV each day should also be considered. Gram-negative bacilli-associated shunt infections should be treated with a systemic third-generation cephalosporin or systemic plus intraventricular aminoglycoside with systemic ticarcillin or piperacillin. Decisions about shunt removal depend on the patient's response to therapy and serial culture results.

c. **The postoperative neurosurgical patient.** Nosocomially acquired pathogens include gram-negative enteric bacilli, *Pseudomonas* spp., *S. aureus, S. epidermidis,* and streptococci.

d. **Head trauma.** Patients are predisposed to acute or recurrent meningitis. *S. pneumoniae,* other streptococci, or gram-negative bacilli are found most frequently.

e. **Recurrent meningitis.** *S. pneumoniae* is the most common causative organism. Also found are *Haemophilus* spp., streptococci, *Neisseria* spp., staphylococci, and, especially after prophylactic antibiotic therapy, gram-negative rods.

f. **The immunosuppressed host.** Potential pathogens include *Listeria monocytogenes, Pseudomonas aeruginosa, S. aureus, S. pneumoniae,* gram-negative enteric bacilli, streptococci, anaerobes, *Acinetobacter* spp., *Cryptococcus neoformans,* and coagulase-negative staphylococci. Patients who are neutropenic (e.g., following chemotherapy) may develop central nervous system infections with any of these pathogens. *Listeria, S. pneumoniae,* and *Cryptococcus* are most commonly found in patients with malignancies who have **normal** neutrophil counts in peripheral blood (e.g., patients with Hodgkin's disease).

2. **THERAPY FOR BACTERIAL MENINGITIS.** When the cerebrospinal fluid gram stain or bacterial culture or both yield positive findings, therapy specific to the infecting organism should be instituted.

a. **Pneumococcal and meningococcal meningitis.** There should be prompt initiation of a 10- to 14-day course of penicillin (18–24 MU/d IV in divided doses every 2 to 4 hours) or ampicillin (12 g/d IV in divided doses every 2 to 4 hours). Chloramphenicol (75–100 mg/kg/d IV in divided doses) or ceftriaxone 1–2 g IV q12h) can be used in the penicillin-allergic patient. Most first- and second-generation cephalosphorins do *not* cross the blood-brain barrier. In cases of meningococcal meningitis, respiratory isolation of the patient is suggested for the first 24 hours of treatment, and prophylaxis of close contacts with rifampin (adult dose 600 mg bid for 2 days) should be given. In areas where high-level resistance to penicillin (MIC ≥1 µg/mL) is prevalent, initial treatment of suspected pneumococcal meningitis should include ceftriaxone or cefotoxime, plus vancomycin.

b. *Haemophilus influenzae* **meningitis.** Ampicillin, 2–4 g IV q4h, plus chloramphenicol, 75–100 mg/kg/d IV q6h, or ceftriaxone, 1–2 g IV q12h, should be initiated for all patients until it has been determined whether the individual isolate produces beta-lactamase. Ampicillin may be continued alone for beta-lactamase-negative strains, for a minimum course of 10 days. Chloramphenicol, ceftriaxone, and cefotaxime are effective for patients with a beta-lactamase-positive isolate. Failure to improve on appropriate therapy may indicate the presence of subdural effusions (especially in children) or a para-meningeal focus of infection (e.g., sinusitis).

c. **Gram-negative bacillary meningitis.** The most likely organisms causing meningitis in adults are *Klebsiella, Escherichia coli,* and *Pseudomonas.* Initial therapy of community-acquired gram-negative meningitis should be a third-generation cephalosporin in high doses (e.g., cefotaxime 50 mg/kg IV q6h). An aminoglycoside should be added (IV and intrathecally) in the severely ill patient or if *Pseudomonas* infection is suspected (0.03 mg of tobramycin or gentamicin or 0.1 mg of amikacin/mL of estimated cerebrospinal fluid volume every 24 hours). The volume of cerebrospinal fluid in adults is estimated at 1 ml per pound of body weight. In hospital-acquired meningitis not involving neurosurgery, a third-generation cephalosporin should be administered. If the meningitis was acquired in the hospital following neurosurgery, nafcillin should be added to a third-generation cephalosporin and aminoglycoside. In the penicillin-allergic patient, vancomycin may be substituted for nafcillin. Therapy should be continued for at least 10 days after the last sterile cerebrospinal fluid culture.

d. *Listeria monocytogenes* **meningitis.** Ampicillin, 2 g IV q4h (or penicillin, 18–24 MU/d IV in divided doses q4h), should be given for at least 3 weeks. In the patient allergic to penicillin, chloramphenicol, 75–100 mg/kg/d in divided doses q6h (or trimethoprim-sulfamethoxazole) may be effective, but there has been little clinical experience with agents other than ampicillin or penicillin.

e. *Staphylococcus aureus* **meningitis.** Nafcillin, 2–3 g IV q4h, may be given, or vancomycin, 1 g q12h, can be used in the penicillin-allergic patient. Vancomycin may also be administered intrathecally at a dose of 20 mg/d. Penicillin may be used for penicillin-susceptible organisms. A careful search for associated abscesses (e.g., para-meningeal) should be considered.

f. *Staphylococcus epidermidis* **meningitis.** Infection with this organism is usually associated with the presence of an infected ventricular shunt. Vancomycin, 1 g IV q12h, is the drug of choice. Rifampin may be added and may improve the possibility of curing this infection without removal of the shunt.

3. THERAPY FOR NONBACTERIAL MENINGITIS

   a. **Tuberculous meningitis.** The clinical presentation of this type of meningitis often includes cranial nerve palsies and is similar to the presentation of cryptococcal meningitis. Treatment is with isoniazid, 600 mg/d (with pyridoxine), and rifampin, 600 mg/d, often with a third agent, pyrazinamide, for the initial 2 months of therapy. The dosage of isoniazid may be reduced after 1 month of therapy. The optimal total duration of therapy has not been well defined, and the use of corticosteroids, especially for basilar meningitis, remains controversial.

   b. **Fungal infections**

      (1) *Cryptococcal meningitis.* Amphotericin B (0.3 mg/kg/d) plus 5-flucytosine (150 mg/kg/d) or amphotericin B alone (0.5–0.8 mg/kg/d) for 6 weeks is the treatment of choice. The level of 5-flucytosine should not exceed 100 µg/mL when measured 1 to 2 hours after oral administration (see Table 3–13 for treatment in patients with AIDS).

      (2) *Coccidioidal meningitis.* Amphotericin B 0.5–0.6 mg/kg/d should be administered IV and intrathecally. Alternatively, fluconazole 400 mg PO qd can be administered indefinitely.

      (3) *Candidal meningitis.* Amphotericin B with 5-flucytosine is the recommended therapy.

   c. **Amebic meningitis.** Though recovery from this type of meningitis is uncommon, systemic and intraventricular administration of high-dose amphotericin B is recommended.

Durand ML, Calderwood SB, Weber DJ, et al. Acute bacterial meningitis in adults—a review of 493 episodes. N Engl J Med 1993;328:21–28.
Schlech WF, Ward JI, Band JD, et al. Bacterial meningitis in the United States, 1978 through 1981. JAMA 1985;253:1749–1754.
Tunkel AR, Scheld WM. Acute bacterial meningitis. Lancet 1995;346:1675–1680.

B. Brain Abscess

Prompt recognition of brain abscess should lead to early administration of parenteral antibiotics and neurosurgical evaluation. Few patients present with the classic triad of fever, headache, and focal neurologic defect, and a high index of suspicion should prompt CT scans of the head in patients with any suggestive symptoms or signs. Physical examination and laboratory findings are often nonspecific. Lumbar puncture is contraindicated when brain abscess is suspected. CT of the head, with contrast enhancement, is the most sensitive diagnostic test. If a CT scan is not immediately available to confirm the diagnosis, appropriate antibiotics should be started without delay.

1. BACTERIOLOGY. When material is available from a brain abscess, gram stain and aerobic, anaerobic, mycobacterial, and fungal cultures should be performed. The most common aerobes isolated are streptococci, followed by organisms of the Enterobacteriaceae family and *Pseudomo-*

nas spp., *Staphylococcus aureus, Haemophilus* spp., and coagulase-negative staphylococci. Anaerobes are usually found in mixed infections, with *Bacteroides* and *Peptostreptococcus* being the most common. Much less common are *Propionibacterium acnes* and others, such as *Veillonella* and *Actinomyces* spp. Some abscesses may appear sterile if the handling of material for anaerobic cultures is not adequate. Fungal and parasitic infections are appearing more frequently in the immunosuppressed patient.

2. **THERAPY.** Studies of antibiotic penetration and activity in brain abscesses are incomplete. Therapy should be parenteral and high dose. Penicillin (20 MU/d) and chloramphenicol (1 g q6h) have been commonly used. However, metronidazole has advantages over chloramphenicol in that it is bactericidal against *Bacteroides fragilis,* attains high concentrations in brain abscess pus, and is not degraded in pus. If gram-negative bacilli are suspected, especially when the patient has a prior history of otic infection, a third-generation cephalosporin should be added.

   If staphylococci are suspected, nafcillin (2 g IV q4h) should be substituted for penicillin. Vancomycin may be used if a methicillin-resistant strain is isolated.

   The duration of parenteral therapy should be at least 4 to 6 weeks, often followed by a prolonged course of oral therapy (2 to 6 months). Sequential CT scans may be helpful in determining the duration of therapy.

   The role of **surgical therapy** must be individualized, and neurosurgical consultation should be obtained early. Recent experience has suggested that some patients may be treated without extensive neurosurgery.

Boom WH, Tuazon CU. Successful treatment of multiple brain abscesses with antibiotics alone. Rev Infect Dis 1985;7:189–199.

Chun CH, Johnson JD, Hofstetter M, et al. Brain abscess—a study of 45 consecutive cases. Medicine 1986;65:415–431.

Kaplan K. Brain abscess. Symposium on infections of the central nervous system. Med Clin North Am 1985;69:345–360.

XV. SEPSIS AND SEPTIC SHOCK

Sepsis refers to a clinical syndrome consisting of the physiologic changes induced by severe systemic inflammation. Although bacterial infection is suspected in most cases, other diseases associated with systemic inflammation can lead to sepsis. Bacteremia is the single leading cause of sepsis in the United States but is documented in fewer than 50% of cases. Although the term "gram-negative sepsis" is engrained in the minds of most clinicians, infections with either gram-negative or gram-positive organisms can be associated with sepsis. A complex network of interacting bacterial components (e.g., endotoxin) and endogenous mediators (e.g., cytokines) has been implicated in mediating this disorder.

   The **sepsis syndrome,** which recently has been renamed "systemic inflammatory response syndrome (SIRS)," is defined as the clinical condition in which infection is suspected and evidence of altered organ perfusion is present in the form of **hypoxemia, tachycardia, acute renal failure,** or **metabolic acidosis.** The core temperature of the patient may be elevated or depressed. (Hypothermia is considered to be a worrisome prognostic sign.) In many cases of sepsis, progressive hypotension ensues, leading to the clinical syndrome known as septic shock, which is associated with a mortality rate of 25%–50%. **Septic shock** develops as a result of an overall **reduction in vascular tone** (decreased systemic vascular resistance [SVR]), **myocardial suppression** (decreased inotropy or stroke volume), **capillary leak,** and **arteriovenous shunting.** Unrelenting sepsis is almost invariably associated with the development of multiple organ dysfunction syndrome (MODS). Common complications include acute (formerly, adult) respiratory distress syndrome (ARDS), disseminated intravascular coagulation (DIC), hepatic dysfunction, mental status changes, and gastrointestinal bleeding.

All patients with suspected sepsis deserve thorough and complete clinical evaluation. Every effort, including bacterial cultures of blood, urine, and sputum, should be made to determine whether a treatable infection is present; if further testing is clinically indicated, cerebrospinal fluid and other normally sterile body fluids also should be obtained for bacterial culture. Patients with septic shock are best managed in an intensive care unit. Physiologic monitoring with arterial catheters, pulmonary arterial (Swan-Ganz) catheters, and pulse oximeters is used for management of unstable patients.

Adequate **volume resuscitation** is critical in the management of a patient with septic shock. Generally, isotonic crystalloid solutions (e.g., **normal saline**) are preferred over colloid solutions for this purpose. Intravenous fluid should be infused to maintain the pulmonary capillary wedge pressure ≥8–12 mm Hg. Vasopressors should be reserved for patients with septic shock refractory to volume infusion. If a vasopressor is required, **dopamine** is the treatment of choice for septic shock. Therapy is usually initiated at a rate of 2–4 µg/min IV and titrated upward to maintain the systolic blood pressure ≥90 mm Hg or the mean arterial pressure ≥70 mm Hg. Dobutamine may be useful for increasing myocardial contractility in selected patients with no evidence of coronary vascular disease or cardiac ischemia. The administration of norepinephrine (Levophed) or phenylephrine (Neo-Synephrine) is usually reserved for patients whose hypotension is refractory to dopamine infusion therapy. Packed red blood cell transfusions should be considered for selected patients to improve oxygen delivery to tissues. Mechanical ventilatory support, often using positive end-expiratory pressure (PEEP), may be required, especially in patients who develop ARDS. Although beneficial in animal models of septic shock, high-dose corticosteroid therapy is contraindicated for the treatment of septic shock in humans. Administration of antiendotoxin antibodies and anticytokine agents (e.g., anti-TNF antibodies, soluble TNF receptor) have not clearly demonstrated benefit in clinical trials.

All patients with suspected sepsis should receive empiric intravenous **broad-spectrum antibiotic therapy.** Appropriate initial regimens include the following:
- The combination of (1) a third-generation cephalosporin (e.g., cefotaxime, ceftriaxone, ceftazidime), or an antipseudomonal penicillin (e.g., mezlocil-

lin, piperacillin, azlocillin, ticarcillin), or ticarcillin-clavulanate, or piperacillin-tazobactam with (2) an aminoglycoside (e.g., gentamicin, tobramycin)
- The combination of (1) ampicillin with (2) an aminoglycoside and (3) either clindamycin or metronidazole
- Imipenem with or without an aminoglycoside

The spectrum of antimicrobial therapy can be narrowed upon identification of a pathogenic bacterial species from clinical specimens.

Bone RC. The pathogenesis of sepsis. Ann Intern Med 1991;115:457.
Bone RC. Sepsis syndrome: new insights into its pathogenesis and treatment. Infect Dis Clin North Am 1991;5:793.
Parillo JE. Management of septic shock: present and future. Ann Intern Med 1991;115:491.
Parillo JE, Parker MM, Natanson C, et al. Septic shock in humans: advances in the understanding of pathogenesis, cardiovascular dysfunction, and therapy. Ann Intern Med 1990;113:227.
Waage A, Brandtzaeg P, Espevik T, Halstensen A. Current understanding of the pathogenesis of gram-negative shock. Infect Dis Clin North Am 1991;5:781.

XVI. THE IMMUNOCOMPROMISED HOST

Fever, particularly in the leukopenic patient, should be presumed due to infection, and therapy should be started immediately after appropriate cultures are obtained. When searching for infection in the neutropenic patient, it is important to remember that local signs of purulence and inflammation may be subtle. If no obvious primary site can be found, bacteremia must be assumed.

The most common causes of bacteremia are *Escherichia coli, Klebsiella* spp., *Pseudomonas aeruginosa,* and *Staphylococcus aureus. Staphylococcus epidermidis* infections are becoming more common, especially in patients with Hickman (or other indwelling) catheters. There is no ideal empiric antibiotic combination. A third-generation cephalosporin with an aminoglycoside or another beta-lactam provides effective initial empiric therapy for most neutropenic patients. Vancomycin may be added to this regimen, especially if a patient has a Hickman catheter. If blood cultures are positive, therapy is usually continued for 14 days, with extension until the neutropenia resolves. If blood cultures are negative, antibiotics may be stopped when the granulocyte count is greater than $500/mm^3$. If a patient remains febrile after 5 to 7 days of antimicrobial therapy, superinfection, particularly with fungi, must be considered. Amphotericin B therapy is often recommended at dosages of 0.5 mg/kg/d, along with antibiotics, until the granulocytopenia resolves.

Treatment recommendations for viral infections are shown in Table 3–6, and recommendations for fungal infections are given in Table 3–10.

Hathron JW, Rubin M, Pizzo PA. Empirical antibiotic therapy in the febrile neutropenic cancer patient: clinical efficacy and impact of monotherapy. Antimicrob Agents Chemother 1987;31: 971–977.
Hughes WT. Guidelines for the use of antimicrobial agents in neutropenic patients with unexplained fever. J Infect Dis 1990;161:381–396.
Masur HM, Shelhamer J, Parrillo JE. The management of pneumonias in immunocompromised patients. JAMA 1985;253:1769–1773.
Schimpff SC. Overview of empiric antibiotic therapy for the febrile neutropenic patient. Rev Infect Dis 1985;7(suppl 4):734–740.

TABLE 3–10. Treatment of Fungal Infections

INFECTION	TREATMENT	COMMENTS
Histoplasmosis		
Immunocompetent		
Acute pulmonary	Itraconazole 400 mg PO qd × 3 mo Fluconazole 400 mg PO qd × 3 mo Amphotericin B 0.5–0.7 mg/kg/d × 3 wk	Usually benign and self-limited unless large inoculum (treat only for severe symptoms)

Disseminated	Initial therapy
	  Amphotericin B 0.5–0.7 mg/kg/d
	  Itraconazole 400 mg PO qd
	Maintenance therapy
	  Itraconazole 400 mg PO qd
	  Amphotericin B 1 mg/kg/wk
		Amphotericin B preferred for severe disease

Chronic pulmonary	Small, thin-walled cavities: observe, or itraconazole 400 mg PO qd for symptoms Large, thick-walled cavities: treat as for disseminated histoplasmosis	
Immunocompromised		

All forms of disease	Initial therapy: amophotericin B 0.5–0.7 mg/kg/d
	Maintenance therapy:
	  Itraconazole 400 mg PO qd
	  Amphotericin B 1 mg/kg/wk
	  Fluconazole 400 mg/PO qd
		Until clinical improvement, at least 7–10 d
		Life-long suppressive therapy usually required

Coccidioidomycosis		
Primary pulmonary	No therapy	No evidence dissemination, negative CF titer
Chronic pulmonary	Amphotericin B 1 mg/kg/d Fluconazole 400 mg PO qd Itraconazole 400 mg PO qd	No treatment for solitary nodule or asymptomatic cavitary disease
Disseminated	Amphotericin B 1 mg/kg/d Fluconazole 400 mg PO qd Itraconazole 400 mg PO qd	Follow CF titers
CNS disease	Systemic amphotericin B 1–1.5 mg/kg/d + intrathecal amphotericin B Fluconazole 400 mg PO qd	

Blastomycosis

Primary pulmonary — Treatment is controversial, may consider itraconazole or ketoconazole

Disseminated (chronic pulmonary, skin, genitourinary, bone, mucosa) — Amphotericin B 0.3–0.6 mg/kg/d (~2–3 g total dose); Itraconazole 400 mg PO qd (for isolated chronic pneumonitis)

Sporotrichosis

Cutaneous, lymphocutaneous — Itraconazole 200–400 mg PO qd; SSKI 2–4 mL PO tid (begin with 1 mL and gradually increase as tolerated)

Pulmonary/disseminated — Amphotericin B 1.5–2.5 g (total dose); Itraconazole 400 mg PO qd

Aspergillosis

Sputum colonization — No treatment for immunocompetent patients — Consider therapy in patients at high risk for dissemination

Allergic bronchopulmonary aspergillosis (ABPA) — Corticosteroids (e.g., prednisone 20–40 mg PO qd), environmental measures to reduce exposure

Aspergilloma — No therapy for asymptomatic disease; For hemoptysis, consider surgery or intracavitary amphotericin

Invasive aspergillosis — Amphotericin B 1–1.2 mg/kg/d (optimal duration unknown); Consider surgical resection for localized disease

Cryptococcosis

Pulmonary only — Generally no therapy in immunocompetent patients; Consider fluconazole 200–400 mg PO qd for compromised hosts

Disseminated (skin, bone, CNS) — Amphotericin B 0.6–1 mg/kg/d ± 5FC — AIDS patients require indefinite maintenance with fluconazole 200–800 mg PO qd; CSF cryptococcal antigen titer and culture qwk until negative; CSF examined q3mo for 1 y after therapy completed (for non-AIDS patients); Consider intrathecal amphotericin B for refractory disease

Mucormycosis

Rhinocerebral or cutaneous — Amphotericin B 1–1.5 mg/kg/d, 3–6 g total dose; Aggressive surgical resection — Consider surgical drainage for synovial or bone disease

Pulmonary or gastrointestinal — Amphotericin B as above

Disseminated — Aggressive use of amphotericin B (as for rhinocerebral)

XVII. INFECTIONS ASSOCIATED WITH INTRAVASCULAR CATHETERS

Long-term vascular access catheters are commonly used in patients requiring prolonged intravenous therapy. Depending on the type of catheter (e.g., tunneled vs. subcutaneous port), infections can be divided into four major types:

- Catheter-associated bacteremia (bacteremia without evidence of primary focus)
- Exit-site infection (focal tenderness or purulence or both at exit site with or without associated bacteremia)
- Tunnel infection (focal tenderness or purulence or both along subcutaneous tunnel site with or without associated bacteremia)
- Septic/suppurative thrombophlebitis

The most frequently encountered organisms include coagulase-negative staphylococci, *Staphylococcus aureus,* aerobic gram-negative bacilli, and *Candida* spp. Each type of infection must be treated with intravenous antibiotics to which the organism is susceptible. General considerations in line removal include site of infection (all tunnel-site infections generally require removal, whereas exit-site and line-associated bacteremia may be treated with the line in place, depending on the organism), patient clinical status (all hemodynamically unstable patients should have the catheter removed), specific organism involved (*Candida* spp., many gram-negative bacilli, including *Pseudomonas, Corynebacterium* JK, and *S. aureus* often necessitate catheter removal). Persistent bacteremia despite antibiotics, infected thrombus/suppurative thrombophlebitis, or evidence of septic embolization also necessitates catheter removal in most instances. Initial empiric therapy for suspected line infection may include vancomycin combined with either an aminoglycoside or third-generation cephalosporin (e.g., ceftazidime or ceftriaxone).

XVIII. ACQUIRED IMMUNODEFICIENCY SYNDROME (AIDS)

The care of HIV-infected patients is undergoing rapid changes with advances in the understanding of the pathophysiology of HIV infection. Viral load quantitation is likely to become an important means of assessing the response to antiviral therapy and the risk of disease progression in HIV-infected individuals. Combination therapy with nucleoside analogs and protease inhibitors shows significant promise in decreasing viral load and slowing CD4 cell decline and may replace monotherapy as first-line antiviral therapy.

Baseline evaluation of HIV-infected individuals should include a detailed history (TB exposure, sexually transmitted diseases, residence in areas where dimorphic fungi are endemic, previous hepatitis), physical examination, and laboratory evaluation (CBC, creatinine, liver panel, RPR or VDRL, *Toxoplasma* serology, hepatitis serologies, PPD skin testing, and chest radiograph). Unless specifically contraindicated, all HIV-infected individuals should receive a dose of the 23-valent pneumococcal vaccine. Hepatitis B vaccine should also be administered to individuals who are antibody negative and are at risk for acquiring infection. Specific prophylaxis for opportunistic infections is dictated by the degree of immunosuppression, as reflected by the CD4 count, and is shown in Table 3–11.

Although there is at present no cure for HIV infection, antiviral therapy has been shown to slow the progression of HIV-related disease, reduce the number of opportunistic infections, and prolong the lives of patients with established AIDS. The recommendations for initiation of antiviral therapy are undergoing continued changes, but many authorities currently recommend antiviral therapy when the CD4 cell count has fallen below $500/mm^3$, when an HIV-infected individual has had an opportunistic infection (even if the CD4 count was greater than $500/mm^3$), or in an individual with a high viral load. With the demonstration of continuous HIV replication following initial infection and the advent of potent newer antiviral agents, earlier therapy with combination regimens may prove to be a more effective strategy. The first-line choice for antiviral therapy is also evolving, with a bias toward initiation with combination therapy rather than a single agent. As results of several ongoing trials become available, optimal antiretroviral therapy recommendations will likely emerge. Table 3–12 lists the currently available antiretroviral agents, their recommended doses, and the more common adverse effects.

Antiretroviral chemotherapy, supportive care, prophylaxis, and treatment of opportunistic infections are the main therapeutic approaches to HIV infection and AIDS. The management of AIDS-related opportunistic infections is complicated by the lack of expected response to treatment, the need for prolonged courses of therapy, simultaneous opportunistic infections, and a high incidence of toxic drug reactions. The treatment recommendations for the more frequently encountered opportunistic infections in HIV-infected individuals are given in Table 3–13.

Bozette SA, et al. A controlled trial of early adjunctive treatment with corticosteroids for *Pneumocystis carinii* in the acquired immunodeficiency syndrome. N Engl J Med 1990;323:1451–1456.

Drugs for AIDS and associated infections. Med Lett 1995;37:87–94.

Gagnon S, et al. Corticosteroids as adjunctive therapy for severe *Pneumocystis carinii* pneumonia in the acquired immunodeficiency syndrome–a double-blind, placebo-controlled trial. N Engl J Med 1990;323:1444–1450.

Lane HC, Laughon BE, Falloon J, et al. Recent advances in the management of AIDS-related opportunistic infections. Ann Intern Med 1994;120:945–955.

Saag MS, Holodniy M, Kuritakes DR, et al. HIV viral load markers in clinical practice. Nature Med 1996;2:625–629.

Sande MA, Volberding PA, eds. The Medical Management of AIDS. Philadelphia: W.B. Saunders Co, 1995.

USPHS/IDSA guidelines for the prevention of opportunistic infections in persons infected with human immunodeficiency virus: a summary. Ann Intern Med 1996;124:349–368.

XIX. TRAVEL AND MALARIA

For the majority of travelers, only routine immunizations are recommended (Table 3–8, p. 109). Information on which immunizations are needed and whether a country requires an International Certificate of Vaccination can be obtained from many sources. *Health Information for International Travel* (published by the CDC yearly) and the "Blue Sheet" (published biweekly by the CDC) are most useful.

Text continued on page 143

TABLE 3-11. Prophylaxis Regimens for Selected Infections in HIV-Infected Adults

PATHOGEN	INDICATION	PROPHYLACTIC REGIMEN
Pneumocystis carinii	Prior *P. carinii* pneumonia (PCP)	TMP-SMX, 1 DS or SS PO qd
	CD4 count <200/µL	TMP-SMX, 1 DS 3×/wk
	Oropharyngeal candidiasis	Dapsone 100 mg PO qd
	Unexplained fevers >2 wk	Aerosolized pentamidine 300 mg each month via Respiragard II nebulizer
Mycobacterium tuberculosis	PPD ≥5 mm	INH sensitive: INH 300 mg PO + pyridoxine 50 mg PO qd × 12 mo
	Prior, untreated positive PPD	INH 900 mg PO + pyridoxine 50 mg PO 2×/wk × 12 mo
	Exposure to active TB	INH resistant: Rifampin 600 mg PO qd × 12 mo
Toxoplasma gondii	Antibody to *T. gondii* and CD4 <100 µL	Primary prophylaxis: TMP-SMX (see doses above)
	Prior toxoplasmosis	Dapsone 50 mg PO qd + pyrimethamine 50 mg PO qwk + folinic acid* 10 mg PO qwk
		Secondary prophylaxis: pyrimethamine 50 mg PO qd + sulfadiazine 1g PO q6h + folinic acid* 10 mg PO qd
		pyrimethamine 50 mg PO qd + clindamycin 300 mg PO q6h + folinic acid* 10 mg PO qd
Mycobacterium avium complex	CD4 count <75–100/mm³	Rifabutin 300 mg PO qd
		or
		Clarithromycin 500 mg PO qd bid
		or
		Azithromycin 250 mg PO qwk

*Leukovorin.

TABLE 3-12. Agents Used to Treat Human Immunodeficiency Virus (HIV)

AGENT	STANDARD DOSAGE	COMMON ADVERSE EFFECTS	COMMENTS
NUCLEOSIDE RT-INHIBITORS			
Zidovudine (AZT)	200 mg PO q8h	Bone marrow suppression, nausea, headache, myalgia, malaise	Decreases mother to child HIV transmission
Didanosine (ddi)	>60 kg: 200 mg tab or 250 mg powder q12h <60 kg: 125 mg tab or 167 mg powder q12h	Pancreatitis, diarrhea, peripheral neuropathy	Decreases absorption of drugs that require acidic pH
Zalcitabine (ddC)	0.75 mg PO q8h	Peripheral neuropathy, oral ulcers, pancreatitis	
Stavudine (d4T)	>60 kg: 40 mg PO q12h <60 kg: 30 mg PO q12h	Peripheral neuropathy, nausea, pancreatitis	
Lamivudine (3TC)	150–300 mg PO q12h	Headache, diarrhea	
PROTEASE INHIBITORS			
Saquinavir	600 mg PO q8h	Headache, diarrhea	Relatively low bioavailability
Ritonavir	600 mg PO q12h	Nausea, paresthesia, aminotransferase elevation	Multiple drug interactions; survival benefit in patients with advanced AIDS
Indinavir	800 mg PO q8h	Renal stones, hyperbilirubinemia	

TABLE 3–13. Treatment of Opportunistic Infections in Patients with AIDS

PATHOGEN	TREATMENT	DURATION	COMMENTS
Pneumocystis carinii			
Mild disease	TMP-SMX 2 DS tabs PO q8h	21 d	
	TMP 15 mg/kg/d (divided into 3 doses) + dapsone 100 mg PO qd	21 d	
	Clindamycin 450 mg PO q6h + primaquine 15 mg PO qd	21 d	
	Atovaquone 750 mg PO q8h (tablets) or q12h (suspension)	21 d	
Acutely ill (Po₂ <70)	TMP-SMX (5 mg/kg q8h) IV	21 d	Combined with steroids
	Pentamidine 4 mg/kg/d IV qd	21 d	Prednisone 40 mg PO bid × 5 d
	Clindamycin 900 mg IV q6h + primaquine 30 mg PO qd	21 d	40 mg PO qd × 5 d
	Trimetrexate 45 mg/m² IV qd + folinic acid (leukovorin) 20 mg/m² IV q6h	21 d	20 mg PO qd × 11 d
Toxoplasmosis	Pyrimethamine 200 mg PO × 1, then 50–75 mg PO qd and folinic acid (leukovorin) 10 mg PO/IV qd		Treat for 3–6 wk; then convert to suppressive doses (see Toxoplasmosis, secondary prophylaxis)
	and		
	either sulfadiazine 1–1.5 g PO q6h		
	or		
	clindamycin 600 mg PO/IV q6h		

Alternatives

Pyrimethamine + folinic acid (as above)
and
Clarithromycin 1 g PO q12h
or
Azithromycin 1 g PO, followed by 0.5 g PO qd
or
Atovaquone 750 mg PO q6h
or
Dapsone 100 mg PO qd

Cryptococcal meningitis
Amphotericin B 0.5–1 mg/kg/d IV until stabilized
Followed by chronic suppression with fluconazole 200–400 mg PO qd

Disseminated *Mycobacterium avium*-complex (MAC)
Clarithromycin 500 mg PO bid or azithromycin 250–500 mg PO qd
and
Ethambutol 15–25 mg/kg/d PO
May consider adding:
Rifabutin 300 mg PO qd
or
Amikacin 7.5 mg/kg/d IV
or
Clofazamine 100–200 mg PO qd
or
Ciprofloxacin 750 mg PO bid

Note: efficacy not definitively established in clinical trials

Table continued on following page

TABLE 3-13. Treatment of Opportunistic Infections in Patients with AIDS *(Continued)*

PATHOGEN	TREATMENT	DURATION	COMMENTS
Cytomegalovirus (CMV) retinitis	Induction with either: Ganciclovir 5 mg/kg IV q12h × 14–21 d *or* Foscarnet 90 mg/kg IV q12h × 14–21 d Followed by chronic suppression: Ganciclovir 5 mg/kg IV 5–7×/wk or 1 g PO tid *or* Foscarnet 90–120 mg IV qd		

Candidiasis
  Oral
	Nystatin solution or tablets
	  500,000–1,000,000 U PO 3–5×/d
	Clotrimazole troches 10 mg 5×/d
	Fluconazole 100–200 mg/d
	Ketoconazole 200 mg PO qd		

Esophageal	Fluconazole 100–200 mg PO qd Amphotericin B 0.3–0.5 mg/kg/d IV Ketoconazole 200–400 mg PO qd		

Disease	Treatment	Duration	Comments
Bacillary angiomatosis (*Bartonella* infection)	Erythromycin 500 mg PO/IV q6h Doxycycline 100 mg PO q12h		
Coccidioidomycosis (pulmonary and extrapulmonary)	Fluconazole 400–600 mg PO qd *or* Itraconazole 200–400 mg PO qd *or* Amphotericin B 0.6–0.8 mg/kg/d IV Followed by chronic suppression with: Fluconazole 200–400 mg PO qd *or* Amphotericin B 1 mg/kg/d IV *or* Itraconazole 200–400 mg PO qd	2–4 wk	Lifelong suppression is probably required Consider addition of intrathecal amphotericin B 0.1–0.3 mg/d for meningitis
Blastomycosis	Amphotericin B 0.5–1 mg/kg/d IV Followed by chronic suppression with: Itraconazole 200–400 mg PO qd		

Table continued on following page

TABLE 3–13. Treatment of Opportunistic Infections in Patients with AIDS *(Continued)*

PATHOGEN	TREATMENT	DURATION	COMMENTS
Histoplasmosis	Amphotericin B 0.6–1 mg/kg/d IV Followed by chronic suppression with: Itraconazole 200–400 mg PO daily *or* Fluconazole 200–400 mg PO qd *or*		
Cryptosporidiosis	Amphotericin B 1 mg/kg IV 1–2×/wk No standardized therapy; consider Paromomycin 500–750 mg PO tid *or* Azithromycin 500–1000 mg PO qd		Symptomatic treatment with imodium, loperamide, tincture of opium, or octreotide
Microsporidiosis	Albendazole 200–400 mg PO bid		Probably useful only for septata intestinalis
Herpes simplex infection			
Mild	Acyclovir 200–400 mg PO 5×/d	7–10 d	
Severe	Acyclovir 5 mg/kg IV q8h		
Chronic suppression	Acyclovir 200–400 mg PO bid–tid	Indefinitely	
Varicella zoster (shingles)			
Mild	Acyclovir 800 mg PO 5×/d Famciclovir 500 mg PO tid	7–10 d	
Severe	Acyclovir 10–12 mg/kg IV q8h		

A. Malaria

Since the risk of acquiring malaria in different areas changes frequently, it is important to obtain recent information from the sources noted, as well as from the *Morbidity and Mortality Weekly Report,* local health departments, and the CDC. In addition to chemoprophylaxis, it is important to reduce exposure to mosquitoes by the use of protective screening, clothing, and mosquito repellent (e.g., N,N-diethylmetatoluamide [DEET]).

1. CHEMOPROPHYLAXIS recommendations are:
   a. **For *Plasmodium ovale, P. vivax, P. malariae,* and chloroquine-sensitive strains of *P. falciparum.*** Chloroquine phosphate, 300 mg PO of base, is recommended once a week on the same day, beginning 1 week prior to travel, continuing every week during travel, and for 4 weeks following departure from the malarious area.
   b. **For a presumed attack of chloroquine-resistant *P. falciparum* malaria.** In addition to the above course of therapy, the traveler should take Fansidar tablets (3 tablets: 75 mg of pyrimethamine and 1500 mg of sulfadoxine PO) or mefloquine 1250 mg PO, as a single dose. Medical attention should be sought immediately. (Note: The combination of chloroquine and Fansidar sometimes causes potentially fatal cutaneous reactions, such as the Stevens-Johnson syndrome; Fansidar should not be taken late in pregnancy or by sulfa-allergic patients.)
   c. **For long-term travel in areas with high risk of chloroquine-resistant *P. falciparum.*** Mefloquine, 250 mg PO once weekly, starting 1 week before entering the endemic area, continuing every week during travel, and for 4 weeks after leaving the endemic region. Alternatively, chloroquine prophylaxis may be combined with doxycycline, 100 mg PO qd starting 1 to 2 days before departure, continuing during travel in an endemic region, and continuing for 4 to 6 weeks following return from an endemic region.

2. THERAPY. Most patients with acute malaria can be treated with oral medications. The initial treatment is the same for all forms of malaria, unless the patient has acquired chloroquine-resistant *P. falciparum* malaria. Even chloroquine-resistant malaria will have some response to chloroquine but will recur. If the patient is seriously ill, treatment should be directed as though the malaria were chloroquine resistant. Oral therapy for chloroquine-sensitive malaria is chloroquine phosphate, 600 mg (active base), followed by 300 mg (base) 6, 24, and 48 hours later. For *P. vivax* and *P. ovale* malaria, chloroquine therapy should be followed by primaquine 15 mg (base) PO qd for 14 days starting around the fourth day. For parenteral therapy of a severe attack, quinidine gluconate should be used, 10 mg/kg (maximum, 600 mg) IV loading dose over 1 hour, followed by continuous administration of 0.02 mg/kg/min IV (maximum, 10 mg/kg q8h) until oral chloroquine therapy is possible. Administration of IV quinidine requires hospitalization in an ICU with continuous hemodynamic and cardiac monitoring. Widening of the QRS interval or significant lengthening of the QT segment requires discontinuation of drug infusion.

Recommended oral therapy for *P. falciparum* (chloroquine-resistant) malaria is quinine sulfate, 540 mg (active base) tid for 3 to 7 days plus one of the following:

- Fansidar, 3 tablets (pyrimethamine 75 mg and sulfadoxine 1500 mg) once; or
- Tetracycline, 250–500 mg qid for 7 days *or*
- Doxycycline, 100 mg bid for 7 days *or*
- Clindamycin, 900 mg tid for 3 days

Alternatively, mefloquine 1250 mg alone may be given once. (Note: mefloquine must not be given with quinine.) For the severely ill patient, IV quinidine gluconate may be given as above, and oral therapy with quinine plus a second drug (as above) begun as soon as possible. For additional information on side effects, contraindications, and alternate agents, *The Travel and Tropical Medicine Manual* (see reference list at end of section) may be consulted. Exchange transfusion therapy should be considered for gravely ill patients with malaria (e.g., cerebral malaria, parasitemia ≥10% of erythrocytes). The Malarial Branch, Centers for Disease Control and Prevention, in Atlanta, Georgia, may be contacted for information regarding the therapy of malaria: for recorded information on prophylaxis, (404) 332-4555; for questions about management of acute attacks or on prophylaxis, (404) 488-4046 [emergency, (404) 639-2888].

B. Traveler's Diarrhea

The majority of cases of traveler's diarrhea are caused by bacteria, such as enteropathogenic *Escherichia coli, Shigella, Salmonella,* and *Campylobacter.* Most of these pathogens can be avoided by the use of only chlorinated, boiled, or carbonated water (and ice). Raw vegetables and fruits may be contaminated when washed in water.

1. **CHEMOPROPHYLAXIS.** Bismuth subsalicylate (Pepto-Bismol), 60 ml PO qid, may prevent symptomatic infection. Prophylactic antibiotics for most travelers have more associated risks than benefits. Trimethoprim-sulfamethoxazole 1 double-strength tablet PO qd bid, or doxycycline 100 mg PO qd bid, or ciprofloxacin 500 mg PO qd bid may be considered for short-term (less than 2 weeks) prophylaxis in special cases. However, it is recommended that antibiotics be taken only when symptoms occur.

2. **THERAPY.** When diarrhea does occur, bismuth subsalicylate (Pepto-Bismol, 30 ml every 30 minutes for 8 doses) or an antimotility agent (diphenoxylate hydrochloride with atropine [Lomotil] or loperamide hydrochloride [Imodium]) may be taken for no longer than 2 days. For **bloody diarrhea with fever, ciprofloxacin, 500 mg PO bid for 5 days, trimethoprim-sulfamethoxazole, 1 double-strength tablet PO bid for 5 days, or trimethoprim, 200 mg PO bid for 5 days,** is suggested.

Other helminthic, protozoal, and arthropod-borne diseases are discussed elsewhere (Med Lett Drugs Ther 1988;30:15–22). Table 3–14 provides a summary of treatment recommendations for some common parasitic infections.

TABLE 3–14. **Treatment Recommendations for Selected Parasitic Infections**

ORGANISM	THERAPY
Entamoeba histolytica (amebiasis)	
Asymptomatic disease	Iodoquinol,* 650 mg PO tid for 20 d
Intestinal disease	
Mild to moderate	Metronidazole, 750 mg PO tid for 5–10 d, plus iodoquinol, as above, or tetracycline, 500 mg PO tid for 5 d
Severe	Above regimen plus emetine, 1 mg/kg/d IM (maximum of 60 mg/d) for up to 5 d
Extraintestinal disease	Metronidazole plus iodoquinol, as above, or chloroquine phosphate, 1 g PO qd for 2 d, then 500 mg PO qd for 4 wk plus emetine, as above, for 10 d
Ascaris lumbricoides (round worm)	Mebendazole, 100 mg PO bid for 3 d, or pyrantel pamoate, 11 mg/kg once (maximum of 1 g)
Enterobius vermicularis (pinworm)	Pyrantel pamoate, 11 mg/kg PO once (maximum of 1 g), or mebendazole, 100 mg PO once†
Giardia lamblia (giardiasis)	Metronidazole,‡ 2 g PO qd for 3 d or 750 mg tid for 5 d, or quinacrine HCl, 100 mg PO tid for 5 d
Strongyloides	Thiabendazole, 25 mg/kg PO bid (maximum of 3 g/d for 2–3 d), or ivermectin, 200 µg/kg/d PO for 2 d, or albendazole, 400 mg/d PO for 3 d
Tapeworms	
Diphyllobothrium latum (fish)	Niclosamide, 2 g chewed thoroughly as a single dose
Taenia saginata (beef)	As above
Taenia solium (pork)	As above; praziquantel for neurocysticercosis, or albendazole, 7.5 mg/kg PO bid for 8–14 d
Trichuris (whipworm)	Mebendazole, 100 mg PO bid for 3 d

*Maximal dose of 2 g/d. Increased dose or duration may result in optic neuritis. Available from Glenwood Laboratories, Inc., 83 North Summit St., Tenafly, NJ 07670.
†Repeat either agent in 2 wk if in heavily contaminated area.
‡Not currently licensed for giardiasis.

Centers for Disease Control. Recommendations for the prevention of malaria among travelers. MMWR 1990;39:1.
Jong EC, ed. The Travel and Tropical Medicine Manual. Philadelphia: W.B. Saunders Co.; 1987.
Medical Letter. Advice for travelers. Med Lett Drugs Ther 1987;29:53–56.
Medical Letter. Drugs for parasitic infections. Med Lett Drugs Ther 1988;30:15–22.
Medical Letter. Mefloquine for malaria. Med Lett Drugs Ther 1990;31:13.

XX. TICK-BORNE DISEASES

Tick-borne diseases can result from infection with pathogens that include bacteria, rickettsia, viruses, and protozoa. Awareness of both the geographic distribution and clinical presentation is critical in determining the probable cause of a tick-borne illness. Because rapid and specific diagnostic tests are often unavailable and delay in treating these infections is associated with significant morbidity and mortality, empiric treatment is often justified. Table 3–15 shows the more common tick-borne illnesses and their appropriate therapy.

TABLE 3–15. Treatment of Tick-Borne Diseases

DISEASE	CAUSATIVE AGENT	REGION	TREATMENT

Lyme disease	*Borrelia burgdorferi*	Northeast, WI, MN, CA	Early: doxycycline 100 mg PO bid × 2–3 wk
			    amoxicillin 500 mg PO tid × 2–3 wk
			Late: ceftriaxone 2 g IV qd × 3 wk
			    penicillin G 3–4 mU IV q4h × 3 wk
			    doxycycline 100 mg PO bid × 30 d

Relapsing fever	*Borrelia* spp.	West	Doxycycline 100 mg PO bid × 7–10 d Erythromycin 500 mg PO qid × 7–10 d
Tularemia	*Francisella tularensis*	AR, MO, OK	Gentamicin 1–1.5 mg/kg IV q8h × 7–10 d Doxycycline 100 mg PO/IV bid × 21 d
Rocky Mountain spotted fever	*Rickettsia rickettsii*	Southeast, Lower Midwest	Doxycycline 100 mg PO/IV bid × 5–7 d Chloramphenicol 500 mg PO/IV q6h × 5–7 d
Ehrlichiosis	*Ehrlichia* spp.	Lower Midwest, Southeast, Northeast, WI, MN	Doxycycline 100 mg PO/IV bid × 7–10 d
Babesiosis	*Babesia* spp.	Northeast, WI, MN	Quinine sulfate 650 mg PO tid × 7 d + Clindamycin 600 mg PO tid × 7 d
Colorado tick fever	Coltivirus species	West	No treatment
Tick paralysis	Toxin-mediated		Remove tick

Spach DS, Liles WC, Campbell GL, et al. Tick-borne diseases in the United States. N Engl J Med 1993;329:936–947.

XXI. FEVER OF UNKNOWN ORIGIN

Infections account for 30% to 40% of fevers of unknown origin (FUO). In one series, the infectious etiologies found were as follows: mycobacterial infection, intraabdominal abscess, UTI, cytomegalovirus infection, sinusitis, osteomyelitis, catheter infections, candidiasis, amebic hepatitis, and wound infection. After a thorough investigation of the FUO, including cultures of blood and other potentially infected sources, drug fever resulting from use of antimicrobial agents should be considered. Likely agents that cause fever include isoniazid, nitrofurantoin, novobiocin, penicillin, streptomycin, sulfonamides, and vaccines.

If no apparent etiology for FUO is found, **symptomatic therapy** may be tried, first with the use of antipyretics, such as acetylsalicylic acid or acetaminophen. If effective, these agents can be continued for a prolonged period. Prostaglandin synthetase inhibitors, such as indomethacin or ibuprofen, are alternatives. Prednisone may also be tried, if no evidence of infectious or neoplastic processes has been found.

There are a few diseases that warrant a therapeutic trial of antimicrobial agents in the absence of a firm diagnosis. If tuberculosis or granulomatous hepatitis is suspected, a short course (2 to 3 weeks) of antimycobacterial chemotherapy can be tried. Penicillin and an aminoglycoside may be used if clinical findings suggest culture-negative endocarditis.

Durack DT, Street AC. Fever of unknown origin—reexamined and redefined. Curr Clin Top Infect Dis 1991;11:35–51.

Jacoby GA, Swartz MN. Fever of undetermined origin. N Engl J Med 1973;289:1407–1410.

Larson EB, Featherstone JH, Petersdorf RG. Fever of undetermined origin: diagnosis and follow-up of 105 cases, 1979–1980. Medicine 1982;61:269–292.

Petersdorf RG, Beeson PB. Fever of unexplained origin: report on 100 cases. Medicine 1961;4:1–30.

4 4 4 4 4 4 4 4 4 4 4 4

CARDIOVASCULAR DISEASES

WILLIAM L. DALEY
RICHARD P. SHANNON

I. ANGINA PECTORIS

Angina pectoris is the clinical term given to the symptoms of **chest discomfort resulting from an imbalance between myocardial oxygen demand and myocardial oxygen supply** (oxygen deficiency). Although angina is usually the presenting symptom of many patients, observations made during coronary angioplasty indicate that angina is usually a late symptom in the sequence of events that occur when myocardial blood flow is reduced from occlusion of a coronary blood vessel. In many cases, angina is not due to a single factor but rather to a combination of factors. Clinically, myocardial oxygen demand correlates with the product of heart rate and systolic blood pressure (double product). This calculation is a useful index to measure myocardial oxygen demand, particularly during exercise.

Patients with fixed coronary artery obstruction may have superimposed vasoconstriction or platelet fibrin deposition that can further compromise flow. At peak exercise, a reduction in luminal diameter of at least 50% to 60% is required before flow is reduced and ischemia develops. A decrease in luminal diameter of approximately 90% is usually needed for ischemia or angina or both to be present at rest.

Angina is usually described by patients as an ache, pressure, tightness, heaviness, squeezing, or crushing discomfort occurring substernally or in the left precordial area. It is similar to the discomfort of myocardial infarction but less severe. The discomfort may involve the epigastrium in addition to the chest and may radiate to the arms (sometimes stopping at the elbow), neck, jaw, teeth, back, abdomen, or on rare occasions the cranium, particularly the occipital area. Other symptoms that may be associated with angina pectoris are shortness of breath or dyspnea, palpitations, and lightheadedness. Although chest discomfort is the most common symptom of ischemia, it may not be the presenting symptom.

Most patients with angina pectoris usually have underlying atherosclerotic coronary artery disease. However, angina pectoris may result from nonatherosclerotic etiology. Thus, the **differential diagnosis of angina pectoris is rather extensive,** including anxiety, hyperventilation, mitral valve prolapse (Barlow's syndrome), Tietz's syndrome, pericarditis, aortic dissection, pulmonary infarction, severe aortic valve regurgitation, aortic stenosis, and hypertrophic cardiomyopathy. In aortic stenosis and hypertrophic cardiomyopathy, the coronary arteries may be normal but demonstrate decreased vasodilator response. In addition, myocardial oxygen demand is enhanced due to increased muscle mass and elevated left ventricular systolic pressure. Furthermore, the flow to subendocardial regions may be reduced because of elevated end-diastolic pressures.

In atherosclerosis, the endothelium is impaired, which results in abnormal vasodilator response. Abnormal vasodilator response to both pharmacologic and physical stimuli contributes to myocardial ischemia through vasoconstriction and thrombus formation. Thus, angina may develop during

149

administration of exogenous catecholamines, exercise, cold exposure, and emotional and mental stress.

A. Treatment

Treatment of angina pectoris should be individualized according to symptoms. The goal of therapy is to modify favorably the relationship between myocardial oxygen supply and demand. Beta-blocking agents, calcium slow channel blocking agents, and nitrates are all useful in reducing episodes of angina and increasing exercise capacity. Comparative effects are shown in Table 4–1.

1. BETA-BLOCKING AGENTS (Table 4–2). Beta-blocking agents are usually the initial therapy for ischemic anginal syndromes. They reduce heart rate both at rest and during exercise. They also lower blood pressure and reduce myocardial contractility. The net result is a reduction in myocardial oxygen demand by reducing the double product (heart rate × blood pressure). Beta-blocking agents may be **nonselective** (affinity for both beta$_1$ and beta$_2$ receptors) or **selective** (affinity for beta$_1$ receptors). Beta$_1$ receptors are located in the myocardium, with small amounts of beta$_2$ in the atrium. Beta$_2$ receptors are located primarily in the bronchioles, peripheral vascular smooth muscles, and other specialized sites, such as pancreatic islet cells. Patients with asthma, chronic obstructive pulmonary disease, diabetes, or intermittent claudication may benefit from a low dose of beta$_1$ selective agents administered with caution. Although beta selectivity does not appear to be important for antianginal efficacy, it is important for the profile of side effects. Some beta blockers have the capacity to activate the receptor—hence the term intrinsic sympathomimetic activity (ISA), as seen with pindolol. This property limits the efficacy for treating patients with angina because, at higher doses, heart rate is not decreased and may even be increased. The major effect of beta blockers with sympathomimetic activity is lowering of blood pressure. Labetolol is a drug that possesses both beta-blocking and alpha-blocking actions. This drug can be used to treat patients with angina as well as patients with significant hypertension.

   Side effects of beta blockers include fatigue, impotence, cold extremities, bronchospasm, worsening claudication, bradycardia, and cardiac conduction disturbances. Central nervous system side effects are based on the lipid solubility property of the agent. Those agents that are lipid soluble readily cross the blood-brain barrier and are more likely to cause insomnia, depression, and nightmares. Patients should be cautioned that sudden discontinuation of beta blocker therapy may precipitate anginal symptoms or lead to myocardial infarction.

2. CALCIUM CHANNEL BLOCKING AGENTS (Table 4–3). Calcium channel blocking agents are standard therapy in the treatment of hypertension and angina pectoris. They selectively inhibit the influx of calcium into the calcium-L channel in both smooth muscle and myocardial cells. All have a peripheral arteriolar and coronary vasodilating effect and a negative inotropic effect, although the latter is modest in the case of nifedipine. **There are two distinct classes of calcium channel antagonists** based

TABLE 4-1. Comparative Effects of Angianginal Agents

AGENT	ARTERIAL DILATOR	VENODILATOR	PREVENTS CORONARY VASOCON-STRICTION	HEART RATE	SYSTOLIC BLOOD PRESSURE	AV* CONDUCTION	TACHYPHYLAXIS
BETA BLOCKERS							
Nonselective	0†	0	–	– – –	– – –	–	No
Selective	0	0	–	– – –	– – –	–	No
Intrinsic sympathomimetic activity	0	0	–	–/0	– – –	0	No
CALCIUM CHANNEL BLOCKERS							
Nifedipine	+ + +	0	+ + +	+ +	– – –	0	No
Nicarpidine	+ + +	0	+ + +	+ +	– – –	0	No
Verapamil	+ +	0	+ + +	–/0	– –	–	No
Diltiazem	+	0	+ + +	– –	–/0	0/–	No
NITRATES	+ +	+ +	+ + +	+	– –	0	Yes (long-acting nitrates)

*AV, atrioventricular.
†+, increase effect; –, decrease/negative effect; 0, no effect.

151

TABLE 4-2. Properties of Various β-Adrenergic Receptor Antagonist Agents

GENERIC (AND TRADE) NAMES	PLASMA HALF-LIFE (H)	LIPID SOLUBILITY	METABOLIZED BY	USUAL ORAL DOSE FOR ANGINA	IV DOSAGE
NONCARDIOSELECTIVE					
Propranolol* (Inderal)	1-6	+++	Liver	20-80 q6-8h; 1-10 mg* start 10-20 mg	1-10 mg* (0.1 mg/kg)
(Inderal-LA)	8-11	+++	Liver	80-320 mg qd	—
Oxprenolol* (Trasicor)	2	++	Liver	As propranolol	1-12 mg
Timolol* (Blocadren)	4-5	+	Liver, kidney	5-20 q12h bid; 15-45 mg tid or qid	0.4-1 mg
Nadolol* (Corgard)	16-24	0	Kidney	40-240 mg qd; mean 100 mg	—
Sotalol (Sotacor) (Betapace)	15-17	0	Kidney	240-480 mg qd in 2 doses for arrhythmias	10-20 mg
Penbutolol* (Levatol)	27	+++	Liver	Not studied	—
CARDIOSELECTIVE					
Acebutolol* (Sectral)	8-12	0	Liver, kidney	200-400 mg PO q8h; 900 mg optimal	12.5-50 mg
Atenolol* (Tenormin)	6-9	0	Kidney	50-100 mg qd up to 200 mg	5-10 mg*
Betaxolol* (Kerlone)	15	++	Liver, kidney	10-20 mg qd†	—
Metoprolol* (Lopressor) (Betaloc)	3	+	Liver	50-100 mg PO q8-12h	5-15 mg*
VASODILATORY BETA BLOCKERS, NONSELECTIVE					
Carteolol* (Cartrol)	5-6	0/+	Kidney	Dose not available for angina	—
Labetalol* (Trandate) (Normodyne)	3-4	+++	Liver	100-200 mg PO tid; max 2400 mg/d	1-2 mg/kg* for severe hypertension
Pindolol* (Visken)	4	+	Liver, kidney	5-15 mg PO tid	—
Carvedilol†	6	+	Kidney, liver	400 mg qd	—
VASODILATORY BETA BLOCKERS, SELECTIVE					
Celiprolol† (Selecor)	6-8	0/+	Chiefly kidney	400 mg qd	—

*Approved by FDA.
†Pending approval by FDA.
Modified from Opie LH. Drugs for the Heart, 4th ed. Philadelphia: W.B. Saunders Co., 1995, pp. 20-21.

TABLE 4–3. Calcium Channel Antagonists: Indications and Dosage

AGENT	INDICATIONS	DOSAGE
FIRST-GENERATION CALCIUM CHANNEL ANTAGONISTS		
Verapamil (Isoptin, Calan)	PSVT with narrow QRS complexes	IV bolus 5–10 mg repeated after 10 min
	Atrial flutter/fibrillation	5–10 mg IV bolus repeated after 10 min; *or* 80–120 mg tid increasing to 80–120 mg qid; beware of digitalis toxicity
	Prophylaxis of PSVT	80–120 mg PO tid
Sustained release	Hypertension	80–120 mg PO tid; *or* 240–360 mg PO qd
	Hypertrophic cardiomyopathy*	240–480 mg PO tid
Diltiazem (Cardizem) (Herbesser) (Tildiem) (Tilazem)	Angina	30–120 mg PO tid or qid
	Prinzmetal's angina	
	Non-Q-wave infarction	60 mg PO qid
IV Diltiazem	Atrial flutter/fibrillation	IV 20–25 mg bolus then 5–15 mg/min infusion
Nifedipine (Procardia) (Adalat) (Procardia SL)	Angina of effort	30–80 mg PO tid or qid Procardia SL 30–150 mg/d
	Prinzmetal's angina	10–20 mg PO tid or qid
	Severe hypertension	10 mg SL (sublingually) or bite and swallow
SECOND-GENERATION CALCIUM CHANNEL ANTAGONISTS†		
Amlodipine (Norvasc)	Hypertension, angina (does not exacerbate CHF)	5–10 mg PO qd
Felodipine SR (Plendil)	Hypertension, angina (may stimulate myocardium)	5–10 mg PO qd (decrease dose in elderly)
Isradipine (DynaCirc)	Hypertension (effects on sinus node)	2.5–10 mg PO bid
Nicardipine (capsules) (Cardene)	Hypertension (minimal cardiodepression)	20–40 mg PO tid
SR	As above	30–60 mg bid
Intravenous	As above (excessive hypotension)	5–15 mg/h
Nimodipine (Nimotop)	Cerebroselective	60 mg q4h

*Not FDA approved.
†All agents have interactions and precautions similar to those of nifedipine.
Modified from Opie LH. Drugs for the Heart, 4th ed. Philadelphia: W.B. Saunders Co., 1995, pp. 74–75.

on molecular structure: the dihydropyridines (DHPs) (related to nifedipine) and the non-DHPs (related to verapamil) (papaverine derivative) and diltiazem (benzothiazine).

The DHPs are more vascular selective. Thus, their dominant effect is peripheral and coronary vasodilation. They have minimal or no effect on the sinus and AV nodes. The rapid vasodilatory effects of these agents lead to reflex tachycardia, exacerbation of CHF, and stimulation of the renin-angiotensin system (RAS). These undesirable effects are more common among the short-acting DHPs. Since the advent of truly long acting agents (nifedipine XL, amlodipine, felodipine) there have been fewer side effects. In a recent clinical trial (PRAISE), amlodipine had no detrimental effect on patients with ischemic class II and III CHF.

The non-DHPs are less vascular selective than the DHPs and predominantly inhibit nodal tissue (decrease sinus rate) and myocardial contraction. These agents should be used with caution in patients taking beta blockers and patients with left ventricular dysfunction. They may be safely used in appropriately selected patients without sinus node or AV node disease.

Calcium antagonists have the ability to prevent coronary vasoconstriction. In general, verapamil or diltiazem is preferred over nifedipine and other DHPs for monotherapy, as agents in the latter group have the potential to cause a reflex tachycardia.

3. NITRATES (Table 4–4). Nitrates have several mechanisms of action. They have both arteriolar and venous dilating effects. The arteriolar dilating effect may, however, produce a reflex tachycardia that may be attenuated by concurrent beta blockade. The venodilating effect is very potent and plays a major role in alleviating pain by decreasing oxygen demand when used in an acute anginal episode. Coronary vasodilation is induced through the exogenous production of nitric oxide (NO·), which is now known to be endothelial-derived relaxing factor (EDRF). Nitrates also play a major role in platelet disaggregation via the same mechanism.

A major drawback to the use of nitrates is the development of **tolerance.** Numerous studies have shown that tolerance develops in a few days with continuous exposure. This explains the lack of efficacy of nitrate patches to provide a sustained antianginal effect after a 24-hour period. One method of overcoming tolerance is to use the drug intermittently. Because of these problems, nitrates are not recommended as primary or monotherapy for patients with angina. Examples of the use of nitrates are the application of paste for 4 to 8 hours in a 24-hour period, the use of a patch overnight, and the use of isosorbide dinitrate (Isordil) tablets on an 8-hour schedule rather than a 6-hour schedule.

Nitrates can be combined with beta blockers very effectively. The combination of nitrates with calcium slow channel blocking agents should be done cautiously, since postural hypotension may be a problem. Table 4–1 shows the comparative effects of antianginal agents.

B. Therapy in Specific Syndromes

1. CHRONIC STABLE ANGINA. Chronic stable angina is an episodic clinical syndrome. A careful and detailed history to evaluate the chest pain is the key to diagnosis. Patients with chronic stable angina usually have angina during periods of exercise, stress (mental or emotional), sexual activity, cold exposure, or anything that increases oxygen demand by raising the heart rate and blood pressure (double product) or has the propensity to produce vasoconstriction of the coronary vasculature.

TABLE 4-4. Nitrates

DRUG	ROUTE	FORMULATION	DOSAGE	DURATION OF ACTION*	SIDE EFFECTS
Nitroglycerin	Sublingual	Nitrostat Tabs	0.3–0.6 mg prn	30 min	All nitrates have the potential to cause side effects related to vasodilating properties, e.g., headaches, flush ing, reflex tachycardia, postural hypotension, dizziness
	Buccal	Nitrogard (sustained-release tablets, capsules)	1–2 mg tid	4–5 h	
	Oral	2.5–6.5 mg tid	4–8 h		
	Transdermal	Ointment (2%)	1.5–2 in q4–6h	3–4 h	Tolerance
		Nitrodisc	8–16 cm²	Up to 24 h	
		Nitro-Dur	5–30 cm²/d		
		Transderm-Nitro	2.5–15 mg/d	Up to 24 hr	Tolerance
		Deponit	16–32 cm²/day	5–10 min	
	Nasal mucosa;	Spray;	0.4 per dose		
	intravenous	solution	10–200 µg/min		
		Sublingual	5–15 mg	Onset 5–10 min, effect up to 60 min	
Isosorbide dinitrate		Oral	5–80 mg bid–tid	2–8 h	
		Spray	1.25 mg on tongue	2–3 min	
		Chewable	5 mg qd	2 min–2½ h	
		Oral/sustained release	40 mg qd–bid	2–6 h	
		Intravenous	1.25–5 mg/h		
		Ointment	100 mg/24 h	Not effective during continuous therapy; tolerance	
Isosorbide-5-mononitrate (ISMO)	oral	Tablets	20 mg bid (7 h apart) 120–240 mg qd (slow release)	12–14 h after 2 wk	Same
Pentarythritol tetranitrate	Oral	Tablets	10–60 mg q6h	4–6 h	Same
Erythrityl tetranitrate	Sublingual	Tablets	5–15 mg q6h	3–6 h	Same
	Oral	Tablets	10–30 mg q6h	4–6 h	

*Period of time that a dose has antianginal effect.

155

The patient usually describes the discomfort as a heaviness, pressure, squeezing sensation, tightness, or choking. The patient rarely describes his or her symptoms as classic pain. Prompt relief with sublingual nitroglycerin or rest is a hallmark of chronic stable angina. When all of these features are present, the pain is typical (definite) angina. If any one of the features is absent, the pain is probably angina. If more than one feature is absent, the pain is considered atypical angina. **A stable pattern of pain in terms of frequency, severity, duration, and provocation is a feature of chronic stable angina.** The classification of pain as atypical, probable, or definite angina defines the likelihood of significant coronary artery disease being present. In men, the presence of angiographically demonstrable coronary artery disease for atypical, probable, or definite angina is 22%, 60%, and 88%, respectively. In women, the incidence is 5%, 35%, and 58%.

The **Canadian Cardiovascular Society Classification** is useful in describing the severity of angina to guide therapy (Table 4–5). Formal assessment of exercise capacity helps define the severity of incapacity as well as identifies factors that may be associated with a poor prognosis. Such factors include short exercise duration, marked ST depression at low workloads, and a hypotensive or poor (failure of systolic pressure to exceed 130 mm Hg) blood pressure response during exercise.

a. Diagnosis. A detailed and systematic history will most often uncover the diagnosis of ischemic heart disease. The physical examination often is normal. The most commonly used test in the diagnosis of ischemic heart disease is the exercise treadmill test. The specificity of exercise testing can be improved by IV administration of thallium-201 or technetium-99m sestamibi (Tc-sestamibi) to determine regional myocardial perfusion. Coronary angiography is indicated in patients with chronic stable and unstable angina who have failed medical therapy and in patients with suspected left main or severe three-vessel disease or both. Other indications for coronary angiography include patients with repeated hospitalizations for anginal symptoms, patients with careers that involve the

TABLE 4–5. **Grading of Angina of Effort by the Canadian Cardiovascular Society**

I. Ordinary physical activity does not cause angina. Angina occurs with unusually strenuous or prolonged exertion at work or recreation.

II. Slight limitation of ordinary activity. Angina may occur with walking or climbing stairs rapidly, walking uphill, walking or stair climbing after meals, in cold, in wind, under emotional stress, or only during the few hours after awakening. Walking more than 2 blocks on the level and climbing more than 1 flight of ordinary stairs at a normal pace and in normal conditions may cause angina.

III. Marked limitation of ordinary physical activity. Walking 1 to 2 blocks on the level and climbing 1 flight of stairs in normal conditions and at normal pace may cause angina.

IV. Inability to carry on any physical activity without discomfort. Anginal syndrome may be present at rest.

safety of others (e.g., airline pilots), and patients who require a definitive diagnosis to guide medical therapy.

b. **Treatment.** Management of patients with ischemic heart disease involves individualized therapy with special emphasis on **risk factor reduction.** Medical therapy includes aspirin 325 mg PO daily for both primary and secondary prevention. Beta blockers reduce the myocardial oxygen demand by inhibiting an increase in heart rate during exercise. Calcium channel antagonists are also recommended to treat angina pectoris and may be the initial drug of choice in certain circumstances. Short-acting calcium channel blockers should be avoided when treating patients with angina pectoris. Nitrates also play an important role in the management of angina pectoris. They reduce myocardial wall tension and oxygen demand by decreasing venous return to the right heart. In addition, nitrates increase coronary blood flow to the subendocardium. A common problem associated with nitrate use is the development of tolerance, which usually develops with 12 to 24 hours of continuous use.

Use of a long-acting medication that requires once-daily administration may improve compliance, but this decision needs to be balanced against the possible increased cost and side effects of long-acting preparations. If symptoms are not adequately controlled, a combination of two or three classes of antianginal agents is recommended. When using combination therapy, it is important to understand the interactions of individual classes of drugs. Verapamil and diltiazem may produce disturbances in cardiac conduction, particularly when used in conjunction with beta blockers.

In addition to antianginal pharmacologic therapy, care should be taken to identify and treat other factors that may alter the supply and demand balance in any given patient, such as anemia, hypoxemia (COPD, sleep apnea, or interstitial pulmonary disease), congestive heart failure, thyroid dysfunction, or use of sympathomimetic drugs.

c. **Indications for mechanical revascularization.** In chronic stable angina, there are three major indications for intervention with mechanical therapy. However, the availability and the safety of these procedures should not replace the continuing need to modify risk factors and change lifestyles.

(1) *Symptoms.* Patients with symptoms not adequately controlled with medical therapy are candidates for intervention with mechanical therapy.

(2) *Functional impairment.* Patients with very abnormal exercise test results may require mechanical therapy depending on their coronary anatomy and response to medical therapy.

(3) *Anatomy.* Patients with left main coronary artery stenosis or patients with three-vessel disease and impaired left ventricular function may benefit from mechanical therapy for improved survival.

2. UNSTABLE ANGINA (CRESCENDO ANGINA). The term *unstable angina* is used to describe a variety of clinical syndromes. There are three distinct

types of patients who fall within the group of unstable angina pectoris: (1) patients without previous anginal symptoms (new onset angina), (2) patients with a history of chronic stable angina in whom the pattern of angina changes in frequency and severity and in whom provoking factors are less than previously noted or less responsive to nitroglycerin, and (3) those with angina at rest. Unstable angina may also occur after MI (post-MI angina) or may even awaken patients from sleep at night (nocturnal angina). The pain of unstable angina may be so prolonged that it may not be distinguishable from that of acute MI. The mechanism responsible for the development of unstable angina usually involves a change in myocardial oxygen supply as a result of progressive atherosclerosis, transient platelet aggregation, thrombus formation or increased coronary vasomotor tone occurring at the site of endothelial injury, or plaque rupture.

a. **Treatment.** Because the symptoms of unstable angina may be similar to those of acute MI, these patients should be admitted to the hospital immediately for observation and monitoring. Acute MI should be ruled out by means of serial ECGs and cardiac enzyme determinations. ECGs recorded during episodes of pain will often show ischemic changes. The presence of transient ST elevation should raise the possibility of a vasospastic element.

Patients with unstable angina often are receiving therapy that will affect treatment choices. Doses of antianginal medications should be adjusted to achieve optimal heart rate and blood pressure control. Concomitant medical problems, anemia, hypertension, tachycardia, arrhythmias, and congestive heart failure should be treated. Chewable aspirin 325 mg should be administered immediately after the diagnosis is made.

In patients whose pain is not initially controlled with bed rest, sedation, and optimization of oral medications, a nitroglycerin infusion and heparinization (to keep partial thromboplastin time 1.5 to 2 times the control value) are advised. Nitroglycerin is administered intravenously with an initial dose of 10 μg/min, which is titrated up every 5 to 10 minutes to control pain or until the systolic blood pressure is less than 110 mm Hg. If the patient becomes hypotensive, **reduce** the infusion rate, **elevate** the foot of the bed, and **give** intravenous fluids if necessary. Reflex tachycardia can be managed by increasing doses of a beta-blocking drug. Nitroglycerin should not be mixed in a plastic bottle, as it is absorbed by polyvinylchloride. When the pain has resolved and while the nitroglycerin infusion is being tapered, treatment with oral medications should be instituted.

If patients fail to respond to nitroglycerin infusion and other pharmacologic interventions, arteriography, with consideration of mechanical intervention, is recommended. The use of the intraaortic balloon pump in refractory cases may be a temporizing measure while arranging for angiography and subsequent surgery or angioplasty. The intraaortic balloon pump decreases the afterload pressure of the heart, thus reducing myocardial oxygen demand. For those patients who respond to pharmacologic interventions, stratification and early cardiac angiography are recommended in the high-risk group. The decision for mechanical intervention should be individualized and based on symptoms and laboratory data.

b. **Thrombolytic agents in unstable angina.** Thrombolytic agents have clearly affected the morbidity and mortality of AMI. However, given the pathophysiology of unstable angina, thrombolytic therapy has no demonstrable benefit and has been shown to actually increase morbidity and mortality.

c. **Thrombin inhibitors.** The thrombin inhibitors (hirulog, hirudin) failed to demonstrate increased efficacy over heparin therapy. Therefore, the use of these agents in unstable angina or MI has not been favored.

d. **New antiplatelet agents: platelet glycoprotein IIb/IIIa inhibitors.** Platelets play an important role in the pathophysiology of unstable angina and MI. Aspirin, the most commonly used antiplatelet agent, inhibits cyclooxygenase and thus prevents the production of thromboxane A_2 but leaves other pathways for platelet aggregation to proceed. Platelet glycoprotein (GP) IIb/IIIa receptor binds fibrinogen and is the final pathway leading to platelet aggregation. The GP IIb/IIIa inhibitors are potent inhibitors of platelet aggregation and are undergoing extensive evaluation at present. Several GP IIb/IIIa inhibitors have been tested in patients with unstable angina and acute MI and have shown favorable results. The GP IIb/IIIa inhibitors undergoing evaluation at present are shown in Table 4–6.

3. SILENT MYOCARDIAL ISCHEMIA. Silent myocardial ischemia occurs when there is objective evidence of ischemia in the absence of symptoms. Since the advent of continuous ambulatory ECG monitoring, many patients with typical stable angina have been found to have frequent episodes of asymptomatic ischemia. Three subsets of these patients have been classified by Cohn: **type I,** patients with coronary artery disease who have never experienced symptoms; **type II,** patients who have had an MI and subsequently exhibit painless ischemia on exercise testing; **type III,** patients with angina pectoris who have intermittent episodes of silent ischemia.

TABLE 4–6. **Glycoprotein IIb/IIIa Inhibitors Recently Evaluated in Clinical Trials**

AGENT	TYPE	STUDY
Abciximal Fab (ReoPro)*	Monoclonal antibody	EPIC, EPILOG TAMI-8
MK-852	Cyclic RGD peptide	
Integrelin	Cyclic KGD peptide	IMPACT-1, II, AND AMI
Lamifiban	Peptide derivative	
Tirofiban	Nonpeptide	RESTORE
Xemlofiban	Orally active agent	

*Licensed for use during angioplasty by the FDA.

The full clinical implications of silent ischemia are not well understood, but several longitudinal studies have demonstrated an increased incidence of ischemia, MI, and sudden death in asymptomatic patients with positive exercise tests. In addition, patients with asymptomatic ischemia who have had an MI are at greater risk for a second coronary event. Ischemia can occur with or without evidence of increased myocardial oxygen demand (increased product of heart rate and blood pressure).

a. **Treatment.** There have been few studies to evaluate if pharmacologic intervention for silent myocardial ischemia has the same effect as seen in patients who manifest symptoms of angina pectoris. It appears that the same principles apply and that all three classes of antianginal drugs may be beneficial. The use of aspirin in patients with asymptomatic ischemia after MI has been shown to reduce coronary events. Because vasoconstriction is thought to be a significant pathophysiologic component of this condition, a calcium channel blocking agent is recommended as first-line therapy. Beta-blocking agents may also be used.

The management of patients with asymptomatic myocardial ischemia must be individualized. Treatment intervention should be based on the following: the degree of positivity of the exercise stress test, with particular attention to the stage at which ECG evidence of ischemia appears, the magnitude and number of perfusion defects seen on thallium scintigraphy (exercise stress test with thallium scintigraphy is recommended), the ECG localization of ischemia, and change in left ventricular function documented on radionuclide ventriculography or echocardiography. Coronary arteriography is recommended in patients with evidence of severe ischemia on noninvasive testing. Asymptomatic patients with silent ischemia and significant left main coronary artery disease or three-vessel coronary artery disease and impaired left ventricular function are appropriate candidates for coronary artery bypass surgery. In the ACIP study, revascularization was better than medical therapy in suppressing ECG changes and reducing hospitalization over a 1-year period of follow-up. Patients with silent myocardial ischemia require close follow-up with noninvasive testing to determine change in left ventricular function and time to positivity of the exercise stress test.

4. VARIANT ANGINA (CORONARY ARTERY SPASM, PRINZMETAL'S ANGINA). The pain associated with coronary artery spasm is similar to that of other forms of angina pectoris and responds to nitroglycerin. A major difference is that the pain is spontaneous. It occurs predominantly at rest, especially in the early hours of the morning. The pain is usually not provoked by exertion.

Coronary artery spasm should be suspected on the basis of the patient's history. Patients sometimes note that beta blockers exacerbate symptoms. Transient elevation of the ST segment on the ECG with an episode of pain is highly suggestive of spasm. Provocation of spasm with intravenous ergonovine is the most effective method for diagnosis. However, acetylcholine, an endothelial cell-dependent vasodilating agent, is now frequently used to demonstrate endothelial cell vasore-activity. Provocation with ergonovine or acetylcholine is not recommended in patients with significant fixed obstructive coronary artery disease. Spasm can occur in any coronary artery, although the right coronary artery is most commonly affected. Multivessel spasm is extremely rare; when it occurs, it is associated with intractable ventricular tachycardia.

a. **Treatment.** The sine qua non of variant angina is a history of spontaneous or unprovoked episodes of typical angina. The differential diagnosis on presentation should be unstable angina until proved otherwise. Acute treatment of the chest pain episode is generally sublingual nitroglycerin. Calcium channel blocking agents are the long-term treatment of choice for this condition. In most cases, a single agent is sufficient, but in resistant cases, combination therapy with diltiazem and nifedipine or verapamil and nifedipine around the clock is useful. Continuous nitrate therapy is not recommended because of problems with tolerance, but targeted nitrates may be helpful in patients with a predictable pattern of pain. Beta-blocking drugs are contraindicated.

The natural history of spasm is one of periods of symptomatic exacerbation followed by periods of relative quiescence. If a patient has been without symptoms for 6 to 12 months on therapy, withdrawal of therapy can be attempted. Patients with spasm who do not have significant fixed coronary stenoses are not candidates for mechanical intervention.

5. **ANGINA WITH NORMAL CORONARY ARTERIES (SYNDROME X, MICROVASCULAR ANGINA).** A diagnosis of angina with normal coronary arteries is suspected when there is a convincing history of anginal chest pain (with or without documented reversible ischemic ECG changes) and when angiography fails to demonstrate obstruction of major coronary vessels or spasm. Other causes of chest pain (esophageal spasm, acid reflux with esophagitis, gallbladder disease, cervical radiculopathy, Tietz's syndrome, and costochrondritis) should be excluded.

The etiology of syndrome X is still not fully understood, although studies have demonstrated that some patients with syndrome X have an abnormal vasodilating response of their small or resistance vessels (diminished coronary reserve), whereas other patients apparently have a low pain threshold or other noncardiac causes of pain.

The clinical features of microvascular angina are similar to those of classic angina, although atypical features are common, including rest pain, prolonged pain, and pain that is less responsive to nitroglycerin. Although there is no apparent gender difference in the perception of angina, the syndrome of microvascular angina is found predominantly in women.

a. **Treatment.** Many patients with microvascular angina respond to beta blockers, calcium channel blockers, and nitrates. However, a large number continue to have pain. The natural history of the disorder is variable. Many patients have resolution of symptoms with time but may have periods of exacerbation. Even in patients with persistent symptoms there does not appear to be a risk for MI or sudden death. Patient reassurance is an important part of therapy.

Bostom AG, Cupples AL, Jenner JL, et al. Elevated plasma lipoprotein (a) and coronary heart disease in men aged 55 years and younger: a retrospective study. JAMA 1996;276:544–548.

Braunwald E, ed. Heart Disease: A Text Book of Cardiovascular Medicine, 4th ed. Philadelphia: W.B. Saunders Co., 1992.

Lobo RA, Notelovitz M, Bernstein L, et al. Lp(a) lipoprotein: relationship to cardiovascular disease risk factors, exercise, and estrogen. Am J Obstet Gynecol 1992;166:1128–1190.

Opie LH, ed. Drugs of the Heart, 4th ed. Philadelphia: W.B. Saunders Co., 1995.

Prospective Randomized Amlodipine Survival Evaluation (PRAISE) Trial. Presented at the American College of Cardiology 45th Annual Scientific Session, March 27, 1996.

Rogers W, Bourassa MG, Andrews T, et al. Asymptomatic Cardiac Ischemia Pilot (ACIP) Study: 1 year follow-up. Circulation 1994;90(part 2):1–17 (abstract).

Willerson JT. Medical treatment of coronary heart disease. In: Willerson JT, ed. Treatment of Heart Disease. New York: Gower Medical Publishing, 1992.

II. MYOCARDIAL INFARCTION

A. General Management of Acute MI

Management of acute myocardial infarction (AMI) has changed considerably in the past several years. The major change has been the use of thrombolytic therapy, antiplatelet agents, and angioplasty to reestablish arterial patency and limit infarct size. Figure 4–1 shows an approach to the **triage** of patients

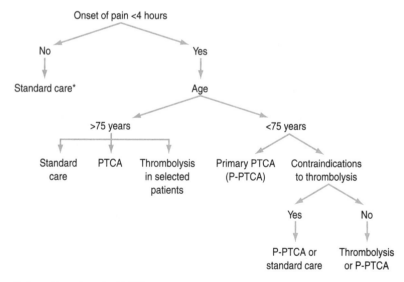

*Patients with ongoing pain with ECG evidence of ongoing ischemia may be candidates for intervention.

FIGURE 4–1. History suggesting acute myocardial infarction and electrocardiographic (ECG) changes with ST elevation. Triage strategy. PTCA, percutaneous transluminal coronary angioplasty.

with acute infarction. The most crucial aspect of intervention management is aimed at preserving myocardium and reestablishment of coronary flow within a critical time frame. Studies indicate that maximum benefit is achieved from lytic therapy when it is initiated within 1 to 3 hours after the onset of symptoms. Modest benefit is attained when therapy is instituted 3 to 6 hours after the onset of infarction, and some benefit is possible up to 12 hours if chest pain is ongoing and ST segment elevation is apparent in ECG leads that do not demonstrate new Q-waves.

General **contraindications to lytic therapy** include recent surgery or head trauma, active internal bleeding, suspected aortic dissection, pregnancy, diabetic hemorrhagic retinopathy, severe hypertension, and history of cerebral vascular accident or previous allergic reaction to the thrombolytic agent. Hemorrhagic stroke is the most frequent complication. The rate increases with advancing age, with patients age >70 years experiencing twice the rate as younger patients. However, several studies have shown that this group of patients benefits from lytic therapy. Decisions about thrombolytic therapy must be made on a case-by-case-basis in these patients.

1. PAIN RELIEF. **Morphine 2–6 mg IV** should be given every 5 to 30 minutes. Many patients require large doses, and a total of up to 15 to 20 mg may be needed. Caution must be used in elderly patients and patients with COPD.

2. NITROGLYCERIN (NTG) paste or infusion is used if patients continue to have ongoing ischemia. NTG reduces systemic vascular resistance and pulmonary capillary wedge pressure and increases collateral coronary blood flow to the subendocardium, thereby protecting ischemic myocardium. When NTG is administered, an adequate coronary perfusion pressure should be maintained (IV NTG 10 µg/min initial dose and up to 200 µg/min for the first 24 to 48 hours is usually administered).

3. OXYGEN THERAPY at 2–3 L/min via nasal prongs and sedation is given as required.

4. Patients should be on a LIGHT DIET during the first 24 hours.

5. ARRHYTHMIA PREVENTION. Studies have failed to demonstrate any survival advantage for patients given prophylactic antiarrhythmic therapy after admission to a monitored unit. Arrhythmias should be promptly diagnosed and treated to prevent further deterioration related to increased myocardial oxygen demands, decreased cardiac output, or electrical instability. The routine use of lidocaine is not recommended.

6. BETA-ADRENERGIC BLOCKERS. The early use of IV beta blockers for patients with increased heart rate in the absence of contraindications (congestive heart failure, hypotension, bradycardia, AV block) has been shown to reduce myocardial oxygen demand, infarct size, and ventricular fibrillation. In addition, beneficial effects of long-term beta blocker use have been well documented in large-scale trials, which have demonstrated reduction in mortality, reinfarction, and sudden death. Caution must be taken when administering beta blockers because of their occasional unpredictable hemodynamic effects. Propranolol (0.5 mg increments IV up to a total of 0.1 mg/kg) and metoprolol (5 mg every 5

minutes to a total of 15 mg IV) are the most commonly used beta blockers at this time.

7. ANTICOAGULANTS AND ANTIPLATELET. Thrombus and platelet aggregation plays an important role in the pathogenesis of AMI. The use of heparin and aspirin to impede the process is indicated. Both heparin and aspirin have been shown to reduce the risk of fatal and nonfatal MI. Unless contraindicated, aspirin 325 mg daily should be given to all patients. This should be started immediately by having the patient chew an aspirin. Heparin is generally administered as a 5000 U bolus IV, followed by a continuous infusion of 1000 U/h and adjusted to keep the partial thromboplastin time 1.5 to 2 times normal. Heparin may also be administered by weight adjustment.

8. CALCIUM CHANNEL BLOCKERS. Calcium channel blockers have been shown to be effective in acute and chronic stable angina, but there have been conflicting reports about their use in AMI. Patients with continued post-MI ischemia caused by coronary vasospasm may benefit from a calcium channel blocker. Diltiazem, in both long-term and short-term studies, has demonstrated beneficial effects (prevention of reinfarction and reduction in mortality) following non–Q-wave MI in patients who do not have CHF.

9. ANGIOTENSIN-CONVERTING ENZYME (ACE) INHIBITORS. ACE inhibitors have demonstrated improvement in mortality as well as the prevention of heart failure and recurrent MI in patients with left ventricular function of 40% or less. ACE inhibitors should be started once the patient is hemodynamically stable.

B. Acute Transmural MI

1. PATHOPHYSIOLOGY. The pathophysiology of AMI has been controversial since Hippocrates first postulated that heart disease can cause sudden death. The causes of MI can be divided into those that decrease myocardial oxygen supply and those that increase myocardial oxygen demand. Atherosclerotic plaque is the most common cause for reduction of coronary blood flow, thereby reducing oxygen supply. These plaques reduce the cross-sectional area of coronary artery lumen, thus reducing coronary perfusion pressure. When a critical stenosis develops, coronary blood flow is adequate at rest but cannot increase to meet metabolic demand. The subendocardium blood reserve becomes much more limited than that of the subepicardium. **In most cases, MI occurs when an atherosclerotic plaque ruptures, leading to thrombus formation with resultant coronary artery occlusion.**

2. SYMPTOMS. Classically, AMI is diagnosed as a constellation of symptoms. Chest pain described as pressure, heaviness, squeezing, crushing, and ache is often associated with nausea, vomiting, diaphoresis, and shortness of breath. Generally, the pain involves the sternum or epigastrium (or both), and in many cases, it may radiate to the arm, elbow, jaw, or neck. Any combination of these symptoms may occur in an individual patient. Epigastrium pain secondary to AMI may be misdiagnosed as indigestion. In the elderly patient, AMI may occur as a

sudden onset of shortness of breath, weakness, loss of consciousness, or confusion. Chest discomfort in AMI may be atypical or may be absent in 15% to 30% of AMI cases (silent AMI).

3. LABORATORY FINDINGS. The initial ECG shows ST elevation in the leads reflecting the area of the myocardium involved. As the ECG changes evolve, the associated T waves may be tall and peaked. Within hours, the T waves usually become inverted, and Q waves develop. In the majority of cases, the ST segment returns to the baseline unless an aneurysm develops (then ST elevation persists). Cardiac enzymes (creatinine phosphokinase, CPK-MB) become elevated within 4 to 6 hours and peak around 18 to 24 hours. Lactic dehydrogenase (LDH) rises in 24 to 48 hours, and LDH_1, the cardiac isoenzyme, rises before total LDH ($LDH_1 > LHD_2$). Troponin-I increases within 4 to 8 hours after angina, peaks at 12 to 16 hours, and remains elevated for 5 to 9 days. It is more sensitive and specific for myocardial injury than CPK-MB. A measurement >1.5 ng/ml is suggestive of myocardial injury. A mild leukocytosis may persist for several days.

4. CARDIAC IMAGING. Myocardial perfusion imaging with thallium-201 or Tc-sestamibi, although very sensitive for the diagnosis of MI, cannot distinguish AMI from old scar. 2-Dimensional echocardiography can be of value to identify wall motion abnormalities, to estimate left ventricular ejection fraction, pericardial effusion, ventricular aneurysm, or left ventricular thrombus, and to coordinate clinical and physical diagnosis of right ventricular infarction. Doppler echocardiography is useful in the detection of mitral and tricuspid regurgitation and ventricular and atrial septal defects (VSD and ASD).

5. REPERFUSION IN ACUTE MYOCARDIAL INFARCTION. Approaches to the management of AMI have changed significantly in the past decade based on a better understanding of the pathophysiologic mechanism involved. The primary goal in the treatment of AMI centers on limiting myocardial damage through early restoration of coronary blood flow. This can be achieved through thrombolytic therapy and mechanical interventions.
   a. **Thrombolytic therapy.** Several large trials have demonstrated that both endogenous and exogenous thrombolytic agents reduce mortality and morbidity from AMI by achieving vascular reperfusion. Thrombolytic agents directly or indirectly activate plasminogen. Table 4–7 describes their characteristics.
      (1) Streptokinase. Streptokinase (SK) is given as a 1-hour IV infusion of 1.5 million units. Aspirin, 324 mg, is also given at this stage. Allergic reactions may be treated with corticosteroids and diphenhydramine. Streptokinase opens vessels in 50% to 60% of cases when given within 6 hours of onset of symptoms. As with any agent that is effective in reestablishing blood flow to ischemic or infarcted myocardium, reperfusion arrhythmias, such as ventricular tachycardia, frequent ventricular ectopy, and various degrees of heart block, may occur.
      Following streptokinase therapy, an **IV heparin** infusion is started to maintain the activated partial thromboplastin time

TABLE 4–7. **Characteristics of Thrombolytic Agents**

	SK	APSAC	t-PA	scu-PA	UK
Fibrin selective	No	No	Yes	Yes	Yes
Plasminogen binding	Indirect	Indirect	Direct	Direct	Direct
Duration of infusion (min)	60	2–5	90–180	90–180	5–15
Half-life (min)	23	90	8	7	16
Fibrinogen breakdown	4+	3+	1–2+	2+	3+
Early heparin required	No	No	Yes	No	Yes
Hypotension	Yes	Yes	No	No	No
Allergic reactions	Yes	Yes	No	No	No
Approximate cost/dose	$200/1.5 MU	$1200/30 U	$2200/100 mg	High	$2200/3 MU
Patency at 90 min	53–65	55–65	69–79	71	66
Patency at 24 h	81–88	88–92	78–85	85	73

Abbreviations: APSAC, anisoylated plasminogen streptokinase activator complex (anistreplase); SK, streptokinase; t-PA, tissue plasminogen activator; UK, urokinase; scu-PA, single-chain urokinase (pro-urokinase) plasminogen activator; MU, million units; U, units.

(PTT) at a level of 1.5 to 2 times the control value. Heparin therapy is maintained for about 48 hours.

(2) **Anisoylated plasminogen-streptokinase activator complex (APSAC, Eminase).** APSAC, a modification of the streptokinase molecule, is administered over 2 to 5 minutes by IV infusion of 30 mg. Plasma half-life is 95 minutes. The reperfusion rate is time dependent and is similar to that of streptokinase. IV heparin infusion is started after infusion of APSAC.

(3) **Urokinase.** This form of lytic therapy has the advantage over SK of not causing an allergic reaction. It is more expensive than streptokinase but less expensive than tissue plasminogen activator (rt-PA). The agent has similar indications, contraindications, and effects to SK. The IV dosage is 3 million units over 45 to 60 minutes. Therapy is followed by heparinization.

(4) **Single-chain urokinase plasminogen activator (scu-PA).** Scu-PA is the precursor of urokinase. Preliminary studies have shown that scu-PA in a dose range of 30 mg to 50 mg has shown a low performance rate and has taken a long time to reperfuse. More recent evidence suggests augmentation of the efficacy of scu-PA when used in combination with urokinase or t-PA.

(5) **Tissue plasminogen activator (rt-PA, Alteplase).** rt-PA is an endogenous plasminogen activator that is secreted by the vascular endothelium. It has a high affinity for specific binding sites. The current recommended dose is 100 mg (60 mg over 1 hour, 40 mg over the next 2 hours). Front-loading of rt-PA (initial bolus of 15 mg, followed by 50 mg over 30 minutes, then 35 mg over 1 hour) is also acceptable. Major bleeding is an infrequent but serious side effect. After use of rt-PA, heparinization for 48 hours and chewable aspirin are recommended. The cost of rt-PA is several times that of SK. Though rt-PA has been demonstrated to have a higher acute patency rate than SK, differences in clinical outcomes in patients treated with SK or rt-PA have not been demonstrated. The choice of thrombolytic agent at the present time must be made on a case-by-case basis.

(6) **New types of t-PA.** In the quest to find a more efficacious thrombolytic agent with less side effects, a mutant or chimeric t-PA is currently undergoing clinical investigation (TIMI 10, TIMI 10B). TNK-t-PA has a longer half-life, is more resistant to plasminogen activator inhibition, and appears to have increased thrombolytic efficacy.

b. **Percutaneous transluminal coronary angioplasty.** Percutaneous transluminal coronary angioplasty (PTCA) is a widely used method of revascularization, especially for severely symptomatic single or two-vessel disease and in selected patients with three-vessel disease with suitable stenoses. Patients with stenosis of the left main coronary artery and those with three-vessel disease and decreased left ventricular function are candidates for revascularization by coronary artery bypass graft (CABG). Studies have shown that in the short-term (1 to 3 years) there are no major differences in survival or MI between PTCA and CABG in appropriately selected patients.

Restenosis (30% to 35%) remains the Achilles heel of PTCA. However, with newer devices (stents) and pharmacologic agents (GP IIb/IIIa) restenosis rates have decreased to 15% to 20%.

The feasibility of performing PTCA as a primary treatment for AMI has been advocated for over a decade. Primary PTCA for AMI without preceding thrombolysis is very effective in restoring coronary perfusion during MI. Although the patency rate is in excess of 90% (compared with 75% to 80% for thrombolysis), the procedure is limited to approximately 15% to 20% of the population. Primary PTCA is limited to those patients who develop AMI in-hospital or those patients who can have the procedure performed within 30 to 45 minutes of presentation. Otherwise, thrombolytic therapy is the mainstay of treatment. Primary PTCA provides a long-term survival advantage, results in shorter hospital stays, and has a lower risk of stroke and bleeding complications than thrombolysis. Indications for primary PTCA in AMI are contraindication to thrombolytics, cardiogenic shock and myocardial ischemia, failure of thrombolysis (rescue PTCA), and recurrent myocardial ischemia postthrombolysis.

The **combination of intravenous thrombolysis and PTCA** has been the subject of a number of major clinical trials. These studies support a more conservative approach to mechanical reperfusion. There are no advantages to combining thrombolytic therapy and PTCA except in patients who demonstrate recurrent ischemia or show evidence of provocable ischemia on a predischarge exercise tolerance test.

C. Acute Nontransmural MI

Patients with MI are usually classified into two groups: **non-Q-wave infarction (nontransmural)** and **Q-wave infarction (transmural).** Classification is based on electrocardiographic findings but, more importantly, represents a difference in pathophysiologic mechanism that may have therapeutic and prognostic significance. Patients with nontransmural infarction may have symptoms similar to those with transmural infarction, although they are more likely to have a stuttering course like patients with unstable angina. The ECG changes are usually ST depression or T-wave inversions, which may persist or worsen over the first 24 to 48 hours. The diagnosis is made on the basis of clinical history, ECG changes, and the characteristic enzyme pattern (similar to that of transmural infarct, though usually with a lower peak CK). The pathophysiology is probably more like that of unstable angina than transmural infarction. Occlusive thrombus is uncommon, but some combination of plaque disruption, change in vasomotor tone, platelet aggregation, and transient subocclusive thrombus followed by reperfusion is likely to be the underlying cause. Many of these patients have diffuse coronary artery disease and may well go on to have unstable courses (hence, the concept of incomplete infarction). The efficacy of thrombolytic agents is unproved in this condition. **Care should be similar to that of transmural infarction.** Some believe that there should be a lower threshold for angiography and invasive therapy because of the high incidence of recurrent ischemia and subsequent infarction. Others believe that the clinical course and the usual stratification strategies are sufficient to select patients for more aggressive therapy.

D. Complications of Q-Wave and Non-Q-Wave MI

Regardless of the type and mechanism of infarction, all patients post-MI must be carefully monitored and managed because of the risk of complications in their course.

1. ACUTE COMPLICATIONS
    a. **Electrical disturbances.** Electrical disturbances are the most frequent complication associated with AMI and vary from premature atrial and ventricular beats to ventricular fibrillation (Table 4–8).
    b. **Conduction disturbances.** Ischemic injury can produce conduction disturbances at any level of the atrioventricular or intraventricular conduction system. **First degree AV block and Mobitz type I block** generally occur in the AV node and are commonly seen in patients with acute inferior MI (IMI). Both are usually transient. **Mobitz type II AV block** is usually associated with anterior MI. It often progresses suddenly to complete atrioventricular block (CHB). Treatment requires insertion of a temporary pacemaker electrode. **Complete AV block** may occur with IMI. In this circumstance, the block progresses from first to second to complete AV block; it is usually transient and may resolve within days. Complete AV block associated with acute anterior MI is generally sudden. Treatment is with a temporary pacemaker and later a permanent transvenous pacemaker if indicated, depending on the patient's subsequent course.
    c. **Intraventricular blocks.** Isolated left anterior fascicular block (LAFB) and left posterior fascicular block (LPFB) rarely progress to CHB. The combination of right bundle branch block (RBBB) with LAFB, LPFB, or first degree AV block (if new) has a high risk of progressing to CHB and constitutes an indication for the insertion of a temporary pacemaker. Similarly, a new LBBB in the setting of an AMI is an indication for a temporary pacemaker. Usually the infarct is anterior and extensive and is associated with a high mortality rate.
    d. **Volume depletion.** Volume depletion as the cause of hypotension should be suspected in patients with hypotension and clear lungs on examination and x-ray. It is particularly common in IMIs. If the patient does not respond promptly to aggressive volume expansion, the diagnosis requires documentation of low filling pressures and low cardiac output by a Swan-Ganz catheter to rule out other causes and guide volume replacement.
    e. **Right ventricular infarction.** Hypoperfusion caused by right ventricular (RV) infarction may be confused with that caused by hypovolemia, as both are associated with low, or normal, PCWP. RV infarction also usually occurs in the setting of inferior wall MI. Vigorous fluid therapy that raises both left and right ventricular filling pressures to an appropriate level is indicated. Patients may require RA pressures in the range of 15 to 20 in order to adequately fill the left ventricle.

TABLE 4–8. Arrhythmias Associated with Acute Myocardial Infarction

ARRHYTHMIA	PRIMARY THERAPY	SECONDARY THERAPY	OTHER
Ventricular fibrillation	Cardioversion, 200–400 Wsec; CPR	Bretylium IV, 5 mg/kg Lidocaine IV, 75–100 mg	
Ventricular tachycardia	Lidocaine IV, 75–100 mg, precordial thump, cardioversion	Procainamide IV, 0.5–1 g loading dose should be given	
Ventricular premature beats (≥6/min, 1–3 mg/min R on T, coupling, multifocal)	Lidocaine IV, 75–100 mg bolus, then 1–3 mg/min infusion	Procainamide IV, 0.5–1 g loading dose; 2–6 mg/min infusion oral quinidine	Exclude other causes, such as low K^+ or Mg^{2+}, digitalis intoxication
Ventricular asystole	CPR	Transthoracic or transvenous pacing	
Accelerated idioventricular rhythm			
Symptomatic	Lidocaine IV, 75–100 mg; pacing if heart block or inappropriate bradycardia is underlying only		
Asymptomatic	None, unless appropriate		
Accelerated junctional rhythm	None	Pacing	R/O digitalis toxicity
Sinus tachycardia	None	None	Seek underlying cause; reflects underlying heart failure requiring treatment; also R/O fever, anemia, hypovolemia
Sinus bradycardia			
Symptomatic	Atropine IV, 0.5–1 mg	Temporary transvenous pacemaker	
Asymptomatic	Atropine		
Atrial premature beats	None		
Paroxysmal supraventricular tachycardia	Carotid sinus massage; Digoxin IV, 0.25 mg	Propranolol IV, 0.5–2 mg; Verapamil IV, 5–10 mg; cardioversion	

Arrhythmia			
Atrial fibrillation	Digoxin IV, 0.25 mg	Propranolol IV, 0.5–2 mg; Verapamil IV, 5–10 mg; diltiazem IV, 20–25 mg bolus, then 5–15 mg/min infusion; cardioverson (synchronized)	May indicate early left ventricular failure
Atrial flutter	Digoxin IV, 0.25 mg	Propranolol IV, 0.5–2 mg; Verapamil IV, 5–10 mg; diltiazem IV, 20–25 mg bolus, then 5–15 mg/min infusion; cardioversion (synchronized)	May indicate early left ventricular failure
First degree	None		
Mobitz type I			
Asymptomatic	None		
Symptomatic	Atropine, temporary transvenous pacing		
Mobitz type II			
Asymptomatic	Temporary pacing		
Symptomatic	Temporary transvenous pacing		
Complete heart block	Temporary transvenous	Atropine IV, 0.5–1 mg; isoproterenol IV, infusion 1–2 µg/min	

f. Infarct extension. Infarct extension occurs in 10% to 30% of patients with AMI. It is diagnosed by reelevation of plasma CPK. New chest pain and new persistent ECG changes frequently but not universally develop. Infarct extension has been reported to occur more frequently in nontransmural MI, suggesting a higher prevalence of subtotal coronary occlusion. Since infarct extension results in further left ventricular dysfunction, aggressive management of post-MI ischemia is essential.

g. Post-MI ischemia. Post-MI ischemia may occur early or late after AMI. It is evidence that additional myocardium is at risk and may represent an incomplete or nontransmural myocardial infarction (non-Q-wave). This may also represent myocardial ischemia at a distance due to critical narrowing of a second coronary artery. Diagnosis may be made by the recurrence of classic angina pectoris with or without ECG changes after a pain-free period. Frequent bouts of CHF secondary to worsening left ventricular function or papillary muscle ischemia may be the only evidence that post-MI ischemia is occurring. In addition to pharmacologic intervention for treatment of ischemia and heart failure, coronary angiography and possible mechanical intervention should be undertaken.

h. Left ventricular failure. Left ventricular function is restricted by the extent of myocardial necrosis; this determines both short-term and long-term prognosis. To establish the prognosis of patients with AMI, Killip categorized patients into four hemodynamic subsets based on admission physical findings. The Cedars-Sinai Hemodynamic characterization is based on hemodynamic features.

Killip class
Class I: No signs of left ventricular failure
Class II: S_3 gallop and/or pulmonary congestion limited to basal lung segments
Class III: Acute pulmonary edema
Class IV: Shock syndrome

Cedars-Sinai hemodynamic class
Class I: PCW ≤ 18; CI > 2.2
Class II: PCW > 18; CI > 2.2
Class III: PCW ≤ 18; CI ≤ 2.2
Class IV: PCW > 18; CI ≤ 2.2

i. Management of pump failure. Invasive monitoring is essential in the management of patients with moderate to severe left ventricular dysfunction in the setting of AMI. This will enable hemodynamic differentiation of the causes of pump failure.

(1) Maintenance of adequate gas exchange requires careful attention. Hypoxemia can precipitate postinfarction ischemia. Supplemental O_2, intubation, or positive end-expiratory pressure (PEEP) may be required. Patients with AMI complicated by mild to moderate heart failure usually respond well to **diuretics.** This results in reduced pulmonary capillary wedge pressure (PCWP) and left ventricular end diastolic pressure (LVEDP), which, in turn, enhance myocardial O_2 perfusion. However, most patients are not total body volume overloaded.

Since the systolic and diastolic dysfunction accompanying MI necessitates relatively high filling pressures to maintain cardiac output, one must be careful not to induce hypovolemic hypotension through excess diuretics.

(2) **Vasodilators** are used in moderate to severe pump failure or in heart failure unresponsive to diuretics (patients with severe mitral regurgitation and ventricular septal defect). These drugs decrease afterload and left ventricular filling pressures, thereby increasing stroke volume and cardiac output. Since vasodilators have a propensity to induce systemic hypotension and decrease coronary perfusion, it is essential that left ventricular filling pressures be maintained at 18 to 20 mm Hg. Short-acting agents are recommended during the early stages of therapy (see Table 4–14, p. 182). After stabilization, long-acting agents may be used.

Administration of **digitalis** to patients with AMI has always been controversial. Digitalis is reserved at present for the treatment of patients with atrial fibrillation or atrial flutter and those with heart failure that persists beyond the acute management phase.

j. **Cardiogenic shock.** Cardiogenic shock is characterized by prolonged tissue hypoperfusion, low arterial blood pressure, markedly reduced cardiac output, and oliguria. The prognosis is extremely poor, with an in-hospital mortality of 80% to 100% in patients who are not candidates for acute mechanical intervention. The cause of cardiogenic shock must be determined in order to plan appropriate intervention. The diagnosis of acute mitral regurgitation secondary to papillary muscle rupture versus ventricular septal defect (VSD) is made by cardiac catheterization and echocardiography. Urgent surgical intervention, usually with intraaortic balloon support, is required. Cardiogenic shock due to pure left ventricular dysfunction may be treated with pharmacologic agents or intraaortic balloon counterpulsation (IABP). If there is an element of ongoing ischemia, some of these patients may be candidates for acute revascularization. Therefore, in appropriate patients, acute angiography should be performed.

2. LATE IN-HOSPITAL COMPLICATIONS OF AMI. Late in-hospital complications include ventricular arrhythmias, CHF, pericarditis, and mural thrombi.

a. **Ventricular arrhythmias** are generally seen in the early phase of AMI. The arrhythmia carries a poor prognosis if observed 4 to 7 days after the event. Long-term antiarrhythmic therapy is often necessary, and electrophysiologic studies may be required to guide therapy.

b. **Congestive heart failure.** Moderate to severe pump failure is usually recognized in the acute phase. However, mild to moderate CHF in some patients is not recognized until the rehabilitation phase. Treatment may only be a diuretic. Digitalis may be indicated if cardiomegaly and S3 gallop persist. Initiation of afterload reduction with an ACE inhibitor not only may improve symptoms but also may improve ventricular geometry and long-term ventricular function.

c. **Pericarditis and Dressler's syndrome.** Acute pericarditis is a frequent complication of AMI occurring within 1 to 4 days after MI. A friction rub can be heard in many cases; it is potentiated by the supine position. One must distinguish acute pericarditis pain from that of recurrent ischemia. This pain may be treated with aspirin.

A delayed form of pericarditis called *Dressler's syndrome* may occur 1 week to several months post-AMI. It is thought to be secondary to an immunologic or autoimmune mechanism. A clinical picture of fever, malaise, anorexia, and arthralgia is often seen. Pleural effusion and even pulmonary infiltration may occur. Treatment is with aspirin or other anti-inflammatory drugs.

d. **Mural thrombi** tend to occur in patients with an acute anterior wall MI with or without aneurysm formation as early as 36 hours after infarction. Systemic embolization is infrequent. Diagnosis may be made by 2-dimensional echocardiography. Immediate anticoagulation with heparin followed by warfarin for 3 to 6 months is indicated if there are no contraindications. In the absence of contraindications, prophylactic anticoagulation should be considered in all patients with large anterior MI, even in the absence of intramural thrombus on 2-D echo. This strategy has not been subjected to prospective randomized study, however.

e. **Ventricular rupture** generally occurs between 5 and 7 days after transmural AMI in approximately 1% of patients. It is usually catastrophic and is associated with electromechanical dissociation. Rarely do patients survive.

E. Rehabilitation

Rehabilitation of the AMI patient occurs in two phases.

1. PHASE I (IN-HOSPITAL). Patients with uncomplicated AMI should stay approximately 24 to 48 hours in a CCU. They should begin leg exercise immediately and progressive ambulation within 48 to 72 hours. Progressive increase in activity is aimed at return to a normal lifestyle.

   Before discharge, most patients should have a **low-level exercise test** for risk stratification. Such testing may show evidence of ischemia, arrhythmia, or hypotension that might not have been observed otherwise. Depending on the data obtained, early invasive intervention may be indicated before discharge. Before leaving the hospital, all patients should be started on aspirin and a beta blocker (if there are no contraindications). Several studies have shown a decrease in mortality and reinfarction when patients with AMI are treated with a beta blocker. In addition, an ACE inhibitor should be initiated if the LVEF is ≤40%.

2. PHASE II (POSTHOSPITAL). This phase of rehabilitation is aimed at conditioning and return to normal function within 2 months and should include an organized program of walking. Later, this should be advanced to jogging as appropriate under supervised conditions. For long-term rehabilitation, a patient may enroll in an individual program. Advancement within rehabilitation depends on individual capabilities.

Over the past decade, several studies have shown that lifestyle intervention programs can have a significant impact on morbidity and mortality post-AMI. Finally, the psychological effects of AMI on patient and family alike can be crippling. Fear of death and hesitation in resuming social and sexual activities are best handled by the physician and family together.

F. Prevention

1. **RISK FACTORS FOR ATHEROSCLEROSIS.** Remediable risk factors are hypercholesterolemia, high blood pressure, and cigarette smoking. Age is a powerful risk factor. Others include diabetes mellitus, stress, family history of coronary artery disease, obesity, and sedentary lifestyle. Obesity has not been proved to be an independent risk factor of coronary artery disease; however, it is associated with hypertension, diabetes, and hypercholesterolemia.

   a. **Hypercholesterolemia.** In general, a cholesterol level less than 200 mg/dL is desirable. It is difficult to designate a limit for cholesterol: elevated serum cholesterol is multifactorial. Serum cholesterol varies from population to population. Atherosclerosis primarily correlates with elevated low-density lipoprotein (LDL) cholesterol. In addition, growing evidence supports the hypothesis that lipoprotein(a) (Lpa) and homocysteine may be a marker for the development of atherosclerosis. Elevation of high-density lipoprotein (HDL > 60 mg/dL) correlates negatively with atherosclerosis. Current guidelines suggest that patients without coronary artery disease and with two or more risk factors benefit when LDL < 130 mg/dL, whereas for those with coronary artery disease an LDL ≤ 100 mg/dL may be advantageous.

   b. **Hypertension.** The role of hypertension in coronary artery disease is twofold: it is a predisposing factor for atherosclerosis, and it increases myocardial O_2 demands in patients with coronary artery disease.

   c. **Cigarette smoking.** Cigarette smoking is related to the development of coronary thrombosis, AMI, and sudden death.

2. **PRIMARY PREVENTION.** Since atherosclerosis is a result of multiple risk factors, it is important to control several risk factors simultaneously (multiple risk factor intervention). The Oslo Study Group Intervention Trial demonstrated a significant reduction in incidence of first-time MI and sudden cardiac death in the trial group. The Multiple Risk Factor Intervention Trial (MRFIT) demonstrated a significantly lower overall mortality in the treatment group when multiple risk factors were addressed simultaneously in the subjects taking aspirin. **Aspirin** is used at present in primary prevention because it inhibits platelet aggregation, thus limiting thrombus formation in atherosclerotic plaques. Several studies have shown a reduction in MI.

3. **SECONDARY PREVENTION.** Secondary prevention is aimed at reducing the risk of complications, recurrence of AMI, or progression of disease in patients who have already had a complication from coronary artery disease. Many studies have confirmed the importance of drugs and

lifestyle changes in reducing the consequences of coronary artery disease. Such measures as the administration of aspirin or beta blockers reduce mortality following an AMI. Modification of factors predisposing to atherosclerosis also influence its progression. In addition, not only may lowering serum cholesterol retard the **progression** of atherosclerosis, but **regression** may occur in some patients. Secondary prevention trials have demonstrated also that exercise reduces weight, modifies the lipoprotein profile, and reduces mortality and morbidity from AMI.

AIMS Trial Study Group. Long-term effects of intravenous anistreplase in acute myocardial infarction: final report of the AIMS study. Lancet 1990;335:427–431.

Antman EM, for the TIMI-9A Investigators. Hirudin in acute myocardial infarction. Safety report from the thrombolysis and thrombin inhibition in myocardial infarction (TIMI) 9A trial. Circulation 1994;90:1624–1630.

Bypass Angioplasty Revascularization Investigation (BARI) Investigators. Comparison of coronary bypass surgery with angioplasty in patients with multivessel disease. N Engl J Med 1996;335:217–225.

Ellis EG, Holmes DR, eds. Strategic Approaches in Coronary Intervention. Baltimore: Williams & Wilkins, 1996.

Grimes CL, Browne KF, Marco J, et al. A comparison of immediate angioplasty with thrombolytic therapy for acute myocardial infarction. N Engl J Med 1993;328:673–679.

ISIS-2 Collaborative Group. Randomized trial of intravenous streptokinase, oral aspirin, both, or neither among 17,187 cases of suspected acute myocardial infarction: ISIS-2. Lancet 1988;2: 349–360.

Simoons MI, Betrin A, Col J. Thrombolysis with tissue plasminogen activator in acute myocardial infarction: no additional benefit from immediate coronary angioplasty. Lancet 1988;1:197–203.

Tcheng JE, et al. Glycoprotein IIb/IIIa receptor inhibitors: putting the EPIC, IMPACT, RESTORE and EPILOG trials into perspective. Am J Cardiol 1996;78(Suppl 3A):35–40.

TIMI Research Group. Comparison of invasive and conservative strategies after treatment with intravenous tissue plasminogen activator in acute myocardial infarction: results of the thrombolysis in myocardial infarction (TIMI) phase II trial. N Engl J Med 1989;320:618–627.

TIMI Research Group. Immediate versus delayed catheterization and coronary angioplasty following thrombotic therapy for acute myocardial infarction: TIMI IIA results. JAMA 1988;260: 2849–2858.

Topol EJ, Califf RM, Weisman HF, et al., on behalf of the EPIC Investigators. Reduction of clinical restenosis following coronary intervention with early administration of platelet IIb/IIIa integrin blocking antibody. Lancet 1994;343:881–886.

III. CONGESTIVE HEART FAILURE (CHF)

A. Pathogenesis and Implications for Treatment

Congestive heart failure (CHF) is a clinical syndrome characterized by pulmonary or systemic congestion or both and limited cardiac output, leading to the symptoms of dyspnea, fatigue, and edema. The proximate cause of this symptom complex is myocardial contractile dysfunction that leads to decreased stroke volume and triggers a series of acute compensatory neurohumoral mechanisms. These include the sympathetic nervous system, which mediates the associated tachycardia, increased inotropy in the residual viable myocardium, and arteriolar constriction to maintain organ perfusion in the face of decreased stroke volume, and the renin-angiotensin system, which mediates arteriolar vasoconstriction and sodium retention. These acute compensations are designed to maintain cardiac output and vital organ perfusion at or near normal resting levels. On a more chronic basis, ventricular remodeling occurs, designed to restore stroke volume through a greater reliance on the Starling mechanism. It is during this chronic phase of adaptation that the double-edged sword of neurohumoral activation and ventricular remodeling becomes manifest, contributing to the progression of the myopathy by the superimposition of increased afterload and fluid retention.

Chronic increases in cardiac filling pressures are the dominant determinants of the commonly encountered pulmonary and systemic venous congestion. The increased left-sided and right-sided filling pressures are a function of both increased cardiac volumes and decreased cardiac chamber compliance. The relative contribution of these two factors to the increases in pressures varies with the etiology of the heart failure syndrome. The decrease in chamber compliance is, in turn, a consequence of functional (impaired isovolumic relaxation, depressed contractility, increased ventricular load) and structural (myocardial fibrosis and scar, ventricular geometry) changes in the injured ventricle. As a consequence, when the increase in cardiac filling pressures is due principally to volume expansion, as in biventricular failure, diuretic therapy is the treatment of choice. However, when the increases in cardiac filling pressures are due to decreases in ventricular compliance, such as seen with myocardial ischemia, the reduction in filling pressures may best be achieved with afterload reduction and relief of myocardial ischemia.

When planning therapy for patients with heart failure, it is important to exclude potentially reversible causes and to identify surgically correctable lesions (valvular disease, ventricular aneurysm, and constrictive pericarditis). Echocardiography is useful to help screen for valvular disease. Coronary artery disease and consequent MI constitute the most common cause of depressed ventricular function in our society. Other causes for cardiomyopathy are listed in Table 4–9. In some patients with heart failure without an obvious cause, detailed cardiovascular evaluation, including catheterization and endomyocardial biopsy, may be appropriate.

The New York Heart Association classification (Table 4–10) is a useful way to stratify patients into a functional class according to the severity of their symptoms. Formal exercise stress testing provides additional functional evaluation.

B. Treatment of Heart Failure

Treatment of a syndrome as variable as CHF must be tailored to the patient. The aim of therapy in CHF is to reduce both preload and afterload, to relieve symptoms of atrial hypertension, and to improve cardiac output. Cardiac glycosides directly affect the myocardium to improve contractility and are useful in short-term but may have less benefit in long-term therapy. Diuretics benefit patients with mild failure (Tables 4–11 and 4–12), but in patients with moderate or severe failure, diuretics alone are insufficient.

In Table 4–13, vasoactive agents that can be used orally are listed. ACE inhibitors have been the mainstay of therapy for long-term use.

Among the drugs that can be used parenterally, direct-acting vasodilators are the mainstay (Table 4–14). Sympathomimetic drugs to improve inotropy and support blood pressure may be necessary in the severely ill patient but may pose a high risk for inducing arrhythmias, myocardial ischemia, or

TABLE 4–9. Common Causes of Cardiomyopathy Other than CAD

INFECTIVE	TOXIC
Viral	Alcohol
Coxsackie B	Bleomycin
Coxsackie A	Doxorubicin (Adriamycin)
ECHO	Lead
HIV	Corticosteroids
CMV	Cocaine
Parasitic	
Bacterial	**INFILTRATIVE**
Spirochetal	Amyloidosis
	Hemochromatosis
METABOLIC	Sarcoidosis
Thiamine deficiency	Neoplastic
Acromegaly	Glycogen storage disorders
Myxedema	
Thyrotoxicosis	**OTHERS**
Diabetes mellitus	Incessant tachycardia
Uremia	Endocardial fibroelastosis
Cushing's disease	Sickle cell anemia
Kwashiorkor	Neuromuscular disorders
Scurvy	Postpartum disorders
	Hypertrophic cardiomyopathy

peripheral vasoconstriction. It is sometimes appropriate to use **combination therapy,** such as dopamine and nitroprusside. The phosphodiesterase inhibitors (PDE), such as amrinone, can be combined with the sympathomimetic drugs. A potential concern about use of phosphodiesterase drugs is the risk of ischemia, arrhythmias, and apparent deterioration in cardiac function when the drugs are discontinued.

1. ACUTE THERAPY. The approach depends on the severity of the failure. Often, patients will be hypoxic, needing supplemental O_2 via nasal prongs, 3–4 L/min. In severe hypoxia and marked respiratory difficulty, intubation and mechanical ventilation may be necessary. In severe failure, particularly with AMI, Swan-Ganz catheter monitoring will help optimize pharmacologic therapy.

Text continued on page 183

TABLE 4–10. New York Heart Association Classification for Severity of Heart Failure

Class I	Ordinary physical activity does not cause undue dyspnea or fatigue.
Class II	Comfort is present at rest, but ordinary physical activity results in dyspnea or fatigue.
Class III	Comfort is present at rest, but less than ordinary physical activity results in dyspnea or fatigue.
Class IV	Dyspnea or fatigue may be present at rest and is made worse by any physical effort.

TABLE 4-11. Thiazide Diuretics: Doses and Duration of Action

GENERIC NAME	TRADE NAME	DOSAGE*	DURATION OF ACTION (h)
Hydrochlorothiazide	HydroDIURIL, Esidrix, Thiuretic	12.5–25 mg (BP) 25–100 mg (CHF)	6–12
Hydroflumethiazide	Saluron, Diucardin	12.5–25 mg (BP) 25–200 mg (CHF)	6–12
Chlorthalidone	Hygroton, Thalitone	12.5–50 mg	48–72
Metolazone	Zaroxolyn, Diulo	1–5 mg (BP) 5–20 mg (CHF)	18–25
Bendrofluazide	Naturetin	1.25–2.5 mg (BP) 10 mg (CHF)	6–12
Bendroflumethiazide			
Polythiazide	Renese	1–2 mg (BP)	24–48
Chlorothiazide	Diuril	250–1000 mg	6–12
Cyclothiazide	Anhydron	1–2 mg	6–12
Trichlormethiazide	Metahydrin, Naqua	1–4 mg	About 24
Indapamide	Lozol	2.5 mg (BP)	16–36

*BP, use for blood pressure lowering; CHF, use for congestive heart failure.

179

TABLE 4–12. Diuretics

DRUG	DOSAGE	ADMINISTRATION	DURATION OF ACTION (h)	SIDE EFFECTS
POTASSIUM-DEPLETING AGENTS				
Furosemide	20–240 mg/d or 2–20 mg/h	Oral IV	6–8 2	Hypokalemia, hypotension, hyperuricemia, skin rash, abnormal liver function
Bumetanide	0.5–2 mg/d	Oral IV	4–6 2–3	Muscle cramps, hypotension, dizziness, encephalopathy in patients wth liver disease
Ethacrynic acid	50–100 mg/d	Oral IV	12 2	Hypotension, hypokalemia
POTASSIUM-SPARING AGENTS				
Amiloride	5–15 mg/d	Oral	24	Hyperkalemia
Triamterene	100–200 mg/d	Oral	24	Hyperkalemia, nausea
Spironolactone	50–200 mg/d	Oral	24	Hyperkalemia, gynecomastia

TABLE 4–13. Nonparenteral Drugs for Congestive Heart Failure

CLASS	DOSAGE	VENODILATOR	ARTERIAL DILATOR	BP	CO	SVR	RAP
DIRECT-ACTING VASODILATORS							
Hydralazine	50–200 mg q6–8h	+/0	+++	0/–	++	–	0
Isosorbide dinitrate	20–60 mg q4–6h	+++	+	0/–	+	0/–	–
Nitroglycerin ointment	1.5–2 in. q6h	+++	+				
Nitroglycerin patches	5–30 cm² q12h	+	+				
ALPHA-RECEPTOR BLOCKADE							
Prazosin q8h	1–5 mg	+	++	–	+	–	–
CONVERTING ENZYME INHIBITORS							
Captopril	6.25–37.5 mg q6–8h	+	+++	–	+	–	–
Enalapril	2.5–10 mg qd or bid	+	+++	–	+	–	–
Lisinopril	5–20 mg qd	+	+++	–	+	–	–

BP, blood pressure; CO, cardiac output; SVR, systemic vascular resistance; RAP, right atrial pressure.
Key: +, increase; 0, no effect; –, moderate decrease; 0/–, no effect to moderate decrease.

TABLE 4-14. Parenteral Drugs for Congestive Heart Failure

CLASS	DOSAGE	VENODILATOR	ARTERIAL DILATOR	INOTROPIC EFFECT
DIRECT-ACTING VASODILATORS				
Nitroprusside	0.5–10 µg/kg/min	+	+++	0
Nitroglycerin	10–200 µg/min	+++	++	0
SYMPATHOMIMETIC AGENTS				
Dopamine	1–20 µg/kg/min	0	0	+++
Dobutamine	2.5–15 µg/kg/min	0	0	+++
PHOSPHODIESTERASE INHIBITORS				
Bipyridine derivatives				
Amrinone	0.5 mg/kg bolus × 2, 40 µg/kg/min infusion	0	+	+++
Milrinone	12.5–75 µg/kg (given as 10-mg boluses)	0	++	+++
DIURETICS				
Furosemide*	2–20 mg/h	+	0	0

*IV furosemide drips are effective parenteral therapy in decompensated CHF.
+, increase; 0, no effect.

a. **Mild failure.** Patients with mild failure can be treated with **diuretics** (Table 4–12) and **digoxin, 0.125–0.25 mg/d,** depending on the patient's size, age, and renal function. Digoxin is particularly effective for a patient with atrial fibrillation with a rapid ventricular response. Digoxin toxicity may be exacerbated by hypokalemia.

b. **Moderate to severe failure.** In this setting, **IV diuretics** are supplemented by afterload-reducing and preload-reducing agents. **IV nitroglycerin** offers both preload and afterload reduction and is the agent of choice in acute myocardial ischemia. **Nitroprusside** is also effective, especially as an afterload-reducing agent. It is the agent of choice if severe hypertension is present. If patients are not responding adequately, the addition of a sympathomimetic agent (dopamine or dobutamine) is appropriate. Inotropic agents increase cardiac output but differ widely in their effects on peripheral vascular resistance. As noted, these agents may induce myocardial ischemia. Therefore a more desirable agent may be necessary (such as a vasodilator). A vasodilator may induce hypotension by decreasing arterial pressure, thereby exacerbating cardiac ischemia. All agents must be used with caution in patients with ischemic heart disease and hypotension. General measures should include bed rest, diet control, and oxygen. Usually Swan-Ganz catheter monitoring at this stage is necessary. If failure persists, phosphodiesterase inhibitors (administered IV) may be added.

2. LONG-TERM THERAPY. Digoxin, diuretics, and ACE inhibitors form the basis for **conventional therapy** in the treatment of chronic CHF. There is overwhelming evidence to indicate that ACE inhibitors are the preferred treatment in chronic symptomatic CHF of any cause because of both improved survival and symptomatic and functional improvements. When ACE inhibitors are poorly tolerated, a combination of isordil and hydralazine is a suitable alternative. Most recently, digoxin was shown to be useful in reducing symptoms without adversely affecting survival in patients with symptomatic CHF, in contrast to other (milrinone, flosequinan, vesnarinone) oral inotropes. Finally, oral diuretics are useful in minimizing fluid retention in patients with CHF. Importantly, oral furosemide should be administered bid to avoid compensatory sodium retention following the 6-hour diuresis.

New evidence suggests that certain classes of agents may offer additional benefits in terms of symptomatic improvement and survival in subsets of patients with CHF. Novel vasodilators with evidence of efficacy in chronic CHF include the angiotensin II receptor antagonists (losartan) and second-generation dihydropyridines, such as amlodipine (PRAISE I), in select patients with idiopathic but not ischemic cardiomyopathy. Finally, there is renewed interest in the use of beta-adrenergic receptor antagonists in combination with alpha-adrenergic receptor antagonists (carvedilol) in the treatment of CHF with associated functional and survival benefits. In contrast to conventional therapies, the use of these **adjuvant therapies** may be limited to certain groups of patients with CHF depending on etiology and tolerance.

Another factor that should be considered in treating patients with dilated cardiomyopathy is the role of **anticoagulation** in preventing systemic emboli. Patients with evidence of myocarditis on biopsy may benefit from steroids and possibly immunosuppressive drugs. However, this has not been proved in prospective randomized studies.

In suitable candidates with refractory failure and severe impairment of cardiac capacity, cardiac transplantation should be considered (see section VI, pp. 198–201 on heart transplants).

C. Other Causes of Heart Failure

1. **CARDIOMYOPATHY ASSOCIATED WITH HYPERTENSION.** Some patients with long-standing hypertension develop marked left ventricular hypertrophy and experience effort-related dyspnea and pulmonary edema secondary to impaired left ventricular relaxation (left ventricular diastolic dysfunction). Evaluation of function with echocardiography or radionuclide scanning usually indicates preserved systolic function, but diastolic abnormalities can be detected. In this situation, **calcium channel blockers (verapamil, slow-release capsule, 240–360 mg/d; diltiazem, slow release 120–300 mg/d, or nifedipine, slow release 10–40 mg/d)** may lower blood pressure and increase ventricular compliance, thus allowing more rapid filling during diastole and reducing wedge pressure. The most important issues in management are careful blood pressure control and control of heart rate, as tachycardia can contribute to impaired LV compliance and increased LA pressure by limiting myocardial perfusion and diastolic filling time. Aggressive diuresis should be avoided.

2. **HYPERTROPHIC CARDIOMYOPATHY.** Hypertrophic cardiomyopathy may occur with or without probable LV outflow obstruction. Patients are at risk of sudden death. Doppler echocardiography is the most useful diagnostic test. Estimates of the left ventricular outflow tract pressure difference can also be made using Doppler echocardiography.

Strenuous physical activity should be avoided. Administration of **beta blockers (propranolol, 80–120 mg qid) or verapamil, 240–480 mg/d,** can lessen symptoms. Diuretics should be avoided. If atrial fibrillation develops, digoxin should be used to control the ventricular response, and patients should receive **anticoagulation** to prevent emboli.

Surgical therapy (myomectomy with or without mitral valve replacement) should be considered only for patients who have significant outflow tract pressure differences and whose conditions are refractory to medical treatment. Recent data suggest that sudden death in hypertrophic cardiomyopathy is often due to ventricular arrhythmia or, less commonly, bradyarrhythmias. Therefore, Holter monitoring and electrophysiologic (EP) studies are indicated in patients with syncope or documented life-threatening arrhythmias. Limited experience with dual chamber pacing has suggested that selected patients may benefit in terms of symptoms referable to outflow tract obstruction, perhaps due to regression of hypertrophy.

The availability of genetic markers now makes it possible to screen siblings and progeny of affected patients to identify those at risk, although these studies do not necessarily predict prognosis.

Cohn JN, Archibald DG, Ziesche S, et al. Effect of vasodilator therapy on mortality in chronic congestive heart failure: results of Veterans Administration Cooperative Trial. N Engl J Med 1986;314:1547–1552.
Cohn JN, Johnson G, Ziesche S, et al. A comparison of enalapril with hydralazine-isosorbide dinitrate in the treatment of chronic congestive heart failure. N Engl J Med 1991;325:303–310.
Consensus Trial Study Group. The effects of enalapril on mortality in severe congestive heart failure. Results of the Cooperative North Scandinavian Enalapril Survival Study (CONSENSUS). N Engl J Med 1987;316:1429–1435.
Packer, M, ed. Physiological determinants of survival in congestive heart failure. Circulation 1987;4:1–111.
Packer M, Bristow MR, Cohn JN, et al. The effects of carvedilol on morbidity and mortality in patients with chronic heart failure. N Engl J Med 1996;334:1349–1355.
SOLVD Investigators. Effects of enalapril on survival in patients with reduced left ventricular ejection fraction and congestive heart failure. N Engl J Med 1991;325:293–302.

IV. VALVULAR HEART DISEASE

A. General Principles of Treatment

Regardless of severity, all patients with valvular heart disease should receive antibiotic prophylaxis for endocarditis (see Chapter 3). In general, valve surgery is not recommended for asymptomatic patients. However, formal evaluation of cardiac function and exercise capacity is recommended in most.

B. Approach to Specific Conditions

1. **AORTIC STENOSIS.** Aortic stenosis (AS) may be due to rheumatic heart disease (RHD), congenital bicuspid valve, or senile calcific changes. AS frequently occurs as a mixed lesion, with some degree of aortic insufficiency. It should be noted that in elderly patients with senile calcific aortic stenosis, modest gradients (20 to 40 mm Hg) may be associated with significant valvular stenosis due to low cardiac outputs, usually associated with coronary artery disease.

    Valve replacement is recommended for patients with symptoms of angina, syncope, or CHF who have severe AS (aortic valve area <1 cm^2). Medical management of symptomatic patients with AS is fraught with difficulty because of the high risk of inducing hypotension, potassium shifts, myocardial ischemia, and worsening LV function with agents usually employed to treat angina or CHF. Echocardiography with Doppler is an excellent screening test for severe AS, but most patients will require cardiac catheterization before valve replacement. Percutaneous transluminal valvuloplasty may be a temporizing measure in severely symptomatic patients who could not tolerate surgery. Although the long-term results of this procedure are not known, studies do indicate a 30% to 50% restenosis rate by 6 to 12 months.

2. **AORTIC REGURGITATION.** Aortic insufficiency (AI) may be due to RHD, arteritis, endocarditis, aortic dissection, or collagen vascular disease. Acute AI (as with endocarditis) is tolerated poorly and often leads

promptly to CHF. Chronic AI may be well tolerated for long periods in spite of impressive peripheral manifestations of acute runoff. The principles of management include afterload reduction using either ACE inhibitors or calcium antagonists.

Chronic aortic regurgitation can lead to irreversible left ventricular dysfunction. Therefore, valve replacement is advised when the first symptoms of CHF develop. In the asymptomatic individual with severe regurgitation who demonstrates deterioration of ventricular function in serial noninvasive studies (increases in LV end systolic volume index ≥ 55 mL/m^2), valve replacement may also be recommended.

3. **MITRAL STENOSIS.** Mitral stenosis (MS) is almost always due to RHD. Less common causes include prosthetic valve dysfunction, left atrial thrombus, and left atrial myxoma.

Mildly symptomatic patients can be improved by **diuretics** and controlling the ventricular response (if they are in atrial fibrillation) with **digoxin or a beta blocker.** Patients with atrial fibrillation should receive **anticoagulation therapy** to prevent systemic emboli. **Surgery** is indicated for symptomatic patients (NYHA class III–IV) who do not respond to a simple drug regimen or who show signs of progressive pulmonary hypertension (valve area ≤ 1 cm^2) or systemic emboli. Concomitant mitral regurgitation may result in an overestimate of the severity of mitral stenosis because of failure to consider the total cardiac output (forward plus regurgitant fraction) in calculating valve area. The symptomatic state of MS tends to progress slowly, so intervention is rarely urgent. Mitral valve balloon valvuloplasty may be performed, but long-term results are not known. Initial reports indicate better long-term results with mitral valvuloplasty than with aortic valvuloplasty.

4. **MITRAL REGURGITATION.** Mitral regurgitation (MR) may be due to RHD, myxomatous mitral valve, endocarditis, dilated cardiomyopathy, or coronary artery disease. The most common cause today is coronary artery disease with papillary muscle dysfunction.

Surgery is recommended when symptoms develop and the regurgitation is moderate to severe. Chronic MR is generally well tolerated for long periods with the use of afterload reduction, but acute or subacute MR (secondary to MI, papillary muscle rupture, chordae tendineae rupture, or endocarditis) may be associated with more acute deterioration. If left ventricular function is severely compromised (ejection fraction <30%), surgery carries an increased risk and may result in little improvement in symptoms. Surgery is also a higher risk in patients with concomitant coronary artery disease, and in general a decision must be made about revascularizing the patient at the same time. Recent surgical advances have led to the use of mitral valve repair as opposed to replacement in selected patients with severe myxomatous degeneration. Maintenance of chordal integrity confers greater improvement in ventricular function by preserving normal patterns of ventricular contraction.

5. **MITRAL VALVE PROLAPSE.** Mitral valve prolapse (MVP) is a myxomatous degenerative change of the valve leaflets and chordae tendineae that

results in displacement (prolapse) of the valve leaflet(s) into the left atrium. Although it is a feature of many connective tissue disorders, it frequently occurs in the absence of any systemic illness. Symptoms include atypical chest pain, dyspnea, palpitation, and dizziness. Common physical signs include a mid-to-late systolic click or systolic murmur or both. Diagnosis is made by 2-D echocardiography (systolic displacement of a leaflet beyond the mitral annulus into the left atrium). For most patients, this is a benign disorder. In a few patients, serious complications may occur, including cardiac arrhythmias, infectious endocarditis, systemic emboli, sudden death, and chordae tendineae rupture with flail leaflet and severe MR.

6. TRICUSPID STENOSIS AND REGURGITATION. Tricuspid regurgitation (TR) usually develops in association with pulmonary hypertension or other causes of a dilated RV. TR may also result from RHD or endocarditis.

Tricuspid stenosis is rare, but when present, it is nearly always rheumatic in origin. In these cases, the left-sided valves are always involved by the rheumatic process. Methysergide and carcinoid tumors may also cause tricuspid stenosis.

7. PROSTHETIC VALVES. The major complications of prosthetic valves are endocarditis, thromboembolism, and valve dysfunction. Endocarditis is the most serious complication. Clinical manifestations of prosthetic valve endocarditis (PVE) can be subtle. Changing murmur, fever, failure to thrive, and heart failure are the most common findings. The mortality rate associated with medically treated PVE is extremely high; therefore, the timing of surgical intervention is crucial.

Thromboembolism remains an important complication of prosthetic valves. Most of the clinically detected emboli are cerebral. Patients with mechanical prosthetic valves must receive anticoagulation. Bioprosthetic valves without anticoagulation have a thrombotic rate equal to that of mechanical valves with anticoagulation. Major drawbacks of bioprosthetic valves are early degeneration, cusp tear, perforation, and flail leaflets. Mechanical valves are much more durable. The use of homografts remains experimental.

V. CARDIAC ARRHYTHMIAS

A. Normal Conduction System Physiology

In the normal heart, the sinus node has the fastest intrinsic rate of depolarization and consequently serves as the pacemaker site. Depolarization spreads across the atria (the P wave on the surface ECG represents this event). The wave of depolarization reaches the specialized conduction tissue in the lower part of the interatrial septum, the atrioventricular (AV) node. Conduction through the AV node is slowed to allow adequate ventricular filling following atrial contraction and to protect the ventricle from too rapid a rate. The bundle of His originates in the AV node and is responsible for conducting the impulse into the ventricle. These events are not seen on the surface ECG and occur during the P-R interval. The wave of depolarization is propagated into the ventricles via three branches of the bundle of His (right, left anterior, and left posterior fascicles). The fascicles branch into an extensive network of fibers, transmitting impulses to the ventricular myocardium (QRS on the surface ECG). Repolarization of the ventricle is represented by the T wave. Repolarization of the atria is usually not seen on the surface ECG.

In the resting state, there is a large electrical gradient between the inside and the outside of the cells (range of −60 to −90 mV). The gradient is maintained because of the difference between intracellular and extracellular potassium concentrations. During depolarization, the gradient becomes less negative owing to the influx of sodium and calcium ions. The initial phase of depolarization is rapid due to the influx of sodium through fast channels. The plateau phase of depolarization lasts much longer and is due primarily to the influx of calcium through the calcium slow channels. After depolarization, cells remain in a refractory state for a variable period of time. During this refractory state, further stimulation will not result in depolarization. **Repolarization** occurs as an active process in which sodium and calcium are exchanged for potassium via an active transport mechanism.

A feature possessed by some of the heart cells is **automaticity.** Cells that have this property are found in the sinus node, atria, AV node, and His-Purkinje system. Automaticity refers to a slow depolarization during electrical diastole. When the membrane potential reaches a threshold level that varies from site to site, an action potential results. In the normal situation, the sinus node has the fastest intrinsic rate of spontaneous depolarization. Consequently, it becomes the pacemaker site for normal sinus rhythm. However, in certain pathologic conditions (i.e., if the sinus node is malfunctioning), other areas may take over the pacemaker function, usually at a slower rate.

B. Tachyarrhythmias

Tachyarrhythmias are rhythms with ventricular rates of more than 100 bpm and can be regular or irregular with a narrow or wide QRS. There are two basic mechanisms for the development of tachyarrhythmias: enhanced automaticity and reentrant arrhythmias.

Enhanced automaticity is due to an increased rate of diastolic depolarization. A variety of potentially reversible causes increase automaticity. These include ischemia, hypoxia, electrolyte abnormalities (hypokalemia or hypomagnesemia), thyroid excess, digitalis toxicity, and use of beta agonists.

Reentrant arrhythmias require the presence of two pathways that have the potential for conduction. In general, there must be a difference in the speed of conduction and refractoriness of the two pathways for tachycardia to develop so that an impulse will encounter a unidirectional block in one of the pathways. By the time the other pathway has conducted the impulse, the pathway that was initially blocked will conduct the impulse in the reverse direction and thus maintain the circuit to conduct the tachycardia.

1. **REGULAR TACHYARRHYTHMIAS WITH NARROW QRS COMPLEXES.** The differential diagnosis of regular tachyarrhythmias with a narrow QRS includes sinus tachycardia, paroxysmal supraventricular tachycardia, atrial flutter, and nonparoxysmal junctional tachycardia. All originate above the bifurcation of the His bundle—thus the name *supraventricular arrhythmia.*

a. **Sinus tachycardia.** Sinus tachycardia is an acceleration of the normal depolarization of the sinus node. The heart rate rarely exceeds 150 bpm except in infants and adults during exercise. **Treatment** is usually directed at the underlying cause. Common causes include fever, sepsis, CHF, hypovolemia, anemia, thyrotoxicosis, pulmonary embolism, anxiety, and abrupt discontinuation of beta-adrenergic blocking agents. If the patient has unstable angina or AMI, direct therapy to lower the heart rate may be indicated.

b. **Paroxysmal supraventricular tachyarrhythmias (PSVTs).** PSVT may be secondary to a reentrant arrhythmia or, less commonly, enhanced automaticity (ectopic tachycardias). When reentry is the mechanism, the AV node is usually involved as one arm of the reentry circuit. The heart rate is usually 150 to 200 bpm but occasionally may be faster. Diagnosis is usually made by the history of abrupt onset and termination. In general, those due to reentry are more responsive to therapy than are the ectopic tachycardias.

Initial **treatment** includes measures to increase vagal tone, such as carotid sinus massage and Valsalva maneuver, which may be both diagnostic and therapeutic. If vagal maneuvers are unsuccessful, pharmacologic agents are used to alter conduction and interrupt a reentry circuit.

Verapamil is the drug of choice, **IV 0.075–0.15 mg/kg (5–10 mg)** given over 2 to 3 minutes. Peak effects occur in 10 minutes. A repeat dose may be given in 30 minutes. Verapamil should be used with caution in the presence of hypotension, severely compromised left ventricular function, or known conduction system disease.

Beta blockers are also used to treat PSVTs. They should be used with caution in patients with hypotension, severe left ventricular dysfunction, and bronchospastic pulmonary disease. Propranolol is administered in increments of 1 mg IV every 5 minutes until either the rate is controlled or a total of 0.1 mg/kg (5–10 mg) is administered. Metoprolol is administered as a 5 mg IV bolus.

Adenosine, a class IV agent with multiple cellular effects, is approved by the FDA for the treatment of PSVT. It has an extremely short half-life of 10 to 30 seconds. Side effects include dyspnea, flushing, and chest pain. Adenosine is given as an initial IV bolus of 6 mg; if no effects occur within 1 to 2 minutes, a 12 mg bolus is given and may be repeated. Contraindications are asthma, second or third degree AV block, and sick sinus syndrome. The effects of adenosine are attenuated by theophylline and potentiated in the presence of persantine.

IV digitalis glycosides are also effective agents through their vagotonic actions on the AV node but have a longer time course of action.

Once normal sinus rhythm (NSR) is achieved, an **antiarrhythmic agent** should be prescribed to prevent recurrence. Digoxin or a beta blocker, particularly propranolol, is most commonly used. Patients should be cautioned about the role that stimulants, such as caffeine, may play in the initiation of paroxysmal supraventricular tachycardia by provoking premature atrial beats, which trigger reentry.

If pharmacologic agents are unsuccessful, either synchronized direct-current countershock or rapid atrial stimulation may be successful. These should be used urgently if the patient is hemodynamically unstable or is having ongoing ischemia. There is increasing enthusiasm for the use of radiofrequency ablation to prevent PSVT, particularly where reentry occurs within the AV node. Although the procedure is curative, there is a 3% to 5% incidence of complete heart block, requiring permanent pacing.

c. **Atrial flutter.** Atrial flutter is commonly seen in patients with valvular heart disease or other structural heart disease. It is due to rapid atrial depolarization at a regular rate of 250 to 300 bpm. Because the AV node cannot conduct atrial impulses at this rate, a 2:1 AV block develops producing a regular ventricular response of one-half the atrial rate. Any regular narrow complex tachycardia at 150 bpm should be assumed to be atrial flutter until proven otherwise. Carotid sinus massage will usually increase the degree of AV block (2:1 to 4:1) without a change in the atrial depolarization rate. Diagnosis is made by observing atrial depolarization appearing as a sawtooth deflection in the inferior leads.

Digoxin, verapamil, diltiazem, or a **beta blocker** alone or in combination remains the mainstay of therapy for atrial flutter. Verapamil and beta blockers are given as above for more rapid control of the ventricular response. IV beta blockers should be given with caution if IV calcium channel blockers have been given. Digoxin may be given as an initial 0.25 mg dose IV.

Cardioversion should be performed if the patient is symptomatic (hypotension, angina, pulmonary congestion) from the arrhythmia. Atrial flutter is usually terminated by low-level energy (20 to 50 joules). Cardioversion is safe with small amounts of digitalis glycoside, but it is not recommended when large amounts must be given. Patients may convert to atrial fibrillation or NSR. Rapid atrial pacing is commonly used in the postcoronary artery bypass patients and in patients resistant to drug therapy. In particularly refractory cases, there is evidence to suggest that radiofrequency ablation within the area between the tricuspid annulus and the coronary sinus may prevent recurrence.

d. **Nonparoxysmal junction tachycardia.** This occurs most commonly with digitalis toxicity, after cardiac operation (particularly mitral valve replacement), and in patients with inflammation close to or involving the AV node. The rate rarely exceeds 140 to 150 bpm. The electrocardiographic morphology reveals regular QRS complexes, and retrograde atrial activity can sometimes be seen. This arrhythmia is generally well tolerated by the patient. Correction of any electrolyte imbalance or withholding digoxin is usually the only intervention required.

2. REGULAR TACHYCARDIA WITH WIDE QRS COMPLEXES. This is one of the most difficult arrhythmias to diagnose. The differential diagnosis is SVT with aberrant conduction or ventricular tachycardia (VT).

a. **SVT with aberrant conduction.** The QRS is usually wide and notched and has a bizarre complex. The abnormal QRS complex may be due to existing bundle branch block. In some instances the aberration is present only in association with the arrhythmia. Diagnosis of SVT with aberration vs. ventricular tachycardia is made by additional features.
   - Evidence of AV dissociation favors ventricular tachycardia.
   - A bundle branch block before or after the tachycardia with identical QRS morphology during the tachycardia favors SVT with aberrancy.
   - A QRS duration of greater than 0.14 favors VT. Although the Wellens criteria for ventricular tachycardia serve as a guideline for the diagnosis of VT, they are not absolute.

   Patients with SVT with aberration are usually more stable than a patient with VT at a similar rate, but this does not reliably distinguish the cause. If one is confident of the diagnosis of SVT with aberration, **therapy** should be initiated as described above for SVT. In any patient with structural heart disease or coronary artery disease, a wide-complex tachycardia should be assumed to be VT, and therapy for presumed VT should be initiated. The mechanisms of VT include **reentry,** particularly in patients with remote MI and myocardial scar, as well as **triggered activity** due to inward calcium current through the sodium-calcium exchanger, particularly during periods of myocardial ischemia. Less commonly, VT may be due to increased automaticity.

b. **Ventricular tachycardia (VT). Cardioversion** is the treatment of choice in the presence of hemodynamic compromise. Cardioversion of ventricular tachycardia is usually accomplished with low energy (50 to 100 joules). A thump to the precordium is successful in some patients in converting VT. **Lidocaine** is usually the drug of choice for VT via an initial bolus of 1 mg/kg. Frequently a second bolus of 0.5–0.75 mg/kg is required within 20 to 30 minutes of the first bolus. A maintenance dose of 1–4 mg/min or 20–55 μg/kg/min is administered to suppress further ventricular activity. Another medication that may be given if lidocaine is ineffective is **procainamide.** An initial bolus of 100 mg over 2 minutes up to 25 mg/min to 1 g in the first hour is followed by an infusion of 20–40 μg/kg/min (1–4 mg/min). **Quinidine** may also be used to suppress recurrent VT. Therapeutic blood levels of quinidine are achieved with doses of 300–600 mg PO or IM every 6 hours. IV quinidine produces severe hypotension and should be avoided. There are several other second-line agents that may be useful in treating or preventing recurrent VT. **Disopyramide** has electrophysiologic properties similar to quinidine and may be used orally (100–300 mg q6h). **Tocainide** (300–600 mg PO q8h) and **mexiletine** (250–300 mg PO q8h) are lidocaine analogs. They have the advantage over procainamide and quinidine of not prolonging the QT interval but are only available in oral preparations and, therefore, have limited utility in acute situations.

Phenytoin is effective in digitalis-toxic arrhythmias. The IV dose is 10–15 mg/kg over 1 hour followed by oral maintenance of 400–600 mg/d.

Bretylium tosylate is used to treat recurrent or resistant ventricular tachycardia. It may be given as an IV bolus of 5–10 mg/kg over 10 minutes followed by a 1–2 mg/min infusion. The major side effect is hypotension from peripheral vasodilation. However, initial sympathomimetic effects may occur.

c. **Torsades de pointes.** This is a form of ventricular tachycardia usually associated with prolongation of the QT interval and caused by pharmacologic agents such as quinidine, procainamide, or disopyramide and by electrolyte abnormalities. Cardioversion is often necessary, but the tachycardia may recur. Correcting the precipitating factors (hypocalcemia, hypomagnesemia) and, in some cases, overdrive pacing and isoproterenol infusion (2–8 μg/min) to shorten the QT interval may be successful in preventing recurrences.

d. **Ventricular flutter and fibrillation.** Both are medical emergencies and require immediate cardioversion.

3. IRREGULAR TACHYCARDIA WITH NARROW OR WIDE COMPLEXES. The differential diagnosis of irregular tachycardia with narrow or wide complex is among atrial fibrillation (AF), multifocal atrial tachycardia (MAT), SVT with varying degrees of AV block, and multiple premature beats originating from the atrium, junction, or ventricle.

a. **Atrial fibrillation** is usually recognized by its irregularly irregular ventricular response and a baseline with no organized atrial activity. Fine atrial fibrillation and coarse atrial fibrillation refer to the amplitude of the fibrillatory waves and have no therapeutic significance. Carotid sinus pressure usually results in slowing of the ventricular response.

The most common underlying heart diseases in patients with AF are atherosclerosis, hypertension, rheumatic heart disease (particularly mitral stenosis), pericarditis, and cardiomyopathy. Noncardiac causes include thyrotoxicosis, COPD, pneumonia, and pulmonary embolism. Elderly patients may have atrial fibrillation as a manifestation of degenerative changes in the conduction system and may have no underlying structural heart disease (see Sick Sinus Syndrome, p. 195).

Digitalis glycosides are used commonly for treating atrial fibrillation. An initial IV loading dose of **0.25–0.5 mg of digoxin** may be given to the patient who has not been receiving digoxin. The loading dose is governed by the lean body weight. IV digoxin begins to exert its effect in 15 to 30 minutes. Additional digoxin may be administered every 2 to 4 hours in increments of 0.125 or 0.25 mg as needed for rate control to a total of 1–1.25 mg in 24 hours.

Diltiazem (20–25 mg IV) is the drug of choice if rapid control of ventricular response is necessary. It is associated with less hypotension compared with verapamil and may be administered as a continuous drip for more sustained control. **Verapamil** is a reasonable alternative but fraught with less predictable hemodynamic responses. Verapamil is administered IV at a dose of 5–10 mg over 1 minute and repeated in 30 minutes if necessary. Effects are seen in 10 minutes. Caution should be used when administering this drug to an elderly patient or when sick sinus syndrome is suspected. **IV beta blockers** (propranolol 0.5–1 mg IV bolus, metoprolol 5 mg IV bolus) may also be used for rapid control of the ventricular response. Esmolol is a short-acting parenteral beta blocker that can be administered as an IV drip for more sustained control. Caution should be exercised in using combinations of beta blockers and calcium antagonists. Patients who are hemodynamically unstable with a rapid ventricular response may require emergency cardioversion. Elective conversion to NSR may be performed in stable patients. It is recommended that patients be given anticoagulants for 2 to 3 weeks before elective cardioversion. Long-term anticoagulation is recommended in patients with chronic or recurrent AF. If the time of onset of atrial fibrillation can be determined accurately to be less than 3 to 5 days, anticoagulation before cardioversion is not necessary.

b. **Multifocal atrial tachycardia.** This arrhythmia is easily confused with atrial fibrillation because it usually has a similar ventricular rate and the rhythm is irregularly irregular. The diagnosis is made by the presence of organized P waves with three or more different morphologies, varying P-P intervals, and varying P-R intervals. The rhythm is generally not responsive to carotid sinus massage. It occurs most frequently in patients with chronic pulmonary disease.

The arrhythmia is **best treated** by correcting the underlying respiratory or metabolic disorder if present. If rate control is necessary, the **treatment of choice is diltiazem** 20–25 mg IV, although this is not uniformly successful.

c. **Atrial or junction premature beats.** Multiple atrial or junction premature beats produce an irregular rhythm. The QRS complex of the premature beat may be similar to or slightly different from the normal sinus beat. If a P wave precedes the QRS complex, it is usually atrial in origin; if a P wave follows the QRS complex, the beat is usually junctional. Atrial and junctional premature beats are benign, and no treatment is required. They sometimes may be harbingers of other atrial arrhythmias.

d. **Ventricular premature beats.** Ventricular premature beats usually produce bizarre QRS complexes, which are usually followed by a compensatory pause. Occasionally there is no compensatory pause, and the premature beat is said to be "interpolated." The morphology of the premature beat varies depending on the site of origin. Premature beats originating from the left ventricle have a RBBB morphology, and those originating from the right ventricle have an LBBB morphology. Treatment depends on the presence or absence of symptoms, the setting, and the frequency. When treatment is indicated on symptomatic grounds, the agents of choice are the same as those used in VT.

C. Bradyarrhythmias

Bradyarrhythmias are rhythms with heart rates of less than 60 bpm and usually indicate pathology of the sinus or AV nodes.

1. **SINUS BRADYCARDIA.** The presence of sinus bradycardia may indicate pathology of the sinus node, may be a normal physiologic response especially in well-trained athletes, or may be the result of pharmacologic agents, such as beta blockers, calcium channel blockers, or amiodarone. Sinus bradycardia may also be seen in patients with a diagnosis of hypothyroidism.

2. **SINUS ARREST AND SINUS EXIT BLOCK.** In sinus arrest, the sinus node stops depolarization instantaneously. In sinus exit block, the sinus node depolarizes normally, but the impulse cannot exit the sinus node. Therefore, in both arrhythmias, P waves are usually absent or intermittent.
    a. **Treatment.** Treatment of either type of block is indicated if the rate is associated with symptoms (hypotension, dizziness, syncope, CHF). Negative chronotropic drugs should be discontinued. Immediate therapy of choice is atropine 0.5–1 mg IV or Isuprel 1–2 µg/min IV. Insertion of a permanent transvenous pacemaker is indicated only if the rhythm is refractory to these measures and the patient remains symptomatic.

D. AV Block

1. **DIAGNOSIS**
    a. **First degree AV block.** This is present if the P-R interval is greater than 0.20 second and all P waves are followed by a QRS complex.
    b. **Second degree AV block.** In second degree AV block, all P waves are not followed by a QRS complex. There are two types of second degree AV block: Wenckebach (or Mobitz type I) is diagnosed by observing progressive prolongation of the P-R interval for each conducted beat until a P wave is not followed by a QRS (blocked beat). The classic features of **Wenckebach periodicity** are not always present on the ECG (atypical Wenckebach). Typically, the first P-R interval of each group is constant and is the shortest interval. The increments in the P-R interval progressively decrease; thus, the R-R interval progressively shortens until the pause. Type I block usually implies disease in the AV node.
    c. **Mobitz type II.** Blocked beats, P waves, occur without progressive prolongation of the P-R interval. Type II block implies disease in the distal His-Purkinje system, making it a more serious arrhythmia than type I because the risk of sudden asystole is greater.
    d. **Third degree AV block.** In contrast to first and second degree AV block, there is no relationship between the P waves and the QRS complexes in third degree AV block. The P-P and R-R intervals are usually regular, and the P waves may precede or follow the QRS or may be found within the QRS complex. The QRS complex may be of junctional or ventricular origin.

e. **Syncope (Adams-Stokes attacks).** These are usually due to profound bradycardia or asystole. The treatment of choice is permanent transvenous pacing, using a rate-responsive, dual-chamber device in otherwise active individuals.

2. TREATMENT. Mobitz type I AV block is usually transient and commonly occurs in the setting of acute inferior wall MI. It is most likely to respond to atropine or isoproterenol if any therapy is needed. **Digitalis toxicity** should always be considered in patients with Mobitz type I AV block who are receiving digoxin therapy. Patients with Mobitz type II have a more serious AV block that is more likely to progress to complete heart block. Patients should be evaluated for a permanent transvenous pacemaker. The treatment of choice for third degree heart block is a **permanent transvenous pacemaker,** unless it occurs in a clearly reversible disorder, such as digitalis toxicity or an acute IMI.

E. Arrhythmia in Special Circumstances

1. WOLFF-PARKINSON-WHITE SYNDROME (WPW). Patients with this syndrome have another bypass tract in addition to conducting via the AV node. When conduction occurs via the bypass tract, it produces a short P-R interval, a delta wave, and a wide QRS complex. During bypass tract conduction, the QRS complex may be similar to that seen in AMI. The two most common arrhythmias that occur in patients with WPW are paroxysmal SVT and atrial fibrillation. Most cases of PSVT involve a narrow complex (antegrade conduction is through the AV node and retrograde via the bypass track). Treatment of paroxysmal SVT is the same as previously described, although radiofrequency ablation is gaining in popularity as a curative procedure, particularly for those with refractory arrhythmia or medication intolerance. Atrial fibrillation may be conducted quite rapidly through the bypass track with wide QRS complexes and rates approaching 300 bpm. Both digoxin and verapamil are contraindicated for control of ventricular response in atrial fibrillation occurring in WPW syndrome, as they may paradoxically accelerate the ventricular response. Patients may require cardioversion and treatment with quinidine or procainamide to prevent recurrence of AF.

2. SICK SINUS SYNDROME (TACHY-BRADY SYNDROME). This syndrome is a constellation of arrhythmias. It occurs most frequently in the elderly. Patients with sick sinus syndrome (SSS) may have periods of sinus bradycardia, sinus arrest, PSVT, atrial flutter, and atrial fibrillation with either rapid or slow ventricular response. In patients with SSS who have atrial tachyarrhythmia, treatment of the tachyarrhythmia may result in symptomatic bradycardia. Therefore, some patients may require a transvenous permanent pacemaker as part of their treatment regimen. Care must be taken during cardioversion, as there is a high likelihood that there may be no spontaneous sinus activity after cardioversion or that the patient may have an extremely slow sinus node response.

TABLE 4–15. Antiarrhythmic Drugs Used in Therapy of Ventricular Arrhythmias

AGENT	DOSAGE	PHARMACOKINETICS	SIDE EFFECTS AND CONTRAINDICATIONS
Quinidine (Class IA)	1.2–1.6 g/d PO in divided doses, q4–12h depending on preparation Not IV; risk of hypotension	$t_{1/2}$ 7–9 h. Level 2.3–5 μg/mL; hepatic metabolism; reduce dose in liver disease	Diarrhea, nausea; torsades de pointes and hypotension; hemolytic anemia
Procainamide (Class IA)	IV 100 mg bolus over 2 min, up to 25 mg/min to 1 g in 1st h; then 2–6 mg/min; PO 1 g, then up to 1000 mg q6h	$t_{1/2}$ 3.5 h. Level 4–10 μg/mL; renal elimination	Hypotension with IV dose; drug induced lupus; torsades de pointes rare
Disopyramide (Class IA)	Oral dose 100–200 mg q6h; loading dose 300 mg (less if CHF)	$t_{1/2}$ 8 h. Level 3–6 μg/mL, toxic >7 μg/mL; hepatic metabolism (50%), unchanged urinary excretion (50%)	Hypotension; QRS or QT prolongation; torsades; negative inotropic effects; urinary retention
Lidocaine (Class IB)	IV 100–200 mg; then 2–4 mg/min for 24–30 h	Effect of single bolus lasts only few min, then $t_{1/2}$ about 2 h, hepatic metabolism. Level 1.4–5 μg/mL; toxic >9 μg/mL	Reduce dose by half if liver blood flow low (shock, β-blockade, cirrhosis, cimetidine, severe heart failure); high-dose CNS effects
Tocainide (Class IB)	Oral loading 400–800 mg; then 400–800 mg PO, then bid-tid	$t_{1/2}$ 13.5 h. Level 4–10 μg/mL; unchanged renal excretion (50%)	CNS, GI side effects; sometimes immune-based problems (lung fibrosis, blood dyscrasias)
Mexiletine (Class IB)	Oral 100–400 mg PO q8h; loading dose 400 mg	$t_{1/2}$ 10–17 h. Level 1–2 μg/mL; hepatic metabolism, inactive metabolites	CNS, GI side effects; bradycardia, hypotension especially during cotherapy
Phenytoin (Class IB)	IV 10–15 mg/kg over 1 h; PO 1 g; 500 mg for 2 d; 400–600 mg qd	$t_{1/2}$ 24 h. Level 10–18 μg/mL; hepatic metabolism; hepatic or renal disease requires reduced doses	Hypotension; vertigo; dysarthria; lethargy; gingivitis; macrocytic anemia; lupus; pulmonary infiltrates

Drug	Dose	Pharmacokinetics	Side Effects
Flecainide (Class IC)	100–400 PO mg bid; hospitalize	$t_{1/2}$ 13–19 h. Hepatic metabolism ($^2/_3$); $^1/_3$ renal excretion, unchanged; 1 μg/mL	QRS prolongation; proarrhythmia; depressed LV function; CNS side effects; increased incidence of death postinfarct
Propafenone (Class IC)	150–300 mg PO tid	$t_{1/2}$ variable 2–10 h, up to 32 h in nonmetabolizers. Level 0.2–3 μg/mL. Variable hepatic metabolism (P-450 deficiency slows)	QRS prolongation; modest negative inotropic effect; GI side effects; proarrhythmia
Sotalol (Class III)	160–640 mg qd, occasionally higher, may divide doses; not approved in use	Not metabolized; renal loss	Myocardial depression; sinus bradycardia; AV block; torsades especially if hypokalemic or if dose too high
Amiodarone (Class III)	PO loading dose 1200–1600 mg/d; maintenance 200–400 mg/d, sometimes less	$t_{1/2}$ 25–110 d. Level 1–2.5 μg/mL; hepatic metabolism; lipid soluble with extensive distribution in body; excretion by skin, biliary tract, lacrimal glands	Pulmonary fibrosis; QT-prolongation; hypothyroidism
Bretylium (Class III)	IV 5–10 mg/kg, lifting arm, repeat to max 30 mg/kg, then IV 1–2 mg/min or IM 5–10 mg/min or IM 5–10 mg/kg q8h at varying sites (local necrosis)	$t_{1/2}$ 7–9 h. Level 0.5–1 μg/mL	IV: hypotension; initial sympathomimetic effects

$t_{1/2}$, plasma half-life.
Modified from Opie LH. Drugs for the Heart, 4th ed. Philadelphia: W.B. Saunders Co., 1995.

F. Classification of Antiarrhythmic Drugs

A useful classification (Vaughn-Williams) based on electrophysiologic properties is shown in Table 4–15. The pharmacologic and electrophysiologic properties of various intravenous and oral antiarrhythmic agents are shown in Tables 4–15 and 4–17. Table 4–16 shows drug interactions.

Mandel WJ. Cardiac Arrhythmias, Their Mechanism, Diagnosis and Management, 2nd ed. Philadelphia: JB Lippincott Co., 1987.
Wilkins EW. Emergency Medicine, 3rd ed. Baltimore: Williams & Wilkins, 1989.

TABLE 4–16. **Interaction of Antiarrhythmic Drugs**

DRUG	INTERACTION WITH	RESULT
Quinidine	Digoxin	Increased digoxin level
	Beta blockers, verapamil	Enhanced hypotension, negative inotropic effect
	Amiodarone, sotalol	Increased risk of torsades
	Diuretics	If hypokalemia, risk of torsades
	Verapamil	Increased quinidine level
	Nifedipine	Decreased quinidine level
	Warfarin	Enhanced anticoagulation
	Cimetidine	Increased blood levels
	Enzyme inducers	Decreased blood levels
Procainamide	Cimetidine	Decreased renal clearance
Disopyramide	Amiodarone, sotalol, beta blockers, verapamil	Torsades Enhanced hypotension, negative inotropic effect
Lidocaine	Beta blockers, cimetidine, halothane	Reduced liver blood flow (increased blood levels)
Mexiletine	Theophylline	Theophylline levels increased
Flecainide	Added SA or AV node inhibition (beta blockers, verapamil, diltiazem, digoxin)	SA and AV nodal depression; depressed myocardium; conduction delay
Encainide	See flecainide	See flecainide
Propafenone	As for flecainide, digoxin, warfarin	Enhanced SA, AV, and myocardial depression; digoxin level increased; anticoagulant effect enhanced
Sotalol	Diuretics, class IA agents, amiodarone, phenothiazines	Risk of proarrhythmia
Amiodarone	As for sotalol, digoxin, flecainide, warfarin	Risk of proarrhythmias; digoxin and flecainide levels increase
Verapamil	Beta blockers, excess digoxin	Increased myocardial or nodal depression

Enzyme inducers: hepatic enzyme inducers, i.e., barbiturates, phenytoin, rifampin.
Modified from Opie LH.: Drugs for the Heart, 4th ed. Philadelphia: W.B. Saunders Co., 1995.

TABLE 4–17. Effects and Side Effects of Some Antiarrhythmic Agents on Electrophysiology and Hemodynamics

AGENT	SINUS NODE	A-HIS	PR	H-P	QRS	QT	RISK OF TORSADES	RISK OF MONOMORPHIC VT
Lidocaine	0	0/↓	0	0	0	0	0?	0?
Quinidine	→	0	0/→	→	↑	↑	++	0,+
Procainamide	0	0/↓	0/→	→	0/→	↑	+	0,+
Disopyramide	→	0	0/→	0/↓	↑	↑	+	0,+
Phenytoin	0	↑/0	0	0	0	↓	0,+	0,+
Mexiletine	0	↑/0	0	→/0	0/→	0	0,+	0,+
Tocainamide	0	↓/0	0	→/0	0	0	0,+	0,+
Flecainide	0/↓	↓↓↓	↑	↓↓	↑	↑ (via QRS)	0	+++
Encainide	0/↓	↓↓↓	↑	↓↓	↑	↑ (via QRS)	0	+++
Sotalol	↓↓	→	↑	0	0	↑	++	0,+
Amiodarone	→	→	0/→	0/↓	0	↑	+	0,+
Bretylium	→	→	↑↑	→	0	–	0,+	0,+
Verapamil	→	→	↑↑	→	0	0	0	0

A-HIS, atria-His conduction; H-P, His-Purkinje conduction; VT, ventricular tachycardia; ↓, depresses; ↑, increases; →, prolongs; ←, shortens.
Modified from Opie LH. Drugs for the Heart, 4th ed. Philadelphia: W.B. Saunders Co., 1995.

VI. SELECTION AND MANAGEMENT OF HEART TRANSPLANT PATIENTS

Cardiac transplantation is performed to improve quality of life and prolong survival. Most people who undergo heart transplantation have a diagnosis of ischemic or idiopathic cardiomyopathy. Other less common diagnoses are postpartum cardiomyopathy and congenital heart disease. The most common indicator for heart transplantation is class IV heart failure.

A. Patient Selection

Patients selected for cardiac transplantation have a poor prognosis and an expected 6- to 12-month survival of less than 50%. Patients deemed appropriate for transplantation on the basis of their prognosis must meet the following selection criteria.

1. AGE. The preferred cutoff age has been 55 years, although there have been no significant differences in incidence of rejection and 1-year survival among younger patients age 19 to 54 versus older patients age 55 to 65. Recently, some transplant centers have liberalized this age limit.

2. PULMONARY VASCULAR RESISTANCE Early data suggest that patients with pulmonary hypertension do poorly after cardiac transplantation, principally because of right heart failure.

3. COMORBID DISEASE. Patients who are candidates for transplantation must be free of other diseases. Diseases that preclude transplantation are malignancy, peripheral vascular disease, collagen vascular disease, renal dysfunction beyond that expected from severe CHF, hepatic dysfunction, diabetes mellitus (a relative contraindication), peptic ulcer disease (a relative contraindication), concurrent infection, marked obesity, and cachexia.

4. PSYCHOSOCIAL BEHAVIOR. Since the stress and demands placed on patients after cardiac transplant are intense, it is imperative that they be emotionally stable. Patients are excluded if there is a history of active drug or alcohol abuse. In addition, mental illness is an absolute contraindication for transplantation.

B. Management of the Postcardiac Transplant Patient

Postoperative immunosuppression therapy has become the mainstay of cardiac transplantation. Immunosuppressive therapy may be divided into three phases. **Early rejection prophylaxis** occurs 2 to 3 weeks after transplantation. **Chronic maintenance therapy** is given chronically throughout the duration of the transplant. Rejection is usually diagnosed by endomyocardial biopsy. Treatment of acute allograft rejection varies in part due to variation in chronic maintenance regimens.

C. Prognosis

Currently, the 1-year survival for cardiac transplant patients is 85% to 90%; the 5-year survival is approximately 70%. The majority of surviving patients lead active lives with few or no cardiac symptoms.

Copeland JG, Emery RW, Levinson MM, et al. Selection of patients for cardiac transplantation. Circulation 1987;75:1.

Kannel WB, Sorlie P, McNamara PM. Prognosis after initial myocardial infarction: The Framingham Study. Am J Cardiol 1979;44:53.

Macoviack JA. Selection and management of heart transplant patients. Cardiol Clin North Am 1990;8:1.

HYPERTENSION

DAVID C. DUGDALE

I. GENERAL PRINCIPLES

Excess morbidity and mortality rise in proportion to blood pressure elevation, and even mild hypertension adds to the risk of atherosclerotic disease. Prospective studies show that lowering blood pressure prevents or delays

- **Cardiac disease** (CHF, left ventricular hypertrophy, aortic dissection, and ischemic heart disease)
- **Cerebrovascular disease** (stroke and transient ischemic attack)
- **Progressive renal insufficiency**
- **Accelerated hypertension**

Benefits of treatment are greatest among patients with severe hypertension. Long-term studies of preventing hypertensive complications have primarily used thiazides, beta-adrenergic blockers, hydralazine, alpha-methyldopa, and reserpine. Newer agents have been tested for efficacy of blood pressure control. The presence of other independent risk factors for atherosclerosis magnifies the detrimental effect of hypertension and may indicate the need for more aggressive attempts at blood pressure control.

Treatment should be considered if blood pressures above 140/90 mm Hg have been documented on at least three occasions. The measurements should be done after 5 minutes of rest and at least 30 minutes after caffeine or cigarette use. The blood pressure cuff should have a rubber bladder that encircles at least 80% of the arm. Two or more readings separated by 2 minutes should be averaged. If the first two readings differ by more than 5 mm Hg, additional readings should be obtained. Patients should be questioned about the use of medications that may raise blood pressure, including nonsteroidal anti-inflammatory drugs (NSAIDs), oral contraceptives, tricyclic antidepressants, decongestants or appetite suppressants, and monoamine oxidase (MAO) inhibitors.

The **target blood pressure** for a patient with hypertension is usually a systolic blood pressure less than 140 mm Hg and a diastolic blood pressure less than 90 mm Hg. The presence of target organ damage, such as renal insufficiency, or additional cardiovascular risk factors, such as diabetes, suggests a lower target blood pressure (120 to 130/80 to 85 mm Hg). There is uncertainty about the degree to which a lower blood pressure target may increase the cardiovascular mortality by excessively lowering diastolic blood pressure in the coronary circulation, especially in those with established coronary artery disease (J Gen Intern Med 1996;11:350–356, and 1996;11:379–380). This concept, commonly called the *J-curve hypothesis* does not apply to the cerebral or renal circulations.

A. Lifestyle Modification

Lifestyle modification (previously called *nonpharmacologic therapy*) is appropriate initial treatment of uncomplicated stage 1 and 2 hypertension (blood pressure less than 180/110 mm Hg). In 1993, the fifth report of the Joint National Commission on Detection, Evaluation, and Treatment of high blood pressure (JNC 5) recommended a 3 to 6 month period of lifestyle modification before initiating drug therapy for this group of patients.

1. WEIGHT REDUCTION causes a fall of 1 to 2 mm Hg/kg of weight loss that is independent of reduced sodium intake (Arch Intern Med 1990;150: 1701–1704). **Reduction of dietary sodium intake** from the American average daily consumption of 150 mmol/d to 100 mmol/d (2.3 g of Na or 6 g of NaCl) lowers systolic blood pressure by 7 mm Hg, although it is effective in only 50% to 60% of patients (Br Med J 1991;302:819–824). Low Na intake also decreases diuretic-induced kaliuresis.

2. REGULAR AEROBIC EXERCISE (e.g., brisk walking for 30 to 45 minutes three to five times per week) reduces systolic and diastolic blood pressure by 7 mm Hg (J Clin Epidemiol 1992;45:439–447). Relaxation techniques lower blood pressure acutely but have no proven benefit for long-term management of hypertension.

3. ALCOHOL intake should be limited to no more than 1 ounce of ethanol (2 ounces of 100-proof liquor, 8 ounces of wine, or 24 ounces of beer) daily. Although alcohol withdrawal often causes significant hypertension, the effect is short-lived (Ann Intern Med 1986;105:124–125).

4. The role of MINERAL SUPPLEMENTATION in the treatment of hypertension remains unclear. A high dietary **potassium** level may protect against the development of hypertension but has not helped in treatment. **Calcium** supplements cause a decrease of systolic blood pressure of 1.6 mm Hg but no significant change in diastolic blood pressure (Ann Intern Med 1996;124:825–831). A low dietary **magnesium** intake is associated with higher blood pressure, but magnesium supplements do not lower blood pressure.

B. Pharmacologic Treatment

The blood pressure at which to begin pharmacologic treatment and the best initial pharmacologic treatment of essential hypertension remain controversial.

If the blood pressure is above the target established for the patient, drug therapy should be initiated after a 3 to 6 month trial of lifestyle modification. In the absence of target organ damage and other cardiovascular disease risk factors, patients with blood pressures in the 140 to 149/90 to 94 mm Hg range may continue with lifestyle modification alone if follow-up every 3 to 6 months can be assured. For patients with isolated systolic hypertension and no target organ damage or additional cardiovascular disease risk factors, the threshold for drug treatment is usually a systolic blood pressure above 160 mm Hg. As many of these patients are elderly, monitoring for side effects, especially those related to postural hypotension and cognitive effects, is vital.

The once-common stepped care approach (a diuretic, followed by a beta blocker, followed by a centrally active sympatholytic or vasodilator) has become less popular, and many newer agents are available outside of these categories. However, JNC 5 emphasized the initial use of diuretics and beta blockers primarily because they have been demonstrated to reduce cardiovascular morbidity and mortality. Alternative agents from the remaining drug classes are equally effective in reducing blood pressure but have not been shown to reduce cardiovascular morbidity and mortality.

Individualization of drug therapy is based on demographic data (older patients and blacks usually respond better to diuretics and calcium channel blockers; younger patients and whites respond better to beta blockers and angiotensin-converting enzyme [ACE] inhibitors) and comorbid conditions (Table 5–1). Although many antihypertensive drugs affect serum lipoprotein levels adversely (Table 5–2) the clinical significance of this effect is not yet defined (Ann Intern Med 1995;122:133–141).

If monotherapy is not effective, a second and then a third drug from different drug classes may be added or substituted. Monotherapy with most agents is effective in 40% to 50% of patients. Blood pressure can be controlled with two drugs in 80% to 90% of patients.

II. SPECIFIC MEDICATIONS

A. Diuretics (Table 5–3)

1. THIAZIDES. Among the diuretics, thiazides remain the cornerstone of antihypertensive therapy. Their metabolic side effects include hypokalemia, hypomagnesemia, hyperuricemia, and hyperlipidemia. The thiazides may promote hyperglycemia when used as part of a multidrug regimen, but thiazide monotherapy does not increase the risk of hyperglycemia requiring treatment (Ann Intern Med 1993;118:273–278). The consequences of mild hypokalemia or hypomagnesemia are uncertain (Ann Intern Med 1995;122:223–226), but only serum potassium levels below 3.1 mEq/L promote cardiac arrhythmias. Adverse effects of hypokalemia are more likely for patients with ischemic heart disease, hepatic insufficiency, diabetes mellitus, and concomitant use of corticosteroids or cardiac glycosides. Daily doses of hydrochlorothiazide greater than 50 mg are associated with an increased risk of cardiac arrest (N Engl J Med 1994;330:1852–1857); addition of a potassium-sparing agent to the drug regimen reduced the risk.

   In patients without edema, thiazides are more effective than loop diuretics, may be given once daily, and are less likely to cause hypokalemia. The antihypertensive effect may require 2 to 4 weeks to develop, although it is often complete in 1 week. Indapamide and metolazone are the only thiazides that are effective when the serum creatinine is above 2.5 mg/dL. For all other patients, the least expensive drugs in this class, hydrochlorothiazide and chlorthalidone, are the drugs of choice.

2. THE LOOP DIURETICS, more potent than the thiazides, are useful in patients with renal insufficiency and in combination with sodium-retaining antihypertensives, such as minoxidil. They should be used twice per day for blood pressure control.

3. POTASSIUM-SPARING DIURETICS are usually used in combination with a thiazide and minimize hypokalemia due to the potassium-wasting diuretics. They should be used with caution in patients with renal disease or at risk for hyperkalemia. **Spironolactone** is as potent as hydrochlorothiazide but has a higher incidence of side effects, particularly at doses above 100 mg/d. **Triamterene** and **amiloride** are not, by themselves, useful antihypertensive agents.

Text continued on page 210

TABLE 5-1. Individualization of Antihypertensive Drug Therapy

CLINICAL SITUATION	PREFERRED	REQUIRES SPECIAL MONITORING	RELATIVELY OR ABSOLUTELY CONTRAINDICATED
CARDIOVASCULAR			
Angina pectoris	Beta blockers, calcium channel blockers	—	Direct vasodilators
After MI	Non-ISA beta blockers	—	Direct vasodilators
CHF	Diuretics, ACE inhibitors	—	Beta blockers, calcium channel blockers, labetalol
RENAL			
Bilateral renal artery stenosis or stenosis to single functioning kidney	—	—	ACE inhibitors
Renal insufficiency (serum creatinine 1.5–2.5 mg/dL)	—	—	Potassium-sparing agents
Renal insufficiency (serum creatinine ≥2.5 mg/dL)	Loop diuretics	ACE inhibitors	Potassium-sparing agents
OTHER			
Obstructive lung disease	—	—	Beta blockers, labetalol
Dyslipidemia	—	Diuretics, beta blockers	—
Diabetes mellitus	—	Diuretics, beta blockers	—
Liver disease	—	Labetalol	Methyldopa
Vascular headache	Beta blockers	—	—
Pregnancy (chronic hypertension)	Methyldopa	—	ACE inhibitors
Pregnancy (preeclampsia)	Methyldopa, hydralazine, nifedipine, labetalol	—	Diuretics, ACE inhibitors
Cyclosporine-associated hypertension	Nifedipine, labetalol	Verapamil, nicardipine, diltiazem	—
Depression	—	Centrally acting sympatholytics	Reserpine

Adapted from the Fifth Report of the Joint National Committee on Detection, Evaluation, and Treatment of High Blood Pressure, 1993. Arch Intern Med 1993;153:154–183.

TABLE 5–2. Changes in Serum Lipid Levels with Antihypertensive Therapy

DRUG CLASS	CHANGE IN TOTAL CHOLESTEROL (mmol/L)*	CHANGE IN HDL CHOLESTEROL (mmol/L)*	CHANGE IN LDL CHOLESTEROL (mmol/L)*	CHANGE IN TRIGLYCERIDES (mmol/L)†
Diuretic	0.29	−0.02	0.24	0.35
Nonselective beta blocker	0.1	−0.11	0.05	0.54
Selective beta blocker	0.06	−0.07	−0.08	0.11
Beta blocker with intrinsic sympathomimetic activity	−0.12	−0.03	−0.19	0.16
Alpha blocker	−0.15	0.01	−0.17	−0.09
Sympatholytic	−0.05	−0.04	−0.06	0.15
ACE inhibitor	−0.01	0.02	−0.05	−0.07
Calcium channel blocker	0.03	0.01	0.12	−0.06

*To convert changes in cholesterol levels from mmol/L to mg/dL, multiply by 39.
†To convert changes in cholesterol levels from mmol/L to mg/dL, multiply by 89.
Data derived from Kasiske BL, Ma JZ, Kalil RSN, Louis TA. Effects of antihypertensive therapy on serum lipids. Ann Intern Med 1995;122:133–141.

TABLE 5–3. Diuretics

AGENT	TRADE NAME	ORAL ADULT DOSE (mg)	DURATION OF DIURETIC EFFECT (h)	COMMENT
THIAZIDES AND RELATED AGENTS				
Chlorothiazide	Diuril	125–500 qd, given bid	PO 6–12 IV 2	Absorption decreased by bile acid binders; decrease lithium clearance and effect of sulfonylureas; associated with photosensitivity, pancreatitis, and interstitial nephritis. Available for IV use; usually 500 mg q12–24h
Chlorthalidone	Hygroton	12.5–50 qd	24–72	In combination therapy, 12.5–25 mg qd usually preferred dose
Hydrochlorothiazide (HCTZ)	Esidrix, Hydrodiuril, Oretic	6.25–50 qd	6–12	In combination therapy, 6.25–25 mg qd usually preferred dose; least expensive thiazide diuretic
Indapamide	Lozol	2.5–5 qd	24–36	May be used in renal insufficiency; limit dose to 2.5 mg qd for hypertension; does not raise serum triglyceride level
Metolazone	Diulo, Mykrox, Zaroxolyn	2.5–20 qd	12–24	May be used in renal insufficiency; limit dose to 5 mg qd for hypertension
LOOP DIURETICS				Agents are chemically dissimilar but cleared hepatically and renally; all increase urinary loss of K, Ca, and Mg; ototoxicity possible at high doses; decrease lithium clearance; onset of action 5 min with IV route
Bumetanide	Bumex	PO 0.5–5 qd, given bid IV/IM 0.5–2 q2–6h	PO 4–6 IV 2–3	1 mg bumetanide equal to 40 mg furosemide
Ethacrynic acid	Edecrin	PO 25–100 qd, given bid IV 0.5–1 mg/kg/dose, q8–12h	PO 12 IV 2	Only diuretic available for patients with allergy to sulfur-containing diuretics

LOOP DIURETICS *Continued*

Furosemide	Lasix	PO 20–320 qd, given bid IV/IM 10–80 q2–6h	PO 6–8 IV 2	Use bid for hypertension; maximum daily dose 600 mg; least expensive of loop diuretics
Torsemide	Demadex	PO 5–10 qd IV 20–80 q2–6h	PO 6–8 IV 1–2	Can be used qd for hypertension

POTASSIUM-SPARING DIURETICS

Amiloride	Midamor, Moduretic	5–10 qd	24	May cause hyperkalemia (see text); decrease lithium clearance; all agents available as fixed-dose combination medication with HCTZ Combination with HCTZ only available containing 50 mg HCTZ
Spironolactone	Aldactone, Aldactazide	25–200 qd, given bid–tid	48–72	Effective as single agent; interferes with digoxin immunoassay; may cause gynecomastia or menstrual irregularity; least expensive K-sparing diuretic
Triamterene	Dyrenium, Dyazide, Maxzide	37.5–100 qd	24	Little intrinsic antihypertensive effect; bioavailability of the HCTZ component of Dyazide capsules is 50% that of Maxzide and plain HCTZ pills; may promote nephrolithiasis with stones containing triamterene

B. Beta-Adrenergic Blockers (Table 5–4)

These drugs are effective in the treatment of hypertension and in prevention or delay of hypertensive complications. **Metoprolol** is significantly more effective than diuretics in primary prevention of coronary heart disease among hypertensive men (JAMA 1988;259:1976–1982). **Propranolol, metoprolol, atenolol, and timolol** reduce the rates of reinfarction and cardiovascular death after MI. Properly titrated, the agents in this class are equally effective in blood pressure reduction.

1. BETA$_1$-SELECTIVE AGENTS vary in the degree of relative beta$_1$ inhibition. Their selectivity is lost at higher doses but may be an important theoretical consideration in choosing therapy for patients with obstructive pulmonary disease and diabetes. **Beta$_2$ blockade** may trigger adverse effects, such as bronchospasm, dampened manifestations of hypoglycemia, and loss of beta$_2$-mediated peripheral vasodilation (which may promote hypertension in patients with pheochromocytoma or taking sympathomimetics, such as phenylpropanolamine or pseudoephedrine).

2. INTRINSIC SYMPATHOMIMETIC ACTIVITY (ISA) occurs with **pindolol, acebutolol,** and others, which are mild sympathetic agonists that block access of more potent circulating catecholamines to beta-adrenergic receptors. They are less likely to affect resting cardiac function than are beta blockers lacking ISA. However, they cause a comparable decrement in maximal heart rate response to exercise.

3. LABETALOL is unique in its ability to block both alpha and beta receptors.

4. ADVERSE EFFECTS. The most common side effects of the beta blockers are fatigue, depression, and impotence. They are contraindicated in patients with severe cardiac conduction defects (greater than first degree AV nodal block with PR interval over 0.24 seconds) or in those using MAO inhibitors. Beta blockers must be used carefully in patients with bronchospastic pulmonary disease, diabetes, or CHF due to systolic dysfunction and in those taking verapamil or diltiazem (additive effects on the cardiac conduction system may occur). After abrupt discontinuation of high doses of propranolol, a withdrawal syndrome including hypertension and cardiac ischemia has been reported; beta blockers should be tapered over 2 to 3 weeks.

C. ACE Inhibitors (Table 5–5)

These agents decrease levels of circulating angiotensin II and aldosterone. Although they are as effective as thiazides and beta blockers for mild hypertension, JNC 5 recommended that they be first-line therapy only in selected situations. In insulin-dependent diabetic patients with microalbuminuria, progressive proteinuria and the progression of renal disease are reduced by ACE inhibitors (N Engl J Med 1993;329:1456–1462). Survival of patients with significant CHF may be improved (N Engl J Med 1996;335:490–498). Although particularly effective in treating renovascular hypertension, ACE inhibitors may cause reversible acute renal failure in such patients, especially those with bilateral renal artery stenosis or a stenotic artery to a single functioning kidney.

TABLE 5-4. Beta Adrenergic Blockers

Most agents are cleared hepatically. For the hepatically metabolized drugs, enzyme inducers (e.g., rifampin, barbiturates) may decrease plasma levels, whereas cimetidine, hydralazine, phenothiazines, propafenone, quinidine, and verapamil may increase them. May reduce plasma clearance of drugs metabolized by the liver (e.g., lidocaine, warfarin). Use cautiously with calcium channel blockers.

AGENT	TRADE NAME	USUAL ADULT DOSE (mg); (MAXIMAL DAILY DOSE)	PLASMA T$_{1/2}$ (h)	BETA$_1$ SELECTIVE	ISA*	COMMENT
Acebutolol	Sectral	100–400 bid (1200)†	3	+	1+	Active metabolite renally excreted
Atenolol	Tenormin	25–100 qd (150)†	6–9	+	—	Excreted unchanged in urine; bioavailability reduced by PO ampicillin; available for IV use
Betaxolol	Kerlone	5–20 qd (40)	14–16	+	—	Most beta$_1$ selective of the beta blockers
Bisoprolol	Zebeta	5–10 qd (20)	9–12	+	—	Beta$_1$ selectivity less at doses above 10 mg qd
Carteolol	Cartrol	2.5–5 qd (10)†	6	—	1+	——
Carvedilol	Coreg	6.25–25 bid (50)	7–10	—	—	Has alpha-adrenergic blocking properties
Labetalol	Normodyne, Trandate	100–600 bid (1200)	4–6	—	—	Has alpha-adrenergic blocking properties; most effective beta blocker for blacks; available for IV use
Metoprolol	Lopressor, Toprol XL	25–100 bid (200)	3–4	+	—	Toprol XL is extended release form for qd administration; available for IV use

Table continued on following page

211

TABLE 5-4. **Beta Adrenergic Blockers** (*Continued*)

AGENT	TRADE NAME	USUAL ADULT DOSE (mg); (MAXIMAL DAILY DOSE)†	PLASMA T₁/₂ (h)	BETA₁ SELECTIVE	ISA*	COMMENT
Nadolol	Corgard	20–320 qd (640)†	14–18	—	—	Excreted unchanged in urine
Penbutolol	Levatol	20–40 qd (80)†	5	—	1+	—
Pindolol	Visken	5–20 bid (60)†	3–4	—	3+	May cause insomnia, nervousness
Propranolol	Inderal, Inderal LA	20–160 bid (640)	3–5	—	—	Used qid for angina pectoris; Inderal LA is extended release form for qd administration; available for IV use; least expensive beta blocker
Timolol	Blocadren	10–20 bid (40)	4	—	—	—

*ISA, intrinsic sympathomimetic activity.
†Reduce dose if serum creatinine greater than 2.5 mg/dL.

TABLE 5-5. Agents Affecting Angiotensin System

ACE inhibitors may cause acute hypotensive response in the elderly and patients taking diuretics. Monitor renal function in patients with congestive heart failure or possible renovascular hypertension. For most ACE inhibitors, decrease dose for patients with renal insufficiency. Hypotensive effect of ACE inhibitors may be blunted by NSAIDs. May cause hyperkalemia.

AGENT	TRADE NAME	USUAL ADULT DOSE (mg); (MAXIMUM DAILY DOSE)	TIME TO PEAK EFFECT (h)	COMMENT
ACE INHIBITORS				
Benazepril	Lotensin	10–40 qd-bid (80)	2–4	Least expensive of ACE inhibitors
Captopril	Capoten	12.5–50 bid-tid (450)	1–1.5	Not a "prodrug"; FDA approved for CHF
Enalapril	Vasotec	2.5–20 qd-bid (40)	4–6	FDA approved for CHF; may be given once daily if daily dose above 5 mg
Enalaprilat	Vasotec IV	1.25 q6h	0.5	Only parenteral ACE inhibitor
Fosinopril	Monopril	10–20 qd-bid (80)	2–6	No dose reduction necessary in patients with renal dysfunction
Lisinopril	Prinivil, Zestril	5–20 qd-bid (80)	6	Not a "prodrug"; FDA approved for CHF; no taste alterations
Quinapril	Accupril	5–20 qd-bid (80)	2	FDA approved for CHF
Ramipril	Altace	1.25–10 qd-bid (20)	3–6	FDA approved for CHF
ANGIOTENSIN RECEPTOR BLOCKER				
Losartan	Cozaar	25–50 qd-bid (150)	1–2	Reduce dose in patients with hepatic disease; may cause hyperkalemia

ACE inhibitors do not affect serum glucose, lipid, or uric acid levels. They can cause hyperkalemia, especially in patients with diabetes, renal disease, or CHF, and should be used cautiously with potassium-sparing diuretics, potassium supplements, and NSAIDs. Adverse effects are rash, dysgeusia, angioedema, and cough (due to reduced bradykinin degradation). Early reports of neutropenia caused by captopril were generally in patients with renal insufficiency or collagen vascular disease during treatment with relatively high doses.

Losartan is not an ACE inhibitor, but it does decrease the effect of circulating angiotensin II. Losartan and its active metabolite (synthesized via the cytochrome P450 system) block the angiotensin$_1$ receptor found in vascular smooth muscle and the adrenal gland, thereby reducing vasoconstriction and aldosterone secretion. Since it is not an ACE inhibitor, bradykinin is not affected and cough is not a side effect. Like ACE inhibitors, it is less effective for the treatment of hypertension in blacks; other precautions appropriate to ACE inhibitors apply to losartan.

D. Calcium Channel Blockers (Table 5–6)

These drugs share a common mechanism, vasodilation with a decrease in peripheral vascular resistance, but their typical effects vary considerably. The **dihydropyridines,** such as **nifedipine,** have vasodilatory effects that occur well before cardiotoxic levels develop, so careful concurrent use with beta blockers is possible. Headache, flushing, and peripheral edema are common side effects. Some patients treated with **nicardipine** experience an aggravation of angina; the mechanism is unknown. **Verapamil** and, to a lesser extent, **diltiazem** have negative inotropic and chronotropic effects, and cardiotoxicity is frequent with concurrent use of beta blockers. They are contraindicated in patients with sinoatrial node dysfunction and AV block greater than first degree. Constipation is the most common side effect. They are less likely than nifedipine to cause peripheral edema and reflex tachycardia. The calcium channel blockers, particularly the short-acting ones, may increase the risk of MI (JAMA 1995;274:620–625), but the data are still inconclusive (JAMA 1995;274:654–655).

E. Peripheral Alpha-Adrenergic Receptor Blockers (Table 5–7)

These agents may cause severe postural hypotension with the first dose, typically 30 to 90 minutes after administration. This effect may be minimized by giving 1 mg at bedtime as the initial dose. It may recur with retreatment after a hiatus of a few days. It is more common in volume-depleted or elderly patients. The alpha blockers may improve symptoms of prostatic obstruction in men but aggravate stress incontinence in women.

F. Centrally Acting Sympatholytics (Table 5–7)

Clonidine, guanabenz, and **alpha-methyldopa** have central alpha$_2$ agonist properties. Sedation, dry mouth, and postural symptoms are common side effects of all three drugs. Clonidine has the most rapid effect and is used in oral treatment of "hypertensive urgencies." A demonstrated lack of adverse fetal effects allows alpha-methyldopa to be used in pregnant patients. Of patients treated with alpha-methyldopa, 10% to 20% develop a positive direct Coombs test, but clinically apparent hemolysis is unusual.

Text continued on page 219

TABLE 5-6. Calcium Channel Blockers

Cleared by the liver; cimetidine may increase the effect of diltiazem, nifedipine, and possibly others by reducing first-pass metabolism. Many are used as antianginals. All may increase the serum digoxin level.

AGENT	TRADE NAME	USUAL ADULT DOSE (mg); (MAXIMUM DAILY DOSE)	ONSET OF EFFECT (min)	TIME TO PEAK EFFECT (h)	HALF-LIFE (h)	COMMENT
BENZOTHIAPINES						
Diltiazem	Cardizem	30–120 qid (480)	30–60	2–3	4–6	Short-acting diltiazem not FDA approved for hypertension; available for IV use
Diltiazem (sustained release)	Cardizem SR	60–180 bid (480)	30–60	6–11	5–7	
Diltiazem (extended release)	Cardizem CD, Dilacor XR, Tiazac	120–360 qd (540)	30–60	6–11	5–7	Novel long-acting formulations give variable drug levels over 24 h period
DIHYDROPYRIDINES						Edema, headache, and dizziness are side effects common to this group; taking these drugs with grapefruit juice doubles (or more) absorption
Amlodipine	Norvasc	2.5–10 qd (10)	360	6–9	34	
Felodipine	Plendil	5–10 qd (20)	240	2.5–5	10–36	
Isradipine	DynaCirc	2.5–5 bid (20)	120	0.5–2.5	8	Least expensive dihydropyridine calcium channel blocker
Nicardipine	Cardene	20–40 tid (120)	20	0.5–2	2–4	Available for IV use

Table continued on following page

215

TABLE 5-6. **Calcium Channel Blockers** *(Continued)*

AGENT	TRADE NAME	USUAL ADULT DOSE (mg); (MAXIMUM DAILY DOSE)	ONSET OF EFFECT (min)	TIME TO PEAK EFFECT (h)	HALF-LIFE (h)	COMMENT
DIHYDROPYRIDINES *(Continued)*						
Nicardipine (extended release)	Cardene SR	30–60 bid (120)	—	—	—	May worsen CHF
Nifedipine	Adalat, Procardia	10–30 tid (180)	20	0.5	2–5	May worsen CHF; Adalat CC less expensive than Procardia XL
Nifedipine (extended release)	Adalat CC, Procardia XL	30–120 qd (180)	—	—	—	
Nisoldipine	Sular	10–40 qd (60)	180	6–12	7–12	Peak plasma concentration tripled by taking this drug with a high-fat meal
PHENYLALKYLAMINES						
Verapamil	Calan, Isoptin	40–120 tid (480)	30	1.2–2	3–7	Constipation most common side effect, least expensive nondihydropyridine calcium channel blocker; available for IV use
Verapamil (long acting)	Calan SR, Isoptin SR, Verelan, Covera HS	120–240 qd–bid (480)	30	1.2–2	3–7	Novel long-acting formulations give variable drug levels over 24 h period; some brands formulated for HS dosing

TABLE 5–7. Antiadrenergic Agents

AGENT	TRADE NAME	ADULT DOSE (mg)	TIME TO PEAK EFFECT (h)	COMMENT
PERIPHERAL ALPHA ANTAGONISTS				
				Cleared by liver and kidneys; first dose postural hypotension; less tachycardia than direct vasodilators; effective for symptoms of prostatic obstruction
Doxazosin	Cardura	1–8 qd (16)	2–3	Less postural effect than prazosin
Prazosin	Minipress	1–5 bid–tid (20)	1–3	Least expensive peripheral alpha antagonist
Terazosin	Hytrin	1–10 qd (20)	2–3	Less postural effect than prazosin
CENTRAL ALPHA AGONISTS				
				All agents may cause sedation, dry mouth, sexual dysfunction; rebound hypertension may occur with abrupt withdrawal; hypotensive effect of these agents decreased by tricyclic antidepressants
Alpha-methyldopa	Aldomet	250–1000 bid–tid (2000)	4–6	Increases risk of lithium toxicity; iron salts decrease effect; may cause chronic active hepatitis; may be given IV (250–500 mg q6h)
Clonidine	Catapres, Catapres-TTS	0.1–0.6 bid–tid (2.4)	1–3	Withdrawal syndrome uncommon if daily dose less than 0.6 mg; available in transdermal form, administered weekly; least expensive drug in this class
Guanabenz	Wytensin	4–32 bid (64)	2–4	Alter dose in patients with hepatic dysfunction
Guanfacine	Tenex	1–3 qd (3)	8–11	Usually given at HS; alter dose in patients with renal dysfunction

Table continued on following page

TABLE 5–7. Antiadrenergic Agents (*Continued*)

AGENT	TRADE NAME	ADULT DOSE (mg)	TIME TO PEAK EFFECT (h)	COMMENT
OTHER AGENTS				
				Increase pressor effect of nonprescription directly acting sympathomimetics; prolonged effect after drug discontinuation
Guanethidine	Ismelin	10–50 qd (100)	6–8	Edema and postural hypotension common side effects
Reserpine	Serpasil	0.05–0.25 qd	72–144	Contraindicated in patients with depression, history of depression, or peptic ulcer disease

G. Direct Vasodilators (Table 5–8)

These drugs act primarily on arteriolar smooth muscle, may lead to reflex tachycardia, and are often combined with beta blockers. **Hydralazine** is often used in pregnant patients and in those with pregnancy-induced hypertension (preeclampsia). It is associated with a lupuslike syndrome that is rare unless the total daily dose is greater than 200 mg. **Minoxidil** is a potent drug usually used only in patients with severe hypertension. It causes significant sodium retention and usually must be given with furosemide, 20–40 mg bid. Abrupt withdrawal may cause rebound hypertension.

H. Cost Considerations

Because hypertension is so common, the cost of an antihypertensive regimen should be considered carefully. Important variables to consider in addition to the cost of the drug are dosing interval, drug potency, and the need for laboratory monitoring. Hydrochlorothiazide is the least expensive single agent. However, if potassium supplements are required, combination with a potassium-sparing diuretic may be less expensive. Propranolol, clonidine, hydralazine, and prazosin are also quite inexpensive.

Because propranolol may be used twice per day, it is usually the cheapest beta blocker. However, drugs given once daily, although more expensive per dose, may have lower daily cost. Many fixed-dose drug combinations are available but are generally inappropriate as initial therapy because they impede individualization of drug regimens.

III. RENOVASCULAR HYPERTENSION

A. General Considerations

One percent of patients with hypertension have renovascular hypertension, the most common type of secondary hypertension. It should be suspected in patients with blood pressure that is difficult to control, particularly if a patient is relatively young or has renal insufficiency.

Renovascular hypertension results from macrovascular stenosis, leading to excess renin production and high plasma aldosterone and angiotensin levels. The most common causes are fibromuscular dysplasia (younger patients, mainly female, 25% of cases) and atherosclerotic disease (75%).

The best sequence of diagnostic testing for renovascular hypertension is controversial (Mayo Clin Proc 1994;69:1172–1181). **Noninvasive screening** is probably best done with **duplex ultrasonic study** of the renal arteries (Ann Intern Med 1995;122:833–838). An alternative noninvasive technique is captopril-stimulated radionuclide renography. Confirmation requires **renal angiography** with measurement of renal vein renin activities.

B. Management

Percutaneous **transluminal angioplasty** is beneficial in 70% of patients with atherosclerotic lesions (although those of the renal artery ostium respond poorly) and 60% of those with fibromuscular dysplasia. The majority of patients who respond to angioplasty have a decrease in their medication requirements and improvement in their blood pressure, but only a minority (8% and 22%, respectively) are cured (Mayo Clin Proc 1995;70:1041–1052).

The rate of cure or improvement is similar for **surgical revascularization,**

TABLE 5-8. Direct Vasodilators

Commonly cause reflex tachycardia, edema, and headache. May precipitate angina in patients with coronary artery disease. Should be used in combination with diuretics and beta blockers.

AGENT	TRADE NAME	USUAL ADULT DOSE (mg); (MAXIMUM DAILY DOSE)	TIME TO PEAK EFFECT	COMMENT
Hydralazine	Apresoline	25–100 bid PO (300) 5–10 q3–6h IV 10–50 q3–6h IM	0.5–2 h PO 10–20 min IV/IM	Drug of choice for pregnancy-induced hypertension; may increase plasma levels of hepatically cleared beta blockers; ingestion with food increases bioavailability; least expensive vasodilator
Minoxidil	Loniten	2.5–20 qd–bid (80)	2–3 h	Reduce dose in patients with renal insufficiency; causes hypertrichosis in 80% of recipients; may cause pleural or pericardial effusions

but it should be considered only when angioplasty is impossible or has failed.

Treatment with an ACE inhibitor, beta blocker, or diuretic is the regimen of choice for nonoperable disease. Acute renal failure may result from ACE inhibitor therapy in patients with bilateral renal artery stenosis or renal artery stenosis in a single functioning kidney. Renal function (creatinine clearance) and size (ultrasound) should be followed, as renal damage can progress even with apparently satisfactory blood pressure control.

IV. HYPERTENSIVE CRISIS

Hypertensive emergencies are clinical situations that require immediate blood pressure reduction to prevent or limit **target organ damage** (e.g., cardiopulmonary symptoms and signs, ECG changes, new retinopathy, azotemia, hematuria, or microangiopathic hemolytic anemia). Most patients have a diastolic blood pressure (DBP) greater than 120 mm Hg, although children and pregnant women may have lower blood pressures. Patients without these findings but with severe hypertension (DBP greater than 120 to 130 mm Hg) have a **hypertensive urgency** and should have their blood pressure lowered within 24 hours. Oral therapy may be sufficient to attain this goal.

The most common cause of hypertensive crisis is an abrupt change in the blood pressure control of a chronic hypertensive already under treatment for hypertension. Sympathomimetic ingestion or dietary indiscretion by a patient taking an MAO inhibitor may be occult causes.

The usual goal of treatment is either a 25% reduction of the mean arterial pressure or reduction to a DBP of 100 mm Hg, whichever is higher. Most patients are already volume depleted, and diuretics should not be used except in pulmonary edema. In patients with **myocardial ischemia, pulmonary edema, or aortic dissection,** the DBP should be reduced below 100 mm Hg in 15 to 30 minutes unless organ perfusion is compromised. Particularly in cases of cerebral ischemia, overzealous therapy can be hazardous, worsening the ischemia. For patients with **hypertensive encephalopathy,** the 25% reduction should be done over 2 to 3 hours, and for those with **acute cerebral ischemia or intracranial bleeding,** the reduction should be over 6 to 12 hours, taking care to not go below a blood pressure of 170/100 mm Hg.

A. Drug Therapy (Tables 5–9 and 5–10)

The most rapidly effective agent is continuous IV **nitroprusside,** although close monitoring is required. It should be avoided in pregnancy-induced

TABLE 5–9. Drugs for Hypertensive Urgencies

AGENT	ORAL DOSE (mg)	FREQUENCY	ONSET (min)	DURATION (h)
Captopril	25	q30min	15	4
Clonidine	0.1–0.2	q1h	30–60	8–12
Nifedipine	10 (break capsule and swallow contents)	q15–30min	10–20	3–6
Prazosin	1–2	q1h	30–120	10

TABLE 5-10. **Drugs for Hypertensive Emergencies**

AGENT	ONSET (min)	DURATION	ROUTE	DOSE	COMMENT
Sodium nitroprusside	Immediate	2-3 min	IV infusion	0.3-10 μg/kg/min	Give maximum dose for no longer than 10 min because of risk of cyanide toxicity, especially with renal insufficiency; may cause reflex tachycardia or oxygen desaturation
Nitroglycerin	1-2	3-5 min	IV infusion	5-100 μg/min	May cause headache; preferred in patients with acute cardiac ischemia
Hydralazine	10-20	3-6 h	IV bolus	5-10 mg q20min	May cause tachycardia; if not effective after 20 mg, choose different drug; may be given IM (dose 10-50 mg)
Labetalol	5-10	3-6 h	IV bolus, then infusion	20-80 mg q10min; 2 mg/min infusion	Risk of heart block, CHF, bronchospasm; useful in patients with aortic dissection or excess catecholamines (e.g., pheochromocytoma, cocaine intoxication)
Phentolamine	1-2	3-10 min	IV bolus	5-10 mg q5-15min	Useful in patients with excess catecholamines (e.g., pheochromocytoma, cocaine intoxication)

hypertension because of the risk of thiocyanate toxicity (indicated by dizziness, ataxia, headache, loss of consciousness, and metabolic acidosis). **IV nitroglycerin** is the drug of choice when cardiac ischemia is present. Treatment may be initiated topically or sublingually while IV access is being established.

Oral nifedipine or **clonidine** may be used for hypertensive urgency. For nifedipine, the sublingual route has no advantage over and may be riskier than the oral route.

B. Special Circumstances

1. **AORTIC DISSECTION.** Blood pressure reduction and decrease of shear forces are the goal. Thus, beta blockers (given first) are combined with vasodilators (usually nitroprusside) (JAMA 1990;264:2537–2541). Labetalol may also be used alone.

2. **PREGNANCY-INDUCED HYPERTENSION.** The goal of therapy is to keep the mean arterial pressure between 105 and 126 mm Hg and the DBP between 90 and 105 mm Hg. Hydralazine is the drug of choice. Labetalol and nifedipine are alternates.

3. **PHEOCHROMOCYTOMA.** Phentolamine, given in intermittent IV boluses, is the drug of choice. Labetalol is an alternative (because it has both alpha and beta blockade). Simple beta blockers are contraindicated.

4. **HYPERTENSIVE CRISIS OF PROGRESSIVE SYSTEMIC SCLEROSIS.** ACE inhibitors are the drugs of choice (Ann Intern Med 1990;113:352–357).

Fifth Report of the Joint National Committee on Detection, Evaluation, and Treatment of High Blood Pressure. Arch Intern Med 1993;153:154–183.

Fries ED. The efficacy and safety of diuretics in treating hypertension. Ann Intern Med 1995; 122:223–226.

Gifford RW Jr. Management of hypertensive crisis. JAMA 1991;266:829–835.

Kasiske BL, Ma JZ, Kalil RSN, Louis TA. Effects of antihypertensive therapy on serum lipids. Ann Intern Med 1995;122:133–141.

Littenberg B, Garber AM, Sox HC. Screening for hypertension. Ann Intern Med 1990;112:192–202.

Mejia AD, Egan BM, Schork NJ, Zweifler AJ. Artefacts in measurement of blood pressure and lack of target organ involvement in the assessment of patients with treatment-resistant hypertension. Ann Intern Med 1990;112:270–277.

Oberman A, Wassertheil-Smoller S, Langford HG, et al. Pharmacologic and nutritional treatment of mild hypertension: changes in cardiovascular risk status. Ann Intern Med 1990;112:89–95.

Sibai BM. Treatment of hypertension in pregnant women. N Engl J Med 1996;335:257–265.

6666666666666

RENAL DISEASES

LESLIE S. T. FANG

I. MANAGEMENT OF PATIENTS WITH ACUTE RENAL FAILURE

A. General Principles

Although the causes of acute renal failure (ARF) are diverse, the complications are similar, and general guidelines are applicable to all patients with acute progressive deterioration of renal function. About 70% of patients with ARF have an oliguric phase; the rest have nonoliguric renal failure. A number of complications can arise during acute renal insufficiency, and patient management depends on the complications.

B. Management During the Oliguric Phase

1. **FLUID MANAGEMENT.** The major goal is to avoid fluid overload and excessive fluid depletion. The patient should be weighed daily, with a weight loss goal of about ¼ pound each day. Intake and output should be carefully monitored, and the patient's fluids should be restricted so that the total intake matches the urine output plus insensible losses. In patients with intractable volume overload and congestive heart failure (CHF), peritoneal dialysis, hemodialysis, or continuous venovenous hemofiltration (CVVH) may be necessary.

2. **MANAGEMENT OF ACIDOSIS.** Metabolic acidosis in acute renal failure is due to accumulation of phosphates, sulfates, and organic and inorganic acids. Initial management should be directed at reversal of hyperphosphatemia. Patients should be given phosphate binders, such as **calcium acetate** (PhosLo 667 mg), with each meal. Patients with acidosis not reversed by calcium acetate should be given **sodium bicarbonate,** starting with oral doses of 600 mg bid, increasing to 1.2 g qid, as necessary. The goal is to give enough sodium bicarbonate to maintain serum bicarbonate levels between 16 and 20 mEq/L. The considerable sodium load will limit sodium bicarbonate use if volume overload is a concern. Hypocalcemia can also limit the use of sodium bicarbonate. Rapid reversal of acidosis may worsen hypocalcemia and induce tetany and seizures.

3. **ELECTROLYTE MANAGEMENT.** The primary concern is the management of hyperkalemia (Table 6–1). Cardiac monitoring is indicated until the serum potassium level has been stabilized. In an acute situation, the serum potassium level can be rapidly lowered by the use of glucose and insulin. Sodium bicarbonate can also shift potassium from the extracellular to the intracellular space on an acute basis. **Sodium polystyrene sulfonate** (Kayexalate), 30–50 g in a sorbitol solution, can be given either orally or as an enema for long-term management. This resin exchanges sodium for potassium, calcium, and magnesium. Protracted use may result in sodium overload, hypocalcemia, or hypomagnesemia. In patients with refractory hyperkalemia, peritoneal dialysis or hemodialysis may be necessary.

TABLE 6–1. **Treatment of Hyperkalemia**

Acute Management	
Sodium bicarbonate	50 mEq IV
$D_{50}W$	1 ampule
Insulin	10 U Regular insulin
Calcium gluconate	1 ampule
Chronic Management	
Low-potassium diet	
Sodium polystyrene sulfonate	50 g PO or PR
Dialysis	

4. MANAGEMENT OF UREMIA. To minimize the degree of uremia, patients should receive adequate caloric intake and a low-protein diet. Usually protein intake should be restricted to 0.5 g/kg/d. Adequate caloric intake should be maintained to minimize catabolism. Maximize the use of high-quality protein, essential amino acids, or alpha-keto analogs of essential amino acids in the diet. Prospective randomized studies have suggested that patients in the postsurgical period who develop ARF and require dialysis have improved survival when given **renal failure fluid,** a glucose solution containing essential amino acids.

5. MANAGEMENT OF CALCIUM AND PHOSPHATE HOMEOSTASIS. Hyperphosphatemia should be corrected before aggressive correction of serum calcium to minimize metastatic calcification. Correction of hyperphosphatemia can be done most easily by dietary restriction and by the use of phosphate binders, such as calcium acetate (PhosLo, 667 mg). Calcium acetate should be given with meals to maximize binding of dietary phosphate (e.g., PhosLo 2 tablets PO before meals). The goal is to bring the serum phosphate to a level less than 5 mg/dL. After optimal adjustment of the serum phosphate level, hypocalcemia can be corrected with calcium supplement and vitamin D. A reasonable starting dose of calcium would be 500 mg of Os-Cal tid. A reasonable starting dose of vitamin D would be 0.25 µg of 1,25-dihydroxycholecalciferol (Rocaltrol) daily. Serum calcium values should be monitored closely to avoid hypercalcemia.

6. MANAGEMENT OF DRUGS THAT ARE EXCRETED RENALLY. In patients with oliguric renal failure, all medications should be reviewed, and doses of renally excreted drugs should be adjusted. Drugs containing magnesium should be avoided, as seemingly innocuous drugs, such as Milk of Magnesia or Mylanta, can cause magnesium accumulation, which can lead to CNS toxicity. Life-threatening drug toxicity can be avoided if a careful review of drugs has been carried out.

7. MANAGEMENT OF CARDIOVASCULAR COMPLICATIONS. Careful attention should be focused on fluid management to minimize the likelihood of fluid overload, hypertension, and CHF. Uremic pericarditis, however, is usually an indication that there has been considerable accumulation of uremic toxins and may force initiation of dialysis.

8. **MANAGEMENT OF NEUROLOGIC COMPLICATIONS.** Dialysis is indicated if conservative management fails to control CNS symptoms.

9. **MANAGEMENT OF HEMATOLOGIC COMPLICATIONS. Erythropoietin** can be given to patients with anemia in the setting of ARF. However, erythropoietin is less effective in the acutely ill patient. The usual starting dose of erythropoietin is 4000 units SC three times a week. Before starting erythropoietin, the patient should have adequate iron stores (determine Fe, TIBC, and ferritin levels). Prolongation of bleeding time should be addressed, particularly if a patient has clinically evident bleeding or if a surgical procedure is planned. Trials should be made with **desmopressin** (DDAVP) (0.4 µg/kg IV about 4 hours before a contemplated procedure) to see if the bleeding time can be reversed. Premarin has also been shown to be effective in correcting bleeding time. However, the effect of Premarin is usually apparent only after 3 to 7 days of therapy. Prolonged bleeding time can also be corrected by dialysis, which should be considered in a patient with significant bleeding and uremia.

C. Management During the Diuretic Phase

After volume overload is corrected, intake should be adjusted to match urine output until renal function is at a reasonable level, with a BUN value less than 40 mg/dL and a serum creatinine value less than 2.5 mg/dL. This goal may require supplementation with 0.45% normal saline with 20 mEq/L potassium chloride. As renal function approaches normal, fluid infusion should be progressively decreased and discontinued. This step will minimize the likelihood of overdiuresis during the diuretic phase, which occurs occasionally. During the diuretic phase, medication doses must be readjusted as the patient's renal function improves.

D. Indications for Dialysis

Dialysis is indicated in patients for whom conservative management has failed. Specific indications include the following:
- Intractable volume overload, causing hypertension and congestive heart failure
- Progressive CNS symptoms
- Clinically significant bleeding in severely azotemic patients not responding to DDAVP
- Uremic pericarditis
- Life-threatening drug toxicity
- Intractable hyperkalemia unresponsive to conservative management
- Intractable acidosis

In practice, intractable volume overload and progressive uremic symptoms are the most likely reasons for initiation of dialysis.

E. Selected Issues

Several issues that arise in the management of patients with ARF remain controversial.

1. **ROLE OF LOOP DIURETICS.** Although **furosemide** given early in its course may convert oliguric renal failure to nonoliguric renal failure in about

25% to 75% of cases, this effect may not be associated with improved renal or patient outcome. However, because the patient with nonoliguric renal failure is much easier to manage, attempts should be made to see if loop diuretics are beneficial. Before a loop diuretic is used, volume status should be carefully adjusted. Diuresis in a patient with prerenal azotemia can markedly aggravate the problem. If the patient is euvolemic or volume overloaded, furosemide can be used in increasing doses for diuresis. The starting dose should be 40 mg IV; increasing doses can be given at hourly intervals to see if diuresis ensues. In general, the dose should not exceed 400 mg in any 24-hour period to avoid ototoxicity. Some authors advocate progressive increase of furosemide to doses of 3600 mg daily, but this program can lead to furosemide accumulation and resultant ototoxicity.

2. ROLE OF MANNITOL. Mannitol is an osmotic diuretic that some believe will convert oliguric to nonoliguric renal failure. However, mannitol can cause volume overload in the oliguric patient and should be used cautiously.

3. CONTINUOUS INFUSION OF FUROSEMIDE-MANNITOL SOLUTION. Combination therapy using a continuous infusion of furosemide and mannitol has gained popularity in some institutions; 1 g furosemide is mixed in 500 mL of 20% mannitol and infused at a rate of 10 mL/h. Usually an effect is observed within 6 hours after initiation of infusion. Since both furosemide and mannitol are infused at a fairly low rate, the toxicity of such an infusion is limited, but hyponatremia still can occur. In general, the continuous infusion should be stopped if no significant diuresis is seen within 12 hours of the initiation of therapy. Again, although continuous infusion of furosemide and mannitol has been associated with conversion of oliguric renal failure to nonoliguric renal failure, such therapy may not affect renal recovery or mortality.

4. ROLE OF LOW-DOSE DOPAMINE. Dopamine, given in low doses (less than 5 µg/kg/min), has been shown to enhance diuresis, natriuresis, and kaliuresis. Therefore, low-dose dopamine may be of benefit in patients with oliguric ARF. Unfortunately, there are few clinical studies to substantiate the benefit of low-dose dopamine. Again, in selected patients, low-dose dopamine can convert oliguric renal failure to nonoliguric renal failure, but it is not clear that the therapy actually improves renal recovery or outcome.

5. ROLE OF EARLY, AGGRESSIVE DIALYSIS. Early, aggressive dialysis has been advocated by some as beneficial in ARF. However, only minimal, conflicting clinical information attempting to address this issue is available. In most instances, dialysis should be reserved for the patient in whom conservative measures have failed.

Brezis M, Rosen S, Epstein FM. Acute renal failure. In: Brenner BM, Rector FC Jr, eds. The Kidney, 4th ed. Philadelphia: W.B. Saunders Co.; 1991, Chapter 24.

Hakim RM, Lazarus JM. Hemodialysis in acute renal failure. In: Brenner BM, Lazarus JM, eds. Acute Renal Failure, 2nd ed. New York: Churchill Livingstone; 1988, pp 767–808.

Hua SH, Bushinsky DA, Wish BB, Cohen JJ, Harrington JT. Hospital acquired renal insufficiency: a prospective study. Am J Med 1983;74:243–250.

Kjellstrand CM, Barsoum R. Management of acute renal failure. In: Jacobsen HR, Striker GE, Klahr S, eds. The Principles and Practice of Nephrology, 2nd ed. St. Louis: Mosby–Year Book, Inc.; 1995, Chapter 88.

II. THERAPY FOR SPECIFIC FORMS OF ACUTE RENAL FAILURE

A. Ischemic ARF (Acute Tubular Necrosis)

Ischemic ARF, often called **acute tubular necrosis,** is the result of prolonged compromise in renal perfusion. It is believed that the blood supply to normal kidneys can be interrupted for up to 30 minutes without damage. However, in critically ill patients with sustained hemodynamic compromise, progressive renal dysfunction that is unresponsive to correction of blood volume and cardiac output can develop even with shorter intervals of compromise in renal blood flow. Ischemic ARF is likely to occur in a number of clinical settings (Table 6–2).

Clinically, acute oliguria and progressive deterioration in renal function coincide with the acute ischemic event. Usually, an oliguric phase lasts hours to 10 days, followed by a diuretic phase. Examination of the urinary sediment reveals cellular debris with many cellular and granular casts. Urinary indices show low urine osmolality, and the urinary osmolality seldom exceeds the serum osmolality by greater than 100 mOsm/kg. The urinary sodium level tends to be high in these patients, and the fractional excretion of sodium is usually greater than 1%. The ratio of urinary creatinine/plasma creatinine is usually less than 20:1. Urinary findings are important in the differentiation of acute tubular necrosis and prerenal azotemia (Table 6–3).

1. CONTRAST AGENT-INDUCED **ARF**
   a. **Clinical course.** After antibiotics, contrast media are the most common causes of nephrotoxic ARF. Clinically, osmotic diuresis occurs during the first 10 to 18 hours after administration of contrast medium, since most available contrast agents are hyperosmolar. In susceptible patients, oliguric, and occasionally anuric, renal failure occurs about 24 hours after the contrast study. In these patients, renal function deterioration occurs over 4 to 10 days.

TABLE 6–2. **Common Causes of Ischemic Acute Tubular Necrosis**

After cardiac surgery, particularly in patients with low cardiac output
After vascular surgery, particularly in procedures with cross-clamping of aorta above renal arteries
Loss of intravascular volume by massive hemorrhage
Crush injury
Sepsis, particularly gram negative
Pancreatitis
Gastroenteritis
Postpartum hemorrhage
Rhabdomyolysis with myoglobinuria
Transfusion reaction

TABLE 6–3. **Renal Indices in Acute Tubular Necrosis and in Prerenal Azotemia**

INDEX	ACUTE TUBULAR NECROSIS	PRERENAL AZOTEMIA
Urinary sediment	Cellular debris Granular and cellular casts	Benign sediment
Blood urea nitrogen/ creatinine ratio	About 10:1	>10:1
Urinary osmolality	About 300 mOsm/kg	>350 mOsm/kg
Urinary Na	>40 mEq/L	<20 mEq/L
Urinary creatinine/plasma creatinine ratio	<20:1	>40:1
Fractional excretion of Na	>1%	<1%

Diuresis begins after the oliguric phase, and renal function recovery begins about 1 to 3 days after the beginning of the diuresis. During the oliguric phase, the urinalysis may be benign, with only an occasional granular cast. The patient often has isosthenuria. The urinary sodium level and fractional excretion of sodium are unusually low during the oliguric phase of contrast medium-induced ARF. This is important, as the clinical syndrome can be mistaken for volume depletion and prerenal azotemia. Fluid challenge in these instances can lead to volume overload. Most patients recover the level of renal function that existed before the contrast study. Some patients may have renal insufficiency severe enough to require dialysis. Rarely, patients fail to recover renal function. Diabetics with preexisting renal dysfunction are at highest risk of developing irreversible renal failure. A number of conditions predispose patients to contrast medium-induced ARF (Table 6–4).

    b. **Management.** Patients at risk for contrast agent-induced renal failure should be **hydrated,** as their clinical status permits, before the contrast study (Table 6–5), and the **amount of contrast medium should be minimized.** Newer contrast agents (nonionic or low-

TABLE 6–4. **Predisposing Factors to Contrast Medium-Induced Acute Renal Failure**

Major Predisposing Factors
Preexisting renal insufficiency
Diabetes mellitus
Minor Predisposing Factors
Dehydration
Amount of contrast administered
Cardiac output
Other Predisposing Factors
Multiple myeloma
Advanced age
Previous episodes of contrast medium-induced ARF

TABLE 6–5. **Management of Contrast Medium-Induced Acute Renal Failure**

Before Contrast Study
Identify patients at risk for contrast medium-induced ARF
Hydrate before contrast study, as patient's clinical status permits
During Contrast Study
Minimize amount of contrast administered
Benefit of nonionic contrast agents over conventional agents
After Contrast Study
Match output with intake for next 24–48 h

osmolarity contrast agents) have been touted to be less nephrotoxic. Although some data in animals indicate less nephrotoxicity, the information in humans is less clear. Prospective, randomized studies have yielded conflicting information with respect to benefits of the newer contrast agents over conventional agents. Similarly, the benefits of furosemide or mannitol (or both) have been controversial, with some studies actually showing that these agents may be detrimental. The best management strategy, therefore, remains optimizing the state of hydration of the patient before, during, and after the contrast study. In some patients, contrast agent-induced ARF may develop either because of failure to identify the risk factor (or factors) or in spite of all appropriate precautions. In these patients, fluids, electrolytes, and acid-base balance should be managed carefully. During the oliguric phase of ARF, fluid challenge, use of diuretics, and mannitol infusion have all been shown to be ineffective. Since most patients will experience spontaneous recovery within 7 to 10 days, dialysis can usually be avoided with meticulous conservative management. In a few patients, peritoneal dialysis or hemodialysis may be necessary.

2. MYOGLOBINURIC ACUTE RENAL FAILURE
   a. **Clinical course.** Rhabdomyolysis with associated myoglobinuric ARF has been described in a number of clinical settings. The manifestations and therapeutic options are sufficiently distinctive to warrant special consideration. Myriad clinical settings can result in myoglobinuria and ARF (Table 6–6). Although trauma and crush injury remain the leading causes of rhabdomyolysis, 50% of cases of rhabdomyolysis are nontraumatic. Some clinical settings can potentiate rhabdomyolysis. Dehydration, hypokalemia, hypophosphatemia, and acidosis predispose the patient to myoglobinuric ARF. The clinical history should alert physicians to the possibility of myoglobinuria. Patients have dark amber urine, and electrophoresis or radioimmunoassay will confirm the presence of myoglobin. Marked elevation of serum potassium, phosphate, creatinine (out of proportion to the elevation of BUN), and uric acid levels can occur. Severe hypocalcemia, secondary to hyperphosphatemia as well as deposition of calcium on damaged muscle surfaces, is also common. The patient may become markedly oliguric, with progressive deterioration of renal function. A diuretic phase occurs 5 to 10 days later,

TABLE 6-6. Causes of Myoglobinuria

Trauma
Exertional rhabdomyolysis
Seizures
Drug-related rhabdomyolysis
  Heroin and barbiturates
  Amphetamine, succinylcholine, amphotericin B
Ischemic injury to muscles
Heat stroke and heat cramps
Malignant hyperthermia
Electrical burns
Infections (influenza, leptospirosis, *Clostridium* and *Shigella* species)
Myopathy
  Hereditary (McArdle's disease, Tarui disease)
  Acquired (alcoholic myopathy, polymyositis, dermatomyositis)
Toxins (sea snake bite, spider bite, hornet bite)

with gradual recovery. During the recovery phase, severe hypercalcemia has been noted and is thought to be secondary to remobilization of calcium from damaged muscles.

   b. **Management.** After careful assessment to rule out the possibility of volume overload, **initial management should be directed at inducing diuresis. Mannitol** (12.5–25 g) can be given IV to induce osmotic diuresis. **Saline** should be infused, together with IV administration of a **loop diuretic,** such as furosemide, bumetanide, or ethacrynic acid. **Alkalinization of urine with sodium bicarbonate** should be attempted only after careful assessment of the patient's volume and calcium status. The patient should be carefully monitored to avoid volume overload. When muscle compartmentalization is a problem, the situation should be promptly corrected by fasciotomy.

   If the initial attempts at inducing diuresis with optimization of volume status and diuretics fail, the patient should be managed in the same fashion as other patients with oliguric renal failure. However, special attention should be paid to the patient's potassium, calcium, and phosphate levels and acid-base balance. **Peritoneal dialysis** or **hemodialysis** may be necessary in cases of severe myoglobinuric renal failure. Most patients who develop ARF from myoglobinuria will eventually recover, with normalization of renal function.

B. Obstructive Uropathy

   1. **CLINICAL COURSE.** Obstruction of the urinary tract is a common and potentially reversible cause of acute and chronic renal failure. Obstructive uropathy occurs whenever flow of urine is obstructed at any level from the renal calyces to the urethral meatus (Table 6–7). With significant and persistent obstruction, the renal pelvis and calyces may become abnormally dilated, resulting in hydronephrosis.

   2. **MANAGEMENT.** Therapeutically, the obstruction must be relieved. In instances of bladder outlet obstruction, the placement of a Foley

TABLE 6–7. Causes of Urinary Tract Obstruction

Urethra and Bladder Neck
Benign prostatic hypertrophy
Urethral stricture
Urethral valves
Meatal stenosis
Phimosis
Bladder
Neurogenic bladder
Blood clot
Calculus
Carcinoma of bladder
Ureter
Intrinsic obstruction (calculus, blood clot, renal papilla, carcinoma of ureter)
Extrinsic obstruction (retroperitoneal or pelvic tumors, strictures, retroperitoneal fibrosis, uterine prolapse, ureterocele)
Reflux (vesicoureteral reflux, megaloureter)
Ureteropelvic Junction
Intrinsic obstruction (calculus, blood clot, renal papilla)
Extrinsic obstruction (stricture, aberrant vessels, fibrous band)
Renal Pelvis
Calculus
Blood clot
Papilla
Carcinoma of renal pelvis
Carcinoma of kidney
Tuberculosis

catheter will allow optimization of metabolic parameters before surgical correction of obstruction. When the ureters are obstructed at the ureteropelvic junction, either retrograde or antegrade urography can be used for the placement of a stent or nephrostomy tube for temporary relief. The patient should have surgical correction of the obstruction, if necessary. During the postobstructive phase, brisk diuresis is often noted. This is due in part to fluid overload during the oliguric period and in part to the accumulation of osmotically active products. The patient should be monitored carefully, and adequate hydration should be maintained until renal function returns to a reasonable level (a serum creatinine value of less than 2.5 mg/dL). Half-normal saline with 20 mEq/L of potassium chloride is an appropriate replacement solution. During the postobstructive phase, patients often have an acidifying defect mimicking distal renal tubular acidosis. The degree of recovery depends on the nature and duration of obstruction, and some degree of renal recovery is expected if the duration of obstruction is less than 6 months.

C. Acute Interstitial Nephritis

In patients with ARF, acute interstitial nephritis induced by drugs should be considered because prompt recognition and intervention can prevent the

TABLE 6–8. Drugs Commonly Associated with Acute Interstitial Nephritis

ANTIBIOTICS	NONSTEROIDAL ANTI-INFLAMMATORY DRUGS
Penicillins	*Diuretics*
Cephalosporins	Thiazides
Sulfonamides	Furosemide
Trimethoprim-sulfamethoxazole	Chlorthalidone
Rifampin	*Miscellaneous*
	Allopurinol
	Phenytoin
	Phenylbutazone

morbidity associated with prolonged renal insufficiency. A number of drugs have been implicated (Table 6–8). Some patients with acute interstitial nephritis may have symptoms of hypersensitivity, such as fever, rash, or arthralgias. On examination of the urine, red cells, white cells, low-grade proteinuria (1+), and white cell casts may be noted. Urinary eosinophils, when present, are particularly helpful in confirming the diagnosis. Peripheral eosinophilia and elevated immunoglobulin E (IgE) levels are sometimes present. Gallium-67 scans may also be useful. Patients often have nonoliguric renal failure, with gradual deterioration of renal function. Nephrotoxicity appears not to be dose related. The deterioration usually reverses with discontinuation of the offending drug. Reexposure to the drug will result in recurrence of nephrotoxicity. In some instances, renal failure may be irreversible, particularly in older patients.

The offending agent should be stopped immediately on recognition of the problem. Some investigators believe that steroids are helpful in hastening renal recovery and in optimizing the return of renal function to baseline levels.

D. Nephrotoxicity and Acute Renal Failure

Nephrotoxins have become increasingly important causes of ARF, especially in critically ill patients. Some drugs cause acute renal deterioration on the basis of allergic interstitial nephritis. Others cause acute renal insufficiency by direct nephrotoxicity. In the latter category of agents, antibiotics (particularly aminoglycosides), heavy metals, organic solvents, and some antineoplastic agents are the usual toxins.

1. **AMINOGLYCOSIDES.** Aminoglycoside nephrotoxicity is encountered in about 7% to 20% of patients receiving aminoglycosides. Different aminoglycosides appear to be associated with slightly different risks of nephrotoxicity. Neomycin is the most nephrotoxic and is, therefore, not used IV. Limited absorption of neomycin from the GI tract can occur, however, and may result in nephrotoxicity in susceptible patients. Gentamicin is less nephrotoxic than neomycin and is a commonly used drug for gram-negative systemic infections. In comparative studies, tobramycin, kanamycin, amikacin, and streptomycin appear to be slightly less nephrotoxic than gentamicin. Aminoglycoside nephrotoxic-

ity is more likely to occur in elderly patients with evidence of preexisting renal dysfunction in whom there is volume contraction. Patients with hepatic dysfunction are particularly susceptible to aminoglycoside nephrotoxicity. Concurrent administration of other nephrotoxins may enhance nephrotoxicity. These patients have nonoliguric ARF. The onset of deterioration of renal function is insidious, usually beginning 5 to 14 days after initiation of aminoglycoside therapy. Renal function may continue to deteriorate for 3 to 10 days after cessation of aminoglycoside therapy. Recovery is slow, and the patient may not return to a baseline level of renal function for several months. Some patients may require dialysis. Preventive measures are important. If clinically feasible, aminoglycosides should be avoided, particularly in elderly patients, those with hepatic dysfunction, and those with preexisting renal insufficiency. In patients with renal insufficiency, the dose interval of aminoglycoside administration should be carefully adjusted. In those receiving aminoglycosides, volume depletion and the concurrent use of other nephrotoxic drugs should be avoided. Once-a-day administration of aminoglycoside appears to be less nephrotoxic than multiple daily doses. Renal function and serum levels of aminoglycosides (peak and trough levels) should be monitored closely. If ARF develops, aminoglycosides should be stopped immediately if acceptable alternative antibiotics are available, and management should be conservative. Dialysis may be necessary if conservative measures fail.

2. **ANTINEOPLASTIC AGENTS**
   a. **Cisplatin.** Cisplatin is excreted renally and can cause nephrotoxicity, which becomes clinically apparent 5 to 7 days after administration of the agent. Patients have nonoliguric renal insufficiency, with gradual deterioration of renal function. The renal dysfunction may persist.

   Cisplatin nephrotoxicity is more common in elderly patients, in those with preexisting renal insufficiency, and in those with volume contraction and acidosis. Nephrotoxicity can be largely avoided if care is taken to assess renal function before administration of the drug. The patient should be prehydrated, and acidosis should be corrected before cisplatin therapy. Urine should be alkalinized with sodium bicarbonate infusion. Diuresis should be sustained with the use of saline hydration and loop diuretics for 24 to 48 hours after cisplatin administration.

   b. **Methotrexate.** Methotrexate, particularly in high doses, is nephrotoxic. Clinically evident deterioration of renal function may occur within 24 to 48 hours after administration. When administering high-dose methotrexate, renal function should be carefully assessed, and the dose of methotrexate should be adjusted according to the level of renal dysfunction. Toxicity can be prevented by vigorous hydration with saline and alkalinization of the patient's urine before administration of the agent. Saline diuresis, alkalinization, and use of a loop diuretic to maintain diuresis should be continued for 48 hours after administration of high-dose methotrexate to minimize toxicity. With preexisting renal dysfunction, diuresis and rescue therapy with citrovorum factor should be continued until the serum level of methotrexate is less than 10^{-7} mmol.

3. HEAVY METALS. Lead, arsenic, gold, mercury, bismuth, uranium, and cadmium are associated with nephrotoxicity. Nephrotoxicity usually occurs following attempted suicide or accidental or industrial exposure. Some metals, such as gold, are used therapeutically. Affected patients develop ARF with clinical evidence of tubular necrosis. In some instances, diverse syndromes, ranging from the nephrotic syndrome to Fanconi's syndrome, have been reported. Dimercaprol sometimes can be used to remove the heavy metal load.

4. ORGANIC SOLVENTS. Organic solvents, including carbon tetrachloride (used in cleaning agents, industrial solvents, antihelmintics, and some fire extinguishers), trichloroethylene (spot remover), tetrachloroethylene (dry cleaning), and other chlorinated hydrocarbon compounds, have been associated with nephrotoxicity. Patients who have been exposed to these solvents (accidentally, in an industrial setting, or as the result of a suicide attempt) can develop oliguric renal failure and abnormal results of liver function tests about a week after exposure. Urinalysis reveals proteinuria, hematuria, pyuria, and granular casts. The usual cause of death is acute hepatic failure. Treatment is primarily supportive.

5. MISCELLANEOUS AGENTS
   a. **Ethylene glycol.** Ethylene glycol (antifreeze) is extremely toxic when ingested; 50 to 100 mL can be lethal. During the first 12 hours after ingestion, patients have GI and CNS symptoms: nausea, vomiting, lethargy, and coma. Between 12 and 24 hours after ingestion, the cardiopulmonary symptoms of hypotension and pulmonary edema can be seen. After 24 hours, evidence of oliguric renal failure is apparent, and severe metabolic acidosis with an increased anion gap may develop. Measured serum osmolality is higher than calculated serum osmolality because of the presence of ethylene glycol in the serum.

   The patient should first be stabilized hemodynamically. Metabolic acidosis should be corrected with sodium bicarbonate infusion. Alcohol should be infused to prevent the metabolism of ethylene glycol (100 mL of 10% ethanol initially and 100 mL/h of continuous infusion, with the intention of keeping the serum ethanol level at around 100 mg/dL). Saline diuresis, if feasible, should be sustained. Thiamine and pyridoxine administration may be helpful. Peritoneal dialysis and hemodialysis may be important for the removal of ethylene glycol and for the correction of metabolic abnormalities of ARF.
   b. **Methoxyflurane and enflurane (Ethrane).** These commonly used anesthetic agents have rarely been associated with ARF. Patients develop slowly progressive renal insufficiency after exposure. The diagnosis is made usually by the exclusion of all other possible causes. Patients should be treated conservatively, with the expectation of slow recovery of renal function.

E. Glomerular Diseases

Diseases affecting the glomeruli and the small vessels can first become evident as acute progressive renal deterioration. Most are associated with systemic diseases, discussed further in "Renal Manifestations of Systemic Diseases."

Prompt recognition of the disease processes is important because a number of the diseases may respond to treatment. A brief description of the various management options is given in Table 6–9.

F. Vascular Diseases

Rarely, occlusion of both renal arteries or both renal veins can result in renal insufficiency. Since the processes are potentially reversible, it is important to include large-vessel disease in the differential diagnosis of progressive renal function deterioration.

1. ARTERIAL OCCLUSION. The most common reason for arterial occlusion is progression of renal artery stenosis, either from atherosclerotic renal artery stenosis or from fibromuscular hyperplasia. Arterial occlusion can also result from emboli to the renal arteries. Necrotizing angiitis secondary to IV drug abuse is a rare cause of renal artery occlusion.

Renal artery occlusion should be suspected in patients with abrupt onset of flank pain and oliguric, progressive deterioration of renal function. Examination of the urine reveals hematuria and cellular casts. The diagnosis can be confirmed by renal scan, renal MRA, or renal arteriography, which demonstrate the absence of flow. Once renal artery occlusion is documented, angioplasty or vascular reconstruction should be promptly done if clinically feasible.

TABLE 6–9. **Therapeutic Interventions in Diseases of the Glomeruli and Small Blood Vessels**

DISEASE	THERAPEUTIC OPTIONS
Poststreptococcal glomerulonephritis	Conservative management
Malignant hypertension	Control of hypertension
Systemic lupus erythematosus	Steroids; cytotoxic drugs, particularly cyclophosphamide given IV in pulse doses; ?plasmapheresis
Subacute bacterial endocarditis	Antibiotics for underlying infection
Wegener's granulomatosis	Cyclophosphamide; steroids; plasmapheresis in severe cases
Goodpasture's syndrome	Steroids; cyclophosphamide; plasmapheresis
Thrombotic thrombocytopenic purpura	Plasmapheresis—fresh frozen plasma; possibly antiplatelet agents; possibly cytotoxic agents
Polyarteritis nodosa	Steroids; cyclophosphamide
Rapidly progressive glomerulonephritis	Steroids; cyclophosphamide; plasmapheresis
Serum sickness	Steroids
Drug-induced vasculitis	Stop offending agent; steroids

2. **CHOLESTEROL EMBOLI.** Cholesterol emboli can cause progressive deterioration of renal function. Cholesterol emboli are seen in four clinical settings: (1) abdominal aortography and angiography performed with catheters passing through the abdominal aorta can result in embolization, (2) resection of an abdominal aortic aneurysm, manipulation of the abdominal aorta during vascular surgery, repair of a thoracic aneurysm, and aortic valve replacement have been associated with cholesterol embolization, (3) administration of thrombolytic agents has been associated with cholesterol embolization, and (4) severe ulcerated atherosclerotic disease of the aorta can result in spontaneous cholesterol emboli.

Patients with cholesterol emboli usually have nonoliguric renal failure, although oliguric renal failure can occur in patients with severe disease. Deterioration of renal function begins immediately after the injury and is usually slow, with continuing renal function deterioration over weeks and months. Renal function may gradually improve; however, renal deterioration progressing to end-stage renal disease may occur. The diagnosis should be suspected in patients with nonspecific GI symptoms, anorexia, nausea, vomiting, crampy abdominal pain, and diarrhea. There are often cutaneous signs of cholesterol emboli, particularly in the toes and in the soles of the feet. Some may have evidence of pancreatitis or rhabdomyolysis. Examination of the urine shows red cells, white cells, white cell casts, and eosinophils. Peripheral eosinophilia has been reported. No specific therapy is available.

G. Hepatorenal Syndrome

1. **CLINICAL COURSE.** The hepatorenal syndrome consists of progressive failure of renal function of unknown etiology in patients with severe liver disease. Factors associated with the precipitation of hepatorenal syndrome include excessive use of diuretics, paracentesis, infection, and GI hemorrhage. Hepatorenal syndrome carries an extremely poor prognosis, with a reported survival rate of less than 5%. Patients experience oliguric renal failure, with slow, progressive renal deterioration. Despite compromises in renal function, these patients usually die of complications from hepatic insufficiency. GI bleeding and infection are the most common causes of death. The urinary sediment is normal in these patients despite progressive renal deterioration. The urinary sodium concentration is invariably less than 10 mEq/L, and the fractional excretion of sodium is usually less than 1%. The urinary osmolality is usually only slightly above the serum osmolality. The diagnosis of hepatorenal syndrome has to be one of exclusion, and care should be taken to rule out prerenal azotemia.

2. **MANAGEMENT.** Therapy for the hepatorenal syndrome has been unsatisfactory. Numerous pharmacologic agents have proved unsuccessful in reversing the functional abnormalities in the syndrome. In certain instances, several surgical procedures, such as orthotopic liver transplantation, have been reported to be successful in reversal of the

hepatorenal syndrome. Peritoneojugular shunts (LeVeen's shunts) also have been beneficial in some cases. Dialysis and hemoperfusion have been employed, but, in general, these have merely delayed the inevitable outcome.

Coggins CH, Fang LSF. Acute renal failure associated with antibiotic, anesthetic agents and radiographic contrast agents. In: Brenner BM, Lazarus JM, eds. Acute Renal Failure, 2nd ed. New York: Churchill Livingstone; 1988, pp 295–352.
Gurwitz JH, Avorn J, Ross-Degnan D, Lipsitz LA. Nonsteroidal anti-inflammatory drug-associated azotemia in the very old. JAMA 1990;264:471–475.
Levy M. Nephrology forum: hepatorenal syndrome. Kidney Int 1993;43:737–753.

III. MANAGEMENT OF PATIENTS WITH CHRONIC RENAL FAILURE (CRF)

The goal of managing the patient with CRF is to optimize the clinical and metabolic status by conservative measures. When these measures fail, dialysis and transplantation should be considered.

A. Fluid Balance

In patients with moderate renal insufficiency there is loss in concentrating ability, and they develop polyuria and polydipsia. They depend on adequate intake for excretion of the solute load, and thus they should not have fluid restriction. Fluid restriction can result in intravascular volume depletion, decreased renal perfusion, and worsening of renal function. For these reasons, diuretics should be used judiciously. With severe renal insufficiency, patients may be oliguric and have symptoms of fluid overload. Fluid restriction and diuretics may be necessary in these patients.

B. Sodium Balance

In some instances, patients with a moderate degree of renal dysfunction may have salt-losing nephropathy. These patients should be encouraged to take in salt, and sodium replacement may be required under certain circumstances. In most patients with CRF, however, there is difficulty in excreting salt, and they have problems with sodium overload. In these patients, salt restriction and diuretics may be necessary.

C. Potassium Balance

Hyperkalemia is the most important electrolyte abnormality to correct in patients with CRF. Dietary restriction of potassium should be reinforced. Sodium polystyrene sulfonate (Kayexalate) 30–50 g in a sorbitol solution can be given PO for long-term management. Rare patients may have potassium-losing nephropathy, and their hypokalemia can be treated with cautious potassium replacement.

D. Calcium and Phosphate Balances

Hyperphosphatemia should be corrected first with the use of calcium carbonate (PhosLo, Tums, Tums E-X Extra Strength). Calcium carbonate should be given shortly before meals to optimize phosphate binding. When the serum phosphate level is less than 5 mg/dL, the hypocalcemia should be corrected with calcium supplements and vitamin D preparations. A reasonable starting dose of calcium carbonate is 500 mg PO tid. 1,25-Dihydroxycholecalciferol (Rocaltrol) can be given in doses of 0.25–0.50 µg/d.

E. Acidosis

Metabolic acidosis should be managed with sodium bicarbonate, starting at 600 mg PO tid. The doses of bicarbonate should be increased until the serum bicarbonate level is between 16 and 20 mEq/L. Hypertension or CHF may limit the ability to use sodium bicarbonate.

F. Nitrogen Balance

Restriction to 0.5 g/kg of protein per day usually allows sufficient amounts for daily requirements while reducing increases in azotemia. Severe restriction of protein is probably not indicated. In all instances, it is important to maintain adequate caloric intake to prevent catabolism and muscle breakdown (30–50 kcal/kg/d, more in critically ill patients).

G. Hematologic Abnormalities

Anemia can be managed by replacement of iron and folate in patients shown to have deficiencies. Blood drawing should be minimized. Drugs that can cause hemolysis should be avoided, as a defect in the hexose monophosphate shunt function can be demonstrated in 10% to 25% of uremic patients. **Erythropoietin** is effective for many patients when given 3 times per week. Transfusions may be necessary for patients with severe and symptomatic anemia. Patients with CRF have abnormal results on platelet function tests and prolonged bleeding time. Antiplatelet drugs, such as aspirin and dipyridamole (Persantine), should be avoided. In patients with clinically evident bleeding, DDAVP (0.4 µg/kg) can be given IV to reverse platelet function abnormalities. Premarin has also been shown to be effective in correcting bleeding time. However, the effect of Premarin usually is apparent only after 3 to 7 days of therapy.

H. Renal Osteodystrophy

Persistent hypocalcemia can result in secondary hyperparathyroidism, which leads to bone demineralization. In patients with mild hyperparathyroidism, vitamin D and calcium therapy may be beneficial in the suppression of parathyroid activity. These have to be used judiciously to avoid hypercalcemia.

I. Cutaneous Symptoms

Severe pruritus can cause significant morbidity in the patient with CRF. Itching may respond to menthol or phenol lotions applied locally and can be treated with antihistamines. Ultraviolet light is also helpful in some patients.

J. Cardiovascular Complications

Patients with CRF can develop CHF, coronary ischemia, and uremic pericarditis. CHF can be managed with fluid and sodium restriction and cautious use of loop diuretics. Transfusions may be required in anemic patients with coronary ischemia. In patients with uremic pericarditis, dialysis should be considered. Instillation of nonabsorbable steroids, such as triamcinolone, 100 mg given intrapericardially via a pericardial catheter q6h, appears to be effective in preventing recurrence of pericardial effusions. In patients with recurrent and refractory pericardial effusions, pericardiectomy may be necessary.

K. Hypertension

It is important to control hypertension in the patient with CRF to avoid further renal damage. However, it is equally important not to overtreat and cause renal hypoperfusion. Since volume overload is present in many patients, a diuretic is a reasonable first-line drug to use. Many diuretics are ineffective in patients with severe renal failure. Others are associated with possible hyperkalemia and should be avoided. Some commonly used diuretics include furosemide, bumetanide, ethacrynic acid, and metolazone. Converting enzyme inhibitors and calcium channel blockers are acceptable drugs to use. In both instances, renal function should be monitored carefully, as there is a chance of acute renal function deterioration with these drugs in patients with preexisting renal insufficiency. Beta blockers, particularly in combination with vasodilators, are often effective. Vasodilators, including hydralazine, prazosin, terazosin, and minoxidil, are also effective in CRF.

L. Drug Therapy

Drugs that are potentially nephrotoxic should be avoided, and drugs that are excreted renally must be adjusted. Conservative management is directed toward prolongation of a symptom-free period. When conservative therapy becomes ineffective, dialysis or transplantation must be considered.

Klahr S, Levey AS, Beck GJ, et al. The effects of dietary protein restriction and blood pressure control in the progression of chronic renal disease. N Engl J Med 1994;330:877–884.

Lakkis FG, Martinez-Maldonadao M. Conservative management of chronic renal failure and its complications. In: Jacobson MR, Striker GE, Klahr S, eds. The Principles and Practice of Nephrology, 2nd ed. St. Louis: Mosby–Year Book; 1995, Chapter 91.

McCarthy JT, Kumar R. Renal osteodystrophy. In: Jacobson HR, Striker GE, Klahr S, eds. The Principles and Practice of Nephrology, 2nd ed. St. Louis: Mosby–Year Book; 1995, Chapter 150.

IV. HEMODIALYSIS

With progressive deterioration, renal performance may be so compromised that mechanical assistance becomes necessary. Hemodialysis is useful in patients with ARF or CRF. The procedure involves the passage of blood across a semipermeable membrane. On the other side of the membrane is a specially prepared dialysate designed to correct the metabolic derangements commonly associated with renal failure. The dialysate is usually made hypertonic with the addition of glucose, which allows correction of fluid overload. Acidosis is corrected by the use of bicarbonate in the dialysate. Calcium is added for correction of hypocalcemia, and the potassium content of the dialysate can be adjusted for correction of hyperkalemia. Nitrogenous wastes are removed along a concentration gradient.

For hemodialysis to be effective, a vascular access is required that permits a rate of blood flow of 200 to 300 mL/min into the dialyzer. In addition, an anticoagulant is needed to avert clotting in the dialyzer.

A. Indications and Contraindications

Uremic symptoms (particularly changes in mental status), refractory volume overload, bleeding secondary to uremic effects on platelet adhesiveness, uremic pericarditis in a patient with progressive renal insufficiency, hyperkalemia or acidosis refractory to conservative measures, and life-threatening overdose of a dialyzable toxin are the most common indications for dialysis. Progressive uremic neuropathy, progressive malnutrition and physical deterioration, and emotional considerations may also lead one to initiate dialysis.

The major contraindications to hemodialysis include concern over the risk of heparinization, hemodynamic instability, and other systemic illnesses with grave prognoses that may preclude the initiation of hemodialysis. Patients with active GI bleeding, intracranial hemorrhage, subdural hematoma, hypotension, and unstable angina should be considered for other methods of dialysis.

B. Medical Therapy for Patients on Hemodialysis

Most patients require 3 to 5 hours of hemodialysis three times weekly. Other measures are necessary to avoid significant metabolic derangements. Patients are usually restricted to 60 to 80 g of protein intake each day. Salt and potassium intake is also restricted, usually to 2 g/d each. Fluid restriction may be necessary to avoid overload. Phosphate binders are generally needed to prevent hyperphosphatemia. Vitamin D or analogs and calcium supplements may be necessary to correct hypocalcemia and to prevent renal osteodystrophy. Water-soluble vitamins and folic acid are dialyzable and need to be supplemented.

C. Complications

1. **MECHANICAL COMPLICATIONS.** In rare instances, leaking of blood from the dialyzer or from the lines can create substantial blood loss. Dialyzers can clot because of inadequate heparinization. Rarely, air entering the dialyzer or lines can cause air embolism.

2. **COMPLICATIONS RELATED TO VASCULAR ACCESSES.** Arteriovenous shunts are seldom used now because they are prone to infection, clotting, bleeding, and erosion of skin around the insertion sites of the shunts. Arteriovenous fistulas are less prone to infections than shunts, but they may fail to mature adequately for dialysis. The fistulas are also prone to thrombosis or stenosis and may create problems with ischemia of an extremity secondary to a steal syndrome. On occasion, aneurysms can develop, particularly at the sites of repeated punctures. An arteriovenous fistula may also result in high-output failure in susceptible patients. Subclavian or internal jugular catheters are used for temporary access to the bloodstream. These are prone to infections and clotting and should not be expected to be functional for more than 6 to 8 weeks.

3. **HEMODYNAMIC COMPLICATIONS.** The most common problem during hemodialysis is hypotension, due in part to excessive volume removal and in part to compromised cardiac contractility during the procedure,

presumably resulting from the cardiosuppressant effect of the dialysate. During dialysis, angina, arrhythmia, and, rarely, cardiac tamponade can complicate the procedure.

4. **PULMONARY COMPLICATIONS.** During the initial 30 to 45 minutes of dialysis, transient hypoxemia is seen, caused partly by diffusion of CO_2 across the dialyzing membrane, resulting in hypoventilation, and partly by microembolization of aggregates of white cells formed as a result of complement activation as the blood passes through the dialyzer. On rare occasions, air embolism can complicate dialysis.

5. **NEUROLOGIC COMPLICATIONS.** A dysequilibrium syndrome, with headache, nausea, vomiting, lethargy, and seizures, can complicate dialysis. This syndrome is of particular concern when there is rapid shifting of fluids and solute. The syndrome can be ameliorated by slower dialyses and by the use of the mannitol procedure. A more worrisome neurologic complication is dialysis dementia. Patients have intermittent symptoms of dysarthria, myoclonus, and apraxia. The symptoms subsequently become persistent, and the condition progressively deteriorates until patients are in a mute, vegetative state. Patients usually die within a year of diagnosis. The syndrome is thought to be related to aluminum excess, with deposition in the brain. With deionization of the water used in dialysis, the syndrome is now uncommon. Deferoxamine and renal transplantation have been reported to be beneficial in anecdotal instances.

6. **MUSCULAR COMPLICATIONS.** Cramping can occur during dialysis, particularly with rapid fluid shifts, and can be treated with hypertonic saline infusion.

7. **METABOLIC COMPLICATIONS.** Rapid fluid and electrolyte shifts and rapid correction of acidosis can create symptoms, particularly in a patient prone to arrhythmias. Hypercholesterolemia and hypertriglyceridemia are common in uremic patients undergoing dialysis. Hyperglycemia is occasionally seen.

8. **HEMATOLOGIC COMPLICATIONS.** Patients with CRF who are undergoing dialysis are more prone to infectious complications because of compromised antibody production and compromised cellular immunity. Septicemia from vascular accesses and infections at skin sites, usually with gram-positive organisms, can be treated readily with vancomycin. Since the drug is excreted renally and is not dialyzable, 1 g of vancomycin given at dialysis weekly would usually be adequate therapy.

Even with meticulous care and marked improvement in technical aspects, the annual mortality is estimated at 7% to 13%. Coronary artery disease and sepsis are the major causes of death. Hemodialysis can dramatically improve the well-being of the patient and prolong life, but the physician should be aware of its many possible complications.

Ahsan N, Cronin RE. Dialysis considerations in the patient with acute renal failure. In: Henrich WL, ed. Principles and Practice of Dialysis. Baltimore: Williams & Wilkins; 1994, Chapter 29.

V. ACUTE PERITONEAL DIALYSIS

Peritoneal dialysis can be used in the management of patients with ARF or CRF. In patients with ARF, a percutaneously placed peritoneal catheter is generally used. Peritoneal dialysis is preferred when the heparinization needed for hemodialysis is contraindicated. It is also preferred in patients with hemodynamic instability. Otherwise, the indications for initiation of peritoneal dialysis are the same as those for hemodialysis.

A. Dialysis Exchanges

Commercially available dialysate solutions are generally used. Available solutions include 1.5%, 2.5%, and 4.25% solutions. The more hypertonic solution should be used in the patient with fluid overload. Potassium must be added to the dialysate because most dialysates are potassium free. Small amounts of heparin (250 to 500 U) may be added to the dialysate to minimize fibrin deposition and clotting of the catheter. The dialysate should be warmed to body temperature and should be infused into the peritoneal cavity over a 10-minute period. The dialysate is then allowed to remain in the peritoneal cavity for varying periods (at least 20 minutes) to allow for exchange. The dialysate is permitted to drain until dry over a 30-minute period. Intake and output should be carefully monitored hourly, and blood chemistry studies, including determination of potassium, BUN, creatinine, and glucose levels, should be performed every 8 hours. The dialysate should be examined and cultured periodically.

B. Complications

Bleeding is a rare complication of peritoneal dialysis. The dialysate may be slightly blood tinged during the first few exchanges. Bleeding is usually from small veins lining the peritoneal cavity, and the bleeding should decrease after the first few exchanges. If it persists, the dialysis catheter should be removed and replaced. Another rare complication of the percutaneously placed catheter is **perforation of a viscus.** This can be avoided if surgical placement is used in the presence of ileus or adhesions from prior lower abdominal surgery. If a viscus is perforated, the catheter should be left in place, and surgical exploration for repair of the viscus should be undertaken as soon as possible. The most common problem with peritoneal dialysis is **fluid drainage.** If difficulties occur with either the infusion or the drainage of dialysis solutions, the patient should be placed in a different body position to determine if the flow can be improved. In general, poor drainage is caused by trapping of the catheter in the mesentery, and changing body position can improve flow. If problems with adequate flow persist, the catheter can be flushed with about 50 mL of heparinized saline to dislodge possible fibrin clots from the end of the catheter. If dialysate flow is still inadequate, the catheter should be removed and replaced. No attempt should be made to reposition the dialysis catheter except at the time of the initial placement, since this procedure markedly increases the possibility of peritonitis. **Leakage** may occur around the insertion site. Small amounts of drainage can be managed with more frequent dressing changes. At times, it may be possible to decrease the amount of leakage by placement of a pursestring suture

TABLE 6–10. Antibiotics Used Intraperitoneally for Treatment of Peritonitis

ANTIBIOTICS	DOSE (mg) ADDED TO EACH 2-L DIALYSATE BAG
Penicillins	
Ampicillin	100
Methicillin	100
Carbenicillin	400
Cephalosporin	
Cephapirin (Cefadyl)	200
Aminoglycosides	
Gentamicin	8–10
Tobramycin	8–10
Clindamycin	20
*Vancomycin**	30
*Amphotericin**	4

*May cause some peritoneal irritation.

at the skin. With leakage, the likelihood of wound infection and peritonitis is markedly increased. If leakage is not stopped by a pursestring suture, the dialysis catheter should be removed and replaced. During peritoneal dialysis, the **fluid and electrolyte balance** should be monitored closely. It is important to assess the blood glucose level frequently, particularly if the 4.25% dialysate is used. In general, avoid using 4.25% dialysate solely but instead alternate 4.25% with 2.5% dialysate in patients with fluid overload.

The major problem with peritoneal dialysis is **peritonitis.** The dialysate should be monitored periodically (every other day) in patients undergoing acute peritoneal dialysis. The dialysate should be closely examined, and cultures should be done whenever patients show clinical signs of peritonitis or if the dialysate is cloudy. The presence of significant numbers of white cells, of organisms detected under microscopic examination, or of bacterial growth mandates treatment with antibiotics. The most common pathogen in dialysis-related peritonitis is *Staphylococcus* (either *S. aureus* or *S. epidermidis*). Cephalosporins can be added to the dialysate for these infections, although *S. epidermidis* may be resistant to penicillins and cephalosporins. For peritonitis caused by gram-negative organisms, an antibiotic (e.g., gentamicin, tobramycin) can be used. The antibiotics and doses most commonly used are listed in Table 6–10. Persistent infection in the presence of appropriate therapy requires removal of the peritoneal dialysis catheter.

VI. CONTINUOUS AMBULATORY PERITONEAL DIALYSIS (CAPD)

To manage patients with chronic renal disease with CAPD, the catheters must be placed surgically, and patients should be instructed how to perform peritoneal dialysis on a continuous outpatient basis. The procedure first came into clinical use in the early 1970s and is gaining popularity because of the convenience and the ease with which it can be mastered.

A. Patient Selection

Because CAPD is designed for patients who can manage the exchanges themselves, it is important to select individuals who are motivated, have reasonable eyesight, and have good manual dexterity. Sometimes, family members can be trained to perform the procedure.

B. Placement of the Dialysis Catheter

The catheter for long-term use should be placed surgically at least 2 weeks before the planned initiation of dialysis.

C. Principles

Since the peritoneal membrane is a rather ineffective exchange membrane, CAPD calls for the continuous use of the membrane to maximize clearances. The patient would usually do 4 exchanges a day. The dialysate is infused into the peritoneal cavity and is left there for 4 to 6 hours and drained at the next exchange. The drained dialysate is discarded, and a new dialysate bag is used for the new exchange. The last exchange of the day occurs at bedtime, and the dialysate is allowed to remain in the peritoneal cavity overnight. With the continuous process, excellent fluid, salt, and metabolic control can be achieved.

D. Advantages

Outpatient CAPD can be performed without the use of machines and thus allows for greater flexibility and mobility. Blood pressure control is usually excellent with CAPD because of the ease with which fluid and salt can be removed throughout the procedure. Therefore, fluid, salt, and potassium restriction may be less stringent for the patient using CAPD. Because there is continuous loss of protein throughout the dialyzing process, dietary protein restriction is also relaxed, and most patients are permitted an intake of 80 g of protein each day. Uremia is ordinarily under adequate control, and anemia is usually less of a problem because of decreased blood loss. Because the procedure proceeds relatively slowly, patients are less likely to experience the dysequilibrium syndrome.

E. Complications

The major problem with CAPD is peritonitis. Patients are taught to monitor the fluid carefully, to obtain fluid for analysis and cultures, and to begin antibiotics on an empiric basis with IV or IP administration of vancomycin (1 g), since the major pathogen in peritonitis is *Staphylococcus* species (*S. aureus* or *S. epidermidis*). If infection is confirmed, the IV or IP administration of antibiotic is continued for 14 days. Follow-up cultures are done a week after termination of therapy to ensure clearance of the infection. If infection is persistent despite adequate therapy, the peritoneal catheter should be removed. Hemodialysis for a short period is necessary before another peritoneal catheter can be placed. Removal of the catheter is particularly important in patients with fungal peritonitis, since the infection is rarely cleared without catheter replacement. Excessive weight gain can be a problem because of the continuous glucose infusion. Glucose intolerance can also result. Patients often have hypercholesterolemia and hypertriglyceridemia.

Eschbach JW. Nephrology forum. The anemia of chronic renal failure: pathophysiology and the effects of recombinant erythropoietin. Kidney Int 1989;35:134–148.
Friedman EA. Outcome and complications of hemodialysis. In: Schrier RW, Gottschalk CW, eds. Diseases of the Kidney, 4th ed. Boston: Little, Brown; 1988, pp 3323–3346.
Mion CM. Chronic ambulatory peritoneal dialysis (CAPD) and chronic cycling peritoneal dialysis. In: Schrier RW, Gottschalk CW, eds. Diseases of the Kidney, 4th ed. Boston: Little, Brown; 1988, pp 3235–3280.

VII. DRUG THERAPY IN PATIENTS WITH RENAL INSUFFICIENCY

One of the most important aspects of patient care with either acute or chronic renal insufficiency is the appropriate management of drug therapy, including avoiding certain drugs (Table 6–11). Drugs and drug metabolites may accumulate in these patients, causing toxicity. In renal insufficiency,

TABLE 6–11. **Drugs to Avoid in Renal Insufficiency**

DRUG	REASON FOR AVOIDING DRUG
Antibiotics	
Tetracycline	Antianabolic and may raise BUN; may potentiate acidosis; nephrotoxic
Nitrofurantoin	Accumulates in renal insufficiency; ineffective for UTI*; peripheral neuropathy
Methenamine mandelate	Ineffective for UTI
Nalidixic acid	Metabolic acidosis
Cardiovascular Agents	
Acetazolamide	Potentiates metabolic acidosis; ineffective in renal failure
Mercurials	Accumulates in renal insufficiency; nephrotoxic
Spironolactone	Hyperkalemia
Triamterene	Hyperkalemia
Amiloride	Hyperkalemia
Analgesics and Narcotics	
Aspirin	Antiplatelet effect; gastrointestinal irritation
Nonsteroidal anti-inflammatory drugs	Antiplatelet effect; gastrointestinal irritation; nephrotoxic
Phenazopyridine	Ineffective in renal failure
Sedatives, Hypnotics, and Tranquilizers	
Lithium carbonate	Nephrogenic diabetes insipidus; lithium toxicity; possible nephrotoxicity
Antineoplastic Agents	
Cisplatin	Nephrotoxic
Miscellaneous Agents	
Phenylbutazone	Gastrointestinal irritation; nephrotoxic
Gold	Accumulates in renal insufficiency; nephrotoxic
Magnesium compounds	Accumulates in renal insufficiency; CNS side effects
Aminosalicylic acid	Potentiates acidosis; GI irritation

*Urinary tract infection.

drug binding may be altered either because of decreased protein available for binding (particularly in patients with the nephrotic syndrome) or because of displacement of the drug from binding sites by uremic toxins. Although a variety of nomograms have been constructed for the commonly used drugs, only careful monitoring of drug levels permits dose adjustments to ensure therapeutic levels. Sometimes drug levels may have to be reinterpreted. For example, the therapeutic level of phenytoin is between 4 and 8 μg/dL in patients with advanced renal insufficiency because of

TABLE 6–12. Drugs Requiring Dose Adjustment in Renal Failure

DRUG	ADJUSTMENT FACTOR	DRUG	ADJUSTMENT FACTOR
Antimicrobial Agents		**Cardiovascular Agents**	
Penicillins		Antiarrhythmics	
Penicillin G	2	Procainamide	4
Ampicillin, amoxicillin	2	Disopyramide	4
Carbenicillin, ticarcillin	2	Flecainide	4
Methicillin	2	Encainide	4
Imipenem	2	Mexilitene	2
Aminoglycosides		Antihypertensive agents	
Gentamicin, tobramycin	4–6	Methyldopa	2
Kanamycin, amikacin	4–6	Guanethidine	2
Streptomycin	4–8	Cardiac glycosides	
Cephalosporins		Digoxin	3–4
Cephalexin, cephalothin,	1–2	Digitoxin	1.5–2
cefazolin, cephapirin		**Analgesics and**	
Cephradine	4	**Narcotics**	
Cefamandole, cefoxitin	1–2	Acetaminophen	2
Cefuroxime	1–2	Meperidine	2
Cefotaxime	1–2	Methadone	2
Ceftriaxone	1–2	**Sedatives, Hypnotics,**	
Ceftazadime	1–2	**and Tranquilizers**	
Sulfonamides		Phenobarbital	2
Sulfisoxazole	2	Meprobamate	2
Trimethoprim-	2	**Antineoplastic and**	
sulfamethoxazole		**Immunosuppressive**	
Minocycline	2	**Agents**	
Antifungal agents		Bleomycin	2
Amphotericin	1.5	Cyclophosphamide	2
5-Flucytosine	4–8	**Miscellaneous**	
Fluconazole	1–2	Hypoglycemic agents	
Antituberculous drugs		Insulin	2
Ethambutol	2	Acetohexamide	2
Others		Chlorpropamide	2
Vancomycin	10	Glyburide	2
Metronidazole	3	Others	
Pentamidine	2	Cimetidine	2
		Ranitidine	2
		Propylthiouracil	2
		Clofibrate	4
		Neostigmine	2

TABLE 6–13. Drugs Not Requiring Dose Adjustment in Renal Insufficiency

Analgesics and Narcotics	*Cardiovascular Agents*
Codeine	Antiarrhythmics
Morphine	Lidocaine
Naloxone	Propranolol
Pentazocine	Quinidine
Propoxyphene	Antihypertensive agents
Sedatives, Hypnotics, and Tranquilizers	Clonidine
Barbiturates	Captopril and enalapril
Phenobarbital	Lisinopril
Secobarbital	Diazoxide
Benzodiazepines	Diltiazem, nifedipine, verapamil
Chlordiazepoxide	Hydralazine and prozosin
Diazepam	Minoxidil
Flurazepam	Nitroprusside
Triazolam	Reserpine
Tricyclic antidepressants	Diuretics
Amitriptyline	Bumetanide, ethacrynic acid, furosemide
Desipramine	Thiazides
Imipramine	Metolazone
Nortriptyline	Anticoagulants
Fluoxetine	Heparin
Haloperidol	Warfarin
Glutethimide	*Antineoplastic and Immunosuppressive Agents*
Ethchlorvynol	Azathioprine
Methaqualone	Cytosine arabinoside
Antimicrobial Agents	Doxorubicin (Adriamycin)
Penicillins	5-Fluorouracil
Cloxacilin, dicloxacillin	Methotrexate
Nafcillin	Vincristine
Oxacillin	*Miscellaneous*
Chloramphenicol	Steroids
Clindamycin	Tolbutamide
Erythromycin	Theophylline
Chloroquine	Tubocurarine
Antituberculous drugs	Succinylcholine
Isoniazid	
Rifampin	

enhanced metabolic rate, compared with 10 to 20 µg/dL in patients with normal renal function. In patients undergoing hemodialysis or peritoneal dialysis, it is important to know whether a drug is cleared by dialysis to be able to adjust doses.

A. Drugs That Require Dose Adjustment

Drugs (or their metabolites) that are renally excreted require dose adjustment (Table 6–12). In most instances, the loading dose of medication does not need to be altered even in severe renal failure. Subsequent doses for maintenance therapy require adjustments. Coggins, Bennett, and Singer advocate the use of an **adjustment factor** in severe renal insufficiency (creatinine clearance of less than 20 mL/min). The adjustment factor can be used either to reduce the dose of medication administered or to increase the intervals between doses. For example, tobramycin has an adjustment factor of 4: in a patient with severe renal failure, the dose of tobramycin can be reduced by a factor of 4 given at normal intervals; alternatively, the patient can be given a normal dose of tobramycin at a dose interval that has been increased by a factor of 4 (i.e., given at 32-hour intervals instead of 8-hour intervals). The adjustment factor applies to patients with severe renal insufficiency. Patients with moderate or mild renal insufficiency should have intermediate dose adjustments. It should be stressed that the **exact doses should be governed by clinical responses and serum levels and not rigidly by these approximations.**

B. Drugs That Do Not Require Dose Adjustment

Some drugs can be used in patients with renal insufficiency without dose adjustment (Table 6–13). These drugs are not excreted renally and do not aggravate uremic symptoms. Consequently, whenever feasible, these drugs are preferred to drugs that require dose adjustments.

C. Drugs That Are Dialyzable by Peritoneal Dialysis

Drugs that can be dialyzed by peritoneal dialysis are listed in Table 6–14. The list is partial because the dialyzability of many drugs has not been

---

TABLE 6–14. Drugs Cleared by Peritoneal Dialysis

Antimicrobial Agents	*Cardiovascular Agents*
Penicillin	Antiarrhythmics
Ticarcillin	Quinidine
Imipenem	Procainamide
Cephalosporins	Antihypertensive agents
Cephalexin	Methyldopa
Cephalothin	Diazoxide
Cephradine	Nitroprusside
Ceftriaxone	*Sedatives, Hypnotics, and Tranquilizers*
Cefuroxime	Phenobarbital
Cefotaxime	Ethchlorvynol
Ceftazadime	Lithium carbonate
Cefoxitin	Meprobamate
Cefamandole	*Miscellaneous*
Aminoglycosides	Phenytoin
Sulfonamides	
Sulfisoxazole	
Trimethoprim-sulfamethoxazole	
Antifungal agents	
Flucytosine	
Antituberculous drugs	
Ethambutol	
Isoniazid	

TABLE 6–15. Drugs Cleared by Hemodialysis

Antimicrobial Agents	*Cardiovascular Agents*
Penicillins	Antiarrhythmics
Penicillin G	Procainamide
Ampicillin, amoxicillin	Quinidine
Carbenicillin, ticarcillin	Antihypertensive agents
Imipenem	Methyldopa
Cephalosporins	Diazoxide
Cephalexin	Nitroprusside
Cephalothin	*Analgesics and Narcotics*
Cefazolin	Acetaminophen
Cephapirin	Pentazocine
Cefoxitin	*Sedatives, Hypnotics, and Tranquilizers*
Cefotaxime	Lithium carbonate
Ceftazadime	Meprobamate
Cefamandole	Methaqualone
Cefuroxime	Phenobarbital
Ceftriaxone	Ethchlorvynol
Cephradine	*Antineoplastic and Immunosuppressive Agents*
Aminoglycosides	Azathioprine
Sulfonamides	Cyclophosphamide
Sulfisoxazole	5-Fluorouracil
Trimethoprim-sulfamethoxazole	*Miscellaneous*
Chloramphenicol	Primidone
Antifungal drugs	
Flucytosine	
Antituberculous drugs	
Isoniazid	
Ethambutol	
Metronidazole	
Quinine	

investigated. Patients who are receiving peritoneal dialysis should have these medications adjusted. Patients with severe overdoses of these medications can be treated with peritoneal dialysis. The clinical responses and the serum levels of these drugs should be monitored closely to ensure therapeutic levels.

D. Drugs That Are Dialyzable by Hemodialysis

Drugs that can be dialyzed by hemodialysis are listed in Table 6–15. The list is partial because the dialyzability of many drugs has not been investigated. In general, patients receiving hemodialysis who require these medications should have supplementation of them at the completion of dialysis. Patients with severe overdoses of these medications can benefit from hemodialysis.

Bennett WM, Aronoff GR, Golper TA, et al. Drug Prescribing in Renal Failure. Dosing Guidelines in Adults, 3rd ed. Philadelphia: American College of Physicians; 1994.

VIII. NEPHROLITHIASIS

The incidence of nephrolithiasis appears to be increasing, and recent studies have estimated that 10% to 25% of the population may have symptomatic nephrolithiasis. Most stones (over 60%) contain calcium. Magnesium ammonium phosphate stones account for 15%. Uric acid, cystine, and other stones are less frequent (Table 6–16). Physicochemical factors increasing urinary concentration of stone constituents are thought to be the cause of stone formation. An acidic pH favors the formation of uric acid, cystine, and xanthine stones. An alkaline pH favors the formation of magnesium ammonium phosphate stones (struvite).

Increased urinary excretion of calcium or oxalate can enhance stone formation in a number of instances. Increased calcium excretion can occur in patients with hyperparathyroidism, vitamin D excess, excessive dietary calcium intake, or idiopathic hypercalciuria. Increased excretion of urinary oxalate can be observed in patients with primary hyperoxaluria or enteric hyperoxaluria. Increased uric acid excretion can result from either greater uric acid production or greater renal uric acid excretion. Cystine stones are formed exclusively in patients with an inherited disorder involving abnormal intestinal and renal transport of cystine, ornithine, lysine, and arginine. Xanthine stones are usually seen in patients with a genetic deficiency of xanthine oxidase, resulting in abnormalities in purine metabolism. Rarely, patients taking xanthine oxidase inhibitors for the treatment of uric acid disorders have xanthine stones.

Patients with distal renal tubular acidosis have increased urinary concentration of calcium and phosphate and are prone to stone formation. Infection in the upper tract with urea-splitting organisms can result in persistently alkaline urine, potentiating formation of magnesium ammonium phosphate stones. A number of substances appear to inhibit stone formation, and these include magnesium, citrate, pyrophosphate, and certain protein peptides. Other factors appear to potentiate stone formation. These include much protein matrix and scar tissue in the kidney.

A. General Treatment Principles

In general, in a patient with acute renal colic, relief should come with generous use of analgesics. Fluids should be forced to ensure diuresis over the entire 24-hour period. If possible, patients can be managed on an

TABLE 6–16. **Incidence of Different Types of Stones**

Calcium stones	
Calcium oxalate	33%
Calcium oxalate and phosphate	34%
Calcium phosphate	6%
Magnesium ammonium phosphate	15%
Uric acid	8%
Cystine	2%
Others	1%

outpatient basis. Patients in severe pain and those who are unable to maintain adequate oral intake because of vomiting may need to be hospitalized for IV hydration and analgesia. Stone passage may take hours to weeks. The patient should be given a strainer and should attempt to retrieve the excreted stone. Knowledge of the stone composition may be critical for appropriate medical management. Surgical intervention should be considered only if conservative measures fail.

Patients with fever, chills, and symptoms of renal colic require hospitalization and prompt intervention. If the presence of an infection behind an obstructed ureter is confirmed, antibiotic coverage and surgical decompression are mandatory.

A 24-hour urine collection should be done after the acute episode, at a time when the patient is back to his or her routine activity and diet. The urine should be sent to a laboratory for analysis of calcium, uric acid, and creatinine content.

B. Treatment for Specific Kinds of Stones

1. CALCIUM STONES. The dietary intake of calcium should be modestly restricted. Severe restriction may be counterproductive because of increases in urinary oxalate levels. **Hydrochlorothiazide** ([HCTZ] 50–100 mg/d), together with a mild degree of salt restriction, is useful, since thiazide inhibits distal tubular sodium reabsorption and causes a mild degree of volume contraction and enhanced proximal reabsorption of sodium, calcium, and uric acid. Before initiation of HCTZ therapy, it is important to rule out hyperparathyroidism as the cause of the hypercalciuria, since HCTZ can cause hypercalcemia. Although HCTZ can potentially lead to hypercalcemia in patients with absorptive hypercalciuria, this is not borne out clinically. **Allopurinol** is useful in some patients with calcium stones, as sodium hydrogen urate crystals may form heterogeneous nuclei for calcium oxalate crystal growth. Allopurinol is customarily used in dosages of 100–300 mg/d and is particularly useful in patients demonstrated to have increased urinary uric acid excretion. **Orthophosphate** may be used, as either neutral or acidic sodium or potassium phosphate, in dosages of elemental phosphorus, 1.5–2 g/d. Orthophosphate can cause significant GI side effects, and its dosage may have to be adjusted. **Cellulose phosphate** has been used to bind calcium in the GI tract. It is, however, bulky and expensive, and efficacy has not been established.

2. URIC ACID STONES. In patients known to form uric acid stones, an attempt should be made to alkalinize the urine, since uric acid has higher solubility in alkaline urine. Allopurinol, in dosages of 100–300 mg/d, should be prescribed for patients demonstrated to have recurrent uric acid stones.

3. STRUVITE (MAGNESIUM AMMONIUM PHOSPHATE). Struvites are formed primarily in alkaline urine and are usually the result of upper urinary tract infections with a urea-splitting organism. It is, therefore, important to eradicate the infection. Since the majority of struvites are in the form of staghorn calculi, surgical intervention may be necessary to remove the stone.

4. **CYSTINE STONES.** A vigorous attempt should be made to alkalinize the urine with oral administration of sodium bicarbonate. Dosages of 2.4 g tid may be necessary to accomplish the alkalinization. D-Penicillamine has been shown to be effective in selected patients.

5. **XANTHINE STONES.** The dietary intake of purines should be limited, and a vigorous attempt should be made to alkalinize the urine. In addition to these measures, several less well evaluated modes of therapy have been advocated. Administration of magnesium oxide may improve the solubility of urinary oxalate. It has been suggested that methylene blue is an effective inhibitor of calcium oxalate stone formation. In an uncontrolled study, the administration of potassium citrate, an inhibitor of calcium stone formation, was associated with a very low incidence of new stone formation.

In recent years, surgical intervention for nephrolithiasis has changed with the introduction of lithotripsy techniques. The stone is shattered by subjecting it to focused ultrasonic shockwaves. Extracorporeal shockwave lithotripsy is quickly becoming the treatment of choice for fragmentation and removal of simple stones in the kidney and upper ureters. Its low complication rate and high efficacy are rapidly eliminating the need for surgical lithotomy in centers where the lithotriptor is available.

Coe FL, Parks JH, Asplin JR. The pathogenesis and treatment of kidney stones. N Engl J Med 1992;327:1141–1152.

Pak CYC. Etiology and treatment of urolithiasis. Am J Kidney Dis 1991;18:624–637.

Smith LH. Urolithiasis. In: Schrier RW, Gottschalk CW, eds. Diseases of the Kidney, 4th ed. Boston: Little, Brown; 1988, pp 785–814.

IX. THE NEPHROTIC SYNDROME

Heavy proteinuria can lead to progressive decline in the serum albumin level, lower plasma oncotic pressure, and formation of edema. When more than 3.5 g of protein are excreted in the urine each day and the serum albumin level falls to less than 3 g/dL, the nephrotic syndrome is said to be present. The serum cholesterol level is often increased, and lipiduria is common. Heavy proteinuria leading to the nephrotic syndrome is usually the result of glomerular disease but can occasionally occur with severe tubular diseases. Intrinsic glomerular diseases account for 75% of the conditions causing the nephrotic syndrome. Among these, membranous nephropathy and focal segmental sclerosis are the most common causes of the nephrotic syndrome in the adult. In children, the nephrotic syndrome is due to minimal-change disease more than 95% of the time. In the remaining 25% of adult cases, the nephrotic syndrome is associated with systemic illnesses that can produce glomerular pathology (Table 6–17). Among these illnesses, diabetes mellitus, SLE, and amyloidosis are the most commonly encountered disorders.

A. General Management Principles

1. **RENAL FUNCTION.** The major goal of managing the nephrotic syndrome is to keep the patient reasonably comfortable without compromising the

TABLE 6–17. **Causes of Nephrotic Syndrome**

Glomerular Diseases
Membranous nephropathy
Focal glomerular sclerosis
Minimal-change disease
Focal and diffuse proliferative glomerulonephritis
Membranoproliferative glomerulonephritis
Systemic Diseases
Diabetes mellitus
Systemic lupus erythematosus
Amyloidosis
Less Common Causes
Infection (subacute bacterial endocarditis, shunt infection, malaria, syphilis, hepatitis,
  schistosomiasis)
Toxins (heroin, mercury, gold, penicillamine, bismuth)
Uncommon Causes
Allergens (bee stings, serum sickness)
Mechanical causes (constrictive pericarditis, renal vein thrombosis, obstruction of the
  inferior vena cava)
Malignant disease (Hodgkin's disease, lymphoma, and other malignant diseases)
Pregnancy
Congenital disorders (Fabry's disease, nail-patella syndrome, Alport's syndrome)

renal function by excessive diuresis. A moderate amount of edema should be tolerated, and aggressive diuretic therapy should be reserved for those with symptomatic edema, particularly if skin breakdown or infection becomes a factor. Fluid and salt restriction should invariably be the first step in treating the patient with fluid retention and symptomatic edema. Fluid restriction to 1000 and 2000 mL is usually well tolerated. Sodium should be limited to 2 g/d.

2. DIET. Because of the continuing losses of protein throughout the urinary tract, patients should be instructed to take in a diet rich in high-quality protein. Adequate caloric intake should be maintained to minimize catabolism. Protein should be limited when uremia accompanies the nephrotic syndrome.

3. DIURETICS should be used judiciously. Patients with hypoalbuminemia have intravascular contraction, and aggressive diuresis can accentuate prerenal azotemia by further contraction of the vascular space. In general, thiazides should be tried first, although they are usually of marginal efficacy. A loop diuretic (furosemide, bumetanide, or ethacrynic acid) is usually necessary. The loop diuretic regimen can be gradually escalated to a three-times-a-day schedule. If diuresis is still suboptimal, metolazone, starting at 5 mg/d, can be added. The combination of a loop diuretic with metolazone is usually effective in promoting diuresis in patients with intractable edema.

B. Specific Therapy

Specific therapy is directed at the underlying glomerular lesion.

1. **MINIMAL-CHANGE DISEASE IN ADULTS.** Minimal-change disease in the adult is reasonably steroid sensitive, although the incidence of steroid resistance is much higher than that in children with minimal-change disease. Patients should be managed with fluid and salt restriction and a defined course of steroids (daily or alternate-day steroids). For symptomatic patients whose condition is refractory to steroid therapy, cytotoxic agents (cyclophosphamide) may be of help. Minimal-change disease in the adult, particularly the elderly, may be associated with a lymphoproliferative disorder, and the possibility of associated malignant disease should be evaluated in the elderly patient with the nephrotic syndrome.

2. **FOCAL GLOMERULAR SCLEROSIS.** Unfortunately, no therapeutic interventions have been proved effective in changing the clinical course of focal glomerular sclerosis. Management should, therefore, focus on conservative measures.

3. **MEMBRANOUS DISEASE.** Young males with high-grade proteinuria due to membranous disease appear to be most prone to renal function deterioration. These patients should be considered for aggressive therapy. A multicenter prospective randomized study suggests that alternate-day steroids in doses of 125 mg of prednisone every other day are effective in minimizing renal difficulties in patients with membranous nephropathy. Cytotoxic medications, such as chlorambucil or Cytoxan, given in combination with prednisone, have also been demonstrated to be efficacious.

4. **FOCAL AND DIFFUSE PROLIFERATIVE DISEASE.** There are few studies examining the efficacy of therapy, but treatment with steroids and treatment with cyclophosphamide appear to be of help.

5. **MEMBRANOPROLIFERATIVE GLOMERULONEPHRITIS.** Few studies have been done on effectiveness of therapy in this condition, but steroid therapy and cyclophosphamide therapy seem to be of some benefit.

Bernard DB, Salant DJ. Clinical approach to the patient with proteinuria and the nephrotic syndrome. In: Jacobson HR, Striker GE, Klahr S, eds. The Principles and Practice of Nephrology. St. Louis: Mosby–Year Book; 1995, Chapter 17.

Glassock RJ. Clinical aspects of glomerular diseases. Am J Kidney Dis 1987;10:181.

Ponticelli C, Passerini P. Treatment of the nephrotic syndrome associated with primary glomerulonephritis. Kidney Int 1994;46:595–604.

X. RENAL MANIFESTATIONS OF SYSTEMIC DISEASES

A number of systemic illnesses have significant renal manifestations, and careful attention to the renal issues is critical for successful management.

A. Diabetic Nephropathy

1. **CLINICAL COURSE.** Fifty percent of patients with juvenile-onset diabetes and 6% to 10% of patients with adult-onset diabetes eventually develop end-stage renal disease requiring dialysis or transplantation. Currently, 25% of all new uremic patients with end-stage renal disease have diabetic nephropathy. Patients with juvenile-onset diabetic nephropathy usually follow a predictable course. Careful measurements have

revealed that early in the disease patients actually have increased glomerular filtration rate. Renal size is correspondingly increased. Urinalysis reveals no abnormal findings, with no proteinuria. About 10 to 12 years into the illness, microalbuminuria is noted in some patients, but the patients continue to have normal renal function. However, the presence of microalbuminuria identifies a group who will eventually develop significant renal disease. About 15 to 17 years after the onset of diabetes, patients may develop the nephrotic syndrome. The onset is often abrupt and is associated with a grave prognosis, with progression to end-stage renal disease usually within 2 to 5 years. With the onset of renal dysfunction, hypertension and CHF become significant problems, and retinopathy is often more difficult to control. Renal function classically deteriorates rapidly.

2. **MANAGEMENT.** Several maneuvers are useful early in the course of the disease to decrease the rate of renal deterioration. Rigid **control of both blood sugar and blood pressure** has been shown to be of benefit. A number of studies are now examining the efficacy of **restricting dietary protein** in controlling the rate of declining renal function. Such dietary restriction can be tried in appropriate patients.

A relatively new and important adjunct in diabetic patients with microalbuminuria is the use of **ACE inhibitors.** Once microalbuminuria is present, ACE inhibitors should be used, with the expectation that they will significantly slow the rate of renal function decline.

For the diabetic patient with end-stage renal disease, **hemodialysis, CAPD, renal transplantation,** and simultaneous transplantation of kidney and pancreas are all options. The outlook for diabetic patients receiving hemodialysis has improved substantially. However, mortality in diabetic patients receiving dialysis is still greater than that in the nondiabetic, although the gap is narrowing. Hemodialysis is associated with a first-year mortality of 15% to 30%. By the fifth year, the survival rate of patients is often down to 30% to 50% (Table 6–18). Morbidity is also high for diabetic patients on hemodialysis.

CAPD is a reasonable treatment for diabetics. Since heparinization is not necessary for the procedures and since hemodynamic fluctuations are less drastic than those in hemodialysis, retinopathy is less of a problem in patients undergoing CAPD. Similarly, the problems with

TABLE 6–18. Survival of Diabetic Patients Receiving Hemodialysis

INVESTIGATOR	NO. OF PATIENTS	SURVIVAL (%)			
		1 y	2 y	3 y	4 y
Rothschild	17	85	66	—	—
Soricelli	25	—	62	—	—
Slifkin	97	78	65	55	50
Totten	27	—	75	—	—
Ma	18	85	85	—	—
Shapiro	198	70	50	45	30

TABLE 6–19. Survival of Diabetic Patients Receiving Transplantation

SERIES	NO. OF PATIENTS	SURVIVAL (%)			
		1 y	2 y	3 y	4 y
Living Related Donors					
Minnesota	196				
HLA identical		90	90	88	80
Non-HLA identical		85	75	68	60
Mayo Clinic	39	80	80	80	80
Scandinavian	25	85	85	66	65
Cadaver Donors					
Minnesota	109	75	70	60	60
Mayo Clinic	22	64	52	52	52
Scandinavian	121	60	50	40	35

construction of vascular accesses are obviated. Nonetheless, cardio-vascular and infectious complications continue to be significant in these patients. Peritonitis is of particular concern. The mortality figures are similar for hemodialysis and CAPD, with a mortality of 15% to 20%/y.

Transplantation, in the appropriate candidate, appears to be the most reasonable option for diabetics with end-stage renal disease (Table 6–19). Graft survival probably is similar to that in nondiabetic patients. The major cause of death after transplantation is MI, accounting for about 40% of deaths. Infectious complications account for 20% to 30%. Peripheral vascular disease remains a problem, but neuropathy and retinopathy are improved by transplantation. Vision is stabilized or improved in 75% to 80% of those with transplants. The rehabilitation potential is far superior to that associated with either hemodialysis or CAPD. In selected patients, the simultaneous transplantation of pancreas and kidneys has been attempted, with reasonable success rates. The procedure should be reserved for carefully selected patients. In general, a fistula should be constructed when the serum creatinine level in the diabetic patient has reached 4 mg/dL, and transplantation should be planned. At a serum creatinine level of 6 mg/dL, transplantation should be considered, and patients without a living related donor should be placed on a cadaveric transplant list.

B. Systemic Lupus Erythematosus (SLE)

1. CLINICAL COURSE. Renal failure is the leading cause of death in patients with SLE. Clinical manifestations of renal disease are usually seen during the first 3 years after diagnosis. Such clinical evidence of renal involvement is observed in 60% to 75% of patients. If renal biopsy is performed, light microscopic examination of the biopsy specimen reveals changes in about 90% of patients, and electron microscopic examination demonstrates abnormalities in virtually 100%. The biopsy finding of renal involvement in an overwhelming majority of patients, as

well as the discrepancy between the clinical and pathologic findings, complicate decisions with regard to the selection of appropriate candidates for biopsy and therapy. The clinical presentation and the prognosis differ, depending, in part, on the underlying pathology. Patients with mesangial proliferative and focal proliferative glomerulonephritis usually have a better prognosis than patients with diffuse proliferative glomerulonephritis. Patients with inflammatory changes as opposed to scarring have better responses to therapy. A small number of patients may have membranous glomerulonephritis or interstitial nephritis.

2. **THERAPY.** In general, therapy is reserved for patients with biopsy evidence of inflammation in the absence of significant scarring and for patients with either deterioration of renal function or an increase in the activity of urinary sediment. **Steroids** are often the first agents used for patients with lupus nephritis. Unfortunately, a prospective, randomized study comparing steroids with placebo is lacking. Uncontrolled, non-randomized studies suggest that high-dose steroids are more beneficial than low-dose steroids. The recommended starting dosage is 60–100 mg/d, with tapering as the disease activity permits. **Pulse therapy with steroids,** using methylprednisone, 1 g/d IV for 3 to 5 days, has been advocated. Alternate-day steroid therapy has low toxicity, but its efficacy has not been uniformly demonstrated. A number of prospective, controlled, randomized studies have shown benefit from using **cyclophosphamide.** IV pulse therapy using cyclophosphamide every third month has been demonstrated to have low toxicity and high efficacy. Five prospective, controlled, randomized trials also indicate that **azathioprine,** although of marginal benefit, may allow faster tapering of steroids. Anecdotal reports suggest that patients with elevated levels of circulating immune complexes may respond to **plasmapheresis,** whereas those without these elevated levels do not respond. Further studies are needed to confirm efficacy. **Transplantation** has been successful in patients with end-stage renal disease secondary to lupus nephritis. Recurrence of lupus nephritis has been reported in the transplanted kidney. In general, it is important to be sure that lupus is clinically and serologically quiescent before transplantation to minimize the likelihood of recurrence in the transplanted kidney.

C. Wegener's Granulomatosis

1. **CLINICAL COURSE.** In a patient with progressive renal failure and respiratory tract symptoms, Wegener's granulomatosis is an important disease to be included in the differential diagnosis. If the disease remains untreated, rapid renal deterioration terminates in death within months. Prompt therapy with cytotoxic drugs, on the other hand, usually results in stabilization and gradual improvement in renal function. The mean age of patients at the onset of the disease is 40 years, and there is a 2:1 male/female ratio. The clinical triad of Wegener's granulomatosis includes (1) necrotizing granulomatous vasculitis of the upper and lower respiratory tracts, (2) necrotizing

glomerulonephritis, and (3) varying degrees of disseminated small-vessel vasculitis. Determination of antineutrophil cytoplasmic antibody (ANCA) has allowed for easier diagnosis of Wegener's granulomatosis. The ANCA assay appears to have a high degree of sensitivity and specificity. Spontaneous remission of renal disease is not known to occur. Before the availability of cytotoxic agents, most patients with Wegener's granulomatosis succumbed to renal disease. Without therapy, the mean survival has been 5 months from the onset of clinically evident renal involvement. As noted before, cytotoxic drug therapy generally results in stabilization and gradual improvement of renal function.

2. THERAPY. **Cyclophosphamide** is now generally regarded as the mainstay of therapy. In clinically toxic states, cyclophosphamide, 2–3 mg/kg/d, can be given IV for several days. This can be followed by PO administration of cyclophosphamide in a dosage of 1–2 mg/kg/d. In less toxic situations, the oral regimen can be started from the outset. The total duration of cyclophosphamide therapy required is unclear, but a course of at least 6 to 12 months is recommended unless severe drug toxicity complicates therapy. The disease can recur after the termination of therapy, but recurrences can be treated successfully.

Temporary remissions, especially of the extrarenal disease manifestations, can be seen with the administration of **steroids** alone. However, the renal disease often progresses despite corticosteroid therapy. Steroids can, therefore, be used only to ameliorate symptoms in toxic states in patients with Wegener's granulomatosis. Prednisone should be started at a dosage of 60–100 mg/d, with rapid tapering as the clinical situation permits.

Some studies have demonstrated that **plasmapheresis,** in combination with steroids and cyclophosphamide, can be helpful, particularly in the patient with advanced renal involvement. A number of patients undergoing dialysis have responded to the combination therapy enough to discontinue dialysis.

D. Goodpasture's Syndrome and Antiglomerular Basement Membrane Nephritis

1. CLINICAL COURSE. Patients may have progressive renal insufficiency resulting from antibodies directed against the glomerular basement membrane. The disease may occur with renal involvement alone (antiglomerular basement membrane nephritis), or it may occur in association with pulmonary involvement (Goodpasture's syndrome). Prompt recognition is vital to treatment. The disease usually affects men between the ages of 20 and 30, and many patients have antecedent upper respiratory tract symptoms. There may be an association of the disease with exposure to hydrocarbons. In patients with Goodpasture's syndrome, pulmonary symptoms may range from cough, dyspnea, and mild blood-tinged sputum to massive pulmonary hemorrhage. Pulmonary symptoms precede or are coincidental with renal manifestations in 70% of cases. In some instances, patients may have symptoms of renal insufficiency and may show no evidence of pulmonary involve-

ment. These patients are said to have antiglomerular basement membrane disease. Classically, renal insufficiency progresses rapidly, and end-stage renal disease may result within weeks to months. The diagnosis can be established by detection of circulating antiglomerular basement membrane antibodies or by renal or lung biopsy.

2. THERAPY. **Plasmapheresis** has been demonstrated to be of benefit in patients with antiglomerular basement membrane disease, presumably by removing circulating antibodies. Plasmapheresis leads to prompt cessation of pulmonary hemorrhage and reversal of renal insufficiency. It is important to note that plasmapheresis is of limited benefit in patients with oliguria and severe renal insufficiency (a serum creatinine level >6.8 mg/dL) at the initiation of therapy. Steroids and cyclophosphamide are usually employed also. In instances of life-threatening pulmonary hemorrhage, **bilateral nephrectomy** has been reported to be effective. In all instances, plasmapheresis should be attempted before consideration of bilateral nephrectomy. **Dialysis** can be used for support of patients who have antiglomerular basement membrane disease with renal insufficiency. Dialysis does not remove the antibodies and is of no use in the control of pulmonary hemorrhage. **Renal transplantation** has been successful in patients with end-stage renal disease. However, recurrence of disease in the transplanted kidney has been reported, and it is important to wait until antiglomerular basement membrane antibody titers are undetectable before transplantation is considered.

E. Multiple Myeloma

1. CLINICAL COURSE. Renal insufficiency is the second most common cause of death, after infection, in patients with multiple myeloma. Renal involvement may occur as a direct result of the disease or may be secondary to complications arising during the course of the disease. Clinically evident renal involvement occurs in about half of the patients with multiple myeloma and is associated with a markedly worse prognosis. In the majority of patients with renal involvement, deterioration of renal function is insidious, with slow progression over months to years. Few patients have ARF. The most important factor contributing to renal dysfunction is the presence of Bence Jones proteinuria. Approximately half of the patients with multiple myeloma have Bence Jones proteins (light-chain immunoglobulins) in the urine. The presence and amount of Bence Jones proteins appear to correlate roughly with degree of renal dysfunction. However, some patients with heavy proteinuria may have no evidence of renal dysfunction, and some may have renal insufficiency with no demonstrable Bence Jones proteinuria. Bence Jones proteins may be directly nephrotoxic or may cause tubular obstruction by precipitation in the distal tubules. Renal insufficiency may be the result of amyloidosis, found in about 10% of patients with multiple myeloma. In these cases, a light-chain immunoglobulin, or a fragment thereof, is the major constituent of the amyloid fibrils deposited. Patients with renal amyloidosis usually have hypertension, the nephrotic syndrome, and progressive renal insufficiency. Hypercal-

cemia is another important contributing factor in the development of renal insufficiency in patients with multiple myeloma. Hypercalcemia can cause compromises in renal concentrating ability, volume contraction, nephrocalcinosis, and nephrolithiasis. Hypercalcemia may also have direct nephrotoxic effects.

Other factors that can contribute to the development of renal failure include infections, particularly pyelonephritis, plasma cell invasion of the renal parenchyma, and the hyperviscosity syndrome, with compromises in renal blood flow. Patients with multiple myeloma are also more prone to contrast agent-induced ARF. Although the exact incidence is not known, patients with multiple myeloma should not be exposed to contrast media unless there is an absolute indication for the study.

2. **MANAGEMENT. Preventive measures** are as important as treatment measures in patients with multiple myeloma. The state of **hydration** should be optimized at all times to prevent dehydration and possible precipitation of Bence Jones proteins in the renal tubules. Use of **contrast agents should be avoided** unless there are absolute indications for contrast studies. If use of these agents is necessary, the patient should be vigorously hydrated before the study. The urine, renal function, serum globulin and viscosity, serum calcium level, and uric acid concentration should all be serially monitored. Hypercalcemia should be aggressively treated. Prolonged immobilization should be avoided to minimize the chance that hypercalcemia will develop. This measure is particularly important for patients with bone pain, in whom aggressive radiation therapy and liberal analgesia may be necessary. **Before the initiation of chemotherapy, prophylactic allopurinol, alkalinization, and saline diuresis should be used.** Unnecessary instrumentation of the genitourinary tract should be avoided to reduce the likelihood of infection. Potentially nephrotoxic drugs should not be used.

F. Progressive Systemic Sclerosis (Scleroderma)

1. **CLINICAL COURSE.** Approximately 40% to 50% of patients with progressive systemic sclerosis have clinically evident renal involvement, which becomes manifest about 2 to 3 years after diagnosis. Patients have proteinuria, hypertension, or renal insufficiency. There are two forms of renal involvement. An indolent form is insidious, with mild proteinuria, hypertension, and azotemia. Physiologic studies indicate decreased renal blood flow. Even patients with indolent renal involvement have a worse prognosis than those without renal involvement, and the mortality rate is 6 times that in patients with no renal involvement. Patients with malignant renal scleroderma have rapid and dramatic deterioration of renal function in the setting of malignant hypertension. Progressive renal insufficiency requires intervention within weeks to months.

2. **MANAGEMENT.** Malignant renal scleroderma constitutes a medical emergency, since patients often have malignant hypertension and rapid deterioration of renal function. The **control of blood pressure** with converting enzyme inhibitors (captopril, enalapril) has been shown to

reverse progressive renal deterioration in a number of cases and should be tried. **Malignant hypertension** should be aggressively treated with IV **nitroprusside.** Malignant hypertension and progressive renal deterioration unresponsive to converting enzyme inhibitors have been successfully managed with bilateral nephrectomy in a number of instances. **Dialysis** and **transplantation** have also been successful in patients with renal scleroderma. Steroids, D-penicillamine, and anticoagulation therapy have been tried but have not been shown to be helpful.

G. Henoch-Schönlein Purpura

1. CLINICAL COURSE. Renal involvement is an important complication in patients with Henoch-Schönlein purpura. The syndrome occurs primarily in young children, with 75% of cases occurring in children under the age of 7. There appears to be some seasonal variation in the occurrence of the disease, with spring and fall being the most common seasons. The salient features of the syndrome include (1) skin manifestation of nonthrombocytopenic purpura, (2) joint manifestation of arthralgia, (3) GI manifestations of abdominal pain and hemorrhage, and (4) renal involvement. Clinical evidence of renal involvement is reported in 30% to 70% of patients with Henoch-Schönlein purpura. Some patients with no signs of renal disease have been reported to have pathologic changes on renal biopsy. Fortunately, fewer than 10% of patients have progressive renal failure. Renal involvement is potentially the most life-threatening complication in Henoch-Schönlein purpura and is of important prognostic value. Renal presentations include hematuria, proteinuria (including the nephrotic syndrome), and renal insufficiency. Pathologically, either focal or diffuse proliferative glomerulonephritis can be seen. Immunoglobulin A (IgA) deposition in the mesangium is classically observed.

2. MANAGEMENT. Several therapeutic measures have been tried, but with limited efficacy.

   a. **Conservative measures.** Supportive care should be undertaken, and drugs such as aspirin should be avoided.

   b. **Steroids.** No controlled trials examining the efficacy of steroids in the management of renal complications are available. Joint and GI complications seem to respond to steroid therapy. However, steroids do not appear to affect skin lesions, duration of illness, or development of renal complications.

   c. **Cytotoxic agents.** There are no available controlled trials investigating the effectiveness of cytotoxic agents, although there are suggestions that the prognosis may be improved in some patients with severe renal disease.

   d. **Plasmapheresis.** No controlled trials have examined the use of plasmapheresis in the management of renal involvement in Henoch-Schönlein purpura.

   e. **Intravenous immunoglobulin.** There is evidence that daily IV administration of immunoglobulin for 14 days may be of benefit in this disease.

H. Hemolytic Uremic Syndrome

1. **CLINICAL COURSE.** The hemolytic uremic syndrome primarily affects young children and infants and is characterized by microangiopathic hemolytic anemia, thrombocytopenia, and ARF. Recently, a strong association between *Escherichia coli* 0157:H7 infection and the hemolytic uremic syndrome has been established. There is no specific treatment for the bloody diarrhea induced by *E. coli* 0157:H7, which is associated with the hemolytic uremic syndrome. Treatment with antibiotics is not indicated. Less commonly, hemolytic uremic syndrome can be associated with *Shigella* infection. The syndrome can also be associated with drugs, such as cyclosporine and mitomicin C.

   Rarely, the syndrome can be seen in adults. Most patients have abdominal pain, vomiting, and bloody diarrhea as a prodromal syndrome. Some patients may have an upper respiratory prodrome. The major morbidity arises from ARF and bleeding complications. On renal biopsy, vasculitic changes and focal segmental proliferative glomerulonephritis are seen.

2. **MANAGEMENT.** Supportive care is usually all that is necessary for mild cases of hemolytic uremic syndrome. The use of steroids and cytotoxic drugs may be of limited help. Plasmapheresis with the use of fresh frozen plasma is indicated in patients with severe disease. Early intervention with dialysis appears to be beneficial. Some patients may develop malignant hypertension and should be aggressively treated. Many patients with the hemolytic uremic syndrome will recover normal renal function.

I. Thrombotic Thrombocytopenic Purpura

1. **CLINICAL COURSE.** Thrombotic thrombocytopenic purpura is a disease of unknown etiology characterized by the clinical triad of hemolytic anemia, thrombocytopenia, and abnormal mental status. In many patients, fever and renal failure are also present. The syndrome occurs predominantly in patients 10 to 40 years of age, with a slight increase in prevalence among females. Many patients have prodromes of nonspecific symptoms, such as arthralgia, pleuritis, and Raynaud's phenomenon. Neurologic symptoms range from paresthesia and changes in mental status to seizures and coma. ARF occurs in approximately 50%. These patients have hematuria, pyuria, active urinary sediment (including red cell casts), and abnormal renal function.

   Two forms of the disease have been identified. In the chronic form, symptoms may wax and wane over a period of months. In its acute form, symptoms begin abruptly and follow a fulminant course, with progressive neurologic and renal disorders, often culminating in death. Patients who have the fulminant type often die within 90 days. Thrombotic thrombocytopenic purpura, like the hemolytic uremic syndrome, has recently been associated with *E. coli* 0157:H7 in some acute cases.

2. **MANAGEMENT.** In patients with severe thrombotic thrombocytopenic purpura, plasmapheresis using fresh frozen plasma as replacement should be initiated.

Balon JE, Austin HA, Tsokos GC, et al. Lupus nephritis. Ann Intern Med 1987;106:79.

Balon JE, Fauci AS. Vasculitic diseases of the kidney. In: Schrier RW, Gottschalk CW, eds. Diseases of the Kidney, 4th ed. Boston: Little, Brown; 1988, pp 2335–2361.

De Fronzo RA, Cooke JR, Wright JR, et al. Renal failure in patients with multiple myeloma. Medicine 1978;57:51.

Rees Al, Lockwood CM. Antiglomerular basement membrane antibody-mediated nephritis. In: Schrier RW, Gottschalk CW, eds. Diseases of the Kidney, 4th ed. Boston: Little, Brown; 1988, pp 2091–2126.

Wardle EN. Diabetic nephropathy. Nephron 1987;45:177.

XI. RENAL TRANSPLANTATION

Considerable advances have been made in transplantation and immunology over the past 25 years to make renal transplantation a safe and logical choice in end-stage renal disease. Transplantation, however, should not be regarded as a panacea, as considerable morbidity and mortality are still associated with it. A number of options are possible for the patient considering renal transplantation. The kidney can come from a cadaver, from a living related donor, and, in very selected instances, from a living unrelated donor. Patients receiving kidneys from a living donor have slightly better graft survival, and the amount of immunosuppression required is usually less. However, with the use of cyclosporine, graft survival, even in cadaveric transplants, is reasonable (Table 6–20). It is important to be familiar with the immunosuppressive agents commonly used for transplantation and to be aware of the possible complications related to the procedure.

A. Maintenance Immunosuppressive Agents

1. **STEROIDS.** Steroids are still an important part of immunosuppressive therapy. With the advent of cyclosporine, steroid doses can be tapered much more rapidly, thereby avoiding some of the complications of steroid therapy. Steroids are often used in relatively high doses immediately after transplantation and tapered rapidly as the clinical setting permits. During the first few days after transplantation, 60–100 mg of prednisone often is necessary. The doses are tapered over the course of the next 6 to 12 weeks to a maintenance dosage of usually 15 mg/d.

2. **AZATHIOPRINE.** Azathioprine is an important immunosuppressant with limited side effects. It is usually given in dosages of 50–150 mg/d,

TABLE 6–20. **Graft and Patient Survival at 1 y with Cyclosporine**

DONOR TYPE	GRAFT SURVIVAL (%)	PATIENT SURVIVAL (%)
Living related donors		
HLA identical	92	95
Non-HLA identical	85	92
Cadaver donor	80	86
Living unrelated donor	85	90

depending on the patient's bone marrow reserve. Its major side effect is bone marrow suppression, making the patient more prone to infections. Anemia and thrombocytopenia can also occur. Rarely, azathioprine may cause liver function abnormalities.

3. **CYCLOPHOSPHAMIDE.** Cyclophosphamide is sometimes used in place of azathioprine. The dosage is similar (50–150 mg/d). Its major side effect is bone marrow suppression.

4. **CYCLOSPORINE.** Cyclosporine has been an important addition to the group of immunosuppressive agents. It has little suppressive effect on bone marrow and has permitted faster tapering of steroid doses during the posttransplant period. However, cyclosporine has a number of side effects, including nephrotoxicity, particularly when excessive cyclosporine doses are employed. The nephrotoxic effect of cyclosporine has complicated treatment, since it is often difficult to differentiate between rejection and cyclosporine nephrotoxicity. Serum cyclosporine levels are of marginal help because toxicity may not correlate with serum levels. Other side effects are hyperkalemia, hypertension, and hirsutism. With long-term immunosuppression, malignant disease increases, and unusual tumors, such as CNS lymphoma, can be seen in these patients. It is, therefore, desirable to use the lowest possible maintenance doses of immunosuppressants that can prevent graft rejection.

B. Treatment of Rejection

Several options are available. Prompt recognition and treatment are essential to prevent loss of the graft.

1. **STEROIDS.** Pulse administration of steroids, with a concomitant increase in steroid dose, is effective in rejection. This measure is often all that is necessary for mild rejection. However, repeated pulse administration of steroids and prolonged treatment with high doses of steroids should be avoided because of the morbidity involved.

2. **ANTILYMPHOCYTE GLOBULIN.** Antilymphocyte globulin (ALG) is an immunoglobulin directed against human lymphocytes that is produced usually in horses and is effective for the treatment of rejection. Side effects include hypersensitivity reactions, particularly with the initial doses, production of antibodies against ALG, thereby precluding a repeat course, and excessive immunosuppression, leading to infectious complications. ALG has to be administered in a large volume of solution, which may be a problem if volume overload is present.

3. **MUROMONAB-CD3 (ORTHOCLONE OKT3).** A monoclonal antibody directed against a selected population of T cells appears to be an extremely powerful agent in the treatment of rejection. More than 95% of patients treated have responded to a course of muromonab-CD3, although some of these patients subsequently had another episode of rejection. Muromonab-CD3 can be given in small volumes and will not aggravate problems with volume overload. Patients may have a hypersensitivity reaction to initial doses and can form antibodies to the drug, thereby precluding a repeated course. Muromonab-CD3 can also cause infec-

tious complications by excessive immunosuppression but appears safer than repeated pulse administration of steroids.

4. **DACTINOMYCIN (ACTINOMYCIN D).** Dactinomycin is usually reserved for patients with chronic rejection in whom the other therapeutic interventions have failed. Its effectiveness appears to be limited.

5. **RADIATION.** Radiation, similarly, is reserved for patients with chronic rejection in whom the other treatments have failed. It, too, is of limited efficacy.

Braun WE. Nephrology forum. Long-term complications of renal transplantations. Kidney Int 1990;37:1363–1378.

7777777777

PULMONARY CONDITIONS

TERRY J. MENGERT

7777777777777

I. PULMONARY TESTS: STRUCTURE AND FUNCTION

Accurate diagnosis of pulmonary disease requires an adequate database, including both a thorough review of the patient's symptoms and any history of exposure to environmental risks that affect pulmonary function. The **physical examination** must include vital signs, skin, nails, accessory muscle use, percussion and auscultation of the lungs, thorough cardiac examination, and evaluation of the other organ systems. Many pulmonary tests are available to add to this database.

A. Arterial Blood Gases

The preferred site for drawing blood for arterial blood gas (ABG) studies is the radial artery; the brachial and femoral arteries are other possibilities. One must be careful to eliminate excess heparin from the syringe, evacuate air bubbles, immediately place the sample in ice, record the temperature of the patient, record the FIO_2, and analyze the specimen promptly.

1. **INDICATIONS.** ABG studies are indicated in the critically ill patient and the patient with a potentially serious O_2, CO_2, or acid-base abnormality. The test is also indicated in chronically or critically ill patients with a change in clinical status or ventilator settings. ABG should **not** be routinely determined in patients with acute asthma (unless clinical status or pulmonary function tests [PFTs] indicate severe obstruction), stable patients in the ICU, or patients receiving prophylactic low-flow oxygen (Ann Intern Med 1986;105:390–398).

2. **RESULTS**
   a. **Normal ABG values** are pH 7.35 to 7.45, PO_2 80 to 105 mm Hg, and PCO_2 35 to 45 mm Hg. Normal PO_2 does decline with age. The equation

   $$PO_2 = 109 - 0.43 \times \text{age (in years)}$$

   may be used to predict the expected PO_2 at sea level in the older patient breathing ambient air.
   b. **Alveolar hypoventilation** is defined as a $PCO_2 > 45$ mm Hg. Its causes include compensation for a metabolic alkalosis, decreased respiratory drive, primary lung disorders (via increased dead space), chest wall disorders, and neuromuscular diseases.
   c. **Hypoxia** is defined as $PO_2 < 60$ mm Hg. The five basic causes are hypoventilation, low inspired concentration of oxygen, diffusion impairment, ventilation-perfusion mismatch, and right-to-left shunt.

B. Oximetry

Oximeters determine the concentration of oxyhemoglobin in the blood by means of a spectrophotometer that measures the absorbance of light by oxyhemoglobin. Advantages over traditional ABG studies include continuous monitoring of O_2 saturation and the noninvasive nature of the test.

Disadvantages include lack of P_{CO_2} and pH determinations and measurement errors secondary to jaundice, carboxyhemoglobin levels over 3%, or poor blood flow. Continuous O_2 saturation monitoring is used in the operating room and ICU, in the emergency department patient with cardiorespiratory symptoms, during cardiopulmonary resuscitation, during bronchoscopy, in exercise studies, and in evaluation of sleep apnea. Under most circumstances, O_2 supplementation should be provided to maintain the patient's hemoglobin saturation $(SaO_2) \geq 95\%$. In the patient with known chronic obstructive pulmonary disease (COPD) who may be at risk for CO_2 retention with high-flow O_2, an SaO_2 of 90% is appropriate.

C. Spirometry

Spirometry measures volumes of inspired or expired gas or both. The test is used to
- Detect early lung disease
- Quantitate current pulmonary dysfunction
- Assist with differential diagnosis of dyspnea, cough, and wheezing
- Follow the course of pulmonary disease
- Monitor patient response to therapy
- Screen for possible toxic injury

The measured volumes may be presented as a resting spirogram (Fig. 7–1), flow-volume loops (Fig. 7–2), or forced spirometry (Fig. 7–3).

1. **MAXIMAL VOLUNTARY VENTILATION.** Maximal voluntary ventilation (MVV) is the greatest volume of air the patient can move per minute. It is a composite measurement that depends on the cooperation, strength, and endurance of the patient as well as the intrinsic mechanical

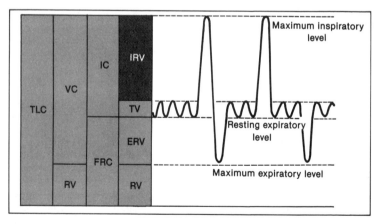

FIGURE 7–1. Static lung volumes are derived from standard spirometry and from a measurement of functional residual capacity either by body plethysmography or by gas dilution. Total lung capacity (TLC), vital capacity (VC), residual volume (RV), functional residual capacity (FRC), tidal volume (TV), inspiratory reserve volume (IRV), expiratory reserve volume (ERV), inspiratory capacity (IC). (From Forster RE II, et al. The Lung: Physiologic Basis of Pulmonary Function Tests, 3rd ed. Chicago: Year Book Medical Publishers, Inc.; 1986.)

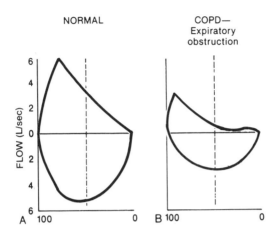

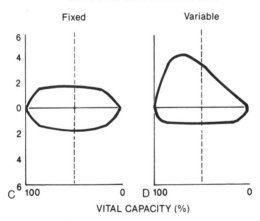

FIGURE 7–2. Flow-volume curves (loops) of maximal forced expiration (upper) and maximal inspiration (lower). Expiratory and inspiratory flow is plotted against lung volume expressed as a percentage of vital capacity. The dashed line can be used to compare flow rates at 50% of the vital capacity, at which point inspiratory flow rates normally exceed expiratory flow rates. **A,** Normal flow-volume curves. **B,** Flow-volume curves illustrating expiratory airflow obstruction showing decreased flow rates at all points in lung volume throughout maximal expiration. **C,** Fixed extrathoracic airway obstruction (cancer or fracture of the larynx). **D,** Variable extrathoracic obstruction (vocal cord paralysis) produces a pattern in which there is a decrease and flattening of maximal inspiratory flow-volume curves. (Modified from Hyatt RE, Black LF. The flow-volume curve: a current perspective. Am Rev Respir Dis 1973;107:191.)

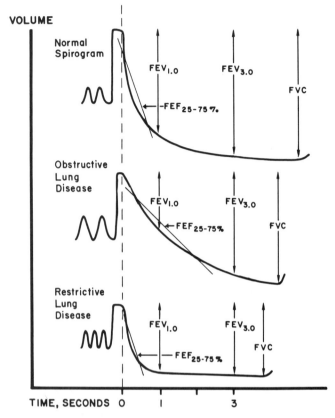

FIGURE 7–3. Simple spirometry usually allows differentiation of obstructive and restrictive patterns. Note that in both patterns, the forced vital capacity (FVC) is reduced; however, flows are reduced in obstruction and are normal or supernormal in restriction. FEV, forced expiratory volume; FEF, forced expiratory flow. (From Slonim NB, Hamilton LH. Respiratory Physiology, 5th ed. St. Louis: C.V. Mosby; 1987.)

properties of the lung. It can be estimated by forced expiratory volume in 1 second (FEV_1) × 35.

2. INTERPRETATION OF SPIROMETRY (TABLE 7–1)
   a. **Obstructive lung disease.** This is indicated spirometrically by an FEV_1/forced vital capacity (FVC) of less than 70% to 75%. Patients with air-flow obstruction are seldom limited in normal activity if FEV_1 is greater than 2 L. Obstruction is severe, and they are symptomatic if FEV_1 is less than 1 L, and conversation can be limited at FEV_1 less than 500 mL.
   In normal individuals, FEV_1 declines with age. In patients who have smoked more than 10 cigarettes per day, the decline in FEV_1 is greater, especially in men, particularly in those between 50 and 70.

In patients younger than 35, smoking cessation is associated with an increase in FEV_1. In individuals older than 35, smoking cessation results in a return to the normal age-related decline in FEV_1 (Am Rev Respir Dis 1987;135:794–799).

b. Restrictive lung disease. This disease may reduce the FEV_1, but in the absence of obstructive disease, the FEV_1/FVC will still be greater than 70% to 75%. Normal FVC rules out significant restrictive lung disease.

c. Bronchodilators. The effectiveness of bronchodilators may be confirmed with spirometry. If after bronchodilator treatment the FEV_1 increases by at least 12% (and an absolute improvement of 200 mL), a significant response has occurred.

d. Postoperative respiratory failure. Postoperative respiratory failure is increased in patients with chronic obstructive pulmonary disease (COPD). Pulmonary function abnormalities that suggest a higher risk of postoperative morbidity and mortality include $FEV_1 < 1.2$ L (or <50% predicted), MVV < 50% predicted, FVC < 2 L, and $Pco_2 > 45$ mm Hg (Am Rev Respir Dis 1979;119:293–310).

e. Pulmonary resection. An MVV less than 50% predicted indicates that the patient is at risk for significant complications. Further assessment of regional lung function is then indicated, using radioisotopic lung scanning techniques. If postoperative FEV_1 is predicted to be less than 800 mL (or <40% predicted), pulmonary resection is generally contraindicated (Am Rev Respir Dis 1975;111:379–387). If the patient has pulmonary hypertension from primary vascular disease or has pulmonary hypertension more severe than would be predicted on the basis of COPD, measurement of unilateral pulmonary artery occlusion pressures may be necessary to estimate the adequacy of the pulmonary vascular bed after resection.

TABLE 7–1. Interpretation of Spirometry*

STATUS	FVC† (%)	FEV$_1$† (%)	FEV$_1$/FVC (%)	D$_{LCO}$† (%)
Normal	≥80	≥80	≥75	≥80
Mildly impaired (usually not related to decreased ability to work)	60–79	60–79	60–74	60–79
Moderately impaired (decreased ability to meet the physical demands of many jobs)	51–59	41–59	41–59	41–59
Severely impaired (unable to meet the physical demands of most jobs)	≤50	≤40	≤40	≤40

*% predicted.

†FVC, forced vital capacity; FEV$_1$, forced expiratory volume in 1 s; D$_{LCO}$, diffusing capacity of the lungs for carbon monoxide.

Adapted from American Thoracic Society. Evaluation of impairment/disability secondary to respiratory disorders. Am Rev Respir Dis 1986;133:1205–1209.

D. Diffusing Capacity

Diffusing capacity of the lung (DLCO) is a measure of its ability to transfer gas across its alveolar surface. The results of the DLCO assessment depend on hemoglobin concentration, area of perfused alveolar membrane, and the resistance of that membrane to carbon monoxide. Diseases that obliterate the alveolocapillary membrane, that recruit or eliminate capillaries, or that change hemoglobin concentration will change the DLCO. The DLCO is decreased in emphysema, restrictive diseases like sarcoidosis, recurrent pulmonary emboli, diffuse interstitial fibrosis, and bleomycin toxicity. The DLCO is increased in erythrocytosis or early CHF.

E. Other Tests

Other tests may be CT of the thorax, esophageal pressure measurement, ventilatory drive assessment, inhalational challenges, scintiscans (including perfusion, ventilation, and gallium scans), pulmonary dead-space determinations, ultrasonography, bronchoalveolar lavage, bronchoscopy, magnetic resonance imaging (MRI), thoracoscopy, mediastinoscopy, and mediastinotomy.

American Thoracic Society. Standardization of spirometry—1987 update. Am Rev Respir Dis 1987;136:1285–1298.

American Thoracic Society. Lung function testing: selection of reference values and interpretive strategies. Am Rev Respir Dis 1991;144:1202–1218.

Burki NK, Albert RK. Noninvasive monitoring of arterial blood gases Chest 1983;83:666–669.

Clawsen JL. Pulmonary function testing. In: Bordow RA, Moser KM, eds. Manual of Clinical Problems in Pulmonary Medicine, 2nd ed. Boston: Little, Brown; 1985, pp 9–17.

Crapo RO. Pulmonary-function testing. N Engl J Med 1994;331:25–30.

Raffin TA. Indications for arterial blood gas analysis. Ann Intern Med 1986;105:390–398.

Tisi GM. Evaluation of pulmonary function before surgery. J Respir Dis 1984;5(1):105–113.

II. OXYGEN THERAPY

Oxygen therapy is used to increase the oxygen delivered to the tissues to improve cellular, tissue, and organ function and thereby avert injury and death of the organism. Oxygen supplementation is justified in a variety of situations. Examples include (1) acute or chronic hypoxia from pulmonary disease, (2) acute myocardial infarction, (3) acute anemia, (4) postoperative care, and (5) CHF. In general, if tissue hypoxia is either suspected clinically or anticipated, it is reasonable to initiate empirically based O_2 supplementation. When O_2 supplementation is expected to exceed 24 to 48 hours, ABG should be measured to document continued need.

A. Oxygen Delivery Systems

The types of oxygen delivery systems, along with their advantages and disadvantages, are given in Table 7–2.

B. Problems with Oxygen Supplementation

Obvious disadvantages of O_2 therapy include cost, fire hazard, infection risk (e.g., from organisms that colonize humidifiers), and development of psychologic dependence on O_2 therapy. Additional problems are described below.

1. **WORSENED RESPIRATORY ACIDOSIS.** Aggressive O_2 supplementation may blunt the hypoxic respiratory drive in COPD patients with chronic CO_2 retention, resulting in increased respiratory acidosis, deteriorating mental status, and worsening respiratory failure. Additional evidence, however, suggests that minute ventilation is only minimally decreased in patients with O_2 supplementation and that the cause of increased CO_2 retention is relaxation of hypoxia-induced vasoconstriction. Oxygen supplementation should always be used judiciously in chronic CO_2 retention. Therapy should be initiated with 1–1.5 L O_2/min via nasal prongs and the clinical status followed closely.

2. **OXYGEN TOXICITY.** High concentrations of FiO_2 over time can injure the lungs. Pulmonary damage depends on FiO_2 and duration of exposure. Opinions vary, but the threshold for clinically significant toxicity is an $FiO_2 \geq 0.6$.

C. Indications for Long-Term Oxygen Supplementation

Some patients with hypoxia and chronic COPD, sleep apnea, and interstitial lung disease will benefit from long-term oxygen use. Benefits may include improved survival, better intellectual function, reduced pulmonary hypertension, and increased exercise tolerance. The following are indications for long-term oxygen therapy.

- Arterial hypoxemia when breathing room air ($PaO_2 \leq 55$ mm Hg or O_2 saturation $\leq 88\%$). The patient's disease should be stable and optimally treated (the decision to prescribe long-term O_2 therapy should not be based on results of ABG determinations obtained during disease exacerbation)
- PaO_2 56 to 59 mm Hg or O_2 saturation 89% accompanied by electrocardiographic evidence of cor pulmonale, dependent edema, or erythrocytosis (hematocrit $> 56\%$)
- Exercise-induced hypoxemia ($PaO_2 < 55$ mm Hg) if O_2 supplementation improves exercise capacity, tolerance, or duration
- Sleep-induced hypoxemia if there is evidence of induced organ dysfunction (e.g., pulmonary hypertension, cardiac arrhythmia, or disturbed sleep pattern) and if nocturnal O_2 supplementation reduces the degree of hemoglobin desaturation
- $PaO_2 > 59$ mm Hg or O_2 saturation $> 89\%$ if medically justified for compelling reasons and other more conservative therapy has failed

D. Additional Concepts

- Low-flow O_2 with nasal prongs at 1–3 L/min is sufficient for most patients.
- The goal is a PaO_2 necessary to maintain hemoglobin at 90% saturation (approximately 60 mm Hg).
- If the patient is chronically hypoxemic, O_2 supplementation is of no benefit if used 12 hours or less per day; in the chronically hypoxemic patient, maximal benefit is realized with continuous therapy.
- Once the supplementation is prescribed, the need for home O_2 should be reevaluated 1, 6, and 12 months after its initiation. Thereafter, the need should be reassessed annually.

TABLE 7-2. Oxygen Delivery Systems*

SYSTEM	ADVANTAGES	DISADVANTAGES	COMMENTS
Nasal cannula (prongs)	Simple; fairly comfortable; can be used during airway care, eating, and drinking	Limited FIO_2 capability; exact FIO_2 quite variable (dependent on inspiratory flow rate and minute ventilation); may dry or irritate mucous membranes	Each L/min raises FIO_2 about 3%; humidify if flow rate >4 L/min (for two prongs); a water-soluble lubricant may help avoid mucous membrane irritation
Simple O_2 mask	Provides higher FIO_2 than nasal cannula	Uncomfortable and must be removed when eating, drinking, and expectorating; FIO_2 is variable, dependent on inspiratory flow and minute ventilation	FIO_2 of about 35% at 6 L/min flow; FIO_2 about 55% at 10 L/min flow; because of CO_2 entrapment, dead space may be increased (with increased work of breathing)
Nonrebreather reservoir mask (the reservoir is attached to the base of the mask, but a one-way valve prevents rebreathing of expired gas)	Provides highest FIO_2 short of intubation (approximately 90-95%)	See Simple O_2 mask above	The reservoir *must* remain filled; because of high FIO_2, absorption atelectasis and O_2 toxicity may occur; if reservoir bag collapse occurs, O_2 delivery will be insufficient to maintain adequate ventilation
Continuous positive airway pressure (CPAP) mask	Increases pulmonary volume, opens previously closed alveoli (reducing shunt); may improve V/Q mismatch	Uncomfortable; risk of aspiration if patient vomits	May improve PaO_2 in intrapulmonary arteriovenous shunt for given FIO_2

Method	Comments	Disadvantages	Notes
Bilevel positive airway pressure (BiPAP) via nasal or facial mask	Provides noninvasive positive pressure ventilation to treat respiratory failure; the ventilator cycles between a higher positive airway pressure with inspiration and a lower positive pressure with expiration	Uncomfortable; aspiration risk; patient may tolerate better with time	Decreased work of breathing; positive pressure during exhalation helps prevent alveolar/small airway collapse; may avoid intubation in select patients
Jet-mixing Venturi mask	Provides more exact FIO_2 than other methods described above	Uncomfortable; must be removed when eating, drinking, and so forth	Most accurate FIO_2 at 24% (flow of 4 L/min) and 28% (flow of 6 L/min); other FIO_2's available (31%, 35%, 40%, and 50%) are less accurate
Open face tent	May be better tolerated in some patients than nasal cannula or face masks; communication and expectoration not impeded	FIO_2 varies with flow rate and minute ventilation; eating impaired	May be able to provide FIO_2 as high as 70%
T tube	Exact FIO_2 possible up to 100%; humidification excellent	Requires endotracheal tube or tracheostomy	Maintain flow rate at least two times minute ventilation; humidification is mandatory because upper airway has been bypassed

*Medical gases do not contain water vapor. Humidification is appropriate at flow rates greater than 4 L/min. Humidification options include passover type, bubble, jet, and heated units. The last-named is the most efficient.

Fulner JD, Snider GL. ACCP–NHLBI National Conference on Oxygen Therapy. Chest 1984;86: 234–247.

Tarpy SP, Celli BR. Long-term oxygen therapy. N Engl J Med 1995;333:710–714.

III. COUGH

Cough is a frequent presenting complaint. The five most common causes of cough are acute respiratory tract infection, asthma, postnasal drip, chronic bronchitis, and gastroesophageal reflux with aspiration. Additional possibilities include cardiac failure, bronchogenic or metastatic carcinoma, sarcoidosis, long uvula, nasal polyps, external auditory canal disorders, and psychogenic cough (J Respir Dis 1986;7(3):21–30). Angiotensin-converting enzyme (ACE) inhibitor drugs (e.g., captopril, enalapril, and cilazapril) are well known to cause a chronic cough in some patients (Ann Intern Med 1992;117:234–242).

Useful points to review in determining the cause of cough include cigarette use, exposure to environmental irritants, duration of cough, whether onset was acute or subacute, circumstances at onset, sputum production, aggravating situations like exercise or cold air exposure, other associated symptoms, and origin of the cough (e.g., pharynx or trachea) (J Respir Dis 1985;6(1):97–107). See Table 7–3 for clues to the etiology of cough, as well as information about specific therapy. In many cases, empiric therapy for a nonsmoking, immunocompetent adult with a chronic cough should begin with an antihistamine-decongestant preparation to treat postnasal drip. Cough is crucial to bronchial hygiene, and it is important to remember this before planning symptomatic therapy. A chronic cough may have associated morbidity: syncope, fractured ribs, costochondral inflammation, costochondral separations, respiratory muscle strain, and abdominal or inguinal hernia formation.

A. Symptomatic Therapy for Chronic Cough

Either of the following may be used for chronic cough: (1) dextromethorphan 20 mg q4–6h or (2) codeine 10–20 mg q4–6h.

Irwin RS, Curley FJ, French CL. Chronic cough: the spectrum and frequency of causes, key components of the diagnostic evaluation, and outcome of specific therapy. Am Rev Respir Dis 1990;141:640–647.

Pratter MR, Bartler T, Akers S, Dubois J. An algorithmic approach to chronic cough. Ann Intern Med 1993;119:977–983.

IV. DYSPNEA

Dyspnea is the subjective sensation of breathlessness. As a presenting complaint, dyspnea usually requires evaluation because it may be associated with life-threatening disorders.

A. Approach to the Patient

Immediate assessment is necessary to rule out life-threatening problems (e.g., upper airway obstruction, myocardial infarction, pulmonary embolism, tension pneumothorax, anaphylactic shock, asthma or COPD exacerbation, noncardiogenic pulmonary edema, and acute paralysis). If needed,

TABLE 7–3. Clues to the Etiology of Cough and Guide to Specific Therapy

DIAGNOSIS	FINDINGS	THERAPY
Asthma	Cough with exercise, cold air exposure, environmental irritant, or wheezing; spirometry may reveal reversible obstruction; if spirometry is normal, consider an inhalational challenge (with methacholine or carbachol)	Bronchodilators; consider corticosteroids if *no* improvement occurs with bronchodilator therapy after several weeks
Postnasal drip and/or sinusitis	Repeated throat clearing; sensation of secretions dropping down back of throat, especially at night; mucoid secretions may be seen in nares or posterior pharynx	Oral antihistamine and/or decongestants; avoid known precipitants; if sinusitis is a good possibility, consider sinus films or CT and empiric oral antibiotic therapy
Postinfection cough	Patient with recent (past 2 to 3 mo) upper respiratory tract infection; often no other cause will be apparent; *do not* perform inhalational challenge in recent upper respiratory tract infection because even normal patients will demonstrate airway hyperactivity	No specific treatment necessary; patient may be given symptomatic treatment; follow-up encouraged until cough resolves
Chronic bronchitis	Patient usually a cigarette smoker; cough accompanied by sputum production daily for 3 mo in 2 consecutive years	*Strongly* recommend stopping cigarette use; bronchodilators reasonable; about 70% of smokers will be free of cough by 6 wk after stopping smoking
Gastroesophageal reflux	Dyspepsia symptoms, heartburn; consider further investigation with upper GI series, endoscopy, esophageal pH monitoring	Dietary change (avoid alcohol, caffeine, fats, and chocolate); elevate head of bed on 6-in. blocks; drug treatment may include antacids, histamine$_2$ (H$_2$) blockers, or metoclopramide
Malignancy	Chest radiograph may reveal mass or infiltrate; further evaluation may include sputum cytology, chest CT and/or bronchoscopy	Depends on exact diagnosis and stage of disease
Interstitial lung disease (including sarcoidosis)	Chest film and pulmonary function testing reveal interstitial disease	Depends on final diagnosis

Adapted from Brown SE. What to do when patients complain of chronic cough. J Respir Dis 1986;7:21–30.

establishing an adequate airway, ventilation, and circulatory support including oxygen treatment are the first priorities. Otherwise, evaluation may proceed more deliberately. When taking the history, one should place particular emphasis on abruptness of onset and duration of dyspnea and its severity (grade 1 = dyspnea when walking up stairs or hills; grade 2 = dyspnea when walking on level ground; grade 3 = dyspnea when walking on level ground ≤ 100 m; grade 4 = dyspnea with routine activities; grade 5 = dyspnea at rest).

B. Therapy

Treatment should always be **specific** to the disease causing dyspnea (described in appropriate sections of this manual). Only rarely can symptomatic treatment be considered (e.g., therapy with benzodiazepines or opioids to reduce respiratory drive).

Manning HL, Schwartzstein RM. Pathophysiology of dyspnea. N Engl J Med 1995;333:1547–1553.
Tobin MJ. Dyspnea: pathophysiologic basis, clinical presentation, and management. Arch Intern Med 1990;150:1604–1613.

V. HEMOPTYSIS

Hemoptysis should alert the physician to a possibly life-threatening disorder.

A. General Approach to the Patient

The goals of therapy are to prevent asphyxia, stop bleeding, and treat the cause of hemorrhage. The ABCs of resuscitation (**A**irway, **B**reathing, **C**irculation) always take priority. The cause of death in massive hemoptysis is **asphyxiation,** not exsanguination. Other sources of hemorrhage, including nasopharyngeal bleeding and GI bleeding (the latter characterized by dark red blood, clots with food particles, history of abdominal symptoms, and acid pH), should be excluded. In true hemoptysis, the blood frequently is alkaline, frothy, and bright red. The quantity and rate of bleeding should be determined as accurately as possible. In most cases, hemoptysis is of short duration and the volume is small, but blood loss greater than 600 mL in 24 to 48 hours defines massive hemoptysis and is a medical or surgical emergency. Thorough history and physical examination are important. Tests may include chest x-ray, CBC, PT, PTT, platelet count, ABG, gram stain and culture of sputum, ECG, and bedside spirometry, if possible. A serum creatinine determination and urinalysis are reasonable if Goodpasture's syndrome or other vasculitis is suspected. Bronchoscopy, rigid or fiberoptic depending on bleeding rate, allows for examination of the larynx and lower respiratory tract.

If there is active bleeding, humidified oxygen should be given, large-bore IV access established, the bleeding lung placed dependent (may be difficult to determine), type and crossmatch blood obtained, and emergent pulmonary, surgical, and anesthesiology consultations obtained. Airway management is crucial.

B. Treatment

When hemoptysis is minor and transient, evaluation need not be emergent. Therapy depends on the specific diagnosis. Antibiotics are often helpful, since bronchitis is the major cause. Elective bronchoscopy is indicated in patients with any of the following: age older than 40 years, abnormal chest radiograph, cigarette use (especially if greater than 40 pack-year history), or suspected foreign body aspiration. In an emergent situation, the guidelines presented should be followed. While awaiting bronchoscopy, one should monitor the patient's status closely with continuous pulse oximetry, frequent ABG determinations, and chest radiographs. In one study, 6% of 123 patients died while awaiting bronchoscopy and definitive therapy (J Thorac Cardiovasc Surg 1983;85:120–124). Fiberoptic bronchoscopy may be used to localize the bleeding site, although if bleeding is particularly active, rigid bronchoscopy will be necessary for adequate suctioning.

Specific treatment of an actively bleeding lesion may include Fogarty balloon catheter inflation proximal to the bleeding site and use of topical vasoconstrictors (epinephrine), coagulants (Gelfoam), or YAG laser–induced coagulation during bronchoscopy. Angiographic embolization of bleeding bronchial arteries may be effective, especially if the patient is not a surgical candidate (Diagn Radiol 1977;122:33–37). Endobronchial irradiation may be useful in stopping bleeding from an endobronchial tumor. Surgery is the treatment of choice for patients with rapid bleeding (≥600 mL/24 h) who are surgical candidates when the bleeding site can be localized and embolization is not a therapeutic option.

Goldman JM. Hemoptysis: emergency assessment and management. Emerg Med Clin North Am 1989;7:325–339.
Rudzinski JP, del Castillo J. Massive hemoptysis. Ann Emerg Med 1987;16:561–564.

VI. PLEURAL EFFUSIONS

Pleural effusion, although the most common clinical manifestation of pleural disease, may occur as a consequence of disease processes far removed from the pleura (e.g., nephrotic syndrome). Normally, the pleural space contains only about 0.1 to 0.2 mL/kg of transudate. This fluid is a result of the balance between hydrostatic and oncotic pressures. The normal flow of fluid is from the parietal to the visceral pleura. Pleural fluid accumulates abnormally when pleural lymphatic drainage is compromised, plasma or pleural space oncotic pressures are shifted, pleural hemodynamics are altered, vascular hydrostatic pressures change, or capillary permeability and surface area are affected by disease.

A. Diagnosis

About 200 to 300 mL of pleural fluid is necessary before costophrenic angle blunting occurs on a PA chest film, but a lateral decubitus radiograph will reveal as little as 150 mL of fluid. A subpulmonic effusion may mimic an elevated hemidiaphragm.

1. THORACENTESIS. Thoracentesis is indicated when the cause of the pleural effusion is uncertain or when the volume of fluid is large and is

inducing such symptoms as dyspnea. In general, thoracentesis can proceed without difficulty if a fluid layer at least 10 mm thick is visualized on a lateral decubitus chest radiograph. Reexpansion pulmonary edema may occur after thoracentesis if too large a volume of pleural fluid is removed too rapidly. Traditionally, no more than 1500 mL of fluid should be removed at one time to avoid this complication.

- **a. Laboratory evaluation.** The first priority is to distinguish an exudate from a transudate, which can be done by determining pleural fluid lactate dehydrogenase (LDH) and protein levels. Additional fluid can be held in the laboratory pending results of these tests. The differential diagnosis of transudates includes atelectasis, cirrhosis, CHF, hypoalbuminemia, nephrotic syndrome, peritoneal dialysis, and urinothorax. The effusions associated with malignancy and pulmonary embolism may also sometimes (<15% to 20%) be transudative. A transudate generally does not require further evaluation; an exudate does. Clinical suspicion of the likely disease or diseases should then guide other tests ordered. Options include the following.

  - *(1)* ***Cell count and differential*** yield useful information. Bloody fluid suggests cancer, pulmonary embolus, trauma, and tuberculosis. Leukocyte count and differential are helpful in distinguishing parapneumonic effusions from tuberculosis or cancer.
  - *(2)* ***Gram stain and culture*** are useful in parapneumonic effusions, in which tuberculosis or other infections are possible.
  - *(3)* ***The pH*** may be useful diagnostically when rheumatoid disease or cancer is suspected, esophageal rupture is suspected, or in evaluation of parapneumonic effusions.
  - *(4)* ***Glucose levels*** may be decreased in cancer, tuberculosis, parapneumonic effusion, and rheumatoid disease.
  - *(5)* ***Cytology*** has variable diagnostic yield but is more useful in detecting malignancy if multiple specimens (from separate thoracenteses) are submitted (Arch Intern Med 1973;132: 854–860).
  - *(6)* ***Amylase levels*** may be helpful in suspected pancreatitis, some malignancies (especially lung and ovary), or esophageal rupture.
  - *(7)* ***Additional tests*** may include hematocrit, triglycerides, and rheumatoid factor.

- 2. TRANSUDATE VERSUS EXUDATE. Any one of the following is sufficient to label pleural fluid as exudative.
  - A pleural fluid/serum protein ratio greater than 0.5:1 (or absolute protein ≥3 g/dL)
  - A pleural fluid/serum LDH ratio greater than 0.6:1
  - An absolute LDH value greater than 200 IU/L

B. Specific Problems

1. PLEURAL EFFUSIONS IN CANCER PATIENTS. The patient with cancer may have fluid accumulation secondary to the disease, but other possibilities

should also be considered: transudates from CHF, hypoalbuminemia, and venous outflow obstruction and exudates from pulmonary embolism with infarction and from pneumonia. The most common malignant diseases associated with pleural effusion are lung cancer (25% to 40%), breast cancer (25%), and lymphoma (10% to 15%).

a. **Pleural fluid characteristics.** Usually, the fluid is exudative (5% to 10% may be transudates) and serosanguineous and has an LDH level of more than 500 IU/L. The leukocyte count is typically 1000 to 5000/L, with mononuclear cells predominating. Cytologic findings are positive 30% to 70% of the time, depending on the pleural tumor burden. Cytologic study and pleural biopsy together will increase the yield. Pleural fluid pH and glucose levels have prognostic significance. If the pH is less than 7.3 and the glucose level is less than 60 mg/dL in a patient having known pleural involvement with cancer, the mean survival is shorter, and the response to tetracycline pleurodesis is poorer (Ann Intern Med 1988;108:345–349).

b. **Management.** When the diagnosis of malignant pleural fluid is confirmed, the rate of fluid reaccumulation will dictate the approach. If reaccumulation occurs over days to a few weeks, palliation should be considered.

c. **Palliation.** Chest tube drainage alone has about a 50% response rate. In the United States, tetracycline (500 mg in 50 mL of saline) is probably the agent of choice for pleurodesis, with reported response rates as high as 83% or more. Other treatments include intrapleural administration of doxycycline, minocycline, chemotherapeutic agents, talc poudrage, and pleurectomy with pleural abrasion. Factors important in considering palliation include the patient's overall condition, symptoms, expected survival, and biochemical characteristics of the pleural fluid (pH and glucose) (Am Rev Respir Dis 1988;138:184–234).

2. **BLOODY PLEURAL EFFUSIONS.** When the pleural fluid is grossly bloody, the effusion may be classified as serosanguineous (5000 to 100,000 RBC/mL), bloody (greater than 100,000 RBC/mL), and a hemothorax (hematocrit of the effusion exceeds 50% of the venous blood hematocrit). Exudative bloody effusions may result from malignant disease, trauma, infection, pulmonary embolism, collagen vascular disease (such as SLE), and contact with asbestos. Traumatic thoracentesis may have occurred. Usually the blood will clear during the course of the tap. Blood from a traumatic tap should also clot.

a. **Management.** In hemothorax, chest tube thoracostomy is appropriate. If hemorrhage continues at the rate of 100 to 200 mL/h, thoracotomy is indicated to ligate the bleeding vessels. If the bleeding has stopped but the hemothorax is incompletely drained, some question the need for thoracotomy. One approach is that if ≥30% of the hemithorax is occupied by undrained clot, thoracotomy is reasonable (J Respir Dis 1986;7(6):18–24).

3. **PLEURAL EFFUSIONS AND PNEUMONIA.** Effusions associated with pneumonia may be **parapneumonic** (secondary to inflammation and increased permeability of the pleura), **complicated parapneumonic** (may or may

not be infected but becomes fibrinopurulent and loculated), **or empyema** (frank pus in the pleural space). A simple parapneumonic effusion will resolve without specific therapy, except that aimed at the pneumonia itself. A complicated parapneumonic effusion may require closed chest tube drainage. Empyema **always** requires chest tube drainage. Thoracentesis should be performed in pneumonia if layering of ≥10 mm of fluid is observed on a lateral decubitus film. If there is concern about the best location to tap the fluid, one should use ultrasound guidance. Pleural fluid should be sent for protein and LDH determinations, in addition to pH, glucose level, gram stain and culture, and total white blood cell count (WBC) with differential. If the fluid is frank pus, however, the only studies necessary are gram stain and culture. Even if there is no growth on culture, many recommend that an effusion with a pH <7.1, a glucose level <40 mg/mL (in the setting of pneumonia), or an LDH level >1000 U/L be treated as an empyema.

a. **Management.** Empyemas require closed chest tube drainage in addition to the antibiotic appropriate for the pneumonia. As mentioned, complicated pleural effusions with low pH or low glucose level or both probably should be treated like empyemas. If the pleural effusion has a pH of 7.1 to 7.2 and a glucose level >40 mg/dL, repeat thoracentesis in 12 to 24 hours may be useful. If the pleural fluid shows a decreasing glucose level or lowered pH or both, closed chest tube drainage may be appropriate. Otherwise, close observation and treatment of pneumonia should be continued.

Sahn SA. The pleura. Am Rev Respir Dis 1988;138:184–234.
Walker-Renard PB, Vaughan LM, Sahn SA. Chemical pleurodesis for malignant pleural effusions. Ann Intern Med 1994;120:56–64.

VII. SOLITARY PULMONARY NODULE

The solitary pulmonary nodule (SPN) is a fairly common problem. It is a lesion no more than 5 to 6 cm in diameter in the lung parenchyma, surrounded by aerated lung tissue. The percentage of pulmonary nodules that are malignant depends on the population base and the size of the nodule (80% to 95% of nodules greater than 3 cm in size are malignant). When possible, resection of the malignant SPN is the treatment of choice. Benign lesions that may manifest as an SPN include hamartomas, granulomas (from tuberculosis or a variety of fungal infections), rheumatoid nodules, sarcoidosis, pulmonary infarction, and arteriovenous malformation.

A. Approach to the Patient

A lesion is more likely to be benign if the patient has no history of cigarette smoking or exposure to other carcinogens, is younger than 35, and/or has a history of tuberculosis or exposure to *Coccidioides, Histoplasma,* or other fungi. Routine workup should include CBC, electrolyte panel, calcium level, urinalysis, and stool Hemoccult.

Chest x-rays should be reviewed thoroughly, and old films should be obtained for comparison. Any of the following calcification patterns strongly suggests a benign lesion: diffuse, clustered or popcorn, dense central nidus, or a concentric or laminated pattern. If diagnosis is still uncertain, chest CT may reveal calcifications and define the relationship of the SPN to nearby thoracic structures and other abnormalities (e.g., enlarged mediastinal lymph nodes). If workup to this point leaves doubt about the potential malignancy of the lesion, a number of approaches may be reasonable.

1. **PERCUTANEOUS NEEDLE ASPIRATION AND BIOPSY.** This procedure is reasonable if clinically the lesion is unlikely to be malignant and if a tissue diagnosis will otherwise influence therapy (e.g., tuberculosis). Contraindications include patient uncooperativeness, a bleeding diathesis, pulmonary hypertension, markedly compromised pulmonary function (e.g., FEV_1 less than 1 L), or surrounding bullous disease. Complications include pneumothorax (11% to 30%) and hemoptysis (10% to 20%).

2. **FIBEROPTIC BRONCHOSCOPY.** Fiberoptic bronchoscopy has an accuracy of less than 30% in the tissue diagnosis of the SPN if the lesion is less than 2 cm in diameter and a diagnostic accuracy of about 50% to 80% for lesions larger than 3 cm. The yield is also better for an endobronchial lesion and a more proximal lesion.

3. **THORACOTOMY.** This procedure should be performed when the lesion is growing, when other approaches have not revealed a benign process, or when malignancy is otherwise likely. The patient must be a surgical candidate. It is contraindicated in the patient with severe COPD, severe CHF, recent MI, or unstable angina. Complications include chest pain, bleeding, and infection. Mortality has been traditionally reported as 3% to 5%.

B. Therapy

A lesion proved to be benign on the basis of a stable appearance on the chest radiograph for 2 or more years, a benign calcification pattern, or a tissue diagnosis confirming granuloma or other nonneoplastic process should be followed. For a suspected malignant SPN, thoracotomy is the treatment of choice in the appropriate surgical candidate. If chest CT shows abnormal mediastinal lymph nodes or mediastinal tumor, mediastinoscopy should be undertaken before surgery. Mediastinoscopy is also appropriate when the SPN is located centrally, when it has a diameter of more than 3 cm, or when biopsy has revealed that it is a small-cell or undifferentiated large-cell carcinoma.

Cummings SR. Monitoring solitary pulmonary nodules. Am Rev Respir Dis 1986;134:453–460.
Khouri NF. The solitary pulmonary nodule: assessment, diagnosis, and management. Chest 1987;91:128–133.
Lillington GA. Management of the solitary pulmonary nodule. Hosp Pract, May 15, 1993, pp 41–48.
Miller KS. Prediction of pneumothorax rate in percutaneous needle aspiration of the lung. Chest 1988;93:742–745.

VIII. PHARMACOLOGY OF AIRWAY DISEASE

Airway abnormalities may include hyperactivity, inflammation, excessive mucus production, and plugging of the airways with mucus and inflammatory debris. Clinically, the patient with airway dysfunction suffers from cough, sputum production, dyspnea, and wheezing. V/Q mismatch may result in hypoxia. Many therapeutic agents are available to combat these problems.

A. Sympathomimetics

The effects of these agents depend on the receptors they stimulate. Alpha receptors mediate vasoconstriction, beta$_1$ receptors mediate cardiac stimulation, and beta$_2$ receptors mediate bronchodilation, hyperglycemia, and muscle tremors.

1. PARENTERAL AGENTS. In some asthmatics, parenteral administration of sympathomimetics results in improved bronchodilation when compared with inhaled agents alone, presumably by delivering medication to airways so constricted that effective delivery is not achieved by the inhaled route (J Allergy Clin Immunol, 1989;84:90–98).

   a. **Epinephrine.** Epinephrine has both alpha and beta agonist effects and short duration of action (15 to 30 minutes). It is available in a nonprescription metered dose inhaler (MDI), injectable solution, or inhaled racemic compound. Epinephrine is crucial in severe allergic reactions, in which its alpha and mast cell stabilizing effects make it the drug of choice. Epinephrine may be administered as follows: 0.3 mL of a 1:1000 solution (0.3 mg) SC q15–30min to a maximum of three doses. Epinephrine should not be used in the patient with recent MI, history of angina, or history of cardiac dysrhythmia. Traditionally, epinephrine use has been avoided in the patient over 40, but age alone should **not** be considered an absolute contraindication (Ann Emerg Med 1988;17:322–326).

   b. **Terbutaline.** Terbutaline is a beta$_2$-selective agent. It is available in tablets, ampules for SC administration, and MDI. It has a longer duration of action than epinephrine and about twice the bronchodilator effect. It also may be better tolerated in the adult but should be used cautiously in the patient with known cardiac disease. An SC dose of terbutaline is 0.25 mg, which may be repeated in 15 to 30 minutes (not to exceed 0.5 mg SC q4h).

2. INHALED AGENTS. Inhaled agents include epinephrine (over the counter), isoproterenol, isoetharine, metaproterenol, albuterol, terbutaline, bitolterol, pirbuterol, and salmeterol. Of these, the most beta$_2$-selective are metaproterenol (Alupent, Metaprel), albuterol (Proventil, Ventolin), terbutaline (Brethine, Brethaire), bitolterol (Tornalate), pirbuterol (Maxair), and salmeterol (Serevent). Salmeterol is the longest-acting agent, with a recommended dosage of 2 puffs via MDI bid. Table 7–4 summarizes available inhaled beta agonists. Generally, oral forms are less well tolerated because they induce more systemic side effects. However, oral agents are added to augment bronchodilation if symptoms remain poorly controlled.

   When prescribing an MDI to a patient, it is the physician's responsibility to review the use of the inhaler with the patient (Table 7–5). As many as one third of patients use MDI incorrectly. In most cases, a spacer device should also be given when prescribing an MDI to improve medication delivery.

TABLE 7–4. The Inhaled Beta Agonists

DRUG	TRADE NAME	BETA SELECTIVITY	DRUG FORM	MDI* DOSE	NEBULIZED DOSE
Isoetharine	Bronkometer Bronkosol	Beta$_1$ and beta$_2$	MDI, nebulized solution	1–2 puffs q4h	0.5–1 mL (5–10 mg) in 1.5 mL NS q15–20min for 3 doses, then q4h
Metaproterenol	Alupent Metaprel	Beta$_2$	Tablets, syrup, MDI, nebulized solution	2–3 puffs q3–4h	0.3–0.5 mL (15–25 mg) in 2.5 mL NS q15–20min up to 3 doses, then q4h
Albuterol	Proventil Ventolin	Beta$_2$	Tablets, syrup, MDI, nebulized solution	2 puffs q4–6h	0.5–1 mL in 2 mL NS q20min for 6 doses then q4–6h
Terbutaline	Brethine Brethaire	Beta$_2$	SC injection, tablets, MDI	2 puffs q4–6h	—
Bitolterol	Tornalate	Beta$_2$	MDI	2–3 puffs q4–6h	—
Pirbuterol	Maxair	Beta$_2$	MDI	2 puffs q4–6h	—
Salmeterol	Serevent	Long-acting beta$_2$	MDI	2 puffs q12h (this dose should not be exceeded)	—

*MDI, metered dose inhaler; NS, normal saline.
Adapted from Webb-Johnson DC, Chin B, Andrews JL. Bronchodilator therapy: Part 1. N Engl J Med 1977;297:476–482.

TABLE 7–5. **How to Use a Metered Dose Inhaler**

Shake cartridge
↓
Take several long breaths in and out
↓
Hold metered dose inhaler 2–4 cm in front of wide-open mouth
↓
Exhale slowly and almost completely
↓
During normal inhalation, deliver single metered dose; deliver dose at start of inhalation
↓
Hold breath for minimum of 5–10 s (if possible)
↓
Wait 1–3 min before taking next puff in same manner
↓
Rinse mouth afterward to minimize systemic effects from medication
↓
Rinse mouthpiece daily with warm water

Adapted from West W. Update on drug therapy for your COPD patient. J Respir Dis 1985; 6(9):44–58.

B. Methylxanthines

Methylxanthines have been reported to stimulate respiratory drive, cause bronchodilation, improve cardiovascular function and ventilation/perfusion matching, increase the endurance and contractile function of the diaphragm, and enhance mucociliary clearance. Their exact mechanism of action remains uncertain. The effectiveness of theophylline in the treatment of acute asthma and COPD has been questioned. Several studies have shown not only no improvement in bronchodilation (when compared with the aggressive use of beta agonists alone), but also an increased incidence of side effects (Ann Intern Med 1987;107:305–309; Am Rev Respir Dis 1985;132:283–286). These studies should not prejudice the clinician against the value of theophylline in the long-term management of the still symptomatic patient with stable asthma or COPD. Double-blind, randomized, controlled studies have demonstrated that theophylline is effective in decreasing the frequency and severity of asthma symptoms when used on a long-term basis, compared with the effectiveness of cromolyn (Lancet 1977;1:381–385), inhaled albuterol (J Allergy Clin Immunol 1987;79:78–85), and oral metaproterenol (J Pediatr 1982;101:281–287). Patients with severe but stable COPD have been shown to have significant improvement in dyspnea, pulmonary gas exchange, vital capacity, and respiratory muscle performance when treated with theophylline as compared with placebo (N Engl J Med 1989;320:1521–1525).

1. **METHYLXANTHINE DOSING.** To achieve optimal benefits from **theophylline,** the plasma level should generally be between 10 and 20 µg/mL. In mild airway disease, some patients still derive benefit with lower serum concentrations. The dose required to produce a particular level varies

widely, and numerous medications affect methylxanthine metabolism (Tables 7–6 and 7–7).

Theophylline toxicity increases when the serum level exceeds 20 µg/mL. Symptoms of toxicity include anorexia, nausea, CNS irritability, tremor, seizures, and cardiac dysrhythmias.

a. **IV aminophylline load. Aminophylline** is 80% anhydrous theophylline. An IV load of 5 to 6 mg/kg is based on the concept that every 1 mg/kg load will increase the serum level 2 µg/mL. If the patient has ingested theophylline in the past 12 hours, one should wait for determination of the serum theophylline level. The IV load should be infused over 20 minutes. The blood level should subsequently be checked 1 to 2 hours after the beginning of the maintenance infusion.

b. **Oral dosage.** At the beginning of oral therapy in the patient in stable condition, the dosage should be titrated slowly over 9 days to achieve the desired serum levels and minimize side effects. The initial dose should be about 400 mg/d (a lower starting dose should

TABLE 7–6. Clinical Situations and Medications Influencing Methylxanthine Metabolism

Serum Levels Increased (Metabolism Decreased)
Infants <1 y old
Elderly patients
Congestive heart failure
COPD
Hepatic dysfunction
Viral or bacterial illness with fever
Cimetidine
Oral contraceptives
Erythromycin
Ciprofloxacin
Allopurinol
Alcohol
Clarithromycin
Methotrexate
Propranolol
Ticlopidine
Verapamil
Serum Levels Decreased (Metabolism Increased)
Children
Cigarette and marijuana smokers
Phenytoin (Dilantin)
Carbamazepine
Barbiturates
Rifampin
Sulfinpyrazone

Data from Hendeles L. Asthma therapy: state of the art, 1988. J Respir Dis 1988;9(3): 82–107; Weinberger M, Hendeles L. Theophylline in asthma. N Engl J Med 1996;334:1380–1388.

TABLE 7-7. Methylxanthine Dosing: Intravenous and Oral

	AMINOPHYLLINE	THEOPHYLLINE
MAINTENANCE INTRAVENOUS INFUSION	mg/kg/h	mg/kg/h
Nonsmokers	0.5–0.7	0.4–0.6
Smokers	0.9	0.75
Cimetidine use	0.3–0.4	0.25–0.3
Cor pulmonale	0.25–0.3	0.2–0.25
Hepatic insufficiency	0.2–0.25	0.18–0.2
EVENTUAL ORAL DOSE* (70-kg PATIENT)	mg/d	mg/d
Nonsmokers	900	800
Smokers	1300	1100
Cimetidine use	600	500
Cor pulmonale	500	400
Hepatic insufficiency	450	350

*Attained over a 9-day period to minimize side effects
Data from Garrity ER Jr, Gross NJ. Prompt management for status asthmaticus. J Respir Dis 1987;8(5):21–32; Hendeles L. Asthma therapy: state of the art, 1988. J Respir Dis 1988;9(3): 82–107; Med Lett Drugs Ther 1987;29:11–16.

be considered in patients with hepatic dysfunction, CHF, or cor pulmonale or in those taking cimetidine). Serum levels should be checked after 3 days and the dose increased every 3 days until therapeutic serum levels are reached. Average eventual oral doses in patients weighing 70 kg are given in Table 7-7.

NOTE: In patients able to take oral medication, there is no good evidence, even in an asthmatic or COPD exacerbation, that IV aminophylline or theophylline is more efficacious than oral delivery of the medication. Strongly consider orally loading the patient and avoiding IV use entirely.

C. Anticholinergic Drugs

Anticholinergic agents have become the drugs of first choice in the management of the stable patient with COPD because they produce bronchodilation as well as or better than beta agonists and have longer duration of action. They are also useful agents in the treatment of a COPD exacerbation. In the asthmatic, however, they appear to be less potent bronchodilators than beta agonists, although in some asthmatics, anticholinergics serve as useful adjunctive therapy.

1. IPRATROPIUM BROMIDE. Ipratropium bromide is available as an MDI and a nebulized solution. The dosage via MDI is 2 to 6 puffs every 6 hours. Sensitivity to the drug is a contraindication to its use. It has a favorable side effect profile and is the preferred anticholinergic. The nebulized solution (0.02%) is supplied in 2.5 mL unit dose vials. The recommended dose is one nebulized treatment every 6 to 8 hours. It may be mixed with albuterol, and both medications may be administered simultaneously via nebulizer as long as the combined solution is used within 1 hour of mixing.

D. Corticosteroids

The mechanism by which these drugs improve limitation of air flow remains unknown. Potential beneficial mechanisms include stabilization of lysosomal membranes, reduced release of cellular mediators of inflammation, decreased mucus secretion, reduction in airway inflammation, and restored beta receptor sensitivity. Corticosteroids have been documented to shorten the duration and severity of severe exacerbations in asthma and to prevent some hospitalizations. Several experts have concluded that the most important intervention that may prevent the several thousand deaths in this country per year from status asthmaticus is earlier and more aggressive use of corticosteroids. The prominent inflammatory component of asthma argues that more aggressive use of inhaled corticosteroids in asthma management is appropriate. Steroids can also play an important role in COPD management. In an acute exacerbation, their early use has been demonstrated to result in more rapid improvement in FEV_1. In chronic, stable COPD (Table 7–8), benefit is seen in relatively few patients (6% to 29%). When corticosteroids are given IV, some benefit is seen in as little as 1 hour, but the full effect is not reached for 6 to 8 hours. The preferred drug for IV use is methylprednisolone (Medrol). Hydrocortisone is more expensive than methylprednisolone at equipotent doses and has a greater mineralocorticoid effect. The IV dose should generally be followed by a tapering oral dose, as outlined in Table 7–9.

The side effects of corticosteroids are numerous, including weight gain, cataracts, osteoporosis, glucose intolerance, aseptic necrosis of femoral heads, capillary fragility, fluid retention, hypokalemia, cushingoid appearance, and suppression of the hypothalamic-pituitary axis. Reactivation of tuberculosis is of concern after a positive purified protein derivative (PPD) tuberculin skin test only if the patient is faced with a prolonged steroid course (months to years). In this circumstance, isoniazid prophylaxis is appropriate. In asthma, aerosol steroids can reduce airway inflammation and hyperreactivity and/or lower the dose of oral corticosteroid needed to maintain airway stability. Most experts consider inhaled steroids to be

---

TABLE 7–8. Clinical Steroid Trial in the Patient with Chronic, Stable COPD but Continued Severe Symptoms

1. Obtain baseline PFTs while patient is optimally and maximally treated.
2. Repeat PFTs on one other occasion before beginning trial to ensure an adequate baseline.
3. Begin patient on 40 mg prednisone per day.
4. Trial should be a minimum of 2 wk and preferably 4 wk.
5. At the end of the trial, repeat PFTs. An increase of FEV_1 by 20% or more (some would use 15%) or a 20% increase in FVC is a significant change.
6. If there is *no improvement* in PFTs, the patient should be tapered slowly off steroids.
7. If the patient responds, attempt to get the patient on an alternate-day regimen or on the lowest dose that maintains functional and PFT improvement.

Adapted from Alberts WM, Corrigan KC. Corticosteroid therapy for chronic obstructive pulmonary disease: is it worth the risks? Postgrad Med 1987;81:131–137.

TABLE 7–9. **Use of Corticosteroids in Acute Asthma or COPD Exacerbation**

ASTHMA

IV loading dose: Methylprednisolone 2 mg/kg or about 125 mg (1 vial) IV
Subsequent doses should be 60–80 mg IV bolus q6–8h until patient is stable. (Optimal dose of corticosteroids is debated.)
Oral therapy: 60–120 mg/d in divided doses, with the dose decreased to a once-a-day morning dose as soon as the clinical condition allows. A steroid taper should not occur until the patient's asthma is well controlled.
When the condition has stabilized, patients should be tapered off corticosteroids in 7–14 d as their clinical condition allows.
Sample steroid taper (every-day regimen): 60 mg × 2 d, 40 mg × 2 d, 30 mg × 2 d, 20 mg × 2 d, 10 mg × 2 d

COPD

IV loading dose: Methylprednisolone 0.5 mg/kg IV q6h for 72 h.
Oral therapy: If possible, corticosteroids should be discontinued after 72 h of IV treatment; if not, begin 60 mg/d and taper as clinical status allows.

ADDITIONAL GENERAL CONCEPTS (ASTHMA OR COPD)

1. Do not begin taper until patient's condition is stable with the initial starting prednisone dose.
2. Search carefully for exacerbating conditions; environmental irritants, suboptimally used medications, poorly tolerated medications (e.g., beta blockers for hypertension management or beta blocker eyedrops for glaucoma).
3. Attempt to get patient on an alternate-day regimen (as dose is reduced on even days, add that dose to odd day, or start taper by tapering dose on even days only).
4. Use inhaled steroids to assist with taper or to help with switching patient to an alternate-day regimen (in the asthmatic).
5. In major stress or surgery, patient will need stress doses of corticosteroids (patient receiving oral steroids longer than 2 wk should be presumed to have hypothalamic-pituitary suppression).

either first- or second-line agents in asthma management. Their role in the management of COPD is not well established, but their use is common and probably beneficial (N Engl J Med 1992;327:1413–1419). Although some minimal systemic absorption occurs when aerosol steroids are used as recommended, the risk of steroid side effects is reduced.

Aerosol steroids may be given as follows:

- Beclomethasone MDI, 2 puffs qid, up to 4 puffs 8 times per day
- Flunisolide MDI, 2 puffs bid, up to 4 puffs bid
- Triamcinolone MDI, 2 puffs tid to qid or 4 puffs bid
- Budesonide MDI, 400–2400 μg/d divided bid to qid

These agents should **not** be used to treat moderate to severe asthma exacerbations. Cough may be prevented by delivering a beta$_2$ agonist via MDI 10 to 15 minutes before use of the aerosol corticosteroid. To avoid oral candidiasis, the mouth and pharynx should be rinsed with water after use. If the voice becomes hoarse, the aerosol steroid should be discontinued for 3 to 5 days. Systemic steroids will generally be necessary during serious illness or surgery (because some suppression of the hypothalamic-pituitary axis still occurs with high-dose aerosol therapy).

E. Cromolyn and Nedocromil

1. **D**ISODIUM **CROMOGLYCATE** is thought to interfere with immunoglobulin E (IgE)-induced release of mediators from mast cells and basophils. It has no bronchodilator activity. Thus, it is an agent for airway hyperactivity prophylaxis. If administered during an asthma exacerbation or COPD flare, it may worsen existing bronchospasm. Cromolyn is available as an inhaled powder, a nebulized solution, and an MDI. Except for causing cough in some patients, it is nearly free of side effects. The use of a beta$_2$ agonist first may prevent cough. Cromolyn is especially effective in treating extrinsic asthma. It is given in a dosage of 2–4 puffs qid or 2 puffs 30 minutes before contact with an asthma-provoking stimulus. This drug should not be used if the patient is wheezing. Cromolyn should be tried for at least 4 weeks before being considered ineffective.

2. **N**EDOCROMIL **SODIUM** is a new agent chemically unrelated to cromolyn but with similar effects. The dose is 2 puffs qid. Side effects may include headache, cough, and pharyngitis.

F. Miscellaneous Agents

1. **S**TEROID-SPARING **AGENTS.** Experience is accumulating in the use of **methotrexate** as a steroid-sparing agent in the patient with asthma who is steroid dependent (N Engl J Med 1988;318:603–607; Lancet 1990; 336:137–140). It should be used only when all other treatment options (e.g., maximal other drug therapy, optimal environmental control) have been exhausted and by pulmonary specialists familiar with its use. The starting dose is 15 mg/wk. Multiple side effects include pulmonary fibrosis. Cyclosporine, gold salts, and troleandomycin are also being studied as potential steroid-sparing agents in chronic asthma.

2. **I**ODINATED **GLYCEROL.** In stable chronic obstructive bronchitis, iodinated glycerol has been shown to improve cough symptoms, patient well-being, and ease in bringing up sputum and to decrease the duration of acute disease exacerbations. The dose is 60 mg qid (Chest 1990; 97:75–83).

3. **M**AGNESIUM **SULFATE.** IV magnesium sulfate (1.2–2 g over 20 min) has been shown in several small studies to increase peak expiratory flow rate (PEFR) and decrease hospital admission in patients with asthma exacerbations who do not respond adequately to aggressive use of beta agonists. Consider using this agent in the asthma patient with normal renal function who is refractory to acute and aggressive asthma management in the emergency department or clinic. Its exact mechanism of action or duration of action is not known (JAMA 1989; 262:1210–1213). It may also provide modest benefit in COPD exacerbations (Arch Intern Med 1995;155:496–500).

4. **P**ARALYSIS AND **SEDATION.** In the **already intubated** asthmatic or COPD patient, paralysis and sedation are frequently necessary. Patients with status asthmaticus who require intubation are usually difficult to manage with the ventilator. When high peak airway pressures and respiratory acidosis continue to be difficult to control, sedation with a

benzodiazepine (e.g., lorazepam) and paralysis (e.g., pancuronium) are of assistance. The dissociative agent ketamine is also a potent bronchodilator and may be a useful adjunct to benzodiazepines for patient sedation. The dose is 2–4.5 mg/kg IV given at the rate of 0.5 mg/kg/min. A continuous infusion may then be required at a dose of 1 mg/kg/h.

5. GENERAL INHALATION ANESTHESIA. All of the commonly used inhalation general anesthetics are powerful bronchodilators (avoid halothane because of arrhythmia risk). In the **intubated** asthmatic who is doing poorly despite maximal conventional bronchodilator management, aggressive sedation, paralysis, and general inhalation anesthesia should be considered.

D'Alonzo GE, Nathan RA, Henochowicz S, Morris RJ, et al. Salmeterol xinafoate as maintenance therapy compared with albuterol in patients with asthma. JAMA 1994;271:1412–1416.
Dompeling E, van Schayck CP, van Grunsven PM, et al. Slowing the deterioration of asthma and chronic obstructive pulmonary disease observed during bronchodilator therapy by adding inhaled corticosteroids. Ann Intern Med 1993;118:770–778.
Drugs for ambulatory asthma. Med Lett 1993;35:11–14.
Huang D, O'Brien RG, Harman E, et al. Does aminophylline benefit adults admitted to the hospital for an acute exacerbation of asthma? Ann Intern Med 1993;119:1155–1160.
McFadden ER Jr, Gilbert IA. Asthma. N Engl J Med 1992;327:1928–1937.
Nelson HS. Beta-adrenergic bronchodilators. N Engl J Med 1995;333:499–506.
Weinberger M, Hendeles L. Theophylline in asthma. N Engl J Med 1996;334:1380–1388.
Weiner C. Ventilatory management of respiratory failure in asthma. JAMA 1993;269:2128–2131.

IX. ASTHMA

The physiologic hallmarks of asthma are airway hyperreactivity and inflammation. Associated airway abnormalities include bronchial wall edema, desquamation of ciliated epithelium, and mucus plugging. The result is pulmonary hyperinflation, increased residual volume, increased functional residual capacity, elevated pulmonary artery pressure, V/Q imbalance, increased work of breathing, and hypoxia. Asthma affects as many as 5% of the US population and results in more than 28 million visits to physicians annually. The prevalence, morbidity, and mortality of asthma are increasing in the United States (MMWR 1990;39:493–497).

Although asthma has been divided into intrinsic and extrinsic types on the basis of whether external agents induced the bronchospastic episodes, most asthmatics have manifestations of both intrinsic and extrinsic disease. Asthma should be considered a syndrome with intrinsic, extrinsic, and occupational aspects. Symptoms include dyspnea, wheezing, and cough. Some asthmatics may have only a chronic cough. Additional characteristics may be seasonal exacerbations, rhinitis, and the triad of chronic sinus disease, nasal polyps, and intolerance of aspirin and other NSAIDs. The differential diagnosis includes anaphylaxis, left ventricular dysfunction, vocal cord abnormalities, upper airway obstruction, cardiac ischemia, and obstructing endobronchial lesions. The results of the physical examination may be normal in patients with cough-variant asthma or in those who are between acute exacerbations. Patients with a severe asthma attack have tachycardia, tachypnea, diaphoresis, accessory muscle use, pulsus paradoxus (if greater than 18 mm Hg, the attack is life threatening), prolonged expiratory phase, and diffuse wheezing.

Asthma severity may be graded as follows:

Mild asthma: Cough and/or wheezing only one to two times per week

Moderate asthma: Cough and/or wheezing greater than two times per week, exercise intolerance, and/or nocturnal asthma compromising sleep two to three times per week

Severe asthma: Daily wheezing, tendency to suffer severe exacerbations, or more than three urgent physician or emergency department visits per year

A. Laboratory Studies

Routine workup may reveal peripheral blood eosinophilia or an elevated total IgE level or both. Other tests that are sometimes useful include skin testing and inhalational challenge.

1. **PULMONARY FUNCTION TESTS (PFTs).** Usually, a reversible air-flow obstruction will be demonstrated. If results of the PFTs are normal, inhalational challenge to methacholine to reveal air-flow obstruction and airway hyperactivity may be necessary. Severe airway obstruction during an asthma attack is characterized by an FEV_1 of <0.8 to 1 L (less than 25% predicted) or a peak expiratory flow rate (PEFR) less than 100 L/min (less than 20% to 25% predicted).

2. **CHEST X-RAYS.** These should be obtained during the initial workup for the new asthmatic and in patients with fever, focal findings on pulmonary auscultation, or failure to respond to appropriate therapy during asthma exacerbations. Routine films are otherwise not required for each asthma exacerbation.

3. **ARTERIAL BLOOD GASES.** With a mild exacerbation, PaO_2 and $PaCO_2$ may be normal or only slightly decreased, but as air-flow obstruction worsens, both hypoxia and hypocarbia occur (with resultant respiratory alkalosis). In a life-threatening attack, the work of breathing further increases, respiratory muscles fatigue, and the PCO_2 starts to rise again. When $PaCO_2$ reaches normal (the crossover point), a dangerous situation exists. Respiratory acidosis will soon follow, and respiratory arrest may be imminent. Nowak et al. (JAMA 1983;249:2043–2046) found that the measurement of PaO_2, PCO_2, and pH could not reliably distinguish patients requiring admission from those who could be discharged from the emergency room. Patients with an FEV_1 of less than 1 L (25% predicted) or a PEFR of less than 200 L/min (30% predicted) were at risk for hypercarbia and marked hypoxia. It is in this group of patients that an ABG measurement is most important.

B. Therapy

The two major components in the treatment of asthma are environmental control and pharmacologic therapy for air-flow obstruction and inflammation. Active patient education is a critical aspect of these components as well. The goal in treatment is to minimize symptoms, manage acute exacerbations aggressively, minimize the number of exacerbations, and minimize the number of medications the patient must take to achieve these ends. Comprehensive asthma treatment has proved successful in patient care (Ann Intern Med 1990;112:864–871).

1. **ENVIRONMENTAL CONTROL.** Possible precipitants include dust, exercise, chemicals, air pollution, occupational irritants, animal danders, environmental antigens (pollens, molds, and so on), and cigarette smoke. Environmental control is based on identifying precipitants and removing them, when possible, from the environment. Any patient who smokes should be strongly encouraged to stop. Other household members who smoke should also stop.

2. **PHARMACOTHERAPY.** See also the preceding section, Pharmacology of Airway Disease.
   a. **Home therapy for acute attacks.** Patients should be instructed in how to manage an asthma exacerbation initially at home. Therapy should start with an inhaled beta$_2$ agonist (not salmeterol) 2–4 puffs q20min for up to 1 hour.
      (1) If there is a ***good response*** (e.g., PEFR > 70% of baseline, no symptoms at rest, patient can climb one flight of stairs) to the therapy, the patient can continue beta$_2$ agonist treatments q3–4h for 24 to 48 hours as required and contact the physician as necessary for follow-up advice.
      (2) If there is only an ***incomplete response*** (e.g., persistent moderate symptoms at rest, inability to climb one flight of stairs without resting, or PEFR 50% to 70% of baseline), the patient should continue with either an inhaled or nebulized beta$_2$ agonist every hour, begin oral corticosteroids (or increase the dose if already taking oral steroids), and contact the health provider if there is no improvement within the next 2 to 6 hours. If, with this therapy, the PEFR persists at 50% to 70% of baseline or deteriorates or if symptoms worsen, the patient should seek care in an emergency department.
      (3) If there is a ***poor response*** (e.g., severe wheezing or breathlessness, severe symptoms at rest, unable to walk 100 feet without stopping, or PEFR < 50% of baseline), the patient should contact the health care provider, begin oral corticosteroids (or increase the dose if already taking oral steroids), and administer 4–6 puffs of a beta$_2$ agonist q10min up to two times or a nebulized solution once. The patient should go to the emergency department if there is not significant improvement within 30 minutes of this therapy, if the PEFR remains <50%, or if inhaled treatments with the beta$_2$ agonist are required (because of persistent symptoms or a PEFR that is declining or remains <70%) every 1 to 3 hours for more than 6 to 12 hours.
   b. **Hospital therapy for acute attacks.** Treatment depends on the severity of the attack. In a mild exacerbation, an inhaled beta agonist may be all that is necessary (in addition to O_2 supplementation and hydration). Table 7–10 presents emergency management of moderate to severe asthma exacerbations. Antibiotics are useful with fever,

TABLE 7-10. **Emergency Management of Severe Asthma Exacerbation**

Patient with moderate to severe wheezing, and/or marked dyspnea, air hunger, diaphoretic skin, accessory muscle use/sitting up and leaning forward/intercostal retractions/etc.

Administer O_2 (4-5 L/min via nasal prongs minimum), cardiac monitor, and pulse oximeter

Obtain vital signs, pulsus paradoxus, and FEV_1 or PEFR (if possible). If FEV_1 less than 1 L (25% predicted), consider ABG. Determine theophylline level if patient is receiving theophylline.

Establish IV access

Beta agonist (first drug of choice):

Albuterol 0.5-1 mL (2.5-5 mg) in 2 mL normal saline (NS) q20min, up to 6 doses (if necessary), then dose q1-2h

or

Metaproterenol 0.3-0.5 mL (15-25 mg) in 2.5 mL NS q15-20min for 3-4 doses (if necessary), then dose q1-2h

or

Terbutaline 0.5 mL (0.5 mg) in 2.5 mL NS q15-20min, up to 3 doses (if necessary), then dose q1-2h

If attack is **moderate or severe,** administer 125 mg of methylprednisolone IV along with inhaled beta agonist.

Consider 0.25 mg terbutaline SC, repeating dose in 15-30 min (maximum dose 0.5 mg q4h). Use terbutaline cautiously in patients with a history of angina or heart disease.

If improvement: Watch serial PFTs and clinical status, and continue beta agonist treatment.

If no improvement: Consider **aminophylline:** Loading dose (if patient not receiving theophylline): 5-6 mg/kg IV infused over 20 min (or oral theophylline 6 mg/kg if patient can take PO medication). If patient has taken theophylline in past 12 h, reduce loading dose by 50-75% or wait for theophylline level while using beta agonist aggressively.

ADDITIONAL CONCEPTS

1. In the **severe exacerbation,** begin O_2 and beta agonist therapy immediately while vital signs are being determined and blood work carried out and IV access is being established.

2. The patient **already receiving steroids** should be given **IV methylprednisolone bolus automatically.** In patient with asthma exacerbation who does not readily respond to beta agonist therapy, methylprednisolone should be given without significant delay. In **moderate to severe asthma** attack, give **methylprednisolone immediately.**

3. In the patient who does not respond to aggressive beta agonist and corticosteroid treatment, consider trying an inhaled anticholinergic agent (e.g., ipratropium bromide) and/or IV magnesium sulfate (1.2-2 g IV over 20 min).

4. Obtain a **chest x-ray** if patient is febrile, has localizing signs, or does not respond to therapy.

5. Check **aminophylline level** 1-2 h after maintenance infusion has started (if aminophylline/theophylline is being tried in the setting of beta agonist/methylprednisolone failure). Current evidence strongly suggests that aminophylline/theophylline is unlikely to help in emergent management of asthma exacerbation.

6. Be **prepared to intubate:** Especially worrisome findings include normal or rising PCO_2, respiratory alternans (alternating ribcage and abdominal breathing), abdominal paradox (inward abdominal motion during inspiration), or apparent exhaustion of patient. The anesthesiologist should be called **early.** Some patients with acute respiratory failure may benefit from noninvasive positive pressure ventilation (with BiPAP).

7. In patient who fails to respond despite maximal medical therapy as outlined above, particularly if fatigue is prominent, intubation is very likely. Do it electively rather than after respiratory arrest!

8. **Admission to hospital** is likely if recurrent failures of outpatient management, lack of subjective improvement, fatigue, failure of posttreatment FEV_1 to increase by greater than 500 mL, or absolute FEV_1 or PEFR remaining less than 60-70% predicted, change in mental status, poor social situation, pneumothorax, worrisome ABG findings, or other complicating factors (e.g., pregnancy or pneumonia).

9. **Do not** manage the patient with acute asthma for prolonged periods in the emergency department. If there is minimal improvement within 1-2 h of arrival, admit to hospital.

purulent sputum, or sinus infection. Choices include trimethoprim-sulfamethoxazole, amoxicillin, amoxicillin-clavulanate, tetracycline, erythromycin, or azithromycin. If the exacerbation requires steroid therapy and the patient has not been taking steroids, oral steroids should be given and the dosage tapered as clinical status allows (ideally in less than 14 days).

  c. **Long-term therapy.** The approach should be stepped care. Routine use of an inhaled corticosteroid with use of an inhaled beta agonist as needed for breakthrough symptoms should be the first-line treatment. Theophylline may also be considered as a second-line or third-line agent. Some patients may even do better with theophylline than with an inhaled beta agonist as a first-line drug. (Theophylline provides more constant 24-hour therapeutic efficacy than an inhaled beta agonist.) If symptoms are still poorly managed, the anticholinergic ipratropium bromide may be added. Cromolyn is an alternative agent to consider, especially in asthma with a strong extrinsic component.

  Oral corticosteroids ultimately may become necessary in the patient with persistent breakthrough symptoms who is taking an inhaled corticosteroid, beta agonist, therapeutic theophylline (as gauged by serum levels), and an inhaled anticholinergic and in whom a 4-week trial of cromolyn has failed. Alternate-day prednisone should be used for maintenance if possible, the dose should be lowered as soon as possible, and trials of inhaled steroids should be used to achieve these ends. Methotrexate or another steroid-sparing agent or both are reserved for the patient whose oral dose of corticosteroids cannot be tapered and who is suffering from steroid side effects. Pulmonary specialist consultation should be obtained.

3. **IMMUNOTHERAPY.** Immunotherapy is a consideration in the asthmatic with significant symptoms who is allergic to specific inhaled allergens that cannot be removed from the environment and in whom pharmacotherapy does not provide good control. Immunotherapy is a possible treatment for allergic asthma caused by house dust, house dust mites, mold spores, and pollens from weeds, trees, and grasses.

Broide DH. Asthma as an inflammatory disease: implications for treatment. Focus & Opinion: Internal Medicine 1995;2:9–16.
Chan-Yeung M, Malo J-L. Occupational asthma. N Engl J Med 1995;333:107–112.
Creticos PS, Reed CE, Norman PS, et al. Ragweed immunotherapy in adult asthma. N Engl J Med 1996;334:501–506.
Expert Panel on the Management of Asthma. Executive Summary: Guidelines for the Diagnosis and Management of Asthma. U.S. Department of Health and Human Services. Publication No. 91-3042A, 1991.
Goldstein RA, Paul WE, Metcalfe DD, Busse WW, Reece ER. Asthma. Ann Intern Med 1994;121:698–708.
McFadden ER Jr, Gilbert IA. Asthma. N Engl J Med 1992;327:1928–1937.
McFadden ER Jr, Gilbert IA. Exercise-induced asthma. N Engl J Med 1994;330:1362–1366.
McNamara RM, Skobeloff EM. Management of asthma. Acad Emerg Med 1994;1:158–161.
Podell RN. National guidelines for the management of asthma in adults. Am Fam Physician 1992;46:1189–1196.

X. CHRONIC OBSTRUCTIVE PULMONARY DISEASE (COPD)

In **chronic bronchitis,** the patient suffers on most days from increased mucus production with chronic or recurrent productive cough that has persisted for at least 3 months per year for at least 2 successive years. **Emphysema** is a pathologic condition in which there are destructive changes in the alveolar walls, with air-space enlargement distal to the nonrespiratory bronchioles. Both disorders are grouped together under the term **chronic obstructive pulmonary disease (COPD),** since both disorders usually are present in the same patient. Both result in expiratory airflow obstruction, cause dyspnea on exertion, and may be complicated by bronchospasm. Smoking is the major risk factor. Additional etiologic agents include recurrent infection, inhaled irritants, environmental factors, and such genetic factors as alpha$_1$-antitrypsin deficiency (to be considered in the patient with a strong family history of emphysema, when COPD occurs at an early age, and if no other risk factors are identified).

A. Laboratory Studies

Chest x-rays are important initially but need be obtained again only if parenchymal infection, neoplasm, or a new cardiopulmonary disorder is suspected. PFTs are useful for diagnosis, prognosis, and assessing response to therapy (see Pulmonary Tests: Structure and Function). Spirometry reveals air-flow obstruction: FEV_1/FVC less than 75% predicted, reduced forced expiratory flow 25%–75% ($FEF_{25\%-75\%}$), increased FRC and RV, and normal or increased total lung capacity (TLC). The D$_{LCO}$ is reduced in patients with emphysema and may be useful in predicting exercise-induced hypoxemia. Spirometry in COPD shows chronic persistent obstructive abnormalities. An alpha$_1$-antitrypsin level should be checked in the initial evaluation of the COPD patient because replacement therapy is now available. This is especially crucial in the patient who develops COPD at a young age, who has no significant cigarette use history, or who has a family history of emphysema.

B. Therapy

The goals of therapy are to alter the natural history of the disease, avoid complications, prevent and treat acute exacerbations, and teach patients to participate in their own management, with special emphasis on rehabilitation.

1. GENERAL PRINCIPLES OF MANAGEMENT. Cessation of smoking is crucial. Physicians should offer to work with patients, counsel them to select a stop date, and make referrals as appropriate. Nicotine gum is sometimes successful; sometimes formal smoking cessation programs are effective. Exacerbating conditions should be identified in the home and workplace. Coexisting problems, including sinusitis, esophageal reflux, and allergic phenomena, should be diagnosed and treated. Annual influenza vaccination is recommended (generally in the fall) because influenza is associated with greater morbidity and mortality in patients with COPD. Amantadine or rimantadine may be used as an adjuvant to late immunization or in the patient in whom immunization is contrain-

dicated. Pneumococcal vaccine is clearly effective when tested in young immunocompetent patients with a high incidence of pneumococcal disease. COPD patients should be vaccinated once (preferably before age 55). Consider revaccinating high-risk patients after 6 years.

Hydration has traditionally been encouraged to prevent the drying of secretions and inspissation of mucus. Excessive polypharmacy should be avoided by routine periodic review of the need for each of a patient's medications.

Exercise will not improve pulmonary function, but it will increase cardiovascular fitness, improve skeletal muscle efficiency, increase exercise tolerance, and boost the patient's morale and sense of well-being. Routine and progressive exercise (generally walking three or four times a week) should be prescribed. Excellent nutritional status and attainment of proper body weight should be encouraged.

The aggressive treatment of bacterial infections, especially pneumonia, is crucial. The role of antibiotics in a COPD exacerbation with purulent sputum but no frank pneumonia has been long debated (West J Med 1988;149:347–351). A recent meta-analysis demonstrated a small but statistically significant improvement when patients with COPD exacerbations were treated with antibiotics (JAMA 1995;273:957–960). Treatment choices (for 10 days to 3 weeks) include amoxicillin, trimethoprim-sulfamethoxazole, doxycycline, tetracycline, and cefaclor. Sputum gram stains and cultures are not necessary in managing acute bronchitis exacerbations.

The complete patient should be considered. Important issues include depression, dependence, impaired sexual function, and psychosocial dysfunction. The physician should be prepared to assist in their management. Oxygen is a drug, and the goal in its use is to maintain $PaO_2 > 55$ mm Hg. See Oxygen Therapy for which patients with COPD are candidates for home oxygen treatment.

2. **MANAGEMENT OF ACUTE EXACERBATIONS OF CHRONIC OBSTRUCTIVE PULMONARY DISEASE.** Acute exacerbations are characterized by increasing purulence of sputum, worsening of airway obstruction, and increased work of breathing. Causes include upper respiratory tract infection, sinusitis, pneumonia, irritant exposure, emotional upset, worsening environmental air, and medication noncompliance. Evaluation should proceed rapidly and include routine blood work, bedside spirometry, ABG determination, ECG, and probably chest x-rays. If the patient is taking theophylline, blood levels should be checked.

   a. **Aggressive bronchodilation.** Beta agonists via nebulizer (e.g., albuterol), combined with ipratropium bromide, are the drugs of choice initially in COPD exacerbations (see Pharmacology of Airway Disease).

   b. **Oxygen supplementation.** This is initiated cautiously, at 1–2 L/min via nasal cannula. Further O_2 supplementation is based on continuous pulse oximetry and ABG analysis, watching for worsening hypercarbia and respiratory failure.

   c. **Pharmacotherapy.** Systemic corticosteroids are also appropriate first-line drugs in the management of an acute COPD exacerbation (see Pharmacology of Airway Disease for dosage and Tables 7–4, 7–9, and 7–10). Although recent studies question the value of **theophylline** compared with beta agonists alone in COPD exacerbation, it is still reasonable to administer theophylline at therapeutic levels (10–20 µg/mL) to patients who do not respond quickly to beta agonist, anticholinergic, and corticosteroid administration.

    Antibiotics may also be helpful.

d. **Respiratory failure.** Many patients with COPD have chronic respiratory failure. Progressive respiratory acidosis or worsening hypoxia, even with aggressive therapy, is an indication for ICU admission and possible endotracheal intubation. In some selected patients, noninvasive positive pressure ventilation may reduce the need for endotracheal intubation (N Engl J Med 1995;333:817–822). Some COPD patients with hypercapnic respiratory failure may benefit from doxapram hydrochloride to stimulate their respiratory drive and thereby avoid endotracheal intubation and mechanical ventilation (Ann Emerg Med 1994;24:701–703). The dose of doxapram is 2 mg/kg IV load, followed by 1–3 mg/min titrated as necessary. The maximum daily dose should not exceed 3 g.

3. LONG-TERM MANAGEMENT OF CHRONIC OBSTRUCTIVE PULMONARY DISEASE
   a. **Anticholinergics.** These drugs are the agents of choice in long-term management of the COPD patient. Ipratropium bromide is preferable to atropine because of a better side effect profile. Advantages over beta agonists include longer duration of action and no evidence of receptor tolerance.
   b. **Beta agonists.** Long-acting and beta$_2$-selective agents are the second-line drugs to consider. Oral agents are less well tolerated than inhaled agents.
   c. **Theophylline.** This agent is only a second-line or third-line drug, and the dosage should always be adjusted carefully. The patient must be instructed never to take the medication "as needed" for worsening dyspnea.
   d. **Corticosteroids** (see Pharmacology of Airway Disease). Some patients will achieve benefit from long-term corticosteroid use. A trial of steroids (2 to 4 weeks) should be considered in the patient whose symptoms and disease are not controlled by maximal doses of an anticholinergic, beta agonist, and theophylline dosed so as to achieve therapeutic levels. The risks of steroids should be reviewed with the patient. The role of inhaled corticosteroids in the care of the COPD patient is still debated. Steroid-induced osteoporosis may be slowed with calcium supplements, an appropriate exercise program, and estrogen in females.
   e. **Antibiotics.** Empiric antibiotic use may be reasonable for some patients when sputum becomes more purulent.
   f. **Iodinated glycerol** (60 mg qid) has recently been shown effective in the management of stable patients with chronic obstructive bronchitis (see Pharmacology of Airway Disease).
   g. **Alpha$_1$-antitrypsin replacement.** Patients with alpha$_1$-antitrypsin deficiency (<11 µmol/L), protease inhibitor phenotype Pi null, Pi Z,

or Pi ZZ, currently nonsmokers, and with airflow obstruction are candidates for enzyme replacement. The recommended dose is 60 mg/kg IV given over 30 minutes every week. Immunization against hepatitis B is recommended before replacement therapy. Replacement is contraindicated in patients with selective IgA deficiencies and antibody against IgA because of the risk of severe anaphylaxis.

h. **Lung reduction surgery.** Patients with diffuse confluent emphysema and severe dyspnea despite maximal medical therapy may benefit from lung reduction surgery. Different techniques available include bilateral resection of diseased upper lobe tissue via median sternotomy, removal of damaged pulmonary tissue in stages, and laser ablation (N Engl J Med 1996;334:1128–1129). Resection of essentially nonfunctional peripheral lung tissue decreases lung size and improves the elastic recoil of the lung (N Engl J Med 1996;334:1095–1099). Beneficial results can include decreased dyspnea, improved overall function, and improved quality of life. The optimal criteria for selecting patients, however, have not yet been determined, and the mortality in some series has been as high as 6%.

i. **Lung transplantation.** Carefully selected patients with severe and end-stage COPD derive benefit from single lung transplantation. In appropriate candidates, postprocedure 1-year survival is about 80%. Criteria for this procedure are currently evolving but probably will include at least the following: failure of maximal medical therapy, age less than 60 to 65 years, life expectancy <3 years without the procedure, absence of other organ failure, absence of significant coronary artery disease, no continued substance abuse (cigarettes, alcohol, drugs), not on long-term high-dose corticosteroids, good medical compliance, appropriate psychosocial support to tolerate the procedure and continued posttransplantation medical care, and otherwise good surgical candidates (J Respir Dis 1996;17:393–412).

Curreri JP, Morley TF, Giudice JC. Noninvasive positive pressure ventilation. Postgrad Med 1996;99:221–230.

Ferguson GT, Cherniack RM. Management of chronic obstructive pulmonary disease. N Engl J Med 1993;328:1017–1022.

Seneff MG, Wagner DP, Wagner RP, Zimmerman JE, Knaus WA. Hospital and 1-year survival of patients admitted to intensive care units with acute exacerbation of chronic obstructive pulmonary disease. JAMA 1995;274:1852–1857.

Shrestha M, O'Brien T, Haddox R, Gourlay HS, Reed G. Decreased duration of emergency department treatment of chronic obstructive pulmonary disease exacerbations with the addition of ipratropium bromide to beta-agonist therapy. Ann Emerg Med 1991;20:1206–1209.

Weinberger SE. Recent advances in pulmonary medicine (Part 1). N Engl J Med 1993;328:1389–1396.

Wulfsberg EA, Hoffmann DE, Cohen MM. Alpha$_1$-antitrypsin deficiency: impact of genetic discovery on medicine and society. JAMA 1994;271:217–222.

XI. BRONCHIECTASIS

Abnormally dilated bronchi (bronchiectasis) are a consequence of severe damage to the bronchial wall. Several forms of bronchiectasis have been described. Cylindric bronchiectasis is the most common, is potentially reversible, and is characterized by failure of the bronchi to taper in diameter as they branch toward the periphery. Varicose bronchiectasis is a more advanced stage of the disease, with further dilation and distortion of the bronchi so that they resemble varicose veins. Saccular bronchiectasis is the worst and most advanced form of the disease. Actual outpouchings (sacs) form in the bronchial walls, and distal bronchi may even be larger than more proximal ones. Mucociliary clearance and cough are ultimately impaired. Once a common disease because of measles, pertussis, tuberculosis, and poorly treated bacterial pneumonias, bronchiectasis is now rare. Currently it is most often found in patients with cystic fibrosis, alpha$_1$-antitrypsin deficiency, complement deficiencies, neutrophil abnormalities, and immotile cilia syndrome.

A. Diagnosis

Bronchiectasis should be suspected in any patient with a chronic productive cough, especially when blood-streaked sputum and purulent sputum occur intermittently. Predisposing conditions or recurrent discrete pulmonary infections in the same lung zone or zones also should suggest the possibility of bronchiectasis. Childhood is the usual time of onset, with most cases diagnosed before the age of 20. Other symptoms may include sinusitis, dyspnea, and fatigue. The chest x-ray may be nondiagnostic or display increased or crowded lung markings, honeycombing, atelectasis, or ringlike shadows. CT can be used to confirm the diagnosis. Bronchography is the definitive procedure but should probably be reserved for surgical candidates only. Anatomic bronchiectasis is common, but symptomatic bronchiectasis is not. Therefore, bronchography should not be performed during an acute pulmonary infection or exacerbation. Bronchoscopy does **not** establish the diagnosis of bronchiectasis.

B. Therapy

All pulmonary irritants, especially cigarette smoking, should be avoided. An influenza vaccination should be provided yearly, and pneumococcal vaccine should be given once. In addition, postural drainage, adequate hydration, optimal nutrition, and bronchodilator therapy in bronchospasm are all important. Antibiotics are indicated for disease exacerbations (e.g., increased cough, purulent sputum, hemoptysis, malaise, and weight loss). Oral antibiotics include trimethoprim-sulfamethoxazole, amoxicillin, amoxicillin-clavulanate, tetracycline, and erythromycin. Choices can be guided by sputum culture. The duration of antibiotic therapy should be 1 to 3 weeks or longer.

Resectional surgery is indicated only in the setting of failed medical therapy, sharply localized bronchiectasis, and no other contraindications to lobectomy. Surgical treatment should not be considered if bronchiectasis is bilateral or involves multiple lobes.

1. CYSTIC FIBROSIS. Mucoid infection with *Pseudomonas aeruginosa* is characteristic of cystic fibrosis (CF), diagnosable with a sweat chloride test. Pulmonary complications, besides recurrent infections and bronchiectasis, include pneumothorax, hemoptysis, and respiratory failure accompanied by pulmonary hypertension and cor pulmonale. In the patient with CF and pulmonary infection, antibiotic choice must

be culture-guided and aggressive (e.g., aminoglycoside and a third-generation cephalosporin or semisynthetic penicillin, or fluoroquinolone). Ciprofloxacin and ofloxacin have been useful as outpatient oral antibiotics after infection has been brought under control with an inpatient IV regimen. Yearly influenza vaccination, pneumococcal vaccination once, hydration, postural drainage, and chest percussion are also helpful. Many CF patients have benefited from recombinant human deoxyribonuclease I (rhDNase, Pulmozyme). rhDNase hydrolyzes the DNA in the sputum and reduces the sputum's viscoelasticity. The result for many patients is improved pulmonary function and decreased relative risk of respiratory tract infections requiring parenteral antibiotic therapy. The usual dose is one 2.5 mg single-use ampule inhaled from a recommended nebulizer every morning. Some patients may benefit from twice-daily administration. This medication is expensive.

Selected patients with advanced disease benefit from bilateral lung transplantation or heart-lung transplantation. Newer therapies (salt transport manipulation, gene therapy) are being studied.

Barker AF, Bardara EJ Jr. Bronchiectasis: update of an orphan disease. Am Rev Respir Dis 1988;137:969–978.
Feil SB. Clinical management of pulmonary disease in cystic fibrosis. Lancet 1993;341:1070–1074.
Kerem E, Reisman J, Corey M, et al. Prediction of mortality in patients with cystic fibrosis. N Engl J Med 1992;326:1187–1191.

XII. SLEEP APNEA

Sleep apnea may be defined as the cessation of respirations lasting ≥10 seconds (per apneic event) and occurring at least five times per hour during sleep. Episodes of hypopnea (ventilation persists, but airflow is decreased by 30% to 50%) lasting 10 seconds or more are also significant. Oxygen desaturation (decrease by ≥4%) occurs during the apneic/hypopneic episodes, with clinical consequences that include increased daytime sleepiness, sleep attacks, morning headaches, and psychosocial dysfunction.

A. Types

Three types of sleep apnea are commonly described.
- **Central apnea** (Ondine's curse) is rare. The apneic episodes are characterized by a lack of respiratory effort. Diseases that may be associated with central apnea include brainstem infarction, encephalitis, myasthenia gravis, bulbar poliomyelitis, and cervical cordotomy.
- **Obstructive apnea** is manifested by occlusion of the upper airway in association with normal or augmented respiratory efforts.
- **Mixed apnea** exists when episodes of central apnea and obstructive apnea occur together.

Sleep apnea is unusual in the otherwise normal patient. Typically, there will be preexisting obesity, a narrowed upper airway, a neuromuscular disorder, or hypothyroidism. Causes of airway narrowing include nasal polyps, chronic rhinitis, macroglossia, and adenotonsillar hypertrophy. The differential diagnosis includes nocturnal myoclonus, narcolepsy, insomnia secondary to anxiety or depression, circadian rhythm disturbance, hypothyroidism, CHF, drug use and abuse (including alcohol), nocturnal asthma, esophageal reflux and aspiration, fibrositis, and inappropriate sleep habits.

B. Diagnosis

A complete sleep history, medical history, and interview with the partner should be obtained, and a physical examination should be performed. An otorhinolaryngologic evaluation is useful for oropharyngeal abnormalities. Sleep laboratory studies may be relatively simple and involve only nighttime recording of respirations and O_2 saturation (using finger or ear oximetry). More complicated sleep studies include continuous ECG monitoring, measurement of respiratory effort, and complete polysomnographic evaluation (with EEG, electrooculogram, and submental electromyogram). Diagnosis requires the documentation of apneic or hypopneic episodes and their clinical consequences.

C. Therapy

Treatment is dependent on the severity of the disease, the type of apnea, and the patient's daytime symptoms.

    1. OBSTRUCTIVE APNEA. Treatment of underlying medical conditions (CHF, COPD, hypertension, and hypothyroidism) and weight reduction are important, but results of voluntary weight reduction are frequently disappointing. Among drugs, alcohol often contributes to the symptomatology of sleep apnea. Additional agents to avoid include barbiturates, narcotics, sedative-hypnotics, and sedating analgesics. Other pharmacologic agents that may complicate the problem are propranolol (decreases the ventilatory response to CO_2), corticosteroids (weight gain), and diuretics (metabolic alkalosis). Patients should be encouraged to sleep in a lateral instead of supine position (a tennis ball can be sewn into the back of night clothes).

        a. **Pharmacologic treatment** may be useful in mild cases, but effectiveness is limited, and no studies have shown long-term benefit. Options include protriptyline (increases muscle tone and decreases rapid eye movement [REM] sleep), medroxyprogesterone (increases ventilatory drive), fluoxetine, and acetazolamide (increases ventilatory drive and corrects metabolic alkalosis). **O_2 supplementation** may prolong apnea episodes, but some patients will benefit. The demonstration of decreased oxygen desaturation during a sleep study with O_2 supplementation is grounds for initiating oxygen therapy. Certain nonpharmacologic treatments may be effective:

           (1) Nasal continuous positive airway pressure will prevent upper airway collapse and has surpassed tracheostomy as the preferred treatment of moderate and severe apnea. Drawbacks, however, include discomfort and noncompliance.

           (2) Nocturnal nasopharyngeal airway produces inconsistent results because the lateral and posterior pharyngeal walls may still collapse and cause obstruction.

           (3) Uvulopalatopharyngoplasty enlarges the pharyngeal space. Only about 50% of patients who undergo the procedure will

benefit, and in some patients, the condition worsens after surgery.

(4) **Tracheostomy** clearly bypasses upper airway obstruction. Drawbacks include the need for an invasive procedure, esthetic considerations, operative morbidity, and postoperative complications.

2. CENTRAL APNEA. Pharmacologic treatment is as described under Obstructive Apnea, but effectiveness is limited. Severe central apnea with associated central alveolar hypoventilation may require aggressive intervention: tracheostomy with nocturnal mechanical ventilation, negative-pressure ventilation, or a diaphragmatic pacer.

Brock ET, Schucard DW. Sleep apnea. Am Fam Phys 1994;49:385–394.
Strollo PJ Jr, Rogers RM. Obstructive sleep apnea. N Engl J Med 1996;334:99–104.

XIII. SARCOIDOSIS

Sarcoidosis is a multisystem disease of unknown cause. Its hallmark is noncaseating granuloma. The lung is most frequently involved. Its clinical course is quite variable: 65% of patients have spontaneous resolution with no permanent loss of pulmonary function, whereas 35% experience tissue destruction and pulmonary fibrosis. Sarcoidosis usually occurs between the ages of 20 and 40 and is 10 times more frequent in African Americans than whites. The estimated incidence is 60 cases per 100,000 population, with 2 to 3 million Americans developing the disease during their lifetime.

A. Clinical Presentation

The disease is often first detected in an asymptomatic patient with an abnormal chest x-ray. These abnormalities are seen in 85% to 90% of patients with this disease. Pulmonary symptoms include cough, wheezing, nonspecific chest pain, and dyspnea on exertion. Extrathoracic manifestations are shown in Table 7–11.

Evaluation includes a complete history and physical examination, chest x-rays, PFTs, baseline ABG determination, PPD and control skin tests, CBC, and determination of calcium, globulin, and alkaline phosphatase levels. Ophthalmology consultation may be useful. Biopsy of easily available extrapulmonary tissue involved in the disease or transbronchial biopsy allows tissue diagnosis. Yield from the latter is 60% when the chest film is normal and >90% if radiographic abnormalities are apparent. Additional studies sometimes helpful in gauging disease activity include bronchoalveolar lavage, serum angiotensin-converting enzyme levels, and gallium lung scans. Chest x-rays are graded as follows.

   0 Normal chest radiographs
   I Lymph node involvement, but no parenchymal abnormalities
   II Lymph node and diffuse parenchymal disease
   III Diffuse parenchymal disease with no lymph node involvement
   IV Chronic disease with pulmonary fibrosis (e.g., honeycombing)

The **activity** of sarcoidosis may be gauged by the clinical features of the disease, the patient's symptoms, worsening radiographic appearance, and declining values on PFTs. Elevated serum angiotensin-converting enzyme

TABLE 7-11. **Extrathoracic Manifestations of Sarcoidosis**

EXTRATHORACIC LOCATION	APPROXIMATE FREQUENCY	MANIFESTATION
Epidermal	20%	Erythema nodosum; plaquelike lesions of trunk and extremities; periorbital or paranasal vesicular lesions or violaceous plaques
Ocular	>20%	Granulomatous uveitis; enlarged lacrimal glands; nodular conjunctiva; retinal involvement (may lead to blindness)
Nasal	1-4%	Severe nasal obstruction; nasal polyps; occasionally destructive lesions of nasal bones and sinuses
Musculoskeletal	5-15%	Arthralgias; arthritis; myopathy; cystic changes of phalanges; osteoporosis
Cardiac	25% (but often clinically silent)	Ventricular ectopy; first degree heart block; supraventricular tachycardia; angina; congestive heart failure; sudden death may occur
Neural	5%	Cranial and peripheral neuropathies; headaches; focal abnormalities; seizures; personality changes
Hepatic	Granulomas are seen in 80%, but clinical manifestations of same in only 5-10%	May be asymptomatic or may include abnormal liver function tests, hepatomegaly, right upper quadrant pain, fever, jaundice
Splenic	Palpable splenomegaly in 3-5%	Splenomegaly, thrombocytopenia
Gastric	Rare	Symptoms of sprue or picture mimicking tuberculous peritonitis; sometimes pancreatitis
Genitourinary	<1%	Renal granulomas are usually asymptomatic; when renal failure occurs, look for another cause; epididymitis, hypercalcemia, and nephrolithiasis may occur

Adapted from Israel HL. Recognizing sarcoidosis outside the lungs. J Respir Dis 1985;6(9):69-87.

levels, positive results on gallium scanning, and bronchoalveolar lavage abnormalities also reflect disease activity. **Prognosis** is highly variable. The following factors favor a better outlook for the patient: white race; age under 40; normocalcemia; no extrathoracic involvement, erythema nodosum, or arthralgia; improvement since the initial diagnosis; radiographic stage 1; and anterior uveitis (as opposed to posterior uveitis).

B. Therapy

Prednisone is the drug of choice for sarcoidosis even though it does not increase the chance of remission. The goal is to reduce symptoms, alleviate organ dysfunction, and lessen the chance of pulmonary fibrosis. One of many recommended treatment strategies follows (J Respir Dis 1985;6(12): 18-22; 1986;7(4):50-58).

Stage I disease: Asymptomatic patients should not be treated (but should be reevaluated in 1 year). If the patient is symptomatic, drug therapy or closer observation (3 to 4 times per year) should be considered.

Stage II disease: Asymptomatic patients should be treated if there is radiographic evidence of disease progression over a 6 to 12 month observation period or if the x-ray appearance does not improve after 1 year and there are no relative or absolute contraindications to corticosteroid therapy. The symptomatic patient should be treated.

Stage III disease: If active alveolitis is present, this stage of the disease should be treated whether the patient is symptomatic or not.

Initial prednisone dosage is 40 to 60 mg qod. Prednisone therapy is also appropriate for uveitis (especially if local therapy has failed), hypercalcemia, myocardial involvement, and neurologic disease. Daily therapy should be started if breakthrough symptoms occur on the off day or if inflammation of extrathoracic organs needs immediate attention. The response to therapy is evaluated by amelioration of symptoms, change in chest x-ray, improvement in PFT values, decrease in elevated serum angiotensin-converting enzyme levels, and/or improved appearance on gallium scans. The dose of prednisone may be increased to as much as 80–120 mg qod if the response to 40–60 mg qod is unsatisfactory. If there is no response in 6 months, the drug dose should be tapered and the drug discontinued. If response has occurred, the dose should be tapered by 10 mg q3mo to the lowest level that continues to suppress granulomatous alveolitis. Every 3 to 6 months, the need for continued prednisone therapy should be reassessed by decreasing the dose while monitoring for increased disease activity.

DeRemee RA. Sarcoidosis. In: Noble J, Greene HL, Levinson W, Modest GA, Young MJ, eds. Textbook of Primary Care Medicine, 2nd ed. St. Louis: Mosby-Year Book; 1996, pp 1591–1594.

Israel HL. Recognizing sarcoidosis outside the lungs. J Respir Dis 1985;6(9):69–87.

Rohatgi PK, Goldstein RA. Does your patient with sarcoidosis require treatment? J Respir Dis 1985;6(12):18–22.

Rohatgi PK, Goldstein RA. Sarcoidosis: treat or leave well enough alone? J Respir Dis 1986;7(4): 50–58.

XIV. PULMONARY THROMBOEMBOLISM

Pulmonary embolism (PE) involves pulmonary vascular obstruction by a displaced thrombus, air bubble, or other particulate matter. The most common precipitant is deep venous thrombosis (DVT). PE is responsible for about 10% to 20% of all hospital deaths, including up to 15% of postoperative deaths, and is the second leading cause of pregnancy-related maternal mortality in the United States. The three major risk factors linked with DVT are blood stasis, endothelial injury, and hypercoagulable states. Patients at increased risk for DVT and PE include those with CHF, trauma, surgery (especially hip, knee, and prostate surgery), age over 60, previous history of thromboembolism, malignant disease, infection, inactivity or obesity, pregnancy, and oral contraceptive use. Hypercoagulable states may be seen with antithrombin III deficiency, protein C deficiency, protein S deficiency, defective fibrinolysis, hyperhomocysteinemia, antiphospholipid antibody syndrome, erythrocytosis, thrombocytosis, or abnormal levels of plasminogen and/or plasminogen activator.

A. Deep Venous Thrombosis

Signs and symptoms include tenderness, leg pain, swelling (a difference in leg circumference of 1.4 cm in men and 1.2 cm in women is significant), and warmth. One also may see a positive Homans' sign, subcutaneous venous distention, discoloration, a palpable cord, and pain on placement of a blood pressure cuff around the calf (considerable pain with the cuff inflated to 160 to 180 mm Hg). Unfortunately, at least one half of the cases of DVT are asymptomatic, and in up to 50% of patients with clinical evidence of DVT, no DVT is demonstrable.

1. DIAGNOSIS. The choice of diagnostic tests depends on the location of the suspected DVT and local experience and expertise.

   a. **Contrast venography** is the diagnostic gold standard. Complications, however, include induced thrombosis in up to 3% to 4% of patients. The postvenographic syndrome (leg pain, swelling, and tenderness) occurs in as many as 24% of patients.

   b. **Doppler ultrasound.** In this operator-dependent study, proximal venous thrombi are detected with an accuracy of >90%, but venous thrombi in the calf are detected only 50% of the time. False-negative studies may occur with nonocclusive proximal thrombi.

   c. **Real-time ultrasound.** Also an operator-dependent study, preliminary data indicate that it is excellent in detecting femoral and popliteal DVTs (mean sensitivity of 96% and mean specificity of 99%). It can also diagnose conditions that may mimic DVT (e.g., Baker's cyst and calf hematoma). It may miss calf DVTs and iliac vein DVTs (Arch Intern Med 1989;149:1731–1734).

   d. **Radioiodinated fibrinogen** has a diagnostic accuracy as high as 92% and is effective in detecting DVTs in the calf. It is not reliable in detecting pelvic DVTs. The test takes 1 to 2 days to perform.

   e. **Impedance plethysmography** has a sensitivity as high as 94% for proximal thrombi, with a specificity as high as 98%. The accuracy for calf thrombi is only about 50%.

   f. **Additional studies** include thermography (high sensitivity but low specificity) and radionuclide venography (good sensitivity but poor specificity and fair effectiveness in detecting calf thrombi).

2. THERAPY

   a. **Heparin.** This remains the treatment of choice in acute DVT. It prevents further propagation of the thrombus, but it probably does not reduce the immediate embolic risk or enhance clot lysis. The therapy for DVT with heparin and warfarin (Coumadin) is described in Table 7–12. Absolute contraindications to heparin include active internal bleeding, intracranial bleeding, intracranial lesions predisposed to bleeding, severe heparin-induced thrombocytopenia, and malignant hypertension.

   Relative contraindications include hemorrhagic diathesis, recent stroke, recent major surgery, severe hypertension, bacterial endocarditis, severe renal failure, severe diabetic retinopathy, thrombocytopenia, peptic ulcer disease, and severe hepatic failure.

   b. **Inferior vena caval barriers.** These are useful if anticoagulation is contraindicated. Possibilities include filters placed by internal

TABLE 7–12. **Therapy for Deep Venous Thrombosis with Heparin and Warfarin (Coumadin)**

Obtain baseline prothrombin time (PT), partial thromboplastin time (PTT), hematocrit, and platelet count
↓
Loading dose of *heparin* 80 U/kg IV, followed by maintenance infusion of 18 U/kg (in obese patients use ideal body weight)
↓
Recheck PTT after 4–6 h and as necessary thereafter (at least once per day); adjust heparin dose to maintain the PTT 1.5–2.5 × control (usual heparin dose is 1200–1500 U/h, but some patients may need 2000 U/h)
↓
Warfarin (Coumadin) should be started the same day as heparin therapy; begin with 5–10 mg/d; the PT must be checked daily, and the goal is a PT 1.2–1.5 × control (total PT, 14–17 s) or INR 2–3
↓
Even when the PT is therapeutic, full anticoagulation effect from warfarin will not be achieved for several more days; heparin, therefore, should not be stopped until 48 h of *joint therapy* have been completed even after the PT is therapeutic
↓
Warfarin should be continued for about 3 mo or until risk factors have been eliminated

ADDITIONAL KEY THERAPEUTIC POINTS
1. The patient should not ambulate for the first 5–7 d of treatment to avoid dislodgment of nonadherent clots.
2. Platelet count should be checked periodically while patient is receiving heparin because about 10% of patients will suffer heparin-induced thrombocytopenia.
3. Multiple drugs can interact with warfarin. All over-the-counter medications and prescription drugs should be checked for a possible interaction before being used. The patient must be cautioned in this regard and should be provided with a Medic Alert bracelet at the time of hospital discharge.
4. Intermittent SC *calcium heparin* q12h can be used instead of continuous IV heparin. Again, PTT should be maintained at 1.5–2.5 × control.

jugular or femoral approach (with fluoroscopic guidance) and actual surgical interruption. The former are preferred. The left ovarian or testicular vein enters the left renal vein, so ligation is necessary if pelvic thrombosis is present.
c. **Thrombolytic therapy.** A controversial option for DVT, this therapy can produce more rapid and complete clot lysis and may reduce the risk of venous hypertension and the postthrombotic syndrome. This treatment should be considered in the setting of an acute massive DVT if there are no contraindications to lytic therapy. Streptokinase, urokinase, or tissue plasminogen activator may be used. See Pulmonary Embolism for dosages and contraindications.

B. Pulmonary Embolism

Signs and symptoms are nonspecific. Dyspnea, pleuritic chest pain, and cough are most common (seen in 81%, 73%, and 60% of patients, respectively). The patient may also suffer from hemoptysis, apprehension, tachypnea (80% of patients), and fever (temperature as high as 39.5°C). Some patients are asymptomatic. As many as one half of patients have no readily apparent predisposing condition.

1. DIAGNOSIS
   a. **Arterial blood gases.** Although ABG determinations are routine, blood gas abnormalities are nonspecific. As many as 13% of patients with confirmed PE will have a PaO_2 greater than 80 mm Hg. Respiratory alkalosis will be seen in more than 80% of patients, and the alveolar – arterial oxygen gradient (A – a gradient) may be helpful. In the normal young person without pulmonary disease, the A – a gradient is 5 to 10 mm Hg. In the elderly patient without known pulmonary disease, an A – a gradient greater than 20 mm Hg is abnormal. If PE is suspected, a normal A – a gradient makes the diagnosis unlikely (Chest 1989;95:48–51).
   b. **Electrocardiogram.** ECG findings are also nonspecific. About 75% of patients with PE will have sinus tachycardia. Other findings include right-sided strain, right-axis deviation, S_I Q_{III} T_{III} pattern (an S-wave in lead I, a Q-wave in lead III, and an inverted T-wave in lead III), right bundle branch block (RBBB), and atrial arrhythmias.
   c. **Pulmonary scintigraphy** is the most useful screening test. A normal or near normal V/Q scan makes the diagnosis of PE unlikely.
   d. **Pulmonary angiography** is the definitive test in the diagnosis of pulmonary thromboembolism. With refinements in use and technique of this test, morbidity is low and mortality is 0.25%. Pulmonary angiography is indicated when anticoagulation has failed and surgical therapy is being considered, in patients with noninvasive studies suggestive of PE but who are not anticoagulation candidates, in patients with a high clinical likelihood for PE but a nonhigh probability V/Q scan, and when lytic therapy is being considered.
   e. **Additional concept.** With V/Q scans of low or intermediate probability, sometimes one can demonstrate a DVT noninvasively before resorting to pulmonary angiography. Approximately 70% of patients with pulmonary thromboembolism will have coexisting thrombi of the deep veins of the thighs or pelvis. The treatment of both DVT and PE is essentially the same: anticoagulation.
   f. **D-dimer levels.** Clot breakdown of a thrombus is associated with elevation of a specific breakdown product of crosslinked fibrin, D-dimer, which in turn can be measured. The sensitivity, specificity, and optimal use of this blood test in the diagnosis of DVT and PE require further study.

2. THERAPY
   a. **Heparin** is the classic treatment of choice in the acute phase of DVT or PE. The approach is outlined in Table 7–12. For an acute PE, some recommend a larger initial bolus of heparin (10,000–20,000 U in an IV bolus) followed 2 hours later by continuous heparin infusion.
   b. **Inferior vena caval barriers.** These should be considered (1) when the diagnosis of PE is confirmed but anticoagulation therapy is contraindicated or has failed or (2) when the patient has already

suffered a massive, life-threatening PE. With devices such as the Greenfield filter, the recurrence rate for PE may be reduced to as low as 5%.

c. **Surgical embolectomy** has a controversial role in the treatment of PE. Mortality is at least 25%.

d. **Thrombolytic therapy.** Hemodynamically unstable patients improve more rapidly with lytic therapy than with heparin. One study demonstrated that capillary blood volume and D$_{LCO}$ were more nearly normal at 2 weeks and at 1 year with thrombolytic therapy than with heparin (mortality was not different between the two groups). Thrombolytic therapy is indicated in confirmed PE with hemodynamic instability in the absence of contraindications.

  (1) *Streptokinase.* Streptokinase is given in an IV load of 250,000 U over 30 minutes, followed by a maintenance infusion of 100,000 U/h for 24 hours (or longer in massive PE with huge DVT—up to 72-hour infusion). Side effects include hemorrhage requiring transfusion in about 4% of patients, oozing from puncture wounds, fever in 20%, and marked allergic reactions in 6%. Some recommend giving 100 mg hydrocortisone IV to minimize allergic phenomena.

  (2) *Urokinase.* Urokinase may be given in an IV load of 4400 U/kg over 10 minutes, followed by a maintenance infusion of 4400 U/kg/h for 12 hours. Side effects include about the same hemorrhage rate as seen with streptokinase, but allergic reactions are rare.

  (3) *Tissue plasminogen activator (tPA).* Dose: 100 mg infused through a peripheral vein over 2 hours (50 mg/h). tPA may also be given directly into the pulmonary arterial system at the time of the pulmonary angiogram.

  (4) *Laboratory monitoring.* With lytic therapy, a bleeding time, thrombin time (TT), PTT, and PT should be checked before the start of treatment. Four hours after the initial bolus, TT should be obtained to confirm the attainment of a lytic state (TT does not need to be checked if tPA is used). All lytic therapy should be followed by administration of a heparin continuous infusion (pushing the PTT to 1.5 to 2 times the control value). For streptokinase and urokinase, however, the heparin infusion should be started only after the postinfusion TT or PTT is <2 × control. For tPA, a heparin bolus and continuous infusion can be started immediately after tPA is administered.

  (5) *Contraindications.* Absolute contraindications include active internal bleeding, altered consciousness, cerebrovascular accident (CVA) in the past 6 months, any history of hemorrhagic CVA or intracranial or intraspinal surgery within the previous 2 months, intracranial or intraspinal neoplasm/aneurysm or AV malformation, known bleeding disorder, persistent severe hypertension, pregnancy, previous allergy to streptokinase product (does not contraindicate tPA administration), head trauma within 1 month, suspected pericarditis, suspected aortic dis-

section, or trauma/surgery within 2 weeks that could result in bleeding into a closed space.

Relative contraindications include active peptic ulcer disease, cardiopulmonary resuscitation for >10 minutes, current use of oral anticoagulants, hemorrhagic ophthalmic conditions, history of chronic uncontrolled hypertension—treated or untreated—history of ischemic or embolic CVA >6 months ago, significant trauma/surgery >2 weeks ago but <2 months ago, and subclavian or internal jugular venous cannulation.

e. **Additional therapeutic concepts.** The patient with suspected acute PE should be administered supplemental oxygen and have continuous pulse oximetry and electrocardiographic monitoring. If the patient is hemodynamically unstable, blood pressure should be supported with IV crystalloid and pressors (e.g., dobutamine, dopamine, or epinephrine continuous infusion) as required. A transesophageal echocardiogram may assist with rapid diagnosis of a large saddle embolus in the unstable patient and obviate the need for studies that require more time (e.g., pulmonary angiogram). Patients who suffer a cardiopulmonary collapse from a suspected massive PE may also be aggressively supported on a cardiopulmonary bypass machine while the diagnosis of PE is confirmed and thrombolysis is accomplished.

f. **Prevention of DVT and PE.** Given the mortality of PE and the difficulties involved in its clinical diagnosis, prevention of DVT and PE is crucial. Fully one third of patients over age 40 who have major surgery or an acute MI will suffer DVT, and this number is even higher following hip, knee, or prostate surgery. Pulmonary thromboembolism occurs in 5% to 10% of patients who have undergone orthopedic procedures of the hip or knee.

(1) *Heparin.* Heparin is the most common and popular agent for prophylaxis. The usual low-dose regimen is 5000 U SC q12h. Heparin is effective in patients undergoing general surgery who are at high risk for DVT or PE and patients with MI or CHF. For general surgery patients, low-dose heparin administration should be started 2 days before the operation. Despite fears regarding this practice, clinically or statistically significant increased bleeding is not seen. This heparin regimen may not be effective in patients with urologic or gynecologic cancer or traumatic hip fracture or in those undergoing major orthopedic surgery or prostatectomy. Adjusted-dose heparin should be considered in the patient undergoing elective total hip replacement. Heparin (3500 U SC tid) should be started 2 days before the operation, and the PTT should be pushed to the upper limit of normal. Apparently, this practice still does not significantly increase the bleeding risk, and it is effective. Heparin should not be used for DVT or PE prophylaxis in patients with a high risk of hemorrhage during general surgery, in patients undergoing intracranial or eye surgery, or in patients with spinal cord trauma.

(2) Graduated compression stockings. These stockings are easily used and are moderately effective. They should be prescribed routinely to medical or surgical patients at risk for DVT, even if another prophylactic regimen is also deemed necessary. The combination of static graduated compression stockings and low-dose heparin is more effective in DVT prophylaxis than the use of low-dose heparin alone.

(3) Dextran probably is effective but is associated with a fairly high risk of inducing pulmonary edema in the elderly, allergic reactions, and excessive bruising. Dextran 40 is administered IV 500 mL preoperatively and then every other day until the patient is ambulatory. Candidates for dextran therapy include patients undergoing surgery for a fractured hip and those having elective total hip replacement.

(4) Two-step warfarin. Oral warfarin should be given 10 days before the planned procedure, prolonging the PT by 1.5 to 3.5 seconds. After surgery, the warfarin dose is increased until the PT is 1.3 to 1.5 times the control value. Candidates include patients undergoing a general surgical procedure who have known malignant disease or a history of prior DVT. Two-step warfarin is also reasonable in patients scheduled for elective total hip replacement and in those with a fractured hip for which surgery is planned.

(5) Pneumatic calf compression. This regimen improves blood flow in the deep veins and enhances blood fibrinolytic activity. It should be begun before surgery and continued until the patient is fully ambulatory. It is the prophylaxis of choice in patients undergoing total hip replacement, major knee surgery, prostate surgery, and neurosurgery and in women undergoing cesarean section. Gradient elastic stockings may be used in conjunction with pneumatic calf compression.

(6) Low-molecular-weight heparins (LMWH). These substances are being studied extensively for both prophylaxis and treatment of DVTs. LMWHs appear to be as safe as and are probably more efficacious than traditional heparin. Advantages include once-a-day administration and fixed dosing not requiring monitoring of the PTT. Dalteperin sodium (Fragmin) and enoxapirin sodium (Lovenox) are two LMWHs currently available for DVT/PE prophylaxis, the former in the setting of general abdominal surgery and the latter in the setting of hip or knee replacement surgery. Although further investigation is required, LMWHs are likely useful in the outpatient treatment of acute DVT (N Engl J Med 1996;334:724–725).

(7) Ineffective methods of prophylaxis include use of aspirin and simple compressive stockings. When prophylaxis is contraindicated, it is appropriate to screen high-risk patients to detect subclinical DVT early. Screening may include impedance plethysmography, Doppler ultrasound, or radiolabeled fibrinogen scanning.

Becker DM, Philbrick JT, Selby B. Inferior vena cava filters indications, safety, effectiveness. Arch Intern Med 1992;152:1985–1994.

Becker DM, Philbrick JT, Walker FB. Axillary and subclavian venous thrombosis prognosis and treatment. Arch Intern Med 1991;151:1934–1943.

Gunnarsson PS, Sawyer WT, Montague D, et al. Appropriate use of heparin. Arch Intern Med 1995;155:526–532.

Hirsh J. Drug therapy: heparin. N Engl J Med 1991;324:1565–1574.

Hull RD, Raskob GE, Ginsberg, et al. A noninvasive strategy for the treatment of patients with suspected pulmonary embolism. Arch Intern Med 1994;154:289–297.

Hull R, Raskob G, Pineo G, et al. A comparison of subcutaneous low-molecular-weight heparin with warfarin sodium for prophylaxis against deep-vein thrombosis after hip or knee implantation. N Engl J Med 1993;329:1370–1376.

King MS. Preventing deep venous thrombosis in hospitalized patients. Am Fam Physician 1994;49:1389–1396.

Moser KM. Venous thromboembolism. Am Rev Respir Dis 1990;141:235–249.

PIOPED Investigators. Value of the ventilation/perfusion scan in acute pulmonary embolism. JAMA 1990;263:2753–2759.

Weinmann EE, Salzman EW. Deep-vein thrombosis. N Engl J Med 1994;331:1630–1641.

XV. ADULT RESPIRATORY DISTRESS SYNDROME

The adult respiratory distress syndrome (ARDS) is a clinical diagnosis based on (1) history of a preceding associated event (pulmonary or nonpulmonary) with rapid onset of respiratory failure, (2) diffuse bilateral pulmonary infiltrates on the frontal chest x-ray, (3) pulmonary capillary wedge pressure ≤18 mm Hg (noncardiogenic pulmonary edema), and (4) decreased PaO_2 refractory to O_2 supplementation (PaO_2/FIO_2 ratio ≤200). ARDS is the end point of a variety of disease processes, including physical trauma, sepsis, aspiration of gastric contents having low pH, drug or toxin exposure, diffuse pneumonia, oxygen toxicity, CNS disease, smoke and irritant gas inhalation, fat embolism, pancreatitis, uremia, burns, cardiopulmonary bypass, and multiple transfusions. Recent studies indicate that the mortality of ARDS has declined in the past several years from 67% to 40% (JAMA 1995;273:306–309).

A. Management

The goals of therapy are to correct hypoxia, to identify and treat the cause of the syndrome, and to prevent complications.

1. CORRECTION OF HYPOXIA. Because of the large shunt fraction, hypoxia is refractory to simple oxygen supplementation in ARDS. Every attempt should be made to maintain the PaO_2 > 55 mm Hg (90% oxyhemoglobin saturation) while keeping the FIO_2 ≤ 0.6. At the same time, an adequate cardiac output (>2.2 L/min/m^2) is essential. To achieve these ends, endotracheal intubation, mechanical ventilation (initially with assist-control mode), and positive end-expiratory pressure (PEEP) are usually necessary.

To avoid **barotrauma,** the minimal level of PEEP that allows an FIO_2 ≤ 0.6 and maintains cardiac output should be used. A decrease in cardiac output of >15% to 20% from the baseline is probably unacceptable. Initial ventilator settings should allow for a tidal volume that prevents atelectasis and worsening shunt yet avoids high peak airway pressures (6 to 10 mL/kg is a reasonable initial tidal volume). Risk factors for pulmonary barotrauma include high tidal volumes, high inflation and inspiratory airway pressures with low lung or chest wall compliance, and PEEP. The lowest level of PEEP necessary to provide adequate tissue oxygenation should be used. With poor pulmonary compliance, inspiratory pressures should be kept <40 to 45 cm H_2O if possible. Some patients with persistent hypoxia may benefit from a different body position than the usual supine position (e.g., lateral decubitus or even prone).

Aggressive sedation (and possibly pharmacologic paralysis) may be needed to optimize mechanical ventilation, reduce airway pressures, and minimize oxygen consumption by the patient. Optimal **volume management** keeps the patient relatively volume restricted without compromising cardiac output, cerebral perfusion, or renal function.

2. SEARCH FOR THE CAUSE OF **ARDS.** One cause of ARDS does not rule out a second or third cause (e.g., the patient with acute pancreatitis, pneumonia, or sepsis). Left ventricular dysfunction as a cause of pulmonary edema and diffuse pulmonary infiltrates should be excluded. Once the cause or causes of ARDS have been determined, specific therapy for each should be implemented.

3. PREVENTION OF COMPLICATIONS. The patient with ARDS may have an ICU course that lasts many weeks. During this time, mortality is usually not directly due to ARDS and hypoxia per se but is secondary to sepsis or multiorgan failure. The following guidelines may be helpful in preventing complications.

   a. **Infection** risk may be reduced by careful handwashing, respiratory equipment care, regular IV access changes, and early use of antibiotics when required.

   b. **GI hemorrhage** may be reduced by using sucralfate. Some authors have suggested that raising the gastric pH (with histamine$_2$ [H_2] blockers or antacids) may increase the risk of nosocomial pneumonia (JAMA 1996;275:308–314).

   c. **Renal failure** risk can be reduced by careful selection and monitoring of drugs (e.g., aminoglycosides), optimal fluid management, and maintenance of adequate oxygenation.

   d. **Prophylaxis of PE** should be implemented.

   e. **Exercise** is important in boosting the patient's morale and in minimizing deconditioning. Regular physical therapy, isometrics, and even assisted walking should probably be used when possible.

   f. **Nutrition** requirements may be high, but supplementation also is associated with complications (Am Rev Respir Dis 1988;137: 1463–1493). When possible, enteral feeding is the method of choice. If carbohydrate intake is too high, however, increased CO_2 production may complicate ventilation and respiratory management. If this becomes a problem, an increasing proportion of fat caloric intake should be provided.

   g. **Emotional support** is crucial. This should be provided not only by family, friends, social workers, and chaplains but also by medical and nursing staff.

h. **Sleep** should be encouraged. A 6-hour period of nighttime rest is necessary. (One may consider using short-acting sedatives, minimizing interruptions, turning down lights, and providing eye shades and ear plugs.)

4. NEWER THERAPIES. Corticosteroids are not helpful in the early management of ARDS, but their role in the late stage of the disease (the fibroproliferative phase) or in certain patient subgroups (e.g., those with increased blood and lung eosinophils) requires further study. Newer therapies that appear promising and are currently being actively investigated include pulmonary surfactant replacement, anti-inflammatory drugs, nitric oxide, ketoconazole, pentoxifylline, and partial liquid ventilation.

5. PROGNOSIS. The course of the patient with ARDS is usually prolonged and plagued by frequent setbacks (e.g., infection, renal and other organ dysfunction, and barotrauma). Of the patients who survive, however, as many as 85% may have nearly normal pulmonary function 1 year later.

Fulkerson WJ, MacIntyre N, Stamler J, Crapo JD. Pathogenesis and treatment of the adult respiratory distress syndrome. Arch Intern Med 1996;156:29–38.
Kollef MH, Schuster DP. The acute respiratory distress syndrome. N Engl J Med 1995;332:27–36.
Matthay MA. The acute respiratory distress syndrome. N Engl J Med 1996;334:1469–1470.

XVI. ACUTE RESPIRATORY FAILURE AND MECHANICAL VENTILATION

Acute respiratory failure (ARF) is characterized by the inability to achieve adequate oxygenation or ventilation or both. PaO_2 less than 60 mm Hg and $PaCO_2$ greater than 50 mm Hg are criteria frequently used to define respiratory failure.

Dysfunction of any component of the ventilatory system may result in respiratory failure: brain, spinal cord, neurovascular system, thorax, pleura, upper airway, cardiovascular system, lower airway, and alveoli. Diseases that may account for respiratory failure include bulbar poliomyelitis, drug overdose, cerebrovascular accident, Guillain-Barré syndrome, spinal cord trauma, multiple sclerosis, myasthenia gravis, pneumothorax, trauma, flail chest, epiglottitis, laryngeal edema, tracheal obstruction from tumor or foreign body, pulmonary contusion, CHF, ARDS, COPD, asthma, pneumonia, and interstitial lung disease.

A. Approach to Treatment

Approach to treatment depends on the underlying pathophysiology. There are five basic mechanisms.

1. DECREASED FIO_2 may occur with exposure to high altitude or suicide attempts.

2. INTRAPULMONARY ARTERIOVENOUS SHUNT occurs with perfusion of nonventilated alveoli. The PaO_2 is decreased. If the shunt is large ($\geq 30\%$), even great increases in supplemental O_2 will not correct the hypoxia (e.g., as seen in ARDS).

3. **ALVEOLAR HYPOVENTILATION** will occur in the setting of decreased tidal volume or increased VD/VT or both. The PaO_2 is decreased, the $PaCO_2$ is increased, and the A – a gradient is normal.

4. **DIFFUSION IMPAIRMENT** as a cause of hypoxemia is unusual. It may be important, however, if the FIO_2 is decreased (e.g., at high altitude) or following extreme physical exertion (e.g., a patient with interstitial lung disease during exercise). The calculated A – a gradient will be abnormal.

5. **V/Q IMBALANCE** is the most common cause of arterial hypoxemia. V/Q imbalance may be divided into low V/Q and high V/Q regions. Low V/Q regions are similar to intrapulmonary arterial-venous shunting, and high V/Q regions are similar to alveolar hypoventilation. Low V/Q abnormalities result in arterial hypoxemia, and the calculated A – a gradient will be increased.

   An important method of determining whether respiratory failure is ventilatory (hypoventilation) or nonventilatory (disease of the lung parenchyma) is the alveolar air equation (Table 7–13). Other useful equations are also given.

B. Clinical Manifestations

Clinical manifestations of respiratory failure depend on the etiology of the disease, on the duration and progression of the failure, and on the degree of concomitant hypoxemia and hypercarbia.

1. **HYPOXEMIA.** Acute symptoms are usually secondary to CNS dysfunction and include dyspnea, disorientation, confusion, delirium, and finally coma and death. Patients may become irritable and restless before loss of consciousness. Signs of hypoxemia include diaphoresis, tachypnea, tachycardia, cyanosis (if severe hypoxemia is present), and cardiac dysrhythmias.

2. **HYPERCARBIA.** Acute symptoms include headache, somnolence, dizziness, and eventually coma. Signs include diaphoresis, hyperventilation or hypoventilation, muscular twitching, tachycardia, and, in some cases, papilledema.

C. Management

1. **GOALS OF TREATMENT**
   - Assure an adequate and patent airway
   - Restore adequate gas exchange (maintain the $PaO_2 \geq 60$ mm Hg, with at least 90% hemoglobin saturation)
   - Achieve the lowest FIO_2 necessary for sufficient oxygenation (keep $FIO_2 \leq 0.6$)
   - Establish an acceptable pH
   - Treat the primary disorder responsible for the respiratory failure
   - Prevent complications

     The $PaCO_2$ should be normalized only in the patient with a usually normal $PaCO_2$. The individual with chronic CO_2 retention and chronic lung disease should be allowed to maintain his or her usual $PaCO_2$. In

TABLE 7–13. **Useful Equations in Pulmonary Medicine**

Alveolar Air Equation

$$P_{AO_2} = F_{IO_2} (P_B - 47) - P_{aCO_2}/0.8$$

where P_{AO_2} = the alveolar pressure of O_2
$\quad$ F_{IO_2} = the fraction inspired concentration of O_2 (0.21–1)
$\quad$ 47 = the pressure of water vapor in mm Hg at 100% saturation
$\quad$ P_B = the atmospheric pressure (at sea level = 760 mm Hg).
With this equation, the A – a gradient can be determined ($P_{AO_2} - P_{aO_2}$). In the normal individual who is young to middle aged, the A – a gradient should be 5–15 mm Hg. With age, the gradient increases.

Dead Space Equation

V_D/V_T (the fraction of each breath wasted in dead space) = $(P_{aCO_2} - P_{ECO_2})/P_{aCO_2}$

where P_{ECO_2} = pressure of CO_2 in mixed exhaled gas. Normally, the V_D/V_T is equal to 24.6 + 0.17 × (age in years).

Shunt Equation

Q_S/Q_T = The percentage of blood flow being shunted
$\quad\quad$ = $(C_{cO_2} - C_{aO_2})/(C_{cO_2} - C_{vO_2}) \times 100$

where C denotes content of O_2 in blood and c, a, and v denote capillary, arterial, and venous, respectively. End-capillary P_{O_2} is estimated by calculated alveolar O_2 (as in the alveolar air equation). The normal shunt fraction is less than 7%. If the P_{aO_2} is greater than 150 mm Hg, a shunt of less than 25% can be approximated when the patient is breathing pure O_2 by dividing the A – a O_2 difference by 20.

Oxygen Content Equation

$$C_{aO_2} = 0.139 \text{ (Hgb) (\% sat)} + 0.003 \text{ (}P_{aO_2}\text{)}$$

where Hgb = grams of hemoglobin per 100 mL of blood and
% sat = percent of hemoglobin saturation.

Compliance Equations

Dynamic compliance =
tidal volume/(peak airway pressure – positive end-expiratory pressure [PEEP])

Peak airway pressure is determined from the ventilator by looking at the maximal airway pressure attained during a ventilated breath. The normal dynamic compliance of a mechanically ventilated patient is 50–80 mL/cm H_2O.

Static compliance = tidal volume/(static pressure – PEEP)

Static (plateau) pressure is determined by momentarily occluding the exhalation tubing of the ventilator before the patient exhales and looking at the airway pressure monitor. Normal static compliance in a mechanically ventilated patient is 60–100 mL/cm H_2O.

some circumstances, tolerating a moderate respiratory acidosis and allowing the pH to run as low as 7.2 to 7.25 may be necessary to avoid high airway pressures (e.g., in a mechanically ventilated asthmatic or COPD patient).

The use of O_2 supplementation, adequate hydration, and bronchodilators and the treatment of the primary problem (e.g., pneumonia, COPD exacerbation, and CHF) have been presented elsewhere in this manual. Criteria for intubation are shown in Table 7–14.

2. **NONINVASIVE POSITIVE PRESSURE VENTILATION (NIPPV).** Some patients with acute respiratory failure may benefit from NIPPV and thereby avoid the risks inherent in endotracheal intubation and mechanical ventilation. With NIPPV, the patient is attached to a ventilator via a nasal mask (or pillow) or a face mask with associated headgear to minimize air leaks. Available ventilator modes include volume-cycled, pressure support, and bilevel positive airway pressure (BiPAP). With BiPAP, the ventilator delivers positive airway pressure during inhalation and a lower level of positive airway pressure during exhalation (similar to PEEP).

Potential candidates for NIPPV should be awake and alert and cooperative, have good airway protective mechanisms, be hemodynamically stable, and not have excessive pulmonary secretions. Uncontrolled studies have demonstrated promising success rates in patients with ARF secondary to COPD exacerbations. Although further studies are necessary, NIPPV may also prove very useful in ARF caused by asthma, CHF, restrictive lung disease, neuromuscular and chest wall disorders, and premature extubation.

3. **MECHANICAL VENTILATION.** Mechanical ventilation provides the bellows function of the respiratory system while the primary disease process is being treated. Most ventilator systems currently in use are positive pressure systems.

TABLE 7–14. **Criteria for Endotracheal Intubation**

Apnea

Inability to clear secretions (intubation may allow for more aggressive and frequent airway suctioning) or an inadequate upper airway

Progressive hypoventilation and worsening respiratory acidosis despite aggressive medical management ($Paco_2 > 50$ mm Hg with a pH < 7.3)

Inability to maintain $Pao_2 \geq 55$ mm Hg despite an $Fio_2 > 0.5$–0.6

Loss of airway protective mechanisms (e.g., absent gag reflex)

When heavy sedation or paralysis of the patient is necessary for treatment (e.g., general surgery) or diagnosis (e.g., pelvic examination performed with the patient under general anesthesia)

When respiratory failure is imminent (patient fatigued or exhausted, respiratory rate <8–10/min or respiratory rate >30–40/min, inspiratory pressure <25 cm H_2O)

Major chest wall trauma

Profound shock

When controlled hyperventilation is required (e.g., in the setting of increased intracranial pressure)

a. **Types of positive-pressure ventilators**
   (1) *Pressure-cycled.* Gas flows into the patient until a predetermined airway pressure is reached. Tidal volume, therefore, is not constant.
   (2) *Time-cycled.* Gas flows for a certain percentage of time during the ventilatory cycle.
   (3) *Volume-cycled* are the most common ventilators in use today. The tidal volume is determined, and a fixed tidal volume is delivered with each breath. The discussion below is limited to volume-cycled ventilators.
b. **Ventilator modes.** Many are used; some of the most common are
   (1) *Controlled.* The machine delivers a breath at a fixed rate irrespective of the patient's effort or demands.
   (2) *Assist-controlled.* The machine senses a patient's efforts to breathe and delivers a fixed tidal volume with each effort, in addition to providing a predetermined backup rate if the patient's inspiratory efforts are infrequent.
   (3) *Intermittent mandatory ventilation (IMV).* Breaths are delivered by the machine, but the patient may also breathe (without machine assistance) spontaneously.
   (4) *Pressure support.* The patient breathes spontaneously and determines ventilator rate. A positive pressure effect is maintained by the ventilator (to compensate for endotracheal tube resistance). Therefore, tidal volume will be determined by inflation pressure and the patient's lung-thorax compliance.
c. **Ventilator settings**
   (1) *Tidal volume.* Tidal volume is the volume of gas delivered with each machine-powered breath. The value set on the machine is greater than the volume of gas the patient actually receives because of the distention of plastic tubing with each breath. A reasonable initial setting is 10 ml/kg. Smaller tidal volumes (5 to 7 mL/kg) may be optimal to avoid high ventilator plateau pressures and the associated complications of ventilator-induced lung injury. Ideally, the plateau pressure (measured in a relaxed patient by momentarily occluding the ventilatory circuit at the end of inspiration) should be maintained at <35 cm H_2O.
   (2) *Sighs* are not used frequently because of the relatively large tidal volumes used (a tidal volume of 10 to 15 ml/kg is about twice a person's normal tidal volume). If a small tidal volume is used (less than 8 ml/kg), a sigh should be set at 1.5 to 2 times the tidal volume every 5 to 10 minutes to prevent atelectasis.
   (3) *Respiratory rate.* Respiratory rate is the guaranteed rate the machine will deliver if the patient is completely apneic. A typical rate is 10 to 14 breaths per minute. Changes in the respiratory rate may be guided by the following equation.

   New respiratory rate = old rate $\times$ (old $Paco_2$/desired $Paco_2$)

   (4) *Flow rates.* Flow rates should be set so that expiratory time exceeds inspiratory time, and a good rule of thumb is to give the patient twice as much time to exhale as to inhale. An

inspiratory flow rate of 60 L/min is a reasonable initial setting for most patients during assist-control or intermittent mandatory ventilation. In the setting of marked air flow obstruction, exhalation time should be increased more.

(5) **Sensitivity.** This is the amount of negative pressure the patient must generate before the machine will deliver an assisted breath in the assist-control mode. The usual initial setting is 1 to 2 cm H_2O.

(6) **Oxygen concentration.** Adjustments to FIO_2 should be guided by blood gas analysis. The FIO_2 should be the lowest necessary to achieve adequate oxygenation. When mechanical ventilation is first instituted, however, 100% O_2 is often administered (unless it is known that a lower FIO_2 will be sufficient).

(7) **Humidifiers.** Gas delivered by the endotracheal route should be 100% humidified.

(8) **Monitors and alarms.** Two of the most important include pressure limit (usually set about 5 to 10 cm H_2O above the pressure necessary to deliver the desired tidal volume) and exhaled tidal volume (to detect decreased tidal volumes being delivered to the patient because of ventilator malfunction or leaks in the circuit). Additional alarms include those that sound with electrical failure or because of inadequate oxygen line pressure.

(9) **PEEP** may be necessary in refractory hypoxemia despite oxygen supplementation. It increases end-expiratory and mean pressure across the walls of airways and alveoli, reexpanding collapsed alveoli and redistributing lung water from alveoli to the perivascular interstitial space, thereby allowing them to participate in gas exchange. PEEP may also have a favorable effect on lung mechanics. The chief disadvantage is decreased cardiac output. Additional potential problems include barotrauma (especially at PEEP ≥ 25 cm H_2O), increased intracranial pressure, decreased renal function from renal vein back pressure, passive hepatic congestion, and exacerbation of intracardiac shunts. PEEP should be considered in the patient with refractory hypoxemia (PaO_2 less than 55 mm Hg despite an $FIO_2 \geq 0.55$) and a **diffuse** pulmonary process. The application of PEEP and additional concepts in its application are presented in Table 7–15. The PEEP weaning process is presented in Table 7–16.

d. **Weaning the patient from mechanical ventilation** (Tables 7–17 and 7–18). Weaning can be a challenging process in certain patients. The physician must deal aggressively with all factors and the disease process responsible for respiratory failure in the first place before the ventilator wean is considered. In particular, the patient should be in optimal electrolyte (including potassium and phosphate) balance, should have a normal pH, and should be in ideal fluid balance (with appropriate management of heart failure and renal or iatrogenic fluid overload).

TABLE 7–15. The Use of PEEP

1. Routine monitors include pulse, blood pressure (BP), respiratory rate (RR), mean arterial pressure, peak inflation pressure, corrected tidal volume, pulse oximetry, and ABGs.
2. If PEEP is to be increased beyond 10 cm H_2O or patient's volume status is uncertain or patient has known left ventricular dysfunction, pulmonary artery (PA) catheter should be inserted. With PA catheter, additional variables to be monitored include wedge pressure, cardiac output, and mixed venous blood gases (optional).
3. Increments in PEEP should be made at 2.5–5 cm H_2O at a time.
4. Risk of significant complications is markedly increased at level of PEEP ≥ 25 cm H_2O.
5. Goal of PEEP is to improve O_2 delivery to tissues, not simply to improve Pao_2. Thus, cardiac output, in addition to Pao_2, must be monitored. O_2 delivery may be calculated by $Cao_2 \times$ cardiac output. Additional factors to consider include risk of barotrauma, change in lung compliance, development of lactic acidosis, and change in mixed venous O_2.
6. Further benefits from PEEP (late PEEP response) may be seen hours after a particular level of PEEP has been achieved.
7. A patient with diffuse pulmonary infiltrates is most likely to benefit from PEEP. If pulmonary process is localized, PEEP may make oxygenation worse by shunting blood away from more compliant (and hence more easily expanded alveoli) lung to less compliant and more diseased lung.

Adapted from Marini JJ. Respiratory Medicine and Intensive Care for the House Officer. Baltimore: Williams & Wilkins; 1981, pp 151–160.

TABLE 7–16. Weaning the Patient from PEEP

1. PEEP reduction should be considered when underlying pulmonary disorder has improved in patients who were responsive to PEEP. If patient is unstable, requires an Fio_2 greater than 0.4–0.5 for adequate oxygenation, or is clinically deteriorating, PEEP withdrawal is unlikely to be successful. Keep in mind that abrupt withdrawal of PEEP may cause deterioration in oxygenation that will not be correctable by returning to previous level of PEEP.
2. Obtain baseline hemodynamic and respiratory parameters, as outlined in Table 7–15.
3. Reduce PEEP by no more than 2.5–5 cm H_2O at single step.
4. After 3 min at new level of PEEP, determine ABG and return patient to previous PEEP level.
5. Compare new ABG with previous ABG to determine if patient will tolerate new level. Keep in mind that deterioration in ABG seen at 3 min will probably be amplified over the next 1–6 h.
6. Perform PEEP reduction no faster than one step every 12 h, as ABG results allow.
7. Monitor patient (including ABGs) several times over the 12 h at the new level of PEEP before a change to the next lower level is contemplated.

Adapted from Marini JJ. Respiratory Medicine and Intensive Care for the House Officer. Baltimore: Williams & Wilkins; 1981, pp 151–160.

TABLE 7-17. General Weaning Parameters

1. Vital capacity >15 mL/kg
2. Inspiratory force more negative than 25 cm H_2O
3. Respiratory rate less than 24 breaths per minute
4. Minute ventilation between 5 and 10 L/min
5. Patient awake and alert, with normal pH, appropriate electrolyte abnormalities (hypokalemia, hypophosphatemia, primary metabolic alkalosis) corrected, hemodynamically stable, and volume status optimal
6. Maximal voluntary ventilation 2 × minute ventilation
7. $Pao_2 \geq 60$ mm Hg with an $FIO_2 < 0.40$
8. Ratio of respiratory frequency/tidal volume during 1 min of spontaneous breathing < 100 breaths per minute per liter

TABLE 7-18. The T Piece Trial

1. Perform trial early in day, with patient alert.
2. Explain procedure to patient.
3. Suction airway and oropharynx.
4. If Pao_2 is marginal, increase the FIO_2 by at least 10%.
5. Have patient sitting or at least semiupright to maximize functional residual capacity (FRC).
6. Place patient on T piece and monitor closely (pulse, BP, RR) q5min and continuously monitor pulse oximetry. Obtain ABG at 20 min. If the patient is tolerating trial well, extubate. If at any time the patient experiences intolerable dyspnea, the RR increases by more than 10/min, the pulse changes by more than 30/min, the BP (diastolic) changes by more than 20 mm Hg, mental status declines, arrhythmias develop, or the ABG is unacceptable, terminate T piece trial.

Adapted from Marini JJ. Respiratory Medicine and Intensive Care for the House Officer. Baltimore: Williams & Wilkins; 1981, pp 146-147.

D. Complications of Respiratory Failure

The complications of respiratory failure were briefly described under Adult Respiratory Distress Syndrome. The clinician must keep in mind that the patient with respiratory failure seldom succumbs because of inability to oxygenate but rather because of the development of a complication while in the ICU. Multiple possibilities include nosocomial infection with sepsis, laryngotracheal injury due to endotracheal intubation, GI hemorrhage, renal impairment or failure, pulmonary thromboembolism, pulmonary barotrauma, and cardiovascular complications.

Curreri JP, Morley TF, Giudice JC. Noninvasive positive pressure ventilation. Postgrad Med 1996;99:221–230.

Dekel B, Segal E, Perel A. Pressure support ventilation. Arch Intern Med 1996;156:369–373.

Esteban A, Frutos F, Tobin MJ, et al. A comparison of four methods of weaning patients from mechanical ventilation. N Engl J Med 1995;332:345–350.

Pingleton SK. Complications of acute respiratory failure. Am Rev Respir Dis 1988;137:1463–1493.

Tobin MJ. Mechanical ventilation. N Engl J Med 1994;330:1056–1060.

XVII. PULMONARY HYPERTENSION

Pulmonary hypertension is a prolonged increase in the pressure of the main pulmonary artery (mean pressure >20 mm Hg). Potential causes are outlined in Table 7–19. Signs and symptoms include exertional dyspnea, chest pain, tachypnea, lightheadedness, syncope, and hemoptysis.

TABLE 7–19. **Causes of Pulmonary Hypertension**

Precapillary
Occlusive pulmonary vascular disease (pulmonary thromboemboli, foreign material [talc, cotton fibers in IV drug users], parasites)
Respiratory disease (obstructive and restrictive lung disease, sleep apnea, and hypoventilation syndromes)
Congenital heart disease (intracardiac septal defects with resultant left-to-right shunt, peripheral pulmonic stenosis)
Pulmonary vasculitis
Primary pulmonary hypertension
Postcapillary
Valvular heart disease (including mitral and aortic valves)
Left atrial myxoma or thrombus
Left-sided cardiac failure
Pulmonary venoocclusive disease
Mediastinal fibrosis
Anomalous pulmonary vein

Data from Rubin LJ. Pulmonary hypertension and cor pulmonale. In: Kelley WN, ed. Textbook of Internal Medicine. Philadelphia: JB Lippincott; 1990, vol. 1; Laor T, DeLuca SA. Pulmonary hypertension. Am Fam Physician 1989;40(5):195–198.

A. Diagnosis

Physical examination may reveal the likely cause (e.g., mitral stenosis murmur). Findings associated with pulmonary hypertension may include a loud pulmonic component of the second heart sound, left parasternal fourth heart sound, tricuspid insufficiency, pulmonic insufficiency, or findings of right-sided heart failure.

Laboratory studies include ECG, ABG, pulmonary function tests (including DLCO), and PA and lateral chest x-rays. Additional studies (echocardiography to evaluate chamber size, wall motion, and valvular abnormalities, ventilation-perfusion lung scanning to evaluate for recurrent or unresolved pulmonary thromboemboli, right-heart catheterization, and pulmonary arteriography) may be helpful. Open lung biopsy in the diagnosis of pulmonary hypertension is controversial.

B. Therapy

Management of pulmonary hypertension begins with the search for the underlying cause and disease-specific therapy, if possible. Additional considerations include

1. OXYGEN SUPPLEMENTATION if PaO_2 is less than 60 mm Hg (less than 90% hemoglobin saturation) or if patient has improved nocturnal desaturation or exercise capacity with supplemental O_2.

2. FUROSEMIDE for treatment of right-sided heart failure as necessary (dose should be increased cautiously to avoid overly aggressive preload reduction and consequent hypotension). Some patients benefit from **digoxin** administration.

3. PHLEBOTOMY (by reducing blood viscosity and improving cardiac output) will benefit the patient whose hematocrit exceeds 50%.

4. VASODILATORS should be used only for selected patients in a controlled setting. Risks with vasodilator therapy include worsened hypoxia, hypotension, and death. Some patients, however, have been shown to benefit from high doses of **calcium channel-blocking agents** (N Engl J Med 1992;327:76–81).

5. SURGICAL THROMBOENDARTERECTOMY is the procedure of choice in patients with accessible thromboemboli who are surgical candidates, whose mean PaO_2 is greater than 30 mm Hg, and who have clinical evidence that the arterial obstruction has been present for at least 6 months.

6. LONG-TERM ANTICOAGULATION with warfarin is appropriate for patients with pulmonary hypertension if there are no contraindications.

7. LUNG TRANSPLANTATION. Patients with end-stage pulmonary vascular disease and an anticipated survival of 12 to 18 months are candidates for lung transplantation. The 2-year postsurgical survival rate in appropriate candidates has been reported to be between 62% and 72%. In the patient with pulmonary vascular disease accompanied by right ventricular failure a combined heart-lung transplant may be the procedure of choice in the appropriate candidate.

Barst RJ, Rubin LJ, McGoon MD, et al. Survival in primary pulmonary hypertension with long-term continuous intravenous prostacyclin. Ann Intern Med 1994;121:409–415.

O'Brien GM, D'Alonzo GE. Pulmonary hypertension: a treatment strategy. J Respir Dis 1996;17:134–142.

Palevsky HI. The management of primary pulmonary hypertension. JAMA 1991;265:1014–1020.

8888888888888

GASTROINTESTINAL DISEASES

KENNETH K. WANG
THOMAS R. VIGGIANO

8888888888888

A. Reflux Esophagitis

1. **RATIONALE FOR THERAPY.** Symptoms of gastroesophageal reflux disease (pyrosis) are common and do not usually warrant therapy unless they are frequent, cause complications such as esophageal strictures or ulcers, or cause inflammatory changes in the esophagus. Therapy for reflux is directed toward the underlying causes, which include a decreased lower esophageal sphincter tone, frequent and prolonged exposure to gastric content, and decreased clearance of gastric acid (N Engl J Med 1994;331:656–660). Gastroesophageal reflux disease has been implicated as a contributing factor in producing atypical symptoms of hoarseness or asthma. Drug treatment has been effective in alleviating these symptoms in selected cases (Am J Med 1995;99: 694–695).

2. **GENERAL THERAPY.** The management of gastroesophageal reflux disease should be approached by first modifying lifestyle factors that may be influencing symptoms (Arch Intern Med 1996;156:477–484). Patients should attempt to
   - Avoid foods that increase the tendency for reflux, including sphincter-relaxing foods (peppermint, chocolate, fatty foods, caffeine, and alcohol) as well as irritant foods (tomato and orange juice)
   - Stop tobacco use
   - Discontinue or modify drugs that lower esophageal sphincter pressure (progesterone-containing birth control pills, aminophylline, anticholinergics, beta-adrenergic agonists, alpha-adrenergic antagonists, calcium channel blockers, and diazepam)

3. **MECHANICAL MEASURES TO DECREASE REFLUX OR INCREASE ESOPHAGEAL CLEARANCE.** In concert with the preceding recommendations, the patient should also be instructed in mechanical measures to decrease esophageal reflux. Patient education is a key component to assuring compliance with these recommendations.
   - Avoid tight-fitting clothes
   - Avoid excessive stooping or bending
   - Elevate the head of the bed at least 6 inches
   - Decrease meal sizes
   - Avoid eating 3 hours before sleep
   - Avoid lying down within 2 hours of eating
   - Weight loss for obese patients

4. **PHARMACOLOGIC THERAPY** (Table 8–1). If the general measures do not result in significant improvement in symptoms or if there are indications of complications of reflux disease (Barrett's esophagus, ulcers, strictures), medications should be added. Recently, it has been found that most reflux occurs after the evening meal rather than at night, and

TABLE 8-1. **Pharmacologic Therapy**

Reflux Esophagitis (Maintenance Therapy Required)

Ranitidine	150 mg PO bid	6–8 wk
Cimetidine	400 mg PO bid	6–8 wk
Nizatidine	150 mg PO bid	6–8 wk
Famotidine	20 mg PO bid	6–8 wk
Omeprazole	20 mg PO qd	6–8 wk
Lansoprazole	30 mg PO qd	6–8 wk
Sucralfate	1 g PO qid	6–8 wk
Metoclopromide	10 mg PO qid	6 wk
Cisapride	10 mg PO qid	6 wk
Bethanecol	25 mg PO qid	6 wk
Peptic Ulcer Disease		
Lansoprazole	30 mg PO qd	6–8 wk
Gastroparesis		
Cisapride	10 mg PO qid	
Crohn's Disease		
Olsalazine	500 mg PO bid	
Mesalamine (Pentasa)	500–1000 mg PO qid	
Mesalamine (Asacol)	800 mg PO tid	
Mesalamine (Rowasa)	4 g PR qhs	
Chronic Ulcerative Colitis		
Olsalazine	500 mg PO bid	
Mesalamine (Pentasa)	500–1000 mg PO qid	
Mesalamine (Asacol)	800 mg PO tid	
Mesalamine (Rowasa)	4 g PR qhs	

therapy needs to be concentrated in this time period, particularly in those individuals with mild esophagitis.

a. **Decreased acid production**

(1) *Antacids.* Liquid antacids, 30 mL 1 and 3 hours after meals and at bedtime, have traditionally been used to neutralize acid and are of considerable value in acutely alleviating symptoms of reflux disease. Antacids can be given in addition to proton pump inhibitors or H_2-receptor antagonists to decrease acute symptoms. Solid tablets, such as calcium carbonate antacids, when dissolved in the mouth may provide as good symptomatic relief. Magnesium-containing antacids may produce diarrheal symptoms, whereas aluminum-containing antacids are constipating. Antacids are only indicated as single therapy in patients without esophagitis.

(2) *H_2-receptor antagonists.* Ranitidine (150 mg bid), cimetidine (300 mg bid), nizatidine (150 mg bid), and famotidine (20 mg bid) are all effective oral agents for decreasing acid production and healing mild to moderate reflux esophagitis. For more intensive therapy, dosages can be increased by giving the medication qid for cimetidine, ranitidine, or nizatidine. For patients with primarily nocturnal symptoms, the total daily dose can be administered primarily at time of sleep. Drug interactions have been reported. Common associations are

increased blood levels of warfarin, theophylline, phenytoin, diazepam, propranolol, lidocaine, and tricyclic antidepressants with the use of cimetidine. All of these medications have also been approved in over-the-counter form at dosages half that of the prescription form. If prescription strength medication is needed, over-the-counter forms are often more expensive given the need for increased dosages. As a maintenance drug, ranitidine has been approved by the FDA at a dose of 150 mg/d to prevent relapse of esophagitis.

(3) ***Proton pump inhibitors.*** Omeprazole (20–40 mg/d) and more recently approved lansoprazole (30–60 mg/d) have been found to be very effective agents in the treatment of severe reflux disease. These medications are more effective than cimetidine in the relief of symptoms and in healing inflammatory changes. Symptoms are usually resolved by 2 weeks after initiation of therapy. Although the standard dose of omeprazole is 20 mg/d, high dosages (40–60 mg) are needed in such conditions as Barrett's esophagus. Lansoprazole may be dispensed as 15 or 30 mg tablets, which are of equal cost. Complications of this form of therapy relate to hypergastrinemia, which has been shown to induce carcinoid tumors in rats but has not been associated with conditions other than chronic gastritis in humans. Intestinal metaplasia of the stomach may develop in patients with *Helicobacter pylori* infection of the stomach treated with long-term proton pump inhibitors. It may be advantageous to treat these patients for *H. pylori* to prevent this premalignant condition from developing. The degree of hypoacidity induced by this class of drugs can interfere with absorption of other medications, including iron and fluconazole. Proton pump inhibitors are more effective than histamine receptor antagonists in decreasing relapse of esophagitis when used as maintenance therapy in severe reflux esophagitis at a dose of 20–40 mg/d of omeprazole and 15–30 mg/d of lansoprazole.

b. **Mucosal protection.** Sucralfate has been found to aid healing of esophagitis when given as a liquid. The liquid form can be dispensed as 30 mL at bedtime or qid. This form can be difficult to carry and is more expensive. It is often more convenient to prepare this slurry by placing one tablet (1 g) in water 1 hour before use. This medication is most useful in severe acute esophagitis or ulceration.

c. **Increasing lower esophageal sphincter tone and esophageal motility.** These agents increase esophageal clearance of acid by increasing peristalsis and decrease reflux by increasing lower esophageal sphincter pressure. Bethanechol, a cholinergic antagonist, is usually well tolerated and can increase salivation to neutralize acid when given at a dose of 25 mg qid. Side effects include increased bronchospasm, diarrhea, increased urination, and blurred vision. Metoclopramide is an antidopaminergic that increases gastric emptying and lower esophageal sphincter pressure when given at a dose of 10 mg qid (before meals and at bedtime). CNS effects often limit its use primarily in older patients who are susceptible to extrapyramidal side effects. Cisapride is the latest addition and the best tolerated agent. It acts primarily at the level of the myenteric plexus. Cisapride is given at a dose of 10–20 mg PO 30 minutes before meals and at bedtime. It is effective in decreasing reflux symptoms and can be used as a single agent in mild esophagitis. However, most commonly, the prokinetic agents are added after failure of first-line agents, such as histamine receptor antagonists and proton pump inhibitors. Cisapride can cause diarrhea, stomach cramps, and headaches.

5. COMPLICATIONS OF GASTROESOPHAGEAL REFLUX DISEASE
   a. **Barrett's esophagus.** The replacement of squamous epithelium by columnar mucosa is thought to be secondary to chronic reflux esophagitis. An esophageal reflux program should be initiated to treat reflux esophagitis. However, the efficacy of antireflux measures in causing regression of a Barrett's esophagus has not been demonstrated (Gastroenterology 1987;92:118). The preferred treatment in Barrett's esophagus has been proton pump inhibitors because of the severe reflux found in these patients. It is an indication for esophagoscopy and biopsy because of its association with esophageal neoplasms. The cost effectiveness of surveillance procedures to detect early neoplasm in Barrett's esophagus is controversial.
   b. **Esophageal strictures, ulcers, asthma, hoarseness, and aspiration pneumonia.** Symptomatic strictures secondary to reflux esophagitis often can be dilated endoscopically. Patients should also be treated for reflux after dilatation with proton pump inhibitors to prevent recurrence of strictures. The combination has been successful in managing most strictures. Surgery may be indicated if endoscopic dilatation provides only short-term improvement. Aspiration pneumonia and pulmonary fibrosis may also result from untreated gastroesophageal reflux. If this recurs despite medical therapy, surgery is indicated. Reflux disease can induce esophageal ulcers, most often in association with Barrett's esophagus. Ulcers usually respond to maximal medical management. Atypical symptoms of reflux disease include hoarseness or asthma. The role of acid reflux in these conditions can be assessed with 24-hour pH monitoring. If reflux is found (>4% reflux over 24 hours), treatment for reflux should be initiated. Surgery may also be indicated for gastroesophageal reflux that has persisted despite intensive medical therapy for at least 4 to 6 months. Before any surgical intervention, 24-hour pH monitoring and esophageal motility studies are essential. Occasionally, bile acid reflux may cause esophagitis as well as gastritis. Bile acid reflux necessitates a surgical drainage procedure different from that for gastric acid reflux. If ineffective esophageal peristalsis is found, surgery should be reconsidered.

B. Nonpeptic Strictures of the Esophagus

Strictures discovered on barium swallow may be asymptomatic but should be investigated by endoscopy and biopsy. Schatzki's rings should be dilated if dysphagia can be attributed to their presence. The cervical Plummer-Vinson's web should have periodic rebiopsy because of a 10% incidence of associated malignant disease. Malignant strictures may also be dilated if symptomatic. If dilatation fails in these patients, esophageal stents or percutaneous gastrostomies may be placed to aid in nutrition.

C. Caustic Ingestions

Ingestion of caustic alkali may cause more severe damage to the esophagus than ingestion of acid. However, neither the type of irritant nor symptoms created by ingestion indicate the actual damage. If patients are seen within 1 hour of ingestion, water lavage of the gastric contents should be done. Endoscopy can assess the extent of damage as soon as possible after ingestion unless esophageal perforation is suspected. A soft-rubber naso-gastric tube can be placed to stent the lumen of the esophagus and to provide decompression of the stomach. Broad-spectrum antibiotics, not routinely necessary, should be given at the first sign of an infection. Steroids have not been shown to prevent stricture formation and are not recommended (N Engl J Med 1990;323:637). Dilatation of caustic strictures may be attempted as early as a week after ingestion.

D. Motility Disorders of the Esophagus

1. PHARYNGEAL DYSPHAGIA. Nasal regurgitation of food, coughing, and other evidence of aspiration are signs of pharyngeal dysphagia. This is often secondary to structural lesions, such as tumors of the posterior pharynx. However, such disorders as hypothyroidism, amyotrophic lateral sclerosis, polymyositis, and Parkinson's disease must be considered.

   Zenker's diverticulum may also cause dysphagia and should be treated surgically if symptoms are severe. Medical management usually involves diet modification to avoid liquids, which commonly are the most difficult to swallow. Endoscopic placement of feeding gastrostomy tubes helps in long-term management of patients with neurologic disorders. Careful assessment should be done to avoid regurgitation and aspiration of enteral feedings.

2. DIFFUSE ESOPHAGEAL SPASM. Diffuse esophageal spasm (DES) often occurs as dysphagia or chest pain and is diagnosed by esophageal manometry and provocative agents, such as edrophonium (Gastroenterology 1981;81:10). Gastroesophageal reflux with secondary esophageal spasm should be carefully excluded. Most patients with DES have prolonged high-amplitude contractions in the body of the esophagus and frequent simultaneous contractions, and approximately a third have elevated lower esophageal sphincter (LES) tone pressures. Pharmacologic therapy should be tailored to the individual patient's tolerance. Anticholinergic agents (dicyclomine hydrochloride 10 mg PO qid), nitrates (isosorbide dinitrate 10–30 mg PO qid), and calcium channel blockers are often good first-line therapy for DES. Nifedipine 10–20 mg PO qid is particularly effective for patients with increased LES tone, but patient tolerance may limit the use of effective dosages. Verapamil 80 mg PO tid or diltiazem 30–60 mg PO qid is most effective

for symptoms that are related to chest pain. Hydralazine can be considered in a dosage of 25–50 mg PO tid. In refractory cases, dilatation may be effective (Gastroenterology 1982;82:1069). Some patients with hypertensive LES pressures and dysphagia may respond to pneumatic dilatations. Occasionally, when medical therapy fails, patients may be referred for a Lowell myotomy. Overall, treatment results for DES have been disappointing.

3. **ACHALASIA.** This progressive denervation of the smooth muscle of the lower two thirds of the esophagus often leads to dysphagia. Patients who have characteristic manometric findings of achalasia should still have esophagoscopy to eliminate the possibility of esophageal tumors that mimic this entity. If symptoms are not severe and changes noted on barium x-ray are slight, pharmacologic therapy with nifedipine 10–20 mg PO qid or isosorbide dinitrate 10–30 mg PO qid may aid in decreasing LES pressure and improve esophageal clearance (Gastroenterology 1981;80:39). Unfortunately, although some symptoms may be relieved with medications, the majority persist (Am J Gastroenterol 1990;84:1259). Botulinum toxin has been used for patients with achalasia. This is administered during endoscopy with the use of a sclerotherapy needle. Pneumatic dilatation often is required for relief of dysphagia. Surgical myotomy should be considered if pneumatic dilatation is unsuccessful on two consecutive attempts. However, myotomy is associated with a high incidence of gastroesophageal reflux.

E. Infectious Esophagitis

Immune suppression caused most commonly by chemotherapy or HIV infection predisposes patients to infection by *Candida albicans* and viruses of the herpes family. Although these often cause oral manifestations and odynophagia, patients may be totally asymptomatic and discovered only at endoscopy to have characteristic discrete punched-out ulcerations or vesicles in herpes virus infection or yellowish white plaques in *Candida* infection. Mild localized *Candida* esophagitis in immunocompetent patients may be treated with nystatin, usually in dosages of 500,000 U PO qid. If this is not successful in relieving symptoms within 48 hours, the dose may be increased to 200,000 U q2h. Clotrimazole may also be used for mild candidiasis as a 10 mg troche dissolved in the mouth qid or as 100 mg tablets tid. Ketoconazole can be used as 200 mg bid in immunocompromised patients. Ketoconazole can have significant side effects, including nausea, vomiting, and hepatotoxicity. Therapy should be continued for 1 to 2 weeks if symptoms disappear and associated problems (e.g., neutropenia) resolve. Fluconazole is an effective drug in immunocompromised hosts at a dose of 100 mg bid but is significantly more expensive. If there is evidence of systemic candidemia or neutropenia in a patient with severe esophagitis, amphotericin B should be used.

Varicella zoster, cytomegalovirus, and herpes simplex may cause viral esophagitis. For varicella zoster, acyclovir may be used (10 mg/kg IV or 800 mg/d PO over a 5-day treatment course). The drug is usually given in a dilute solution to avoid possible crystallization in the kidneys. Coadministration of other nephrotoxic drugs should be avoided. Acyclovir infusion has been

TABLE 8–2. **Screening for Gastrointestinal Carcinoma**

CONDITION	CANCER TYPE	PROCEDURE	INTERVAL
Barrett's esophagus	Esophageal	EGD*	
No dysplasia			3 y
Low-grade dysplasia			1 y
High-grade dysplasia			3–6 mo
Achalasia	Esophageal	EGD	3 y
Gastric adenomas	Gastric	EGD	1–3 y
Familial polyposis	Gastric	EGD	1–3 y
	Papilla of Vater	EGD	1–3 y
	Colon (residual)	Flexible sigmoidoscopy	1 y
Colonic adenomas	Colon	Colonoscopy	1–5 y
Ulcerative colitis	Colon	Colonoscopy	1–3 y

*EGD, esophagogastroduodenoscopy.

associated with femoral phlebitis, reversible CNS side effects, and reduced renal clearance. Ganciclovir is recommended for systemic cytomegalovirus infections at a dosage of 5 mg/kg bid for 5 days. Ganciclovir causes nephrotoxicity and leukopenia.

F. Esophageal Cancer

Medical management of esophageal carcinoma consists primarily of screening for premalignant lesions (Table 8–2). Although screening standards have not yet been established, many gastroenterologists recommend periodic screening of patients with lesions that have a greater disposition to development of carcinoma. Such lesions include strictures from caustic ingestions, Plummer-Vinson's webs, Barrett's esophagus, achalasia, and tylosis palmaris et plantaris. Although peptic esophagitis may be associated with a small increase in incidence of esophageal carcinoma, screening is probably not indicated. Palliative therapy for esophageal carcinoma is nutritional support via percutaneous gastrostomies, laser photoablation of the tumor, dilatation of esophageal strictures, or placement of a stent. Stents have also been used to treat tracheoesophageal fistulas.

Achem SR, Kolts BE. Current medical therapy for esophageal motility disorders. Am J Med 1992;92:98S.

Anderson KD, Rouse TM, Randolf JG. A controlled trial of corticosteroids in children with corrosive injury of the esophagus. N Engl J Med 1990;323:637.

Dehn TC, Shepherd HA, Colin-Jones D, et al. Double blind comparison of omeprazole (40 mg od) versus cimetidine (400 mg qd) in the treatment of symptomatic erosive reflux oesophagitis, assessed endoscopically, histologically and by 24 h pH monitoring. Gut 1990;31:509.

DeVault KR, Castell DO. Current diagnosis and treatment of gastroesophageal reflux disease. Mayo Clin Proc 1994;69:867.

Fennerty MB, Castell D, Fendrick AM, et al. The diagnosis and treatment of gastroesophageal reflux disease in a managed care environment: suggested disease management guidelines. Arch Intern Med 1996;156:477.

Goldin MR, Burns TW, Herrington JP. Treatment of nonspecific esophageal motor disorders: beneficial effects of bougienage. Gastroenterology 1982;82:1069.

London RL, Ouyand A, Snape WJ, et al. Provocation of esophageal pain by ergonovine or edrophonium. Gastroenterology 1981;81:10.

Pera M, Trastek VF, Pairolero PC, et al. Barrett's disease: pathophysiology of metaplasia and adenocarcinoma. Ann Thorac Surg 1993;56:1191.

Ros E, Pujol A, Bordas JM, Grande L. Efficacy of sucralfate in refractory reflux esophagitis. Results of a pilot study. Scand J Gastroenterol 1989;156(Suppl):49.

Traube M, Dubovik S, Lange RC, McCallum RW. The role of nifedipine therapy in achalasia: results of a randomized, double-blind, placebo-controlled study. Am J Gastroenterol 1989;84:1259.

II. STOMACH DISORDERS

A. Peptic Ulcer Disease

Recent advances in our understanding of the pathogenesis of peptic ulcer disease have changed the approach to treatment. Previously, we presumed that idiopathic acid hypersecretion was a common etiologic factor, and our treatment strategies were largely acid suppression or neutralization ("no acid, no ulcer"). We now categorize peptic ulcers as being associated with three major possible etiologic factors: (1) *Helicobacter pylori,* (2) nonsteroidal anti-inflammatory drugs (NSAIDs) or aspirin, and (3) miscellaneous causes. The miscellaneous causes include idiopathic hypersecretion, hypersecretory syndromes (Zollinger-Ellison syndrome), and duodenogastric reflux of gastric mucosal barrier breaking agents, such as bile salts or lysolecithin. Current estimates are that at least 95% of peptic ulcers are due to either *H. pylori* infection or the use of NSAIDs or aspirin. The most common cause of duodenal ulcers is *H. pylori* infection, and almost all duodenal ulcers are benign. The most common cause of gastric ulcer disease is the use of NSAIDs, particularly among older patients, but approximately 5% of gastric ulcers are malignant. In patients who are not infected with *H. pylori* and who are not taking NSAIDs or aspirin, a gastric ulcer should raise suspicion of malignancy (gastroscopy is indicated), and a duodenal ulcer should raise suspicion of a hypersecretory syndrome (check serum gastrin).

    1. HELICOBACTER PYLORI. *H. pylori* is a gram-negative, spiral, microaerophilic bacillus that produces multiple enzymes, including a urease that is important for its pathogenesis. After ingestion, this fastidious organism moves into and through the mucous layer of the stomach and remains in the gastric mucous layer for life unless treated.

       Worldwide, *H. pylori* is one of the most common bacterial infections. In developing countries the prevalence rate is greater than 80%. In the United States, *H. pylori* is present in 40% to 50% of the general population and is more prevalent in the elderly, blacks, and Hispanics, poorer socioeconomic groups, and institutionalized people. The general consensus is that *H. pylori* infection is spread by a fecal-oral or oral-oral route. *H. pylori* is found in 90% to 95% of patients with duodenal ulcers and in approximately 80% of patients with gastric ulcers. If ulcers associated with NSAIDs or aspirin are excluded, the prevalence of *H. pylori* infection in patients with gastric ulcer is similar to that of patients with duodenal ulcer. It is important to emphasize, however, that *H. pylori* infection is not associated with nonulcer dyspepsia or gastroesophageal reflux disease. Treatment of *H. pylori*-positive patients with these conditions is unlikely to result in clinical improvement.

The majority of ulcer patients who are not taking NSAIDs or aspirin will be *H. pylori* positive. Although experts currently recommend routine testing for *H. pylori* in ulcer patients, many practicing physicians will treat ulcers not related to NSAIDs empirically for *H. pylori.* Serologic tests measure antibodies and are useful to diagnose a primary infection. These antibodies remain elevated over time, but a decrease in antibody titer is thought to be suggestive of cure after antibiotic therapy. Breath tests employ a radiolabeled dose of urea, which is split by the bacterial urease in *H. pylori*-positive patients, and then radiolabeled carbon dioxide is exhaled. This is a good noninvasive test for follow-up after treatment. Tests that require endoscopy include the biopsy urease test and histologic analysis, with special routine or tissue stains. Recent cost-effective analyses concluded that cost savings and lower recurrence rates justify initial empiric treatment for *H. pylori* (Ann Intern Med 1995;123:260–268, 665–672).

a. **Treatment of Helicobacter pylori.** The goal of treatment of an *H. pylori*-positive duodenal or gastric ulcer is to heal the ulcer and to eradicate the bacteria. Eradication of *H. pylori* dramatically reduces the recurrence rate for both duodenal and gastric ulcers. Current recommendations are that all patients who have peptic ulcer disease and who are infected with *H. pylori* should receive treatment to eradicate the bacteria (Am J Med 1996;100:42S–51S). Although there is no consensus on the optimal treatment regimen at this time, there is consensus about some guidelines for treating *H. pylori*-positive patients. An important factor that reduces the eradication rate of *H. pylori* is the presence of a metronidazole-resistant strain. Metronidazole resistance occurs in 20% to 30% of *H. pylori* strains and is much more common in underdeveloped countries (>80%) than in the United States (<20%). We know that treatment with one or two antibiotics alone is not effective. Acceptable regimens at this time include dual therapy, bismuth-based triple antibiotic therapy, triple therapy with a proton pump inhibitor, and quadruple therapy (Table 8–3). The duration of these treatment regimens has traditionally been 2 weeks, but recent reports demonstrate successful treatment after several days to 1 week of therapy. Assessment of treatment success is based on the presence of the organism 4 weeks after cessation of therapy. The most common causes of failure to eradicate the bacteria are poor patient compliance or metronidazole resistance. If a patient fails a treatment regimen, a different treatment regimen should be tried, and if compliance is not the problem, eradication should be achieved in approximately 50% of the retreated patients. There is extensive current investigation seeking more simple, inexpensive, and effective treatment regimens.

2. NONSTEROIDAL ANTI-INFLAMMATORY DRUGS. The stomach protects itself from its acid by synthesizing a mucopolysaccharide gel that traps bicarbonate and coats the gastric epithelium. Gastric prostaglandin production is important for gastric mucus synthesis and bicarbonate production. NSAIDs inhibit gastroduodenal prostaglandin synthesis, which causes a decrease in the secretion of mucus and bicarbonate and

TABLE 8–3. Treatment Regimens for *Helicobacter pylori*

TREATMENT REGIMEN	EFFECTIVENESS MEAN ERADICATION RATE	COST	COMMENTS
Dual Therapy			
Omeprazole 20 mg bid Amoxicillin 500 mg qid	57–66%	+++	2 wk Compliance is simpler Variable reports of effectiveness
Omeprazole 20 mg bid Clarithromycin 500 mg tid	66–76%	++++	2 wk Compliance is simpler
Triple Antibiotic Therapy			
Bismuth 2 tab qid Metronidazole 500 mg tid Amoxicillin 500 mg qid	73%	++	2 wk Compliance is difficult
Bismuth 2 tab qid Metronidazole 500 mg tid Tetracycline 500 mg qid	94%	++	2 wk Effective, less expensive Compliance is difficult
Triple Therapy with Proton Pump Inhibitor			
Omeprazole 20 mg bid Metronidazole 500 mg tid Clarithromycin 500 mg tid	90%	++++	7–10 d Compliance moderately difficult
Omeprazole 20 mg bid Amoxicillin 500 mg qid Metronidazole 500 mg tid	84%	+++	7–10 d Compliance moderately difficult
Quadruple Therapy			
Omeprazole 20 mg bid Bismuth 2 tab qid Metronidazole 500 mg tid Tetracycline 500 mg qid	98%	++++	Omeprazole for 10 d Antibiotics for 7 d Compliance is difficult

disrupts the gastric mucosal protective barrier. The risk of peptic ulcer disease with NSAID use is maximal in the first 3 months of treatment and is highest in the elderly and in patients with a previous history of peptic ulcer disease.

It is important for clinicians to remember that NSAIDs have both analgesic and anti-inflammatory properties. The anti-inflammatory properties of NSAIDs are mediated by prostaglandin inhibition and are associated with risk for peptic ulcer disease. Many patients take NSAIDs for pain relief of noninflammatory conditions, such as osteoarthritis, and many do not need the anti-inflammatory properties of NSAIDs. The clinician should decide whether simple analgesic treatment (e.g., acetaminophen) could be substituted for NSAIDs. Patients who require the anti-inflammatory properties of NSAIDs and who are at risk for peptic ulcer disease could be tried on misoprostol (Cytotec), a prostaglandin analog. Because many patients develop diarrhea, the lowest possible effective dose should be used. However, most patients require 200–400 µg of misoprostol tid for a beneficial effect. Current studies are evaluating combinations of misoprostol with either H_2-receptor antagonists, omeprazole, or sucralfate, although none of these agents has been shown to be effective when used alone.

B. Gastritis

1. ACUTE GASTRITIS. Acute gastritis results from mucosal injury that allows backdiffusion of acid. Certain drugs—especially aspirin, alcohol, and NSAIDs—disrupt the mucosal barrier. Stress ulcers, commonly seen in trauma or surgery, are thought to result from ischemia. Gastritis can sometimes be attributed to such events as irradiation, ingestion of alkali, or, rarely, bacterial infection (phlegmonous gastritis).

   a. **Prevention of acute erosive gastritis.** Erosive gastritis can be prevented by increasing gastric pH to greater than 4 with a proton pump inhibitor, H_2-blocker, or a combination of these with antacids. Patients at highest risk of ulceration (with severe burns, trauma, septicemia, CNS damage, respiratory failure, or renal failure) should receive prophylaxis.

   b. **Therapy of acute erosive gastritis.** After initial lavage with tap water, endoscopy should be performed. If diffuse bleeding is seen from superficial erosions, infusion of a solution made from 12 mg of norepinephrine ditartrate in 200 mL normal saline into the stomach for 15 minutes may be helpful. If bleeding is from discrete ulcerations, endoscopic cautery can be performed. If bleeding continues, angiography can be done with the selective infusion of vasopressin. Bleeding does not respond to medical therapy in approximately 20% of patients and may require surgical intervention.

   c. **Therapy of alkaline reflux gastritis.** Although diagnosis is difficult, once it is established this entity generally can be managed by antacids, 30 mL 2 to 3 hours after meals and 60 mL at bedtime. Antacids appear to have significant ability to absorb bile salts. Cholestyramine can also be used at a dosage of 1 package 2 to 3 hours after meals and at bedtime. Surgery is seldom successful in relieving pain in these patients and should be attempted only if additional symptoms are present.

   d. **Therapy of NSAID-related conditions.** For bleeding with significant lesions in the stomach, such as erosions or small ulcers, therapy can be initiated as with gastric ulcer disease. Misoprostol, 200 mg qid, can be given as a preventive agent but may cause loose stools or diarrhea.

2. CHRONIC GASTRITIS. Chronic gastritis can be classified by histologic appearance (superficial versus atrophic) and by the anatomic location of the inflammation (type A, fundus and body; type B, antrum). In type A atrophic gastritis, circulating antibodies against parietal cells and pernicious anemia are often present. In type B atrophic gastritis, antibodies against gastrin-producing cells have been reported. *H. pylori* is the most common etiologic agent for chronic active gastritis. The organism is thought to initially cause a type B form of gastritis involving the antrum and causing hypochlorhydria. In chronic infection, type A pattern may appear. No specific treatment is currently indicated for idiopathic chronic gastritis.

3. ZOLLINGER-ELLISON SYNDROME. This consists of peptic ulceration, acid hypersecretion, the presence of a non–islet cell tumor, and increased serum gastrin. Its treatment should be surgical excision if a tumor mass can be defined. Patients with multiple endocrine neoplasia I usually

have multifocal disease and are not candidates for resection. If tumors cannot be localized, medical therapy should be instituted. Proton pump inhibitors are the treatment of choice for this condition. Octreotide, a somatostatin analog, has been effective in decreasing symptoms and may decrease tumor growth.

C. Motility Disorders

1. **GASTROPARESIS.** This diagnosis is made by the exclusion of obstructing lesions in the stomach and duodenum and demonstration of delayed emptying of either solid or liquid material by radionuclide scintigraphy. Therapy is concentrated on the underlying disorder, including electrolyte abnormalities, diabetes mellitus, and medications (anticholinergics, antidopaminergics, beta-adrenergic agonists, calcium channel blockers). Dietary manipulation is often necessary, with the use of liquid supplements if tolerated. Bypassing the stomach with nasaljejunal or percutaneous jejunal feeding tubes may be effective if the small bowel is not involved. Bethanechol is often used as a prokinetic agent, but it is not well tolerated. Metoclopramide may be used in dosages of 10–20 mg 30 minutes before meals and at bedtime. Side effects include akathisias, oculogyral crisis, increased prolactin secretion, agitation, and sedation. Cisapride is effective and has fewer side effects than metoclopramide at dosages of 10 mg 30 minutes before meals and before sleep. It may be associated with diarrhea, cramps, and seizures. Erythromycin increases gastric emptying at a dose of 250 mg 30 minutes before meals in patients with diabetic or postvagotomy gastroparesis.

2. **NAUSEA AND VOMITING.** After identification of the cause of vomiting, therapy can be initiated. With peripheral vestibular dysfunction, 25 mg of meclizine hydrochloride may be used bid or qid or 50 mg PO before activity. Diphenhydramine hydrochloride can also be used in a dosage of 25–50 mg qid. Both are antihistamines that can cause sedation. Scopolamine transdermal patches applied 4 hours before a provocative event and every 3 days afterward can be effective. Nausea postoperatively or due to gastroenteritis responds well to prochlorperazine, 5–10 mg PO tid or 25 mg bid to qid PR as a suppository. Butyrophenones are also useful in dosages of 2.5–5 mg IM bid but may cause extrapyramidal side effects. Trimethobenzamide hydrochloride is used in dosages of 250 mg PO bid or qid or 200 mg PR as suppositories bid to qid. High-dose metoclopramide 1–2 mg/kg IV has been particularly effective in decreasing nausea due to chemotherapeutic agents. Ondansetron is a new serotonin receptor antagonist given IV at a dose of 4–8 mg to prevent chemotherapy-induced vomiting.

3. **HICCUPS.** This nonspecific symptom should be evaluated for possible causes, such as diaphragmatic irritation and medication effects. Symptomatic therapy with chlorpromazine 25–50 mg IV or metoclopramide 10 mg IV can be helpful.

Driks MR, Craven DE, Celli BR, et al. Nosocomial pneumonia in intubated patients given sucralfate as compared with antacids or histamine type 2 blockers: the role of gastric colonization. N Engl J Med 1987;317:1376.

Hopkins RJ, Girardi LS, Turney EA. Relationship between *Helicobacter pylori* eradication and reduced duodenal and gastric ulcer recurrence: a review. Gastroenterology 1996;110:1244.

Marshall BJ. *Campylobacter pylori:* its link to gastritis and peptic ulcer disease. Rev Infect Dis 1990;12(Suppl 1):S87–93.

Soll AH. Consensus conference. Medical treatment of peptic ulcer disease. Practice guidelines. Practice Parameters Committee of the American College of Gastroenterology. JAMA 1996; 275:622.

Wolfe MM, Jensen RT. Zollinger-Ellison syndrome. N Engl J Med 1987;317:1200–1209.

III. SMALL-BOWEL DISEASE

A. Crohn's Disease

This is an idiopathic inflammatory bowel disease that discontinuously involves the entire GI tract. It is characterized by a cobblestone appearance to the mucosa and the formation of deep linear ulcers. Transmural bowel wall involvement distinguishes it from idiopathic ulcerative colitis and predisposes patients to fistula formation and anal fissures. Efforts should be made to counsel patients regarding disease chronicity and supportive counseling.

1. DRUGS

   a. **Sulfasalazine.** This drug consists of sulfapyridine linked to 5-aminosalicylic acid, which is thought to be the active ingredient. Most of the drug reaches the colon unchanged until the 5-ASA is released by action of bacterial azoreductase. The principal side effects are secondary to the sulfapyridine moiety, which is readily absorbed in the colon. These include nausea, anorexia, dyspepsia , headache, reticulocytosis, rash, oligospermia, bronchospasm, neutropenia, and aplastic anemias. This drug is believed to exert its primary effect on arachidonic acid metabolism. Sulfasalazine has been used at a dosage of 1 g/15 kg to treat mild to moderate Crohn's colitis and ileocolitis. However, evidence concerning its efficacy in ileitis alone is conflicting. It has not been demonstrated to be effective in preventing relapse of Crohn's disease.

   b. **Aminosalicylic acid.** Since up to one third of patients with inflammatory bowel disease are unable to tolerate sulfasalazine because of reactions to the sulfa component, several new drugs have been developed that are constructed solely of 5-ASA. Differences in these drugs are mainly in their coatings, which determine where the drug is released. Currently, osalazine (Dipentum) has been released at a dosage of 500 mg bid for ulcerative colitis in patients intolerant of sulfasalazine. Taken orally, it is released primarily in the colon and would not be useful in ileitis. Mesalamine (Pentasa) is designed to be released in the small bowel and, therefore, is better suited for treating Crohn's disease. It is usually given at a dose of 2–4 g/d in divided doses in 250 mg capsules. The most common side effects are headaches, diarrhea, nausea, and rash. Asacol (400 mg timed-release tablets) is recommended for colonic and distal ileal disease and is given at a dose of 2.4 g/d in three divided doses. Mesalamine (Rowasa) is available as a rectal suppository (4 g/60 mL) to be used at bedtime and retained for 8 hours in patients with proctosigmoiditis.

c. **Corticosteroids.** Corticosteroids have long been recognized as effective in severe Crohn's disease. At doses of 0.25 mg/kg–0.75 mg/kg, depending on severity, **prednisolone** has been effective in treating ileal disease (Gastroenterology 1979;77:847). Therapy with corticosteroids does not prevent relapse.

d. **Antibiotics.** Metronidazole has been shown in European studies to be as effective as sulfasalazine in the treatment of colonic Crohn's disease and more effective in ileal and perianal disease. In the dosages used (10–20 mg/kg/d), however, it often induces nausea, a metallic taste, alcohol intolerance, and a peripheral neuropathy that requires discontinuation of therapy. Almost half the patients treated with this drug complain of numbness and tingling in their fingers and toes. Nonetheless, this drug may be substituted for sulfasalazine in appropriate cases. If metronidazole is not tolerated, ciprofloxacin has been used in fistulizing Crohn's disease at a dose of 500 mg bid.

e. **Immunosuppressive agents.** Immunosuppressive agents, such as azathioprine or its active metabolite 6-mercaptopurine, have been used successfully in the treatment of Crohn's disease, although azathioprine is generally reserved for those who suffer from refractory steroid-dependent disease with severe steroid side effects, postsurgical patients with rapid recurrence of disease, diffuse jejunoileitis with severe symptoms, and intractable perianal disease or fistulas not amenable to surgery. Azathioprine is slowly effective in treating active Crohn's disease, and it must be given for 3 months to achieve results. Azathioprine therapy is usually begun at a dose of 50 mg/d and gradually increased to 2.5 mg/kg. Blood counts should be followed weekly during initiation of therapy and, if they remain stable, may be followed monthly. Cyclosporine has been used in acute flares of Crohn's disease at a dose of 5–7.5 mg/kg/d. Overall, this agent is used in refractory disease as a temporizing measure until azathioprine takes effect. Cyclosporine does not appear to be as effective in Crohn's disease as it is in ulcerative colitis. Methotrexate (25 mg IM every week) with prednisone has also been used (N Engl J Med 1995;332:330).

2. **TREATMENT STRATEGY.** Medical therapy should be dictated by the disease severity. New-onset Crohn's disease with symptoms solely of diarrhea and abdominal cramping without weight loss or evidence of abdominal masses should be treated with sulfasalazine, 500 mg bid increased gradually over a week to 500–1000 mg qid. If mild symptoms persist, a trial of antispasmodic agents for relief of cramping, such as dicyclomine hydrochloride 20 mg qid, or antidiarrheal agents, such as diphenoxylate and atropine 2.5–5 mg q6h, may be added. Tapering to a maintenance dose of sulfasalazine of 2 g/d should not be attempted unless symptoms are relieved and the original dose has been given at least 3 months. For patients intolerant of higher doses of sulfasalazine, the mesalamine compounds can be used. Pentasa is more effective for proximal bowel disease, whereas Asacol and Dipentum are effective for

colonic diseases. Patients with more active inflammation involving significant weight loss, fever, severe diarrhea, or abdominal pain should be treated initially with steroids, beginning with 40–60 mg/d of prednisone in a single dose. Sulfasalazine or mesalamine can be started simultaneously at a dosage of 500 mg bid if colonic involvement is found. After symptom abatement, the steroid dosage may be tapered by 5 mg/wk until the patient is receiving no more than 20 mg/d. Then, the tapering should be done more slowly, at a rate of 5 mg/mo until prednisone can be discontinued. During this time, sulfasalazine should be continued at a maintenance dose of 2 g/d.

Patients with active Crohn's disease involving an inflammatory mass, abscesses, or evidence of malnutrition should be hospitalized and parenteral nutrition and antibiotic therapy started. Parenteral steroids may be started in these patients at a dosage of 40–60 mg/d once an infectious process can be excluded. Patients with recurrent Crohn's disease should be assessed for severity of recurrence, appearance of *Clostridium difficile,* and development of malabsorption as a result of short-bowel syndrome, bacterial overgrowth, or bile salt-induced diarrhea. If recurrent disease is a cause of the patient's symptoms, treatment may be instituted as for new disease. The clinician must always be alert for extraintestinal complications of Crohn's disease, such as iritis, uveitis, peripheral arthritis, erythema nodosum, pyoderma gangrenosum, sclerosing cholangitis, cholelithiasis, and cholecystitis.

a. **Nutritional therapy.** Nutritional support is essential in patients with Crohn's disease. Assessment of nutritional deficiencies should be made and replacements given as needed. Elemental diets have even been found to lead to remissions as often as steroid usage has in selected patients. Total parenteral nutrition should be considered in presurgical candidates, children with growth failure, and patients with malnutrition unable to tolerate oral feedings. Fistula outputs will decrease with total parenteral nutrition, but complete closure is unlikely. Vitamin B_{12} deficiency may occur with extreme ileal disease. Folate deficiency is seen with long-term sulfasalazine use.

b. **Surgical treatment of Crohn's disease.** Approximately 78% of Crohn's disease patients have a surgical resection within 20 years of onset of symptoms. However, surgery should be a last resort, and the minimal amount of bowel should be resected to relieve symptoms. The most common indications for surgery are bowel obstruction, fistula unresponsive to medical therapy, and abscesses. Abscesses usually will not respond to simple drainage and will require surgery. Toxic megacolon occurs less frequently in Crohn's disease than in chronic ulcerative colitis and usually responds better to conservative measures.

B. Malabsorption

Fat malabsorption is best defined as greater than 7 g of fat in a 24-hour stool collection while the patient is receiving a 100-g/d fat diet. Fat malabsorption may occur with factors that impair lipolysis (rapid intestinal transit, decreased bile circulation from bowel resection or liver disease), pancreatic insufficiency, or decreased absorptive area (Crohn's disease). Protein digestion depends on pancreatic enzymes as well as mucosal peptidases. Only in rare disorders, such as Hartnup's disease or cystinuria, is there preferential malabsorption of amino acids. Carbohydrate malabsorption may occur because of decreased pancreatic amylase, decreased mucosal disaccharidases, or general dysfunction of the brush border. Although certain nutritional deficiencies may predominate, most common malabsorptive syndromes affect absorption of a variety of minerals and vitamins. Excess fat in the stool contributes to increased diarrhea secondary to stimulation of colonic secretion by fatty acids. Fatty acids also form a complex with calcium, leaving oxalate to be absorbed, thus causing renal stone formation. Deficiencies of fat-soluble vitamins may lead to secondary hyperparathyroidism and osteoporosis with vitamin D deficiency and increased bleeding with vitamin K deficiency secondary to deficits of factors II, VII, IX, and X. Demyelination of the CNS with vitamin E deficiency has been reported. Disaccharidase deficiencies more commonly cause watery acidic diarrhea and increased flatulence.

1. CELIAC SPRUE. This disorder is caused by increased sensitivity of the small-bowel mucosa to gliadin proteins found in grains such as barley, oats, wheat, and rye. It has been reported that beer should also be excluded because of the hordein contained in malt (Clin Chim Acta 1990;189:123–130). Although celiac sprue may occur as a selective deficiency in iron (anemia), vitamin K (coagulopathy), or vitamin D (osteoporosis), it most commonly occurs as a cause of moderate steatorrhea and weight loss. Diagnosis can be established only by histologic demonstration of blunted small-bowel villi with recovery of the villi after gluten withdrawal (Clin Chim Acta 1987;163:1). Although patients usually recover within 2 months of therapy, some require up to a year.

    Complications of celiac sprue include small-bowel lymphoma in up to 13% of patients. There has also been an increased incidence of malignant GI disease, small-bowel ulcerations, and a syndrome similar to subacute combined degeneration of the spinal column. Vitamin supplementation should be considered in very ill patients. The most common reason for lack of response to gluten-free diets is the difficulty in eliminating sources of dietary gluten. In patients with unresponsive celiac sprue, after exclusion of tropical sprue, lymphoma, bacterial overgrowth syndromes, and Zollinger-Ellison syndrome, the use of steroids may be indicated. Prednisone should be given, 40 mg/d, and then decreased to a maintenance dosage of 10 mg/d to sustain near-normal serum protein levels.

2. INFECTIOUS CAUSES OF MALABSORPTION
    a. **Tropical sprue** occurs in patients who have recently visited tropical areas, such as the Far East, the Caribbean, or the Middle East (Gastroenterology 1981;80:590). The histologic appearance of the small bowel is identical to that in celiac sprue. However, these patients should be treated with vitamin supplementation (folate, 10 mg/d and vitamin B_{12}, 100 µg/d IM) as well as tetracycline, 250 mg qid. In patients unable to tolerate tetracycline, either sulfamethazine

2 g/d or chloramphenicol 500 mg qid may be used until nutritional parameters and small-intestinal villi improve (approximately 3 to 4 weeks).

b. **Bacterial overgrowth** may cause malabsorption by deconjugation of bile salts or direct utilization of vitamins. This spectrum of diseases may be caused by motility disturbances, such as scleroderma or pseudoobstruction, or by disturbances of the anatomy of the small intestine, as occurs in Crohn's disease, small-bowel diverticula, fistula formation, or creation of afferent loops. Careful culturing of aerobic organisms of at least 10^6/mL or 10^4 anerobes from the small intestine is diagnostic. Broad-spectrum antibiotics can be used to suppress bacterial overgrowth. Tetracycline 250 mg qid for a course of 1 to 2 weeks should be used. Patients may require repeated courses of therapy, alternating antibiotics such as metronidazole, ampicillin, trimethoprim-sulfamethoxazole, or neomycin. Some gastroenterologists have advocated C14-glycocholate breath tests to monitor treatment success.

c. **Whipple's disease** is a systemic bacterial infection that causes hyperpigmentation, fever, arthralgias, diarrhea, and confusion (Mayo Clin Proc 1988;63:539–551). Although the organism has not been cultured, it can be observed in the intestinal mucosa, peripheral lymph nodes, cardiovascular system, pulmonary system, and CNS. Recently, PCR has been used to identify the organism. Recommended therapy is trimethoprim-sulfamethoxazole 1 double-strength tablet bid for at least 1 year. If CNS involvement is evident at initiation of therapy, use of penicillin and streptomycin IM for the first 2 weeks of therapy has been associated with fewer relapses. Nutritional supplementation is given as folic acid 2 mg/d. Alternatives to trimethoprim-sulfamethoxazole are chloramphenicol 250 mg qid for 6 to 12 months, oral penicillin 250 mg qid, or oral tetracycline 250 mg qid. Long-term therapy for at least 2 years with tetracycline has been suggested to reduce the number of relapses.

d. *Giardia lamblia* is one of the most common parasitic infections causing malabsorption and may be seen in either stool or duodenal aspirates. Therapy should begin with either metronidazole 250 mg tid for 1 week or quinacrine hydrochloride 100 mg tid for 5 days. A second course may be necessary in up to 10% of patients. Other protozoan causes of malabsorption include *Cryptosporidium* species and *Isospora belli*, which are currently being found as a cause of malabsorption in immunosuppressed patients. No current therapy has been demonstrated to be successful in the eradication of *Cryptosporidium*. Trimethoprim-sulfamethoxazole one double-strength tablet PO qid for 1 week and then bid for 3 weeks is currently recommended for the treatment of *I. belli*.

3. **DISACCHARIDASE DEFICIENCIES.** Lactose intolerance due to the brush border deficiency of lactase is a common cause of bloating and diarrhea. It may be diagnosed by oral administration of lactose or by hydrogen breath tests. Deficiency of lactase activity may also be secondary to diseases that injure the brush border mucosal cells, such

as infectious diarrheas, Crohn's disease, and celiac disease. Treatment is either avoidance of lactose-containing foods or use of lactase packets added to milk products to predigest the lactose.

4. **SHORT-BOWEL SYNDROME.** The loss of more than 100 cm of terminal ileum is associated with malabsorption of fat. However, a small bowel that is 100 cm or longer will still allow oral nutrition with supplementation. Patients with resection of the terminal ileum should receive supplementary vitamin B_{12} 100 µg IM each month. Cholestyramine can be titrated to control diarrhea if less than 100 cm of terminal ileum has been removed. The use of pancreatic extracts, such as Viokase or Pancrease 3 or 4 capsules with each meal, may aid in fatty digestion. H_2-receptor antagonists may be useful in the first month after lengthy small-bowel resections because of the hyperacidity that occurs in this period. Antidiarrheal agents, such as loperamide or diphenoxylate, and atropine may help decrease dumping and increase mucosal contact time with nutrients. Use of medium-chain triglycerides (6–10 carbon fatty acids) bypasses the need for micellar formation and supplies vital calories. Fat-soluble (A, D, K, E) and water-soluble (B, C, folate) vitamins and minerals (calcium, magnesium, iron, zinc) should also be supplemented as needed. Somatostatin analogs (100 µg SC bid) have been shown to decrease the volume of diarrhea and the amount of fluid needed for maintenance in these patients (Digestion 1990;45 (suppl 1):77–83).

C. Intestinal Ischemia and Obstruction

For management purposes, small-bowel obstruction should be divided into mechanical obstruction and ileus. Ileus may be treated with fluid resuscitation and stomach decompression using suction. If symptoms are chronic, intestinal pseudoobstruction should be considered after drug effect is excluded. Mechanical small-bowel obstructions must be divided further into partial small-bowel obstruction (which is treated like an ileus) and complete mechanical small-bowel obstruction (which should be managed surgically because of the high incidence of small-bowel ischemia). With mechanical small-bowel obstruction, a tube should be placed beyond the ligament of Treitz for intermittent suction and decompression. Small-bowel ischemia may be caused by embolism or thrombosis and should be treated either by surgery or angiography with angioplasty. Nonocclusive mesenteric insufficiency may be treated with arteriographic infusion of papavarine. Despite these measures, the mortality in mesenteric ischemia approaches 50%.

Brandt LJ, Berstein LH, Boley SJ, et al. Metronidazole therapy for perineal Crohn's disease: a follow-up study. Gastroenterology 1982;83:383.

Clinical Conference. Tropical sprue in travelers and expatriates living abroad. Gastroenterology 1981;80:590.

Davidson AG, Bridges MA. Coeliac disease: a critical review of aetiology and pathogenesis. Clin Chim Acta 1987;163:1.

Fleming JL, Wiesner RH, Shorter RG. Whipple's disease: clinical, biochemical, and histopathologic features and assessment of treatment in 29 patients. Mayo Clin Proc 1988;63:539–551.

Linn FV, Peppercorn MA. Drug therapy for inflammatory bowel disease: Part II. Am J Surg 1992;164:178–185.

Nightingale JM, Walker ER, Burnham WR, et al. Short bowel syndrome. Digestion 1990;45(Suppl 1):77–83.

Shanbhogue LK, Molenaar JC. Short bowel syndrome: metabolic and surgical management. Br J Surg 1994;81:486–499.

Summers RW, Switz DM, Sessions JT, et al. National Cooperative Crohn's Disease Study: results of drug treatment. Gastroenterology 1987;77:847.

Stokes MA. Crohn's disease and nutrition. Br J Surg 1992;79:391–394.

IV. COLONIC DISEASES

A. Chronic Ulcerative Colitis

This is an idiopathic inflammatory disease of the colonic mucosa and submucosa that causes symptoms of tenesmus, pain, and repeated episodes of bloody diarrhea. Its peak incidence is in the 20- to 40-year-old age group. It has been associated with an increased risk of colon cancer and development of primary sclerosing cholangitis. Treatment depends on its extent and severity.

1. **THERAPY**
   a. **Disease assessment.** Extent is best established with colonoscopy during a period of relative quiescence. Involvement may be purely distal as in ulcerative proctitis (disease limited to the distal 12 cm of the colon), proctosigmoiditis, or any proximal extension of disease including the entire colon. Primarily left-sided disease (proctitis or proctosigmoiditis) may respond to topical agents. Severity is generally established by clinical parameters.
      (1) *Mild disease* usually implies fewer than 4 bowel movements a day with minimal systemic symptoms (fever, weight loss) and very little hematochezia.
      (2) *Moderate disease* involves approximately 4–10 bowel movements a day, with low-grade fever (not exceeding 101°F [38.3°C]), mild abdominal pain, and no evidence of nutritional deficiencies.
      (3) *Severe disease* usually involves high fever, severe abdominal pain, evidence of nutritional compromise, severe GI bleeding requiring transfusions, or evidence of toxic megacolon. Generally, moderate to severe disease should be treated in the hospital with parenteral anti-inflammatory agents.
   b. **Sulfasalazine.** Sulfasalazine is a first-line agent in treatment of chronic ulcerative colitis, in disease of any severity with involvement of more than the rectum. Sulfasalazine, as in Crohn's disease, is usually given in a dosage of 3–4 g/d in 2 to 4 divided doses. Administration should be gradually increased to therapeutic dosages over a 1-week period, starting from 500 mg bid. Dosages higher than 4 g/d rarely prove beneficial. There is usually a response to sulfasalazine within a 2-week period. If no response occurs, sulfasalazine should still be continued with the addition of other agents. If there is response to sulfasalazine, therapy should be continued until clinical and endoscopic evidence of remission is seen. Then the drug may be decreased to 2 g/d for maintenance. Patients with limited proctitis or proctosigmoiditis on initial treatment may not need maintenance therapy. If maintenance therapy is begun, it should be continued for at least 3 years. Sulfasalazine may cause exacerbation

of ulcerative colitis, nausea, headache, rashes, myeloblastic anemia, pancreatitis, alveolitis, and oligospermia.

c. **5-Aminosalicylic acid.** 5-ASA (mesalamine) is thought to be the active moiety in sulfasalazine. Osalazine (Dipentum) is available (500 mg bid) for ulcerative colitis in patients intolerant of sulfasalazine. Asacol (400 mg, two tablets tid) can also be used for colonic disease. Mesalamine (Rowasa) is available as a rectal suppository (4 g/60 mL) to be used at bedtime and retained for 8 hours in patients with proctosigmoiditis. The role of oral 5-ASA at a dose of 0.8 g/d would be as a second-line agent after failure of or intolerance to sulfasalazine. The enema form should be used as a substitute for cortisone enemas or as treatment in those cases unresponsive to corticosteroid enemas.

d. **Corticosteroids.** Cortisone enemas can be given as first-line therapy for left-sided disease. Ulcerative proctosigmoiditis or proctitis can be treated with a once-a-night steroid enema (100 mg hydrocortisone HS), which should be retained for 8 hours. This is usually initiated for a 2-week trial period that may be increased to a twice-daily regimen. It should not be continued longer than a month without response. Oral steroids can be used in mild to moderate colitis that does not respond to sulfasalazine. Prednisone is usually started at 30–60 mg/d and continued for about a 2-week period. If a response is noted, the dosage can be withdrawn at a rate of approximately 5 mg/wk. Limited distal colitis that is unresponsive to local therapy and sulfasalazine usually is unresponsive to systemic steroids as well. Therefore, therapeutic trials of oral prednisone in these patients should be kept brief. Severe ulcerative colitis should be treated with systemic steroids, usually given as a bolus of prednisolone 60–80 mg/d or methylprednisolone 40–60 mg/d in divided doses. Corticotropin has been advocated by some authorities as more efficacious in patients who have not had steroids in the past. The dosage is 120 U/d. Patients should be gradually weaned from corticosteroids if possible, and a maintenance dosage of sulfasalazine (500 mg qid) should be continued to prevent relapse.

e. **Immunosuppressive agents.** Azathioprine and its metabolite, 6-mercaptopurine, have been used in therapy of refractory ulcerative colitis. Most often, azathioprine is administered in a dosage of 2 mg/kg/d and will permit a decrease in steroid use. Mean time of onset of symptomatic relief is 3 months after initiation of therapy. Monthly monitoring of blood counts is necessary because of possible bone marrow suppression. Drug therapy should be halted if leukocyte counts fall below 4000. Side effects of medication include rash, fever, joint pain, hepatitis, pancreatitis, and immune suppression. Cyclosporine has been shown to be of benefit in severe disease at a dose of 2.5–5 mg/kg/d. It will induce and maintain disease remission, although usage must be carefully monitored because of renal toxicity, hypertension, and CNS effects.

f. **Antidiarrheal agents.** These may be used in patients with minimally active disease to control symptoms of diarrhea. Loperamide, tincture of opium, belladonna, and diphenoxylate with atropine have all been used to decrease the number of bowel movements. These agents may be used for patients who have episodes of nocturnal diarrhea that cannot be controlled with other methods but should not be used in any patient with acute moderate to severe symptoms because of the risk of precipitating toxic megacolon.

g. **Nutrition.** Although no specific diet has been found to be helpful in ulcerative colitis, it is important for patients to avoid foods that seem to create increased diarrhea, bloating, and flatulence. Calcium supplementation should be considered in patients receiving steroids. Iron and folate replacement is sometimes necessary in patients with chronic disease. For the seriously ill, TPN should be used to improve overall status if oral intake is going to be restricted for longer than 2 weeks.

2. COMPLICATIONS
   a. **Toxic megacolon.** Toxic megacolon occurs in severe colitis with fever, tachycardia, abdominal pain, abdominal distention, and radiologic evidence of dilatation of the transverse colon greater than 6 cm in diameter. It is usually found in recurrent ulcerative colitis as opposed to the initial presentation. Other causes of fulminant colitis, such as *Clostridium difficile, Salmonella, Shigella,* and *Campylobacter* should be excluded. Supportive care is extremely important, with careful management of fluid and electrolyte balances, blood transfusions, broad-spectrum antibiotics, and large doses of prednisolone (100–200 mg IV). Any anticholinergics or opiates should be discontinued.

   Patients should be kept NPO, with nasogastric tube placement and suction to help decompress the GI tract. Abdominal flat plates should be taken every day for the first 3 days to determine whether the colon is decreasing in diameter. If the colon continues to distend or does not shrink after 3 days, colectomy is generally recommended because of the high incidence of perforation. If the patient responds to these measures, steroids should be continued at high dosage for another 2 weeks. Some believe that Crohn's disease has a decreased incidence of perforation in toxic megacolon than with chronic ulcerative colitis and that it should be treated medically for a longer period. Patients responding to medical therapy are more prone to redevelop toxic megacolon in later flares of colitis and require colectomy (Am J Surg 1984;147:106).

   b. **Colon cancer risks.** Colon cancer rates in ulcerative colitis are highest in those who were less than 20 years of age at disease onset, in pancolitis, and in disease of more than 8 years duration. The incidence of colon cancer has been estimated at 1.4% after 14 years. Colon cancer associated with ulcerative colitis appears endoscopically to be flatter than cancers in the general population, thereby making diagnosis more difficult. *Surveillance colonoscopy is usually recommended after disease has been present longer than 8 years* (Med Clin North Am 1990;74:189). If no dysplasia is found, barium enema study can be alternated with colonoscopy and multiple biopsies on a yearly basis for continued surveillance. If moderate to severe dysplasia is found, colonoscopy with multiple biopsies should be done within 3 months. The area of dysplasia should be carefully identified, and colectomy should be performed because of the high association of occult malignancy with dysplasia.

  c. **Indications for surgery.** Colectomy generally should be recommended in patients with refractory toxic megacolon, suspected colon perforation, uncontrollable colonic hemorrhage, and severe ulcerative colitis that does not improve despite 2 weeks of intensive therapy. Other indications are dictated by the functional abilities of the patient, toxicities of medical therapy, and the long-term risk of malignant disease. Patients with long-standing disease would be considered for colectomy despite mild symptoms because of the increasing malignancy risk. It is useful to note that the operative mortality is approximately 3% in elective colectomy. Younger patients are candidates for ileal pouch anal anastomosis, which preserves bowel continuity and can provide long-term benefits. Pouchitis occurs in 10% to 45% of patients with a pouch and is manifested by bloody stools, increased stool frequency, fever, and malaise. Treatment is usually with metronidazole, topical steroids, or mesalamine.

B. Pseudomembranous Colitis

Pseudomembranous colitis is most commonly found as a sequela of prior antibiotic therapy (ampicillin, clindamycin, cephalosporins, penicillin), usually occurring a week after administration (Rev Infect Dis 1990;12 [Suppl 2]:S243). In the absence of antibiotic exposure, the disease is usually more difficult to eradicate and has a higher relapse incidence. Symptoms generally are fever, bloody diarrhea, and abdominal pain. Although the disease is produced by proliferation of *Clostridium difficile,* it can be diagnosed by detection of the toxin in the stool as well as by culture. Endoscopic evaluation may reveal small yellowish white plaquelike pseudomembranes.

Vancomycin is highly effective in the therapy of pseudomembranous colitis when given orally 125–500 mg qid. Although it is poorly absorbed, it should be carefully monitored when given in the presence of renal failure (Med Clin North Am 1982;66:655). Metronidazole, 500 mg qid, has been found to be equally effective and much less expensive, although a few resistant strains of *C. difficile* have been reported. Bacitracin is also used as treatment (25,000 U qid). Generally these regimens should be continued for 1 to 2 weeks. Ion exchange resins, such as cholestyramine, have been used to bind the toxin of *C. difficile* and decrease diarrhea. Cholestyramine may be given in dosages of 3 g qid. Unfortunately, relapses may occur in as many as 20% of the patients within 3 weeks of discontinuing therapy. Several methods have been advocated to deal with such relapses, including reinstituting a course of metronidazole and adding cholestyramine during the last days of therapy and continuing it for another week after discontinuing antibiotic therapy.

C. Diverticular Disease

This is diagnosed by the presence of multiple herniations of the colonic mucosa through the muscular colonic wall. Diverticuli are associated with increasing age and long exposure to a Western diet. It is generally believed that diverticuli occur secondary to high intraluminal pressure caused by colonic hypermotility and decreased intraluminal mass resulting from lack of dietary fiber. Patients are usually asymptomatic; however, spasmodic left lower quadrant pain may be present. Therapy involves increasing stool bulk with such agents as psyllium, methylcellulose, and bran. In patients with abdominal pain, antispasmodics such as probanthine bromide 15 mg 3 tid have been found effective.

Diverticulitis occurs in approximately one fifth of patients with diverticulosis. Most commonly, pain and fever are the presenting symptoms. This may be associated with upper GI upset as well as changes in bowel habits. The diagnosis is most often made clinically with the prior diagnosis of diverticulosis. However, careful flexible sigmoidoscopy can be valuable in diagnosing acute diverticulitis. If the pain is localized and there are no peritoneal symptoms, broad-spectrum antibiotics, such as ampicillin or a cephalosporin, can be used. However, if there is high fever, leukocytosis, or evidence of peritoneal irritation, the patient should be admitted to the hospital, and broad-spectrum parenteral antibiotics should be given, with anaerobic coverage. Antibiotics should be given for approximately 1 week to 10 days unless there is perforation of the colon. Complications from diverticulitis include the formation of enteroperitoneal abscesses and bowel obstruction secondary to stricture. Fistulas may form between the colon and any adjacent organ, including the bladder, vagina, or small bowel. Fistulas to the bladder are the most common and are difficult to identify. However, computed tomography of the bladder appears to be very sensitive in demonstrating air in the bladder, confirming the presence of a fistula. Surgical resection is necessary when abscesses, fistulas, or strictures appear.

D. Irritable Bowel Syndrome

Irritable bowel syndrome (IBS) is the most common GI disorder faced by the practitioner. Its cardinal manifestations are abdominal pain and either constipation or diarrhea. IBS generally occurs in the 20- to 30-year-old age group and should be diagnosed only when other conditions are excluded. Its cause is unknown; however, several studies have indicated that patients have an increased response to colonic distention in terms of pain perception. There may also be a relationship between increased cluster contractions in the small bowel and the pain. Patients need to be educated about the excellent prognosis of this disorder but should also be reminded of its chronic nature. Diagnostic criteria for IBS are listed in Table 8–4. High-fiber diets should be initiated in most patients, while recognizing that most will have some exacerbation within the first month of therapy. Bulking agents also should be added, with increased liquid intake to prevent stools from becoming too dehydrated from the stool softener's hydrophilic properties. Antispasmodic anticholinergic agents, such as dicyclomine hydrochloride, may be used, starting at 10 mg qid, with gradual increases to as high as 40 mg qid. Newer antimuscarinic agents, such as cimetropium bromide (50 mg PO tid), are under study. Patients primarily with diarrhea may respond to the addition of either diphenoxylate and atropine 2.5–5 mg qid or loperamide 2–4 mg tid. Analgesics, such as pentazocine 50–100 mg qid, may be prescribed for short periods. Antiflatulents may also provide some relief in

TABLE 8-4. Diagnostic Criteria for Irritable Bowel Syndrome

The following symptoms should be present for more than 3 mo:
1. Abdominal pain or discomfort that is relieved with defecation, associated with a change in the frequency of the stool, or associated with a change in stool consistency
2. Two or more of the following present at least 25% of the time
   a. More than three bowel movements a day or less than three bowel movements a week
   b. Altered stool shape
   c. Altered stool passage
   d. Passage of mucus
   e. Bloating or abdominal distention

patients who complain of bloating. Simethicone 2–4 tablets qid or activated charcoal 4 tablets qid supplies some gas relief. Depression may be present in these patients and can be treated with a single bedtime dose of amitriptyline 25–50 mg. If diarrhea is present, imipramine can be used to take advantage of anticholinergic effects. Paroxetine can decrease intestinal transit and may be of use in constipation-predominant IBS. There is no convincing evidence that any therapy is uniformly effective in IBS (Gastroenterology 1988;95:232).

E. Constipation

Constipation is a common symptom reported by 21% of American women (Dig Dis Sci 1989;34:1153). It is difficult to define and is usually related to the individual's expectations. However, two or fewer stools per week is generally considered evidence of constipation. Constipated stools are hard and contain less than 50% water. Constipation may be caused by any mechanism that increases stool transit time, increases colonic absorption of fluid, or disturbs the bacterial content of the colon. Lesions such as anal fissures or hemorrhoids may cause pain and decreased evacuation of the colon. Hirschsprung's disease is usually detected in childhood but may be diagnosed in adults by anal manometry and a rectal biopsy showing aganglionosis. When the cause is idiopathic, several modifications may be made. Increasing dietary bulk corrects constipation in about two thirds of patients (Clin Ther 1989;11:572). Some patients feel less urge to defecate and require modification of their daily schedule in an attempt to defecate at least once a day. Glycerin suppositories may help them by lubricating the stool, thus assisting in emptying the rectum. Inability to relax the rectosigmoid angle during defecation may require the use of biofeedback techniques to retrain rectal reflexes. Some patients, predominately female, have markedly increased colonic transit times, symptoms of abdominal bloating, pain, and a history of laxative abuse. Their symptoms may be aggravated by increased dietary fiber.

F. Chronic Diarrhea

This is defined as diarrhea of longer than 6 weeks duration. It may be divided into two subgroups: osmotic and secretory, based on stool osmolality and persistence of diarrhea with fasting. The osmolar gap found in chronic osmotic diarrheas is most often secondary to either factitial causes with unabsorbed cations, such as magnesium, or disaccharidase deficiencies, such as lactose intolerance. Chronic secretory diarrhea persists with fasting and most commonly is due to bile salt and fatty acid malabsorption. Factitial diarrhea from laxative abuse is common when there are no other detectable causes. Endocrine tumors, such as VIPoma (VIP, vasoactive intestinal peptide), and carcinoid syndrome also produce secretory diarrhea. Collagenous or lymphocytic colitis is a cause of secretory diarrhea, which can be diagnosed only by colonic biopsy.

Therapy consists primarily of careful fluid management, especially with stool outputs greater than 1 L/d. Various oral rehydration solutions are available that primarily supply glucose in combination with sodium, taking advantage of their cotransport mechanism in the small intestine. Opiates, diphenoxylate and atropine 1–2 tablets qid, loperamide 2–4 mg bid, and codeine 30–60 mg qid can be used to decrease the symptoms of chronic diarrheas. Most of these have side effects, such as drowsiness, nausea and vomiting, and respiratory depression. However, loperamide can be used in dosages up to 35 mg/d without significant toxicity. Alpha-adrenergics such as clonidine may be used for chronic diabetic diarrheas in particular. It should be started at 0.1 mg/d and gradually increased to 0.3–0.4 mg/d as tolerated. Patients often develop postural hypotension and drowsiness at high dosages.

In patients with VIPomas, such medications as lithium 300 mg/d and prednisone 60 mg/d are helpful in controlling diarrhea. Lithium has well-known hematologic, CNS, and cardiovascular side effects. Prednisone should be started at 60 mg/d but should be decreased as soon as possible to decrease side effects. Somatostatin, given as 100 µg SC bid, has been found to decrease diarrhea secondary to endocrine tumors but produces steatorrhea and decreased glucose tolerance as its side effects.

G. Colonic Polyps

Small colonic polyps discovered on colon x-ray should generally be followed by colonoscopy for surveillance for additional polyps. A 50% chance of discovering synchronous adenomatous polyps exists. If histologically the polyp is a tubular, tubulovillous, or villous adenoma, the patient should undergo colonic surveillance. If more than three polyps or a large adenomatous polyp (>3 cm) is found or if poor preparation is found, colonoscopy can be repeated in 1 year. If localized carcinoma is found, the patient should be reexamined in 3 months. Otherwise, patients need only be reexamined with colonoscopy in 3 years unless other medical conditions modify this need. Polyps larger than 1 cm have at least a 1% chance of malignancy, and they should be removed and examined histologically. The need for polyp removal is increased based on size and the patient's history. If adenomatous polyps are found, surveillance should be instituted as with small adenomatous polyps. Patients with a family history of hereditary colon cancer require early colonoscopy starting by age 18. In familial polyposis syndromes, screening should begin at age 10 with flexible sigmoidoscopy and be continued until at least age 40 to be certain that polyps do not develop.

Camilleri M, Prather CM. The irritable bowel syndrome: mechanisms and a practical approach to management. Ann Intern Med 1992;116(Pt 1):1001–1008.
Choi PM, Targan SR. Immunomodulator therapy in inflammatory bowel disease. Dig Dis Sci 1994;39:1885–1892.

Fekety R, Shah AB. Diagnosis and treatment of *Clostridium difficile* colitis. JAMA 1993;269:71–75.

Grant CS, Dozois RR. Toxic megacolon: ultimate fate of patients after successful medical management. Am J Surg 1984;147:106–110.

Grotz RL, Pemberton JH. The ileal pouch operation for ulcerative colitis. Surg Clin North Am 1993;73:909–932.

Hanauer SB, Baert F. Medical therapy of inflammatory bowel disease. Med Clin North Am 1994;78:1413–1426.

Katz J. The course of inflammatory bowel disease. Med Clin North Am 1994;78:1275–1280.

Klein KB. Controlled treatment trials in the irritable bowel syndrome: a critique. Gastroenterology 1988;95:232–241.

Korelitz BI. Considerations of surveillance, dysplasia, and carcinoma of the colon in the management of ulcerative colitis and Crohn's disease. Med Clin North Am 1990;74:189–199.

Lewis JD, Fisher RL. Nutrition support in inflammatory bowel disease. Med Clin North Am 1994;78:1443–1456.

Lynn RB, Friedman LS. Irritable bowel syndrome. Managing the patient with abdominal pain and altered bowel habits. Med Clin North Am 1995;79:373–390.

Mills LR, Schuman BM, Thompson WO. Lymphocytic colitis. A definable clinical and histological diagnosis. Dig Dis Sci 1993;38:1147–1151.

Schroeder KW, Tremaine WJ, Ilstrup DM. Coated oral 5-aminosalicyclic acid therapy for mildly to moderately active ulcerative colitis: a randomized study. N Engl J Med 1987;317:1625.

Snape WJ Jr. The effect of methylcellulose on symptoms of constipation. Clin Ther 1989;11:572–579.

Thompson WG. Irritable bowel syndrome: pathogenesis and management. Lancet 1993;341:1569–1572.

Winawer SJ, Zauber AG, O'Brien MJ, et al. Randomized comparison of surveillance intervals after colonoscopic removal of newly diagnosed adenomatous polyps. The National Polyp Study Workgroup. N Engl J Med 1993;328:901–906.

V. ANORECTAL DISORDERS

A. Hemorrhoids

Hemorrhoids are a submucosal venous plexus found in the upper anal canal. External hemorrhoids are those dilated veins that are found below the dentate line. External hemorrhoids usually cause pain only when thrombosed. Frequently this pain persists only for the first 48 hours. If the patient is seen within that time, excision of the clot is the treatment of choice. If the pain has already begun to subside, sitz baths are usually sufficient.

Internal hemorrhoids are the dilated venous plexus found above the dentate line. These are usually responsible for the rectal outlet bleeding the patient experiences and are treated by decreasing abdominal straining and by fixing the prolapsing hemorrhoidal tissue. Decreased abdominal straining can be accomplished by giving bulk-forming agents and thereby decreasing strain in defecation. If substantial prolapse of internal hemorrhoids exists, the tissue may be fixed by rubber band ligation, injection, or hemorrhoidectomy. Infrared or laser coagulation can be used but may be associated with a greater risk of recurrent hemorrhoids. Treatment of hemorrhoids in HIV-positive patients should be as conservative as possible, as there have been recent reports of abscess formation after rubber band ligation.

B. Anal Fissure

An anal fissure is a tear of the squamous cell-lined portion of the anal canal. It is generally less than 1 cm in size and produces severe burning pain during bowel movements. It may also be a cause of rectal outlet bleeding. Most anal fissures are secondary to passage of very firm and large stools. Acute anal fissures should be treated with sitz baths, topical anesthetics, and stool bulking agents. Patients should be able to pass stools without discomfort if this therapy is to succeed. If the fissure becomes chronic, surgical intervention, usually in the form of a lateral sphincterotomy, is indicated.

C. Rectal Abscesses and Fistulas

Rectal abscesses are generally characterized by severe rectal pain, tenderness, and high fever. Suspected abscesses should be surgically evaluated and drained. Fistulas are most often secondary to prior incompletely healed rectal abscesses. They usually begin in the anal canal crypt and extend into the perianal skin region. Fistulas rarely heal by themselves, requiring surgical intervention.

D. Infectious Proctitis

Most cases of infectious proctitis are sexually transmitted. *Chlamydia trachomatis,* probably the most common cause of sexually transmitted disease, can now be easily cultured. Therapy is usually tetracycline 500 mg qid for 1 week. Gonococcal proctitis may occur in homosexual males or in females, spreading from gonococcal cervical disease. Penicillin therapy is recommended unless a resistant strain of organism is present. Then treatment with ceftriaxone 250 mg IM can eradicate the organism. In homosexuals, empiric therapy with penicillin (4.8 million U procaine penicillin IM and probenecid 1 g PO) followed by tetracycline 100 mg PO bid may be beneficial for early relief of symptoms pending cultures (JAMA 1988;260:348). Herpetic rectal infections cause severe pain and may lead to constipation. The presence of characteristic erythematous grouped vesicles usually confirms the diagnosis. Topical acyclovir ointment may decrease the duration of viral replication. Oral acyclovir 400 mg 5 times per day also decreases viral replication and formation of new lesions and leads to earlier resolution of symptoms.

E. Pruritus Ani

Pruritus ani is common but may be a symptom of many systemic illnesses, such as diabetes mellitus, jaundice, or lymphomas. *Candida* may involve this region and can be treated by topical 1% clotrimazole cream. A program of anal hygiene by careful cleansing of the region with a moist towel can decrease symptoms. Contact dermatitis may also be the cause of pruritus ani, from scented toilet paper, bath soaps, or laundry detergents. Removal of the agent and application of 1% topical hydrocortisone can speed relief.

Mazier WP. Hemorrhoids, fissures, and pruritus ani. Surg Clin North Am 1994;74:1277–1292.

VI. PANCREATIC DISEASES

A. Sphincter of Oddi Dysfunction

The sphincter of Oddi is thought to cause biliary colic by either stenosis of the lumen or hypertonicity of the sphincter (dyskinesia). The diagnosis can be established by endoscopic retrograde cholangiopancreatography (ERCP) and biliary manometry. Dysfunction is suggested by the elevation of serum alkaline phosphatase on at least two occasions. Both stenosis and dyskinesia of the sphincter can be treated with sphincterotomy (N Engl J Med 1989;320:82).

B. Acute Pancreatitis

This is known to occur in association with alcohol ingestion, gallstones, trauma to the pancreas, viral infections (mumps, herpes viruses, coxsackie, hepatitis), ischemia, hypertriglyceridemia, hypercalcemia, drugs (steroids, diuretics, sulfas, alpha methyldopa, and azathioprine), collagen vascular diseases, malignant disease, penetrating ulcers, and ERCP. The process is perpetuated by inappropriate activation of pancreatic enzymes and decreased inactivation by trypsin inhibitors. Therapy for acute alcoholic pancreatitis is determined by the severity of the disease. This can be established by using the Ranson criteria (Am J Gastroenterol 1982;77:633), which consist of:

- Criteria on entry: Age greater than 55; WBC greater than $16,000/mm^3$; blood sugar greater than 200 mg/dL; LDH greater than 350 IU/dL; SGOT greater than 250 IU/dL
- Criteria present during the first 48 hours: 10% or more decrease in hematocrit; 5 mg/dL rise in BUN; calcium below 8 mg/dL; >6 L of fluid retention; arterial Pao_2 less than 60 mm Hg; and a base deficit of more than 4 mEq/L

If fewer than 3 criteria are present, pancreatitis may be classified as mild; if more than 4 are present, severe pancreatitis with a poor prognosis is suggested. The degree of pancreatic necrosis may be correlated to the number of Ranson criteria present.

Computed tomography (CT) has been used to supply immediate staging information. A proposed classification based on the degree of inflammatory changes is presented in Table 8–5.

1. TREATMENT OF MILD PANCREATITIS
   a. **Rehydration** should be given immediately, with careful attention to fluid and electrolyte balance.
   b. **Nasogastric suction** should be used only if ileus or nausea and vomiting are present.
   c. **Analgesia** should be supplied with meperidine, 50–75 mg IM q4h prn, or via a patient-controlled anesthesia (PCA) pump.
   d. **Food** should be reinitiated after pain subsides and the patient's appetite returns. This should occur within the first week of

---

TABLE 8–5. **Classification of Pancreatitis Based on Inflammatory Changes Found on CT**

GRADE	FINDINGS ON CT OF THE PANCREAS
A	Normal pancreas
B	Enlargement of the pancreas without peripancreatic disease
C	Pancreatic changes with peripancreatic disease
D	Presence of solitary mass or phlegmon
E	Two or more phlegmon or masses

hospitalization, with serum amylases approaching normal levels. Liquids should be given initially as six small meals per day to reduce acid secretion, which in turn decreases pancreatic secretion. During this time, acid should be suppressed by giving antacids 1 hour postprandially or by an H_2-receptor blocker.

2. THERAPY FOR SEVERE PANCREATITIS
   a. Severe pancreatitis warrants **ICU admission** and careful fluid management with either wedged pulmonary artery pressures or a central venous pressure monitor. If fluid loss exceeds 5 L, colloid replacement should be initiated.
   b. **Nasogastric tube placement** should be instituted, with antacids given every hour as needed to keep the gastric pH greater than 4. IV H_2-receptor antagonists can also be used, as well as sucralfate, to prevent stress ulcer.
   c. **Meperidine** may be given for pain in dosages of 50–100 mg IM q4h or via a PCA pump.
   d. **Cardiac, renal, and pulmonary function** should be monitored for evidence of congestive heart failure, arrhythmias, acute tubular necrosis, atelectasis, pneumonia, pleural effusions, and ARDS.
   e. **Metabolic complications,** for example, **hyperglycemia,** may necessitate institution of insulin therapy early in the disease. **Hypocalcemia** may occur secondary to loss of serum albumin. If loss is severe, calcium can be replaced with 10 mL (1 g) of 10% calcium gluconate, which provides only 93 mg of elemental calcium. IV calcium should be administered over 10 to 15 minutes, with careful monitoring for cardiac arrythmias. Calcium should not be administered until hypokalemia is corrected. **Magnesium may be depleted concomitantly** with hypocalcemia and can be replaced by providing 8–40 mEq/L of fluid given over 4 to 6 hours.
   f. **Parenteral nutrition** should be instituted within 2 days of admission if nutritional intake is expected to be curtailed for a prolonged period. Standard parenteral nutrition formulas may be used. No deleterious effects have been ascribed to IV lipids.
   g. **Prophylactic antibiotics** are generally not indicated in acute pancreatitis unless it is thought to be due to biliary obstruction. Then, ciprofloxacin has been proposed to be the best agent because of its ability to cross the blood-pancreas barrier (Am J Surg 1989;158:472).
   h. **ERCP** should be performed in cases of biliary pancreatitis to remove the common bile duct stone as soon as possible. Sphincterotomy appears to decrease complications and decrease mortality.
   i. **Inhibitors of pancreatic secretions,** such as somatostatin, glucagon, or anticholinergics, or anti-inflammatory drugs, such as steroids, have not been shown to improve survival.

3. COMPLICATIONS. Disseminated intravascular coagulation may occur and should be treated by replacement of blood factors with fresh frozen plasma. Bleeding may appear secondary to stress ulceration, esophageal varices, and bowel infarctions due to vascular thrombosis from pancreatic inflammation. Acidosis may be secondary to ketoacidosis

from hyperglycemic or alcoholic causes, lactic acidosis resulting from decreased perfusion, or ingestion of salicylate-containing or ethylene glycol-containing drugs. Jaundice may be intrahepatic, secondary to the disease process, or extrahepatic, due to retained common bile duct stones or edema of the head of the pancreas. Pancreatic abscess is a dreaded complication, with almost 100% mortality if not surgically debrided. Diagnosis should be established by CT scan to look for gas in either pseudocysts or a pancreatic phlegmon. If infection is suspected, some authors suggest that aspiration of pancreatic fluid via CT-guided biopsy and culturing for bacteria may be beneficial. Use of peritoneal lavage in patients with severe pancreatitis is controversial. Some believe that in patients with profound pancreatitis with pancreatic ascites and evidence of shock, peritoneal lavage may be instituted with a peritoneal dialysis catheter and infusion of standard dialysis fluids into the abdomen (N Engl J Med 1985;312:399). This fluid can be gravity drained continuously to wash out toxic pancreatic substances. Recent studies have advocated the combination of surgical debridement with local lavage (World J Surg 1988;12:255).

C. Chronic Pancreatitis

This diagnosis implies end-stage organ failure with endocrine insufficiency (diabetes mellitus) or exocrine insufficiency with steatorrhea. Chronic pain is also present in approximately 85% of patients. The diagnosis is most reliably made by duodenal intubation and collection of stimulated pancreatic secretions that are analyzed for bicarbonate and pancreatic enzyme content (Gastroenterology 1985;88:1973). Distortion of pancreatic structure can also be seen by ERCP or CT scan.

1. **THERAPY FOR PAIN.** Treatable causes of chronic pancreatitis, such as hypercalcemia, hypertriglyceridemia, and hemochromatosis, should be ruled out. Use of alcohol should be discontinued. Anatomic lesions, such as localized strictures of the pancreatic duct or pancreatic pseudocysts, should be sought. Surgical drainage procedures for pseudocysts are usually reserved for enlarging cysts (>6 cm), bleeding, or infection. CT or ultrasound-guided needle aspiration of pseudocysts may lead to their resolution. Some authorities believe pancreas divisum to be a cause of chronic pancreatitis (Gastroenterology 1985;89:1431). Sphincterotomy should be considered with caution in these patients. Narcotic analgesics should be used sparingly because of the high potential of addiction. Celiac ganglion blocks usually are ineffective unless in the setting of pancreatic cancer. Surgical options include total pancreatectomy and ligation of the pancreatic duct. Some authorities have advocated enzyme replacement with dosages similar to those used for pancreatic exocrine insufficiency to inhibit pancreatic secretion and decrease pain (Gastroenterology 1984;87:44). This is usually given for a period of 1 month.

2. **THERAPY FOR EXOCRINE INSUFFICIENCY.** Dietary modifications should be begun early in pancreatic insufficiency. These include increasing protein intake and decreasing fat to less than 20% of daily calories. Medium-chain triglycerides that do not require pancreatic digestion for

absorption should be the major source of fat calories. Enzymes can be replaced with supplements such as Viokase 8 tablets with each meal, Creon 10 3 capsules with each meal, Cotazym 6 capsules with each meal, or Pancrease MT10 (microencapsulated) 3 capsules with each meal. Enzyme supplements should be divided to give one third of the dose before eating, one third during the meal, and one third after the meal. If supplementation fails to correct the steatorrhea, other causes of malabsorption should be sought. If none are found, the addition of bicarbonate (650 mg with meals) or H_2-receptor antagonists may be necessary.

3. **THERAPY FOR ENDOCRINE INSUFFICIENCY.** Insulin therapy in chronic pancreatitis must be carefully monitored because of the lability of glucose absorption secondary to exocrine insufficiency and the absence of counterregulatory peptides, such as glucagon, during periods of hypoglycemia. Systems of insulin administration that increase flexibility and monitoring are advised.

D. Cystic Fibrosis

Sweat sodium and chloride secretion more than 60 mEq/L with appropriate clinical findings is diagnostic of this autosomal recessive illness. The genetic abnormality has been identified, and gene therapy may someday correct the disease. Nutritional supplementation is the primary GI management problem with this disease, which causes pancreatic insufficiency. Intestinal obstruction may occur secondary to viscous intestinal secretions mixed with partially digested food. This may result from noncompliance or overcompliance with pancreatic enzyme supplementation; 1 tablespoonful of mineral oil given with each meal usually relieves this problem. If it persists, a Gastrografin enema diluted with water to one-third strength is usually successful. Rectal prolapse occurs in 20% of patients but is usually amenable to increased pancreatic enzyme supplementation. Abnormal gallbladder function leading to a microgallbladder or cholelithiasis is found in upward of 40% of patients. Surgery is generally not indicated unless the patient has symptoms. Fatty liver is also commonly found in up to 30%. Liver disease may lead to cirrhosis and portal hypertension in as many as 5% of patients. Bleeding esophageal varices should be treated initially with sclerotherapy. Shunt procedures should be considered if the patient has sufficient pulmonary reserve.

Baker CC, Huynh T. Acute pancreatitis. Surgical management. Crit Care Clin 1995;11:311–322.
Balthazar EJ, Freeny PC, vanSonnenberg E. Imaging and intervention in acute pancreatitis. Radiology 1994;193:297–306.
Bank S, Chow KW. Diagnostic tests in chronic pancreatitis. Gastroenterologist 1994;2:224–232.
Buchler MW, Binder M, Friess H. Role of somatostatin and its analogues in the treatment of acute and chronic pancreatitis. Gut 1994;35(3 Suppl):S15–19.
Calleja GA, Barkin JS. Acute pancreatitis. Med Clin North Am 1993;77:1037–1056.
Cotton PB. Pancreas divisum—curiosity or culprit. Gastroenterology 1985;89:1431.
Geenen JE, Hogan WJ, Dodds WJ, et al. The efficacy of endoscopic sphincterotomy after cholecystectomy in patients with spincter-of-Oddi dysfunction. N Engl J Med 1989;320:82–87.
Keogan MT, Baker ME. Computed tomography and magnetic resonance imaging in the assessment of pancreatic disease. Gastrointest Endosc Clin North Am 1995;5:31–59.
Marshall JB. Acute pancreatitis. A review with an emphasis on new developments. Arch Intern Med 1993;153:1185–1198.

Ranson JHC. Etiological and prognostic factors in human acute pancreatitis. Am J Gastroenterol 1982;77:633.

VII. MISCELLANEOUS

A. Chronic Idiopathic Abdominal Pain

By definition, chronic idiopathic abdominal pain consists of pain of more than 6 months duration, absence of physical or laboratory abnormalities, lack of response to symptomatic therapy, and deterioration of functional status. Treatment should be based on the understanding that chronic pain primarily comes from the evaluative brain centers rather than the peripheral nerves. Therapy should be based on

- Confirmation of the reality of the pain to the patient
- Careful explanation of the chronic nature of the pain and the likelihood that the pain will persist
- Behavior modification techniques to increase physical activity and the patient's coping skills with the assistance of psychiatric consultation
- Avoidance of such medications as aspirin, narcotics, and benzodiazepines, as these are primarily effective only with acute pain
- Use of tricyclic antidepressants in patients with depressive symptoms

Treatment of chronic pain depends on the combined efforts of primary care physicians, physical therapists, and psychiatrists to bring patients to a functional level.

B. Gastrointestinal Bleeding

1. **UPPER GASTROINTESTINAL BLEEDING.** Upper GI bleeding remains a diagnostic and therapeutic challenge because its 10% mortality rate has not decreased in the past 30 years. Any degree of upper GI bleeding must be considered major until proved otherwise. The patient's hemodynamic status must be assessed. Orthostatic changes in blood pressure (a decrease in diastolic blood pressure of more than 15 mm Hg or an increase in pulse rate of 20 beats/min) indicate a 15% loss of blood volume. Hypotension at rest indicates a blood volume loss of at least 25%. Large-bore IV lines should be established and crystalloid given immediately. Laboratory tests should investigate the presence of chronic anemia, hemolysis, coagulation abnormalities, liver dysfunction, or renal dysfunction. Packed red blood cells may be used for blood replacement. Gastric lavage should be instituted with a large-bore tube and infusion of about 200–300 mL of tap water. There is no evidence that lavage with vasoconstrictive agents or cold water is routinely effective. Because 85% to 90% of upper GI bleeding stops on its own in the first 24 hours, endoscopy of all patients is not necessary. If gastric lavage reveals no evidence of active bleeding, patients may be carefully monitored and treated with either antacids, H_2-receptor blockers, or a proton pump inhibitor. There is currently no evidence to suggest that medical therapy for active GI bleeding is effective. However, common practice is to start acid suppression in hopes of preventing future rebleeding. Patients who are actively bleeding or who are not actively bleeding but are older than 60, hemodynamically unstable, require

more than 3 U of blood, have a coagulopathy, or have bleeding while hospitalized should have endoscopy at the earliest opportunity. Depending on the results of this procedure, therapy can be instituted as follows.

a. **Gastric or duodenal ulcer** (40% of hemorrhages). Antacids, H_2-receptor blockers, sucralfate, or proton pump inhibitor may be used if there are no active signs of bleeding. If bleeding is present or a vessel is visible at the base of the ulcer (associated with more than 5 units of blood loss within 24 hours and a 50% chance of emergency surgery), the use of electrocoagulation, heater probe, injection therapy, or laser therapy is indicated (Gastroenterology 1986; 90:217). If bleeding continues, surgical intervention is warranted. If no active bleeding is seen, medical therapy, including treatment of *H. pylori* if present, may be sufficient unless bleeding recurs. Treatment of *H. pylori* is associated with a 90% decrease in ulcer recurrence.

b. **Gastritis and duodenitis** (25% of hemorrhages). These usually respond to removal of the irritating drug and administration of antacids, IV H_2-receptor blockers, omeprazole, lansoprazole, or sucralfate. In stress-related gastritis (severe trauma, CNS injury, or hepatic coma), IV H_2-receptor blocker therapy and antacids should be used to keep the pH greater than 4. Although there has been evidence that decreased gastric acidity may lead to increasing morbidity and mortality from bacterial colonization, the severity of the hemorrhage should determine the agents of choice (N Engl J Med 1987;317:1376).

c. **Variceal bleeding.** If active variceal bleeding is present, IV administration of vasopressin at a rate of 0.2–0.9 U/min and balloon tamponade with a Sengstaken-Blakemore tube or Minnesota tube should be initiated. Evidence exists that the addition of nitroglycerin, either sublingual or IV, may potentiate the effects of vasopressin and decrease its side effects. Balloon tamponade should generally be withdrawn within 24 hours to prevent pressure necrosis of the esophagus. Banding of varices or sclerotherapy should be initiated at the earliest opportunity. Somatostatin (4.2 µg/min) or octreotide (50 µg/h) has been used to treat variceal hemorrhage and has been successful in initially stopping bleeding (Am J Gastroenterol 1990;85:804). Surgical intervention is reserved for those patients who have either bled repeatedly despite sclerotherapy or are continuously hemorrhaging. Propranolol has been used in the prevention of rebleeding after initial variceal bleeding has not been established. Transjugular intrahepatic shunts are of value in the prevention of recurrent bleeding from varices.

d. **Esophagitis.** Antacids and omeprazole 20 mg qAM or lansoprazole 30 mg qAM for 4 to 6 weeks should be used to treat esophagitis or esophageal ulcers. Additional medication (40–60 mg of omeprazole or 60–90 mg of lansoprazole) may be necessary if inflammatory change persists.

e. **Mallory-Weiss tear.** This usually occurs at the gastroesophageal junction and may be treated initially with antacids, H_2-receptor blockers, or protein pump inhibitor. If the patient is vomiting, antiemetics can be given. In 90%, bleeding stops spontaneously. However, continued bleeding may necessitate the use of endoscopic therapy. Rarely, surgical intervention is necessary.

f. **Aortoenteric fistula.** If this is identified on endoscopy, surgery should be undertaken immediately. If massive hemorrhage is continuing despite normal results of upper GI endoscopy and an aortic graft is present, surgery is indicated. If no GI bleeding is noted, CT with IV contrast medium is sensitive for detecting aortic enteric fistulas.

g. **Bleeding neoplasms.** If hemorrhage continues, electrocoagulation, heater probe, or laser therapy is indicated. Resection of the tumor should be undertaken if this is thought to be possible.

2. LOWER GASTROINTESTINAL BLEEDING. Initial evaluation of lower GI bleeding should begin by excluding the presence of upper GI bleeding. Resuscitation and laboratory tests are similar to those in upper GI bleeding. Evaluation of major active bleeding should consist of a careful anal examination. This will usually detect rectal varices, rectal ulcers, and inflammatory bowel disease. If rapid bleeding persists, arteriography is the procedure of choice. This can localize the source of bleeding and also provide a method of therapy with intraarterial vasopressin administration or injection of thrombotic material. Bleeding scans have been controversial because of their low yield but may be valuable before arteriography to establish the presence of profuse bleeding. If the bleeding scan is positive, arteriography should be done immediately. If major bleeding has ceased, colonoscopy can be performed with a rapid preparation. If the GI bleeding is chronic and minimal, full evaluation should again begin with careful anal examination, proctoscopy followed by colonoscopy, and then upper GI endoscopy. If all of these fail to reveal a bleeding source, small-bowel x-rays may be obtained. Enteroclysis has been found by some investigators to be of greater sensitivity in detecting bleeding lesions. Radionuclide scans are usually not useful in chronic bleeding because of the variability of active bleeding. Angiography may be of value in detecting arteriovenous malformations when results of all other studies have been negative. Small-bowel endoscopy has been used with some success in this situation.

a. **Diverticular bleeding.** Diverticular bleeding most commonly occurs from diverticula in the right colon (60%). It is usually secondary to arterial bleeding and is most often self-limited. It recurs in less than half the patients. If bleeding is major or recurrent, angiography is the best means to document the site. Emergency colonoscopy can often be deceived by the presence of clots in nonbleeding diverticula. If the site of bleeding is found, intraarterial vasopressin can be given. Definitive therapy is usually surgical resection of the involved diverticula.

b. **Arteriovenous malformations.** These are becoming increasingly recognized as a cause of chronic GI bleeding. Usually, they appear as a discrete erythematous mucosal lesion on the right side of the colon. Endoscopy is the initial diagnostic procedure of choice and may be useful in treatment of limited lesions with BICAP, heater probe, or laser photocoagulation. Careful and repeated endoscopic evaluation is usually necessary to discover these lesions. Angiography may be useful for continued occult bleeding. Estrogen-progesterone therapy (0.05 mg ethinylestradiol and 1 mg norethisterone qd PO) has been found to be effective in severe bleeding from vascular malformations (Lancet 1990;335:953).

c. **Colonic ulcers.** Solitary ulcers with arterial bleeding are very uncommon but may be associated with massive hemorrhage. Treatment is by endoscopic coagulation or surgical oversewing of the ulcer if endoscopy is not possible.

d. **Colonic varices.** These form in portal hypertension and may be managed with injection sclerotherapy. If this is unsuccessful, portal systemic shunt procedures are used.

e. **Meckel's diverticulum.** This should be a consideration in lower GI hemorrhage in any young person. Technetium-99m pertechnetate or Meckel's scans are useful in demonstrating this diverticulum. Surgical resection is indicated.

f. **Postpolypectomy bleeding.** Commonly, immediately after polypectomy, the bleeding stalk can be resnared, tamponaded, and cauterized. If delayed hemorrhage occurs, usually an ulcer site is present, and either injection sclerotherapy or coagulation with a heater probe is necessary.

g. **Radiation colitis.** This usually causes minor GI bleeding but may bring continuous discomfort to a patient. It can respond to cortisone enemas, but if bleeding points can be seen, endoscopic therapy with heater probe or electrocoagulation may be tried. Laser coagulation may be more useful if involvement is diffuse and surgery is not contemplated.

h. **Hemorrhoids.** If hemorrhoids are a cause of continuous bleeding, injection sclerotherapy or rubber band ligation is usually effective.

Gupta PK, Fleischer DE. Nonvariceal upper gastrointestinal bleeding. Med Clin North Am 1993;77:973–992.

Manten HD, Green JA. Acute lower gastrointestinal bleeding. A guide to initial management. Postgrad Med 1995;97:154–157.

Rosen RJ, Sanchez G. Angiographic diagnosis and management of gastrointestinal hemorrhage. Current concepts. Radiol Clin North Am 1994;32:951–967.

Saari A, Klvilaakso E, Inberg M, et al. Comparison of somatostatin and vasopressin in bleeding esophageal varices. Am J Gastroenterol 1990;85:804–807.

Sharma R, Gorbien MJ. Angiodysplasia and lower gastrointestinal tract bleeding in elderly patients. Arch Intern Med 1995;155:807–812.

van Cutsem E, Rutgeerts P, Vantrappen G. Treatment of bleeding gastrointestinal vascular malformations with oestrogen-progesterone. Lancet 1990;335:953–955.

9999999999999

LIVER DISEASES

ROBERT L. CARITHERS, JR.

I. ACUTE LIVER DISEASE

The major causes of acute hepatocellular injury include **viral hepatitis, drug-induced hepatitis,** and **ingestion of toxins.** Patients with mild to moderate acute hepatitis rarely require hospitalization. The emphasis in these patients is preventing spread of infectious agents and avoiding further liver damage when the underlying etiology is drug-induced or toxic hepatitis. Patients with fulminant hepatic failure (FHF) require special management because of rapid progression of disease and the potential need for urgent liver transplantation.

A. Viral Hepatitis

Six hepatitis viruses have been identified: hepatitis A, B, C, D, E, and G. **Hepatitis A and E** often are contracted through ingestion of water or food contaminated with the viruses or through close contact with infected patients. Travelers to underdeveloped countries are at high risk for infection with these viruses. Hepatitis A also is endemic in the United States and is most commonly found in children in day care centers, homosexuals, and family members of patients with acute hepatitis A. **Transmission of hepatitis A can be prevented by prophylaxis with immune serum globulin. Family members and sexual contacts of patients with acute hepatitis A should receive 0.02 mL/kg** as soon as possible after identification of the index case. **Vaccination should be considered in individuals planning to travel to underdeveloped countries. Primary immunization in adults consists of a single IM injection of hepatitis A vaccine,** which provides protection within 4 weeks. A booster dose in 12 months is recommended for long-term protection. Hepatitis B, C, D, and G virus infections are blood-borne. Infection can follow transfusion of contaminated blood products, intravenous drug abuse, and exposure of health care workers to blood and blood products of infected individuals. Sexual contact and maternal-fetal transfer from a chronically infected mother to her newborn are other possible modes of transmission of hepatitis B and C. Transmission of hepatitis B can be prevented by vaccination or by use of hepatitis B immune globulin (HBIG). The current recommendations for hepatitis B virus prophylaxis are outlined in Table 9–1. Since hepatitis D occurs only in patients infected with hepatitis B, this prophylaxis also is effective in preventing transmission of hepatitis D. The prophylactic use of **immune serum globulin** for prevention of hepatitis C virus infection following needlestick accidents **is not recommended.**

B. Drug-Induced Hepatitis

A variety of drugs can cause hepatocellular injury. Evidence of liver injury is most common 4 to 6 weeks after initiation of treatment. If injury is identified early and the drug is discontinued, complete recovery is the rule. Once hepatocellular injury is recognized, a patient should never receive the offending medication again. Table 9–2 lists commonly used agents that can cause severe hepatocellular injury.

TABLE 9-1. **Prophylaxis for Hepatitis B Virus Infection**

	HBIG*	VACCINE
Newborn of HBsAG carrier	0.5 mL at birth	1 wk, 1 mo, 6 mo
Sexual contact	0.06 mL/kg within 14 d	Immediately, 1 mo, 6 mo
Health care worker	0.06 mL/kg within 7 d	Immediately, 1 mo, 6 mo

*Hepatitis B immune globulin.

1. ISONIAZID. Of patients receiving isoniazid, 10% to 15% develop mild aminotransferase elevation 3 to 4 weeks after initiation of therapy, which resolves despite continuation of the drug. However, prolonged elevation of aminotransferase levels should be followed carefully, and the drug should be discontinued if there is evidence of synthetic dysfunction because of the potential risk of FHF from isoniazid hepatotoxicity. Combined use of isoniazid and rifampin appears to enhance the risk of hepatotoxicity.

2. PHENYTOIN hepatotoxicity is seen most frequently after 4 to 6 weeks of treatment and is associated with fever, diffuse lymphadenopathy, maculopapular rash, splenomegaly, leukocytosis, and atypical lymphocytosis, suggesting infectious mononucleosis or lymphoma. Continuation of therapy despite these symptoms can result in FHF.

3. ALLOPURINOL therapy occasionally results in a systemic vasculitis manifested by fever, rash, eosinophilia, hepatitis, and renal failure.

4. ACETAMINOPHEN. Suicidal overdose with acetaminophen is a common cause of severe liver injury. Ingestion of 10 to 15 g of the drug is usually required for significant hepatotoxicity. However, **chronic alcoholics** and patients receiving **isoniazid** can develop severe liver injury after exposure to much lower doses of acetaminophen. Plasma acetaminophen levels greater than 200 mg/L 4 hours after ingestion or 50 mg/L 12 hours after ingestion suggest a high likelihood of severe liver damage. *N*-Acetylcysteine (Mucomyst) is effective in preventing or limiting the degree of liver damage if given within 12 hours of acetaminophen ingestion. The recommended **initial dose is 140 mg/kg PO followed by 70 mg/kg PO every q4h for a total of 72 hours.** Charcoal infusion

TABLE 9-2. **Drugs Associated with Acute Hepatitis**

Allopurinol	Doxapram
Phenylbutazone	Disulfiram
Indomethacin, ibuprofen, naproxen	Dantrolene
Chlorzoxazone	Halothane
Phenytoin	Valproic acid
Oxacillin, carbenicillin, cloxacillin	Sulfonamides
Isoniazid, rifampin	Mithramycin, L-asparaginase, streptozocin
Aprindine	Propylthiouracil
Cimetidine	

should be avoided because it can interfere with absorption of *N*-acetylcysteine. Signs most predictive of a poor prognosis and the need for urgent liver transplantation following acetaminophen overdose are metabolic acidosis, the development of hepatic encephalopathy, marked elevation of prothrombin time values, and elevated serum creatinine.

C. Toxins

Liver injury also can result from ingestion of hepatotoxins, such as carbon tetrachloride, *Amanita* mushrooms, and herbal remedies such as germander, comfrey, chaparral, and Jin Bu Huan.

D. Management of Fulminant Hepatic Failure (FHF)

There are an estimated 2000 cases of FHF in the United States annually. The early features of FHF are indistinguishable from those of uncomplicated hepatitis. However, patients with FHF develop hepatic encephalopathy and marked prolongation of prothrombin time values within 8 weeks of the onset of acute liver disease. Classification of various stages of encephalopathy is helpful in understanding the clinical features of these patients (Table 9–3).

Various medical treatments have been touted to improve survival in patients with FHF. These include total body plasma exchange, charcoal hemoperfusion, corticosteroids, HBIG for patients with FHF B, and prostaglandins. However, none have been proven in randomized controlled trials to improve survival. The most impressive recent results have been reported in patients who have undergone liver transplantation. Thus, the emphasis in managing patients with FHF currently is oriented toward keeping them in the best possible condition for urgent transplantation.

Most patients with FHF are young and have few other medical problems. Nevertheless, within hours, a number of devastating complications can occur. Successful prevention and management of these complications are the cornerstones of modern management of FHF. This can best be accomplished in an intensive care unit with experienced physicians and nurses in a center with liver transplantation readily available. The most common potential complications of patients with FHF include respiratory depression, hypoglycemia, gastrointestinal bleeding, renal failure, infections, and cerebral edema.

Patients with FHF have a complex coagulopathy that includes diminished synthesis of coagulation factors, impaired fibrinolysis, and diminished number and function of platelets. The usual cause of **bleeding** is **stress**

TABLE 9–3. **Stages of Hepatic Encephalopathy**

STAGE	MENTAL CHANGES	REFLEXES
I	Disorientation	Mild increase; no asterixis
II	Confusion	Increased; asterixis
III	Stupor	Clonus; asterixis
IVa	Comatose	Decreased; flaccid
IVb	Unresponsive	Decerebrate

ulceration. This can be prevented by **aggressive management of gastric pH with H$_2$ blockers or sucralfate.** Maintenance of electrolyte balance, normotension, and reasonable nutritional input also help to prevent this often devastating complication.

Patients with FHF often have profound hemodynamic changes. Many are volume depleted with borderline hypotension and oliguria on admission to the intensive care unit. Placement of a Swan-Ganz catheter to monitor wedge pressure, pulmonary artery pressure, and cardiac output is essential to maintain optimum hemodynamic parameters and to prevent acute tubular necrosis. When renal insufficiency persists despite maximization of intravascular hemodynamics, the etiology is **usually hepatorenal syndrome,** the underlying pathogenesis of which appears to be extreme peripheral vasodilatation with secondary selective vasoconstriction of the renal vasculature. The overall prognosis of patients with the hepatorenal syndrome is dismal, with survival rates less than 10%. However, the syndrome is reversed by successful liver transplantation.

Infection can be another rapidly evolving and devastating complication in patients with FHF. Evidence of bacterial and fungal infections has been found in as many as 90% of patients with FHF. Prophylactic antibiotics appear to be useful in decreasing infections and maximizing the chance of successful transplantation.

The final and most devastating complication of FHF is **cerebral edema,** which is a frequent cause of death in patients awaiting transplantation. Furthermore, a significant number of patients who have successful transplants suffer perioperative brain damage due to cerebral edema. The first sign of incipient cerebral edema is increased intracranial pressure (ICP). A number of transplant units directly monitor ICP in all patients with stage III or IV encephalopathy, despite the hazards of infection and bleeding. With such monitoring, sudden changes in ICP can be detected early and can be effectively controlled by hyperventilation, bolus infusions of mannitol, hypothermia, or continuous arteriovenous hemofiltration. ICP monitoring also can be useful in determining which patients have progressed too far to undergo successful transplantation.

Gordon DW, Rosenthal G, Hart J, Sirota R, Baker AL. Chaparral ingestion: the broadening spectrum of liver injury caused by herbal medications. JAMA 1995;273:489–490.

Hoofnagle JH, Carithers RL, Jr, Shapiro C, Ascher N. Fulminant hepatic failure: summary of a workshop. Hepatology 1995;21:240–252.

Immunization Practices Advisory Committee. Licensure of inactivated hepatitis A vaccine and recommendations for use among international travelers. MMWR 1995;44:559–560.

Lidofsky SD, Bass NM, Prager MC, et al. Intracranial pressure monitoring and liver transplantation for fulminant hepatic failure. Hepatology 1992;16:1–7.

Linnen J, Wages J, Jr, Zhang-Keck Z, et al. Molecular cloning and disease association of hepatitis G virus: a transfusion-transmissible agent. Science 1996;271:505–509.

Mitchell I, Wendon J, Fitts S, Williams R. Anti-tuberculous therapy and acute liver failure. Lancet 1995;345:555–556.

Murphy R, Swartz R, Watkins PB. Severe acetaminophen toxicity in a patient receiving isoniazid. Ann Intern Med 1990;113:799–800.

O'Grady JG, Alexander GJM, Hayllar KM, Williams R. Early indicators of prognosis in fulminant hepatic failure. Gastroenterology 1989;97:439–445.

Rolando N, Gimson A, Wade J, Philpott-Howard J, Casewell M, Williams R. Prospective controlled trial of selective parenteral and enteral antimicrobial regimen in fulminant liver failure. Hepatology 1993;17:196–201.

Rolando N, Harvey F, Brahm J, et al. Prospective study of bacterial infection in acute liver failure: an analysis of 50 patients. Hepatology 1990;11:49–53.

Woolf GM, Petrovic LM, Rojter SE, et al. Acute hepatitis associated with the Chinese herbal product Jin Bu Huan. Ann Intern Med 1994;121:729–735.

Zimmerman HJ, Maddrey WC. Acetaminophen (paracetemol) hepatotoxicity with regular intake of alcohol: analysis of instances of therapeutic misadventure. Hepatology 1995;22:767–773.

II. CHRONIC LIVER DISEASE

A number of liver diseases can cause progressive hepatocellular injury and cirrhosis. Appropriate treatment can arrest the progression of disease and result in normal or near normal life expectancy for patients with many of these diseases. Patients with diseases for which no medical therapy is available may require liver transplantation.

A. Alcoholic Liver Disease

1. **CLINICAL FEATURES.** Symptomatic patients with alcoholic hepatitis and cirrhosis describe a variety of complaints, including vague abdominal pain, anorexia, nausea and vomiting, weakness, diarrhea, weight loss, and fever. The most common physical finding is hepatomegaly. Other findings include hepatic tenderness, an audible bruit over the liver, jaundice, spider angiomas, splenomegaly, ascites, edema, and, in more severe cases, the presence of varying degrees of hepatic encephalopathy. Fever as high as 104°F to 105°F is seen in many patients, and prolonged fever lasting for weeks is not unusual. Other common physical findings include testicular atrophy, peripheral neuropathy, and Dupuytren's contractures. Only modest elevations of aminotransferase values are seen, even when the disease is severe. AST levels are usually less than 300 to 500 IU and are associated with trivial elevation of ALT levels, resulting in the increased AST/ALT ratio characteristic of alcoholic liver disease.

2. **PROGNOSIS.** Because patients with alcoholic hepatitis can experience a wide spectrum of liver injury, the prognosis can vary dramatically. Patients with severe disease have high short-term mortality, approaching that of patients with FHF. In contrast, patients with mild disease are primarily at risk for developing alcoholic cirrhosis. The clinical features indicating severe disease include the presence of hepatic encephalopathy, marked prolongation of prothrombin time, elevation of serum bilirubin above 25 mg/dL, depressed serum albumin, elevated serum creatinine, and older age. The prognosis in patients with alcoholic cirrhosis depends on the degree and number of complications experienced and whether they can abstain from alcohol. Individuals with alcoholic cirrhosis who abstain can often return to full function. Those who have experienced no major complications have a 5-year survival rate of almost 90%, whereas patients who have previously experienced jaundice, ascites, or hematemesis have a 60% chance of surviving 5 years.

3. **MANAGEMENT.** Clinical and biochemical signs of protein-calorie **malnutrition** are seen in 75% of patients hospitalized with moderate to severe alcoholic hepatitis or cirrhosis. Particular attention should be paid to

vitamin and mineral deficiencies, including vitamins A and D, vitamin B_{12}, folic acid, thiamine, pyridoxine, zinc, magnesium, and phosphorus. A conscientious dietitian often can find foods that are palatable. Positive nitrogen balance can be achieved and encephalopathy avoided in patients with cirrhosis by the use of oral branched-chain amino acids, but these supplements are very expensive. The role of hyperalimentation for patients with alcoholic hepatitis and cirrhosis remains controversial. Branched-chain amino acids and other special hyperalimentation preparations have not been shown to increase survival or to speed recovery. Therapy with prophylthiouracil, anabolic steroids, and colchicine has not been shown to improve survival in patients with alcoholic hepatitis or cirrhosis. However, patients with severe alcoholic hepatitis with hepatic encephalopathy, marked prolongation of prothrombin values, and high serum bilirubin may benefit from treatment with prednisone, 40 mg/d for 1 month followed by 20 mg for 1 week and 10 mg for 1 week. No benefit has been shown in patients with milder disease.

B. Chronic Hepatitis

Chronic hepatitis is defined by continued elevation of aminotransferase values for 6 months or longer. A variety of clinical conditions can produce the clinical syndrome of chronic hepatitis, including autoimmune hepatitis, chronic viral hepatitis, drug-induced liver disease, and a number of metabolic diseases. Differentiating these causes is important because the treatment of each is quite different.

1. AUTOIMMUNE HEPATITIS. Classic autoimmune hepatitis (type I) is most commonly seen in young girls and postmenopausal women. Most patients have positive antinuclear and antismooth muscle antibodies and hyperglobinemia. A second type of autoimmune hepatitis, seen primarily in Europe (type II), is characterized by the presence of antiliver kidney microsomal antibodies and appears to be more severe. Patients with progressive liver disease manifested by histologic features of bridging fibrosis, submassive necrosis, or active cirrhosis have a poor prognosis. In these patients, **corticosteroid therapy** usually results in marked improvement in survival. **The usual starting dose is 60 mg/d for 1 week followed by 40 mg/d for 2 weeks, 30 mg/d for 2 weeks, and then 20 mg/d.** Most patients respond dramatically, with resolution of symptoms, normalization of aminotransferase values, and improvement in synthetic function within 2 to 3 months. There is a high complication rate with long-term corticosteroid therapy, especially in patients who receive more than 20 mg/d for extended periods. Therefore, only patients with severe disease should be treated. Liver biopsy is essential in selecting appropriate patients for therapy. In patients who require extended therapy, an attempt should be made to reduce the corticosteroid dose to 5–10 mg/d. Addition of azathioprine, 1.5 mg/kg/d, can be helpful in minimizing the dose of corticosteroids. Remission can be maintained in many patients with azathioprine therapy alone.

2. **CHRONIC VIRAL HEPATITIS.** Ninety percent of infants and 3% to 5% of adults infected with the hepatitis B (HBV) virus develop chronic infection and are at risk for progression to cirrhosis and hepatocellular carcinoma. Forty percent of patients with chronic HBV infection have a good response to interferon-alpha therapy, with disappearance of HBeAg and significant reduction in viral replication within 6 months. With longer follow-up, many of these patients also lose HBsAg. During treatment there is often a flare of disease, with increased aminotransferase values. Interferon should not be administered to patients with evidence of decompensated liver disease because of the risk of precipitating FHF. The recommended dosage of interferon is 5 million U administered SC daily for 4 months. Side effects include malaise, flu-like symptoms, depression, and occasionally hypothyroidism or hyperthyroidism. TSH values should be determined before treatment, and blood counts should be monitored during therapy for evidence of significant leukopenia and thrombocytopenia. Patients infected with chronic hepatitis C virus have a 60% chance of developing chronic liver disease. There is often insidious progression to cirrhosis, and patients are at risk for the development of hepatocellular carcinoma. Interferon-alpha, 3 million U three times a week for 6 months, is effective in normalizing aminotransferase values and eradicating circulating virus in 30% to 40% of patients. However, the relapse rate is high following cessation of treatment. Prolonged administration of interferon therapy for 12 to 18 months appears to increase the response rate in patients with chronic hepatitis C.

3. **DRUG-INDUCED CHRONIC HEPATITIS.** Liver injury from continued use of hepatotoxic drugs can produce a picture indistinguishable from autoimmune chronic hepatitis. Patients may or may not have positive antinuclear or antismooth muscle antibodies. The most common offending agents include alpha-methyldopa, dantrolene sodium, isoniazid, nitrofurantoin, and nonsteroidal anti-inflammatory drugs. If the etiology of chronic hepatitis can be identified before the development of cirrhosis, complete resolution usually occurs with discontinuation of the offending drug.

4. **METABOLIC DISEASE.** The most common metabolic diseases causing chronic hepatitis are Wilson's disease, alpha$_1$-antitrypsin deficiency, and hemochromatosis.
   a. **Wilson's disease.** This is an autosomal recessive disorder manifested by deficient biliary copper elimination. Patients gradually accumulate copper in the liver during the first two to three decades of life. At some point, usually between ages 15 and 25, patients develop hepatitis, which can be accompanied by hemolysis and renal tubular abnormalities. Occasional patients have acute or FHF, although a more common manifestation is chronic hepatitis. There may be mild neurologic dysfunction with loss of concentration or emotional outbursts, which may lead to psychiatric intervention. Clinical diagnosis is based on depressed ceruloplasmin levels (<20 mg/dL), increased urinary copper excretion (>100 µg/d), the pres-

ence of Kayser-Fleischer rings, and detection of abnormally high hepatic copper levels (>250 µg/g). Diagnosis during the hepatic phase is essential because both the hepatic and neurologic sequelae can be prevented by administration of 1–2 g of **penicillamine**/d. Common side effects include fever, pruritus, and a rash. Less common are leukopenia and thrombocytopenia. Patients who develop severe toxic reactions to penicillamine can be treated effectively with **trientine,** in doses of 1–2 g/d.

b. **Alpha₁-antitrypsin deficiency.** The most common clinical presentations of homozygous alpha₁-antitrypsin deficiency (PiZZ) are (1) chronic obstructive pulmonary disease affecting primarily the lower lobes, (2) cholestatic jaundice in infants often progressing to cirrhosis before age 10, and (3) chronic hepatitis and cirrhosis in adults. Depressed serum alpha₁-antitrypsin levels and demonstration of sequestered alpha₁-antitrypsin granules within hepatocytes on liver biopsy establish the diagnosis. Liver transplantation is the only effective therapy.

c. **Hemochromatosis.** Hemochromatosis is the most common genetic disorder causing liver failure. This autosomal recessive defect in iron absorption results in slowly progressive accumulation of iron in the liver, pancreas, heart, and brain. Patients often do not develop symptoms until age 50 or 60. Hepatomegaly is the most common physical finding. If the disease is not recognized, progression to diabetes, cardiomyopathy, and pituitary failure often occurs. Hemochromatosis should be suspected in patients with transferrin saturation greater than 50% who have marked elevation of serum ferritin levels. Younger patients with hemochromatosis may not have elevated ferritin values. For this reason, transferrin saturation is a better screening strategy. The diagnosis is confirmed by documenting markedly elevated hepatic iron concentration. If detected before the development of cirrhosis, all manifestations of hemochromatosis can be prevented by regular phlebotomy.

Adams PC, Gregor JC, Kertesz AE, Valberg LS. Screening blood donors for hereditary hemochromatosis: decision analysis model based on a 30-year database. Gastroenterology 1995;109:177–188.

Carithers RL, Jr, Herlong HF, Diehl AM, et al. Methylprednisolone therapy in patients with severe alcoholic hepatitis: a randomized multicenter trial. Ann Intern Med 1989;110:685–690.

Davis GL, Balart LA, Schiff ER, et al. Treatment of chronic hepatitis C with recombinant interferon alfa: a multicenter randomized, controlled trial. N Engl J Med 1989;321:1501–1506.

Johnson PJ, McFarlane IG, Williams R. Azathioprine for long-term maintenance of remission in autoimmune hepatitis. N Engl J Med 1996;333:958–963.

Krawitt EL. Medical progress: autoimmune hepatitis. N Engl J Med 1996;334:897–903.

Niederau C, Fischer R, Purschel A, Stremmel W, Haussinger D, Strohmeyer G. Long-term survival in patients with hereditary hemochromatosis. Gastroenterology 1996;110:1107–1119.

Perrillo RP, Schiff ER, Davis GL, et al. A randomized, controlled trial of interferon alfa-2b alone and after prednisone withdrawal for the treatment of chronic hepatitis B. N Engl J Med 1990;323:295–301.

Powell WJ, Klatskin G. Duration and survival in patients with Laennec's cirrhosis. Am J Med 1968;44:406–420.

Poynard R, Bedossa P, Chevallier M, et al. A comparison of three interferon alfa-2b regimens for the long-term treatment of chronic non-A, non-B hepatitis. N Engl J Med 1995; 332:1457–1462.

Ramond M, Poynard T, Rueff B, et al. A randomized trial of prednisolone in patients with severe alcoholic hepatitis. N Engl J Med 1992;326:507–512.

Schilsky ML, Scheinberg IH, Sternlieb I. Prognosis of wilsonian chronic active hepatitis. Gastroenterology 1991;100:762–767.

III. CHOLESTATIC LIVER DISEASES

Cholestatic hepatobiliary disorders are characterized by marked elevation in alkaline phosphatase values with or without jaundice. Major causes include extrahepatic biliary obstruction, cholestatic drug reactions, primary biliary cirrhosis, and sclerosing cholangitis.

A. Extrahepatic Biliary Obstruction

Mechanical extrahepatic obstruction most commonly results from malignancy or gallstones. Malignant biliary obstruction usually occurs in older patients. Characteristic clinical features include painless jaundice and weight loss. Ultrasound examination reveals dilated intrahepatic ducts. Except when the tumor is resectable, treatment is palliative, achieved by endoscopic placement of a biliary stent or by bypassing the obstruction through percutaneous insertion of a drainage catheter. The former is preferred because patients do not require a percutaneous catheter. However, endoscopically placed stents have to be replaced periodically because of obstruction. Biliary obstruction due to gallstones usually is accompanied by right upper quadrant pain, fever, and jaundice. The diagnosis is suspected by finding dilated intrahepatic biliary radicals on ultrasound and may be confirmed by percutaneous or endoscopic cholangiography. Most patients respond clinically to treatment with nasogastric suction, intravenous fluids, and antibiotics. Extrahepatic biliary stones can be removed endoscopically. This can be combined with laparoscopic cholecystectomy to prevent recurrence.

B. Cholestatic Drug Reactions

The agents most commonly associated with cholestatic reactions include chlorpromazine and other phenothiazines, gold, chlorpropamide, oral contraceptives, androgens, tolbutamide, and erythromycin. Although resolution may be slow, complete recovery usually occurs after discontinuation of the offending agent.

C. Primary Biliary Cirrhosis

Primary biliary cirrhosis (PBC) occurs most often in middle-aged women. Patients frequently complain of pruritus. There is marked elevation of alkaline phosphatase levels. Associated biochemical features include elevated IgM levels and positive antimitochondrial antibodies. Many patients have associated autoimmune features, particularly Sjögren's syndrome, autoimmune thyroiditis, and renal tubular acidosis. Liver biopsy typically shows inflammation around small bile ducts and nonsuppurative cholangitis. With advancing disease there is ongoing fibrosis and progression to cirrhosis. Severe pruritus can be a significant clinical problem, and these patients are at risk for malabsorption of fat-soluble vitamins and zinc.

Vitamin A, E, and K levels should be measured, and deficiencies should be replaced. However, the most significant clinical problem for patients with PBC is bone disease characterized by impaired osteoblastic activity and accelerated osteoclastic activity. Calcium and vitamin D should be carefully monitored, and appropriate replacement should be instituted. In addition, vigorous physical activity should be encouraged.

Pruritus can be relieved with cholestyramine or, in intractable cases, administration of rifampin. Ursodeoxycholic acid therapy (13–15 mg/kg/d) has resulted in dramatic improvement in liver function tests and a trend toward enhanced survival in patients with PBC. A number of other agents, including penicillamine, cholchicine, chlorambucil, corticosteroids, cyclosporine, methotrexate, and azathioprine, have been studied in controlled clinical trials. None have been shown to prevent progression of the disease, and many have unacceptable side effects. For patients with advanced disease, the only option is liver transplantation.

D. Primary Sclerosing Cholangitis

Primary sclerosing cholangitis (PSC) is characterized by inflammation and fibrosis of the biliary tree, often in patients with ulcerative colitis. Involvement can include the extrahepatic bile ducts, the intrahepatic ducts, or both. Young men are most commonly affected. Symptoms include fatigue, pruritus, jaundice, abdominal pain, and recurrent fever due to repeated episodes of bacterial cholangitis. Biochemical findings include marked elevations in alkaline phosphatase, intermittent elevations in bilirubin, and minimal increases in aminotransferase values. The diagnosis is confirmed by endoscopic cholangiography, which reveals multifocal areas of stricture and dilatation, giving a beaded appearance to the involved portions of the extrahepatic and intrahepatic biliary tree. The clinical course is quite variable. Although many patients remain asymptomatic for long periods, most ultimately become symptomatic and develop liver failure, leading to death or the need for liver transplantation. Age, bilirubin and hemoglobin concentrations, presence of ulcerative colitis, and histologic stage on liver biopsy are independent predictors of a poor prognosis. Patients with PSC have a high risk for cholangiocarcinoma. Because those with associated ulcerative colitis are strongly predisposed to colon cancer, screening colonoscopy at regular intervals is important.

Bachs L, Pares A, Elena M, Piera C, Rodes J. Effects of long-term rifampicin administration in primary biliary cirrhosis. Gastroenterology 1992;102:2077–2080.

Brentnall TA, Haggitt RC, Rabinovitch PS, et al. Risk and natural history of colonic neoplasia in patients with primary sclerosing cholangitis and ulcerative colitis. Gastroenterology 1996;110: 331–338.

Combes B, Carithers RL, Jr, Maddrey WC, et al. A randomized, double-blind, placebo-controlled trial of ursodeoxycholic acid in primary biliary cirrhosis. Hepatology 1995;22:759–766.

Lee Y-M, Kaplan MM. Primary sclerosing cholangitis. N Engl J Med 1995;332:924–933.

Poupon RE, Poupon R, Balkau B, et al. Ursodiol for the long-term treatment of primary biliary cirrhosis. N Engl J Med 1994;330:1342–1347.

Rosen H. Primary biliary cirrhosis and bone disease. Hepatology 1995;21:253–255.

Wiesner RH, Grambsch PM, Lindor KD, Ludwig J, Dickson ER. Clinical and statistical analyses of new and evolving therapies for primary biliary cirrhosis. Hepatology 1988;8:668–676.

IV. MAJOR COMPLICATIONS OF CHRONIC LIVER DISEASES

Patients with chronic liver disease are prone to a number of potentially life-threatening complications. Included among these are variceal hemorrhage, ascites, spontaneous bacterial peritonitis, and hepatic encephalopathy. The opportunity for the patient to undergo successful transplantation often rests on effective management of these complications.

A. Variceal Hemorrhage

Bleeding from esophageal varices is particularly common in patients with decompensated cirrhosis who have large varices and red wales observed on endoscopic examination. **Beta blockers** are effective in reducing the risk of variceal hemorrhage and in preventing rebleeding. Treatment should be started with 40 mg bid of propranolol, with a goal of reducing the pulse rate by 25%.

When a patient with cirrhosis has upper GI hemorrhage, a large-bore IV line should be placed, and replacement with packed red cells should be immediately instituted. **Early endoscopy** is essential, for over 50% of upper GI hemorrhages originate from sites other than esophageal varices, including Mallory-Weiss tears, diffuse gastritis, portal gastropathy, and duodenal ulcers.

If bleeding from esophageal varices is confirmed, IV vasopressin (Pitressin), 20 U in 200 mL of saline at 0.25–0.5 U/min, should be initiated with simultaneous IV infusion of nitroglycerin. As an alternative, octreotide, the long-acting analog of somatostatin, at a continuous IV infusion of 20–50 µg/h, can be used. Sclerotherapy and banding ligation of varices are effective in controlling bleeding in 75% of cases; complications appear to be fewer and rebleeding less with banding. If bleeding continues, hemorrhage can be controlled by placement of a Sengstaken-Blakemore or Minnesota tube. However, patients should be intubated and treated in specialized intensive care units where the nursing personnel are well trained in the use of these tubes and potential complications. Some patients have recurrent episodes of variceal bleeding. **Repeated sclerotherapy or banding** can eradicate varices and prevent recurrent hemorrhage. Patients who fail sclerotherapy should be considered for surgery. The choice of operation depends on the stage of the patient's liver disease and local surgical expertise. Child's classification and its various modifications (Table 9–4) provide the best means for preoperative assessment of surgical risk. Patients with well-compensated disease (scores of 5–8) are good candidates for distal splenorenal shunt. This technically difficult operation does not increase the risk of subsequent liver transplantation. In patients with uncontrolled variceal hemorrhage who have poor synthetic function (scores ≥10), transjugular intrahepatic portosystemic shunts (TIPS) often control bleeding and serve as an effective bridge to transplantation.

B. Ascites

Although the pathogenesis is controversial, avid renal sodium retention is an essential feature of ascites formation. Dietary sodium restriction is a basic ingredient of any effective treatment program. A **2-g sodium diet** is the

TABLE 9-4. Pugh's Modification of Child's Classification

	POINT SCORE FOR INCREASING ABNORMALITY		
	1	2	3
Encephalopathy (grade)	None	1 or 2	3 or 4
Ascites	Absent	Slight	Moderate
Bilirubin	1-2	2-3	>3
Albumin (g/dL)	>3.5	2.8-3.5	<2.8
Protime (sec > control)	1-4	4-6	>6

Adapted from Pugh RNH, Murray-Lyon IM, Dawson JL. Transection of the oesophagus for oesophageal varices. Br J Surg 1973;60:646–649.

minimum tolerable for outpatients. Diuretic therapy can be quite effective in treating **mild to moderate ascites. Spironolactone** (200–400 mg/d) is the most commonly used diuretic. Because spironolactone causes potassium retention, *salt substitutes should be avoided.* Furosemide and other loop diuretics are useful in patients who fail to respond adequately to spironolactone therapy. When used to treat patients with **severe ascites,** diuretics result in a high incidence of hyponatremia, volume depletion, precipitation of hepatic encephalopathy, and renal insufficiency. Vigorous **paracentesis** is safer and more cost effective in such patients. Three to five liters of fluid can be removed daily without deleterious hemodynamic changes. Peritoneovenous shunts have fallen into disfavor because of the high incidence of occlusion and recurrent infection. However, in selected patients, they can be beneficial as a short-term bridge while hepatic function recovers or until transplantation can be performed. TIPS also can be effective in patients with ascites refractory to diuretic therapy. Furthermore, as the 12-month survival of patients with refractory ascites is only 25%, these patients should be considered for liver transplantation.

C. Bacterial Peritonitis

One of the major life-threatening complications of ascites is spontaneous bacterial peritonitis (SBP). Common symptoms include diffuse abdominal pain, fever, and the unexplained onset of hepatic encephalopathy. However, many patients are asymptomatic. Any patient hospitalized with ascites should have a diagnostic paracentesis to rule out the possibility of SBP. Gram stains of ascitic fluid are rarely positive. The presence of more than 250 white cells, particularly when the percentage of polymorphonuclear leukocytes is greater than 75%, should raise the possibility of SBP, and antibiotic therapy should be initiated until ascitic fluid culture results return. The most common organisms causing spontaneous peritonitis are *Escherichia coli, Klebsiella,* and nonenterococcal streptococci. Placing ascitic fluid in blood culture bottles at the bedside significantly increases the yield of bacteria successfully cultured. In presumptive cases of SBP, antibiotic therapy should include coverage against gram-negative and gram-positive organisms. However, aminoglycosides should be avoided because of the high risk of nephrotoxicity in liver disease patients. Cefotaxime, 2 g IV q8h, is more effective than ampicillin and aminoglycosides and is not nephrotoxic. A 5-day course of treatment is as effective as 10 to 14 days. Unfortunately, 75% of patients successfully treated for SBP have recurrence within a year. Prophylactic therapy with norfloxacin (400 mg/d) reduces the incidence of recurrent infection; nevertheless, transplant candidates who develop SBP should have surgery as soon as possible.

D. Hepatic Encephalopathy

Hepatic encephalopathy is a neuropsychiatric syndrome that can occur in patients with acute or chronic liver disease. Accumulation of ammonia, interaction between ammonia, mercaptans, and fatty acids, and false neurotransmitter-induced neural inhibition have all been implicated as causes. The **stage of encephalopathy** (Table 9–3) is a sensitive measure of hepatocellular injury in patients with acute liver failure. In patients with chronic liver disease, encephalopathy generally occurs more gradually, is more commonly associated with extrahepatic precipitating factors, and is more easily reversed. The most common **precipitating factors** are the use of sedative drugs, GI bleeding or excessive protein ingestion, hypokalemia, volume depletion, and infection, particularly SBP. These precipitating causes should be searched for whenever a patient develops encephalopathy.

Once the precipitating factors have been addressed, effective management of encephalopathy consists of cleansing the gut with **sorbitol** or another purgative, restricting protein intake, and initiation of therapy with lactulose. The usual starting dose of **lactulose** is **30 mL qid.** The objective of therapy is to eliminate the encephalopathy and for the patient to have one or two soft formed stools daily while avoiding diarrhea. The best measure of the effectiveness of therapy is the number connection test in which a patient is asked to connect 25 numbered circles as quickly as possible. The test can be repeated periodically, and diet and lactulose therapy can be modified accordingly. Vancomycin and metronidazole can be used in resistant cases of encephalopathy.

Burroughs AK. Octreotide in variceal bleeding. Gut 1994;Suppl 3:S23–S27.

Burroughs AK, Panagou E. Pharmacological therapy for portal hypertension: rationale and results. Semin Gastrointest Dis 1995;6:148–164.

Felisart L, Rimola A, Arroyo V, et al. Cefotaxime is more effective than is ampicillin-tobramycin in cirrhotics with severe infections. Hepatology 1985;5:457–462.

Gimson AES, Westaby D, Hegarty J, Watson A, Williams R. A randomized trial of vasopressin and vasopressin plus nitroglycerin in the control of acute variceal hemorrhage. Hepatology 1986;6:410–413.

Gines P, Arroyo V, Vargas V, et al. Paracentesis with intravenous infusion of albumin as compared with peritoneovenous shunting in cirrhosis with refractory ascites. N Engl J Med 1991;325:829–835.

Gines P, Rimola A, Planas R, et al. Norfloxacin prevents spontaneous bacterial peritonitis recurrence in cirrhosis: results of a double-blind, placebo-controlled trial. Hepatology 1990;12:716–724.

Henderson JM. Role of distal splenorenal shunt for long-term management of variceal bleeding. World J Surg 1994;18:205–210.

Hoefs JC. Spontaneous bacterial peritonitis: prevention and therapy. Hepatology 1990;12:776.

Kellerman PS, Linas SL. Large-volume paracentesis in treatment of ascites. Ann Intern Med 1990;112:889–891.

Laine L, Cook D. Endoscopic ligation, compared with sclerotherapy for variceal bleeding. Ann Intern Med 1995;123:280–287.

Ochs A, Rössle M, Haag K, et al. The transjugular intrahepatic portosystemic stent-shunt procedure for refractory ascites. N Engl J Med 1995;332:1192–1197.

Rössle M, Haag K, Ochs A, et al. The transjugular intrahepatic portosystemic stent-shunt procedure for variceal bleeding. N Engl J Med 1994;330:165–171.

Runyon BA. Care of patients with ascites. N Engl J Med 1994;330:337–342.

Runyon BA, Canawati HN, Akriviadis EA. Optimization of ascitic fluid culture technique. Gastroenterology 1988;95:1351–1355.

Runyon BA, McHutchison JG, Antillon MR, et al. Short-course versus long-course antibiotic treatment of spontaneous bacterial peritonitis. A randomized controlled study of 100 patients. Gastroenterology 1991;100:1737–1742.

V. LIVER TRANSPLANTATION

Liver transplantation is the treatment of choice for patients with end-stage liver disease from a variety of causes (Table 9–5). However, patients must be in suitable physiologic condition to undergo major surgery and must have the ability to comply with the complex medical regimen required following surgery. The operation's timing influences survival and postoperative complications following liver transplantation. Moribund patients who are referred to a transplant center have little possibility of survival. In contrast, patients who are referred in good physiologic condition have an excellent chance of achieving long-term good quality of life.

A. Indications

Liver transplantation is the only effective treatment for patients with cirrhosis due to hepatitis C virus infection, alpha$_1$-antitrypsin deficiency, primary biliary cirrhosis, and sclerosing cholangitis. Patients with autoimmune chronic hepatitis in whom there is decompensation with ascites, jaundice, or variceal bleeding also are excellent candidates. Patients with alcoholic cirrhosis being considered for transplantation should have abstained from alcohol for 6 to 12 months to maximize the potential for spontaneous recovery. In addition, these patients should have effectively dealt with their alcoholism through a successful treatment program before

TABLE 9–5. Indications for Liver Transplantation

Fulminant hepatitis
Chronic hepatitis with cirrhosis
Autoimmune hepatitis
Chronic hepatitis C
Alcoholic cirrhosis
Cryptogenic cirrhosis
Metabolic disorders causing cirrhosis
Alpha$_1$-antitrypsin deficiency
Hemochromatosis
Wilson's disease
Biliary cirrhosis
Primary biliary cirrhosis
Sclerosing cholangitis
Controversial indications
Chronic hepatitis B
Hepatobiliary cancer

being considered for transplantation. Many patients who undergo transplantation have cirrhosis for which no cause can be found. Patients with cirrhosis secondary to hepatitis B virus infection have a high incidence of severe recurrent disease following the operation, although excellent results can be obtained if high-dose hepatitis B immune globulin (HBIG), lamivudine, or famciclovir are given perioperatively and then as needed after surgery. Patients with unresectable hepatocellular carcinoma and cholangiocarcinoma are generally poor candidates for transplantation because of possible recurrent and metastatic tumor.

B. Timing

In many instances the most difficult decision is **the best time for transplantation.** Any patient with chronic liver disease who develops hepatic encephalopathy or ascites should be considered for transplantation. The prognosis of patients with PBC can be determined by their age, serum bilirubin, albumin, and prothrombin values, and the presence of peripheral edema. Unfortunately, for patients with other liver diseases, there are no clearly defined means for selecting the best time for transplantation. Child's classification (Table 9–4) offers helpful information. For example, patients with scores of 5–8 have excellent survival for 5 to 10 years without transplantation. In contrast, those with scores over 12 have less than a 50% chance of surviving 6 months unless transplantation is performed.

C. Postoperative Management

After successful liver transplantation, there is rapid recovery of liver function. Early indications of graft function include prompt bile flow, spontaneous correction of coagulation factors within 48 to 72 hours, and steady improvement in aminotransferase and bilirubin values. In the first 48 hours after liver transplantation, the most common serious complications are **primary graft failure** and **intraabdominal hemorrhage** requiring reoperation. Signs of primary graft failure are persistent jaundice and coagulopathy associated with poor bile flow, metabolic acidosis, and renal insufficiency. Urgent retransplantation is the only option for these patients. Surgery is required for intraabdominal hemorrhage when there is a persistent need for large-volume transfusions and difficulty maintaining hemodynamic stability. Fortunately, these patients do well if they can be returned to the operating room in good physiologic condition.

1. EARLY MANAGEMENT. In the first 2 weeks after liver transplantation, the major concerns are **infection, hepatic artery thrombosis, and allograft rejection.** Most liver transplant recipients receive aggressive prophylactic therapy with acyclovir or ganciclovir to prevent herpes simplex, herpes zoster, and cytomegalovirus (CMV) infections and trimethoprim-sulfamethoxazole to prevent *Pneumocystis carinii* infections. Early infectious complications are usually due to nosocomial infections associated with indwelling lines and catheters. The most common organism is *Staphylococcus epidermidis.* Treatment consists of removal of potentially infected lines and antibiotic treatment with vancomycin. Hepatic artery thrombosis can occur either as massive hepatic necrosis or as a silent occlusion. The diagnosis is suspected

from Doppler sonography showing absence of hepatic artery flow and is confirmed by angiography. If the diagnosis can be made early, revascularization can be performed successfully. Otherwise, retransplantation often is required. Rejection, which occurs in 60% to 70% of patients, typically results in modest nonspecific increases in serum bilirubin and aminotransferase values. The diagnosis is made by liver biopsy, which reveals lymphocytic invasion of biliary endothelium and vascular epithelium. Most rejection episodes respond to bolus corticosteroid treatment daily for 3 to 5 days or monoclonal OKT3 antibody therapy.

2. LATE COMPLICATIONS. Later complications include **infection, rejection, biliary tract complications, portal vein thrombosis,** and **complications of immunosuppressive therapy.** Infection is the leading cause of death after liver transplantation. Late infections, including CMV and fungal infections, are primarily due to opportunistic organisms. CMV infection occurs in more than half of patients after transplantation. Hepatitis due to CMV can be confused with rejection because of nonspecific changes in bilirubin and aminotransferase values. However, liver biopsy shows focal inflammation surrounding CMV inclusion bodies. Most patients respond well to reduction in immunosuppressive therapy plus IV **ganciclovir therapy** (5 mg/kg/d) for 10 to 14 days. Fungal infections, particularly *Candida* and *Aspergillus,* are major causes of death after liver transplantation. If the diagnosis is established early, treatment with amphotericin or fluconazole can be life saving. The most common surgical complications after liver transplantation involve the biliary tract. Diagnosis is usually established by cholangiography. Although surgical intervention may be required, many biliary complications can be effectively treated with radiographic or endoscopic placement of biliary stents.

After hospital discharge of liver transplant recipients, most complications result from **side effects of immunosuppressive therapy.** Hypertension, excessive hair growth, gingival hyperplasia, and renal insufficiency are common side effects of cyclosporine therapy. Complications can be minimized by careful monitoring of cyclosporine levels and appropriate dosage adjustment, particularly in patients with early signs of hypertension and azotemia. Patients bothered by gingival hyperplasia and excessive hair growth can be switched to tacrolimus. Cyclosporine and tacrolimus-induced hypertension can be effectively treated with calcium channel blockers, such as nifedipine (30–60 mg qid), and beta blockers, such as metoprolol (50–100 mg qd). Side effects of prolonged corticosteroid therapy include truncal obesity, bone loss with pathologic fractures, diabetes, cataracts, and aseptic necrosis of the femoral heads. Minimization of dosage levels over time is the best preventive treatment, but oral calcium replacement and avoidance of diuretics also are helpful in reducing osteoporosis. Azathioprine is associated with leukopenia and thrombocytopenia. Thus, any patient treated with this agent requires careful monitoring of blood counts. Late complications of immunosuppressive therapy include malignant disease, particularly lymphomas and skin cancer.

De Man RA, Heijtink RA, Niesters HG, Schalm SW. New developments in antiviral therapy for chronic hepatitis B virus infection. Scand J Gastroenterol 1995;Suppl 12:100–104.

Dickson ER, Grambsch PM, Fleming TR, Fisher LD, Langworthy A. Prognosis in primary biliary cirrhosis: model for decision making. Hepatology 1989;10:1–7.

Oellerich M, Burdelski M, Lautz H, Binder L, Pichlmayr R. Predictors of one-year pretransplant survival in patients with cirrhosis. Hepatology 1991;14:1029–1034.

Samuel D, Muller R, Alexander G, et al. Liver transplantation in European patients with the hepatitis B surface antigen. N Engl J Med 1993;329:1842–1847.

Starzl TE, Demetris AJ, Van Thiel DH. Medical progress: liver transplantation. N Engl J Med 1989;321:1092–1099.

10 10 10 10 10 10 10 10

HEMATOLOGY AND TRANSFUSION MEDICINE

THOMAS H. PRICE
LAWRENCE R. SOLOMON

I. RED CELL DISORDERS

A. Anemia

1. **DEFINITION.** Hemoglobin is under 14 g/dL for men or under 12 g/dL for women, *but* **"low" levels may be appropriate** if tissue oxygen requirements are decreased (e.g., hypothyroidism) or if tissue oxygen delivery is enhanced by a decrease in hemoglobin oxygen affinity. **"Normal" levels may be inadequate** if tissue oxygen delivery is impaired by pulmonary insufficiency, cardiac disorders, or an increase in hemoglobin oxygen affinity.

2. **CLASSIFICATION** (TABLE 10–1)

   a. **Kinetic: decreased red cell production or increased red cell destruction** is distinguished by the **reticulocyte index** (a measure of the number of young red cells released by the marrow relative to normal each day) calculated as follows.

   $$\text{Reticulocyte count (\%)} \times \text{hematocrit}/45 \times 1/\text{shift factor}$$

   The ratio of the patient's hematocrit to the normal value of 45 corrects for anemia severity, whereas the shift factor (2 for anemia of moderate severity) adjusts for the increased life span of the reticulocyte in the blood due to increased erythropoietin levels (indicated by polychromatophilic red cells on the peripheral smear). In the steady state, values over 3 indicate increased destruction or blood loss, and values under 2 indicate decreased production. **The ratio of erythroid to myeloid precursors in the marrow (E/G ratio)** separates production defects into **hypoproliferative** disorders (E/G ratio normal or low) and disorders characterized by **ineffective erythropoiesis** due to intramedullary destruction of marrow erythroid precursors (E/G ratio high).

   b. **Morphologic: normocytic, macrocytic, or microcytic** is distinguished by the **mean corpuscular volume (MCV).** Most anemias are normocytic; microcytosis suggests a cytoplasmic maturation disorder, and macrocytosis suggests a nuclear maturation disorder. A high MCV also occurs with reticulocytosis, thyroid disorders, alcohol abuse, marrow damage, multiple myeloma, and hyperosmolar states. Regardless of the MCV, the **peripheral blood smear** should be examined for mixtures of red cells of different sizes, abnormal red cell shapes, red cell inclusions, and abnormal white cells and platelets.

3. **THE DIAGNOSTIC APPROACH** involves reticulocyte count, MCV, and examination of the peripheral smear initially, followed, if appropriate, by measures of nutrients in blood or serum and by a therapeutic trial. A bone marrow aspirate defines the E/G ratio, the type of maturation, the presence of iron stores, and the presence of abnormal cells. A bone

---

TABLE 10–1. **Kinetic Classification of Anemia**

DECREASED RED CELL PRODUCTION (reticulocyte index <2%)
Hypoproliferative (E/G < 1/2) (MCV *usually* normal)
  Marrow damage (aplasia; hypoplasia): drugs, tumor, immune, toxins, fibrosis,
    idiopathic, radiation, infection, congenital
  Decreased marrow stimulation
    Decreased oxygen requirement: hypothyroidism, hypopituitarism
    Increased oxygen release to tissues: low-affinity hemoglobins, hyperphosphatemia
    Decreased erythropoietin production: chronic renal failure, anemia of chronic disease
  Decreased iron supply or utilization: iron deficiency, anemia of chronic disease, copper
    deficiency
Ineffective (E/G > 1/1)
  Nuclear maturation defects (MCV *usually* high): vitamin B_{12} deficiency,
    myelodysplastic disorders, folate deficiency, cytotoxic drugs
  Cytoplasmic maturation defects (MCV *usually* low): iron deficiency, thalassemias,
    sideroblastic anemias, hemoglobin E

INCREASED RED CELL DESTRUCTION (reticulocyte index > 3%) (MCV normal or high)
  Membrane abnormalities (e.g., hereditary spherocytosis; PNH)
  Enzyme defects (e.g., G6PD deficiency)
  Hemoglobin abnormalities (e.g., sickle cell disease)
  Intracellular parasites (e.g., malaria, babesiosis, bartonella)
  Hypersplenism
  Immune (e.g., idiopathic, drugs, infections, lymphoproliferative or rheumatologic
    disorders)
  Microangiopathic (e.g., vasculitis, intravascular prostheses, TTP, DIC)
  Physical and chemical agents (e.g., bacterial toxins, snake and insect venoms, fresh
    water drowning, marching or jogging)

---

marrow biopsy provides complementary information on marrow cellularity and on the presence of fibrosis, granulomas, vasculitis, or tumor.
Since anemia is often a secondary process, studies to define an
underlying disorder are usually also required.

4. HYPOPROLIFERATIVE ANEMIAS

  a. **Aplastic anemia** is characterized by persistent pancytopenia with
    decreased marrow hematopoietic cells. It may be congenital, idio-
    pathic, or secondary to drugs, toxins, radiation, viral infections, or
    immune dysfunction.
    (1) Diagnosis is by bone marrow biopsy.
    (2) Therapy begins with stopping of all suspect drug or chemical
      exposures. Supportive care includes **red cell transfusion** for
      symptomatic anemia (p. 406), platelet transfusion for active
      bleeding (p. 396), and antibiotics for infections. Transfusions
      should be given sparingly to improve prospects for marrow
      transplantation and to limit transfusion reactions, iron over-
      load, and platelet sensitization. Good dental and body hygiene
      decreases infection risk. Bone marrow transplantation (BMT)
      cures 50% to 80% of patients under age 40 with severe aplasia
      (i.e., reticulocyte index <1%; granulocytes <500/µL; platelets

<20,000/μL; marrow cellularity <25%), and an HLA-identical sibling. Results are better if performed before transfusion or significant infection. Patients and their families should be HLA-typed at diagnosis, and conditioning should begin within 72 hours of initial administration of blood products. Transfusions from family members should be avoided. Risks include death within 3 months after transplant (10% to 25%) and chronic graft-versus-host disease (35%). Antithymocyte globulin (ATG) (40 mg/kg/d for 4 d) benefits 40% to 80% of patients. Toxicity includes phlebitis, fever, skin rash, anaphylaxis, serum sickness, neutropenia, and thrombocytopenia. Corticosteroids are usually given with ATG and for 7 days thereafter to minimize local and systemic reactions. Although response often occurs within 6 weeks, maximum benefit may not occur for 3 to 6 months. Relapse occurs in 35%. A second course may benefit 50% of nonresponding or relapsing patients. Cyclosporine, 12 mg/kg/d, may be as effective as ATG and can improve hematopoiesis in 50% of ATG failures, but continued therapy is needed in some patients to maintain response. Toxicity includes hypertension, hypomagnesemia and opportunistic infections.

Recombinant erythropoietin (EPO), granulocyte colony-stimulating factor (G-CSF), and granulocyte-macrophage colony-stimulating factor (GM-CSF) may improve blood counts in selected patients, but their use should not delay BMT or ATG therapy.

Androgens can benefit patients with less severe aplasia. Therapy for 4 to 6 months is often required, and relapse may follow drug withdrawal. Oral agents (e.g., fluoxymesterone 1 mg/kg/d; oxymetholone 2–5 mg/kg/d) are used in patients with severe thrombocytopenia. IM agents (e.g., testosterone propionate or nandrolone decanoate, 2–4 mg/kg/wk) are more effective and less hepatotoxic. Patients refractory to one androgen may respond to another.

b. **Iron deficiency anemia** is initially normochromic/normocytic, but hypochromia/microcytosis develops with increasing severity and duration. In adult males or postmenopausal females, it is most often due to GI bleeding, and the **GI tract should be studied even when tests for occult blood are negative.** Other causes include malabsorption, pulmonary hemosiderosis, chronic intravascular hemolysis (urinary iron loss), relatively inadequate intake (pregnancy, infancy), heavy uterine bleeding, blood donation, long-distance running (intravascular hemolysis), and vegetarian macrobiotic diets (low intake and absorption).

(1) *Diagnostic tests.* Low serum iron and increased serum iron-binding capacity and red cell protoporphyrin. A low serum ferritin value confirms the diagnosis, but the value may be normal if inflammation, malignant disease, uremia, or liver disease is present. Since inflammation and malignant disease also lower serum iron and raise red cell protoporphyrin values, histologic assessment of marrow iron stores may be required.

(2) ***Therapy.*** **Ferrous sulfate** PO (300 mg tid) increases hemoglobin at least 2 g/dL in 4 weeks and should be continued for 6 months after hemoglobin is normal to replenish stores. Absorption is better if ferrous sulfate is taken when fasting. Side effects (nausea, epigastric discomfort, constipation, diarrhea) may abate if the dose is decreased or given with meals. Parenteral iron dextran (50 mg/mL of iron) is given if oral iron is malabsorbed, poorly tolerated, or insufficient to keep up with continuing iron losses. The dose is calculated as follows.

$$\text{mg iron} = \frac{(\text{hematocrit deficit})(\text{total blood volume})}{(\text{RBC iron content})}$$

$$= \frac{(0.45 - \text{patient hematocrit})(70 \text{ mL/kg} \times \text{kg body wt})}{(0.7 \text{ mg/mL RBC})}$$

An additional 500 mg of iron is needed to replace stores. Doses of 100–200 mg are given by deep zigzag IM injection into the upper outer quadrant of the buttock, but this requires repeated injections, leads to skin staining, and, rarely, causes tumors at the injection site. Alternatively, the total dose can be diluted into 500 mL of 0.9 N saline and given as a single IV infusion over 4 to 6 hours. Since anaphylaxis can occur with either route, a 0.5-mL test dose is given 30 minutes before the treatment dose. Other side effects include headache, malaise, fever, arthralgias, and lymphadenopathy.

c. Anemia of chronic disease. This accompanies overt malignant disease and inflammatory disorders but may be the presenting feature of an otherwise occult process. The MCV is usually normal but may be low. Both serum iron and iron-binding capacity are decreased, whereas serum ferritin and red cell protoporphyrin are high. Histologic evaluation of marrow iron stores may be required to exclude iron deficiency. Iron therapy should be avoided, and the underlying disorder should be treated. Serum erythropoietin levels may be low relative to the severity of anemia, but EPO should only be used in selected patients with symptomatic anemia (e.g., multiple myeloma, HIV patients on AZT).

d. Anemia of chronic renal disease. This condition is due primarily to decreased erythropoietin production; MCV is normal. Acidosis and hyperphosphatemia lower hemoglobin-oxygen affinity and improve tissue oxygen delivery. Thus, symptoms, rather than the hemoglobin level, should be used as an indication for red cell transfusion.

(1) ***Diagnostic tests.*** Low serum erythropoietin levels exclude folate or iron deficiency that may accompany hemodialysis and the presence of other disorders.

(2) ***Therapy.*** EPO (30–150 U/kg 3 times per week IV or SC) is effective in almost all patients. Side effects include hypertension, hyperkalemia, seizures, and clotting of dialysis fistulas. Androgens may potentiate EPO, permitting use of lower doses (10–25 U/kg). Parenteral androgens (nandrolone decanoate 100 mg/wk or testosterone propionate 200 mg/wk IM) are given for 3 to 6 months. Oral androgens are less effective and more hepatotoxic.

(3) *Aluminum toxicity* occurs mainly in hemodialysis patients. MCV may be normal or low. Diagnosis involves assessing aluminum in bone biopsy specimens. Serum aluminum determination before and after deferoxamine infusion is less reliable. Aluminum-containing drugs are discontinued, aluminum-free water is used for dialysis, and deferoxamine is administered (p. 395).

5. NUCLEAR MATURATION DISORDERS (MEGALOBLASTIC ANEMIAS)

a. **General considerations in vitamin B$_{12}$ and folic acid deficiencies.** Macrocytosis and hypersegmented granulocytes are common, but the MCV may be normal, particularly if iron deficiency or thalassemia coexist. Folate doses over 0.5 mg/d are effective in vitamin B$_{12}$ deficiency, but improvement of anemia is incomplete, and neurologic symptoms may develop and progress. Vitamin B$_{12}$ doses over 100 μg/d also are effective in folate deficiency. Thus, these disorders must be distinguished before vitamin therapy is begun. Therapy produces brisk reticulocytosis in 4 to 7 days followed by a rapid increase in hemoglobin, but the MCV can remain high for 2 to 3 months. Further evaluation is needed if hemoglobin levels fail to become normal. Red cell transfusions are needed only for severe symptomatic anemia, and small volumes should be infused slowly to avoid volume overload.

b. **Vitamin B$_{12}$ deficiency** most often results from malabsorption due to gastric disorders (e.g., pernicious anemia, *Helicobacter pylori* gastritis), pancreatic insufficiency, disorders of the terminal ileum, certain infections (e.g., *Diphyllobothrium latum,* bacterial overgrowth, HIV) and some drugs (e.g., cholestyramine, colchicine, high-dose vitamin C, cimetidine, omeprazole, possibly ethanol). Decreased dietary intake occurs in strict vegetarians. Elderly subjects have marginal diets and may malabsorb food vitamin B$_{12}$ (atrophic gastritis). Neurologic symptoms (dementia, personality change, impaired vibratory sense and proprioception, and spastic paraparesis) can dominate the clinical picture and may occur without either anemia or a high MCV. Diagnosis is by low serum vitamin B$_{12}$ levels (also seen in primary folate deficiency, myeloma, other gammopathies), high urine methylmalonic acid excretion and serum homocysteine levels, and reticulocyte response to low-dose vitamin B$_{12}$ (1–2 μg/d). A Schilling test identifies malabsorption of crystalline or protein-bound vitamin B$_{12}$ and distinguishes gastric disorders from disorders of the terminal ileum. Cyanocobalamin or hydroxocobalamin 1 mg is given IM or SC three times per week for 4 to 6 weeks then 1 mg/mo for life. Oral doses of 1 mg/d may also be effective in pernicious anemia. Patients with pernicious anemia and atrophic gastritis should be screened regularly for gastric cancer.

c. **Folic acid deficiency** usually results from poor dietary intake or alcohol abuse, or both. Less common causes include malabsorption due to inflammatory small-bowel disease, altered metabolism due to certain drugs (e.g., oral contraceptives, diphenylhydantoin, methotrexate, trimethoprim, pentamidine), and increased requirements due to pregnancy, hemolytic anemia, hyperthyroidism, and some malignant diseases. Deficiency can cause fetal neural tube defects during pregnancy and may contribute to neuropsychiatric dysfunction. Diagnosis is made by low serum folate level (indicates limited delivery to marrow at the time of evaluation; most sensitive to early depletion; corrects rapidly with food or vitamin intake), low red cell folate value (indicates limited delivery to marrow in the preceding 2 to 3 months; may be normal in early deficiency and in transfused patients; also low in primary vitamin B_{12} deficiency), and reticulocyte response to low-dose folate (0.1–0.2 mg/d). To treat this deficiency, 1 mg/d of folic acid PO (or parenterally in patients with malabsorption) is given.

d. **Refractory anemia and idiopathic sideroblastic anemia.** Clonal myelodysplastic disorders, particularly in the elderly or after exposure to drugs or toxins (e.g., alkylating agents, organic solvents). Sideroblastic anemia may also be hereditary or secondary to drugs (e.g., ethanol, isoniazid, chloramphenicol, lead), chronic inflammation, or malignant or other hematologic disorders. Thrombocytopenia and granulocytopenia are common, and the MCV may be high, normal, or low. Leukemia may develop, but morbidity more often results from infection, bleeding, and iron overload. Diagnostic tests exclude vitamin B_{12} and folate deficiencies and identify associated disorders and drug exposures. Suspect drugs should be stopped, and underlying disorders should be treated. No treatment or only occasional red cell transfusions for symptomatic anemia may be needed. Folic acid (1–2 mg/d PO) prevents deficiency, but improvement in anemia is unlikely. Iron stores should be quantitated, and deferoxamine therapy may be needed to prevent or treat symptomatic iron overload. Efforts to improve cytopenias are seldom effective and include androgens, differentiation therapy with low-dose cytosine arabinoside (10 mg/m^2 SC q12h or 20 mg/m^2/d by continuous IV infusion for 7 to 21 days) or *cis*-retinoic acid, immunosuppression with corticosteroids, cyclophosphamide, or azathioprine, splenectomy (may cause postoperative thrombocytosis and thrombosis), and bone marrow transplantation for young patients. **Pyridoxine** (100 mg PO tid for 3 to 4 months), pyridoxal 5′-phosphate, L-tryptophan, and vitamin C benefit occasional patients with hereditary or idiopathic sideroblastic anemias. Selected patients with symptomatic anemia or severe neutropenia may benefit from treatment with EPO (60–300 U/kg/d SC) and G-CSF (1 μg/kg/d SC) or GM-CSF (1.5 μg/kg/d SC) or both, but G-CSF may decrease survival, whereas GM-CSF may increase evolution to leukemia and lower platelet counts. Chemotherapy is appropriate for overt leukemia, but success is limited by patient age and refractoriness of leukemias induced by chemical carcinogens.

6. CYTOPLASMIC MATURATION DISORDERS
   a. **The thalassemias.** Hereditary defects in synthesis of α or β chains of hemoglobin, primarily in Mediterranean, African, and Asian populations. Microcytosis and hypochromia are prominent, even when anemia is mild and splenomegaly is common, but severity of anemia depends on the number of globin chain genes affected. A thalassemia phenotype may also result from structurally abnormal hemoglobins, such as hemoglobin E in Southeast Asian subjects. Anemia may increase during pregnancy, infection, or use of oxidant drugs (hemoglobin H disease, hemoglobin E).
      (1) Diagnostic tests. Elevated hemoglobin A_2 or F levels or both on hemoglobin electrophoresis (β-thalassemia trait, β-thalassemia [thalassemia major]), hemoglobin H (tetramers of excess β chains) on hemoglobin electrophoresis or Heinz body preparations (α-thalassemia, hemoglobin H disease), in vitro studies of reticulocyte and marrow globin chain synthesis, family studies, tests to exclude iron deficiency, which can suppress hemoglobin A_2 synthesis. If anemia is severe, the presence of unrelated complicating disorders should be considered.
      (2) Therapy. Genetic counseling is provided, as is monitoring for iron overload and avoiding iron therapy. Folate supplements are given. Oxidant drugs (hemoglobin H disease, hemoglobin E) must be avoided. Splenectomy benefits selected patients with hemoglobin H disease or thalassemia major but should be preceded by polyvalent pneumococcal vaccine. Deferoxamine infusions are given prophylactically in thalassemia major and therapeutically when iron overload develops in other forms of thalassemia. The purpose of chronic red cell hypertransfusion is to maintain hemoglobin levels of 10 to 12 g/dL in children with thalassemia major (suppresses erythropoiesis, limits marrow expansion, and prevents bone deformities). High-dose EPO (750 U/kg SC 3 times per week) may improve anemia in splenectomized subjects, but stimulation of Hgb F synthesis with hydroxyurea (10–20 mg/kg/d) is minimally effective. Allogenic BMT can cure 60% to 90% of children below age 14, but 5% to 10% die, and thalassemia may relapse in 20%.

7. HEMOLYTIC ANEMIAS
   a. **Hemolytic anemia** is defined as a rapid fall in hematocrit (acute) or a stable hematocrit with sustained reticulocytosis (chronic) in the absence of bleeding. Reticulocytosis begins 3 to 7 days after onset of hemolysis. Low serum haptoglobin and elevated serum LDH and bilirubin levels occur with both intravascular and extravascular destruction but are insensitive and nonspecific. Intravascular hemolysis causes hemoglobinemia and hemoglobinuria (often transient), and hemosiderinuria develops 4 to 14 days later. All patients with chronic hemolysis require **folate therapy (1 mg/d)** and monitoring for cholelithiasis, iron overload (if extravascular), and iron depletion (if intravascular). Hemolysis may increase with infections

(e.g., sickle cell disease) or the use of oxidant drugs (e.g., G6PD deficiency). Aplastic crises may result from parvovirus infections and require intensive transfusion support.

b. **Sickle cell disorders** are due to inheritance of a structurally abnormal β chain that forms insoluble polymers under hypoxic conditions. **Heterozygotes** are not anemic, and symptoms are rare, but microscopic hematuria and impaired renal concentrating ability may occur, and genetic counseling is needed. **Homozygotes** have chronic intravascular hemolysis and recurrent vasoocclusive events leading to infarctive crises characterized by bone, chest, and abdominal pain, fever, and neurologic and visual changes that are difficult to distinguish from complicating disorders, such as osteomyelitis, cholecystitis, hepatitis, appendicitis, pneumonia, marrow emboli, and meningitis. Diagnosis is made by hemoglobin electrophoresis. Treatment involves avoidance of dehydration and cold exposure, analgesics, correction of hypoxemia and acidosis, incentive spirometry, and treatment of infections. Exchange transfusions to reduce hemoglobin S levels below 40% may be used therapeutically (for neurologic, cardiac, or retinal symptoms, hypoxemia, priapism, severe prolonged or infarctive crises, acute splenic sequestration [infants], and chronic leg ulcers) or prophylactically (during pregnancy or before general anesthesia). Long-term exchange/transfusion may be useful in selected patients with severe neurologic, retinal, or cardiac symptoms. Attempts to modify sickling with urea, cyanate, and induced hyponatremia have had little success. Stimulation of hemoglobin F synthesis with hydroxyurea (15–30 mg/kg/d) decreases the frequency and severity of crises in selected patients, but monitoring for myelosuppression every 1 to 2 weeks is needed, and long-term sequelae remain to be defined.

c. **Hereditary deficiencies of red cell enzymes of glycolysis, the hexose monophosphate shunt, or nucleotide metabolism.** Extravascular hemolysis is diagnosed by specific enzyme assays. In X-linked G6PD deficiency, self-limited hemolysis occurs with infection or the use of oxidant drugs (Table 10–2) if enzyme deficiency is limited to older red cells, and chronic hemolysis occurs if both young and old red cells are affected. Diagnosis may require measuring G6PD activity 3 to 4 months after recovery. **Splenectomy** can benefit patients with severe hemolysis due to pyruvate kinase, hexokinase, glucose phosphate isomerase, or G6PD deficiency. **Vaccinations** for pneumococcus, meningococcus and *Haemophilus influenzae* b should be given several weeks before splenectomy, and long-term postsplenectomy penicillin prophylaxis should be considered.

d. **Hereditary spherocytosis.** Extravascular hemolysis is due to hereditary defects of red cell membrane proteins. Hyperchromic microspherocytes on the peripheral smear may be infrequent and also occur with autoimmune hemolytic anemia. The diagnosis is indicated by increased sensitivity to hypotonic lysis on the incubated osmotic fragility test. Treatment with splenectomy may benefit patients with severe hemolysis or chronic leg ulcers.

TABLE 10–2. **Some Hemolytic Oxidant Drugs and Chemicals in G6PD-Deficient Patients**

ANTIBIOTICS	ANTIPYRETICS	MISCELLANEOUS
Primaquine	Phenacetin	Acetanilid
Quinacrine		Naphthalene
Nalidixic acid		Phenylhydrazine
Nitrofurantoin		Toluidine blue
Sulfonamides (sulfanilamide,		Methylene blue
sulfacetamide, sulfapyridine,		Trinitrotoluene
salicylazosulfapyridine,		High-dose vitamin C
sulfamethoxazole)		
Diaminodiphenylsulfone		
Niridazole		

e. **Paroxysmal nocturnal hemoglobinuria (PNH)** is an acquired clonal myeloproliferative disorder characterized by defective glycosylphosphatidylinositol (GPI), a membrane protein anchor molecule, which leads to intermittent intravascular hemolysis due to complement-mediated membrane damage, a thrombotic diathesis, thrombocytopenia, and neutropenia. PNH may arise from or occur as aplastic anemia. Hemolysis increases during correction of iron deficiency or the administration of blood products, whereas thrombosis increases during surgery or pregnancy. Increased sensitivity of red cells to lysis on incubation with sucrose or acidified serum (Ham test), low leukocyte alkaline phosphatase, and flow cytometry with monoclonal antibodies to GPI-linked proteins establish the diagnosis. Therapy of anemia involves androgens, steroids (prednisone 60 mg at night tapered to 10–40 mg qod), hypertransfusion (hemoglobin >10 g/dL), particularly perioperatively and during pregnancy or iron replacement. Therapy or prevention of thrombosis is done with prednisone, heparin, and Coumadin. The roles of antiplatelet and fibrinolytic agents have not been established. Bone marrow transplant is an option for young patients with severe disease, but up to 15% of patients may have spontaneous long-term remissions.

f. **Immune hemolytic anemia (IHA).** This is due to binding of immunoglobulin or complement to red cells and is characterized by microspherocytes on the peripheral smear. The condition may be idiopathic or secondary to drugs (Table 10–3), infection, malignant disease, lymphoproliferative diseases, or rheumatologic disorders. Reticulocytopenia occurs if antibody binds to reticulocytes or red cell precursors. Warm-reactive antibodies (often IgG) are most active at 37°C and cause extravascular hemolysis. Cold-reactive antibodies (often IgM) are most active below 37°C, bind transiently, fix complement, and cause intravascular hemolysis. Cold agglutinins may react with red cell I or i antigens and cause hemolysis when present in high titers. Drugs or drug metabolites may bind to red cells to form new antigens (haptenic mechanism), or they may

TABLE 10-3. Some Drugs Associated with Immune Hemolytic Anemia

HAPTEN MECHANISM (Strong Drug-RBC Binding)

Penicillins	Tetracycline	
Cephalosporins	Streptomycin	

HAPTEN MECHANISM (Weak Drug-RBC Binding)

Quinine	Sulfonamides	p-aminosalicylic acid
Quinidine	Sulfonylureas	Chlorpromazine
Phenacetin	Thiazides	Nonsteroidal anti-inflammatory drugs
Rifampicin	Isoniazid	

AUTOIMMUNE MECHANISM

Aldomet	Mefenamic acid	Procainamide
Levodopa	Ibuprofen	Fludarabine

modify red cell membranes, permitting autoantibody formation (autoimmune mechanism). Drugs may also cause nonspecific binding of immunoglobulin or complement or both, leading to a positive Coombs' test without hemolysis (e.g., cephalosporins). The direct antiglobulin (Coombs') test is used for diagnosis; it is negative in 5% to 10% of cases. The first step in therapy is to identify associated disorders and stop suspect drugs. Therapy of warm IHA is **prednisone** (40–60 mg/m^2/d—up to 21 days to respond), splenectomy (response **not** predicted by splenic red cell uptake studies; presplenectomy vaccination for encapsulated organisms is indicated and postsplenectomy antibiotic prophylaxis may be given), immunosuppressive agents (cyclophosphamide or azathioprine 1–2 mg/kg/d for 3 to 4 months, but marrow suppression may worsen anemia), and danazol (200 mg tid or qid; 60% to 80% response). IV immunoglobin (0.4 g/kg/d for 4 to 5 days infused over 1 hour) transiently improves anemia in 30% of cases. Rare side effects include acute aseptic meningitis. Plasma change is rarely helpful. Therapy of cold IHA begins with keeping the patient warm. Immunosuppressive agents and plasma exchange may be of benefit; steroids and splenectomy are rarely effective. Identifying compatible blood may be difficult, but transfusions are indicated when anemia is life threatening.

B. Erythrocytosis

1. **DEFINITION.** Hemoglobin >17.5 g/dL in men, >16 g/dL in women.

2. **CLASSIFICATION** (Table 10-4). A high red cell mass (>36 mL/kg for men, >32 mL/kg for women) distinguishes **absolute** from **relative** (low plasma volume) erythrocytosis. Low serum erythropoietin levels distinguish primary marrow proliferative disorders from disorders secondary to systemic hypoxia, renal hypoxia, or autonomous erythropoietin production (high values).

3. **RELATIVE ERYTHROCYTOSIS.** Only associated disorders (e.g., hypertension) are treated.

4. **ERYTHROCYTOSIS DUE TO SYSTEMIC HYPOXIA** (Table 10–4). High red cell mass compensates for increased oxygen needs.

   a. **Diagnostic tests. Arterial blood gases** (Po_2 <60 mm Hg; measured hemoglobin-oxygen saturations <92%, but may fall only during sleep or when patient is supine); P_{50} (<20 mm Hg with high-oxygen affinity hemoglobin); carboxyhemoglobin (>4% in smokers); hemoglobin electrophoresis (rarely useful).

   b. **Therapy** includes continuous or nocturnal oxygen for hypoxemia, surgery for intracardiac shunts, weight loss, and cessation of smoking. Phlebotomy can improve mental alertness, work performance, and headache by increasing blood flow, but blood oxygen-carrying capacity decreases. Thus, the optimum hematocrit must be empirically derived for each patient.

5. **ERYTHROCYTOSIS DUE TO RENAL DISEASES OR NONHYPOXIC DISORDERS.** Red cell mass exceeds tissue oxygen demands. Treatment of underlying disorder and phlebotomy can improve symptoms.

TABLE 10–4. **Classification of Erythrocytosis**

RELATIVE ERYTHROCYTOSIS (normal red cell mass, low plasma volume)
ABSOLUTE ERYTHROCYTOSIS (high red cell mass)
  Erythropoietin independent (autonomous)
    Polycythemia vera
  Erythropoietin dependent (secondary)
    Systemic Hypoxia
      Hypoxemic disorders (Low *measured* hemoglobin-oxygen saturation)
        High altitude
        Pulmonary insufficiency
        Intrapulmonary shunts (cirrhosis, hereditary telangiectasia)
        Alveolar hypoventilation (obesity)
        Cardiac disorders (right-to-left shunts)
      Nonhypoxemic disorders (normal hemoglobin-oxygen saturations)
        Increased hemoglobin-oxygen affinity (low P_{50})
          Abnormal hemoglobins: hereditary (autosomal dominant), acquired
            (carboxyhemoglobin, methemoglobin)
          Decreased 2,3-DPG
    Renal hypoxia
      Cysts
      Tumors
      Hydronephrosis
      Renal artery stenosis
      Chronic pyelonephritis
      Renal transplant rejection
    Nonhypoxic (autonomous erythropoietin production)
      Idiopathic
      Familial (autosomal recessive)
      Ectopic erythropoietin production: hypernephroma, hepatoma, uterine leiomyoma, cerebellar hemangioblastoma

6. **POLYCYTHEMIA VERA** is an acquired clonal myeloproliferative disorder characterized by erythrocytosis, granulocytosis, thrombocytosis, splenomegaly, and thrombosis. Iron deficiency, basophilia, pruritus, and hyperuricemia are also common, and acute leukemia or myeloid metaplasia may develop later.

   a. **Diagnostic indications** include high leukocyte alkaline phosphatase, increased serum vitamin B_{12} binding proteins, abnormal marrow cytogenetics, and autonomous in vitro erythroid colony growth. Causes of secondary erythrocytosis should be excluded.

   b. **Therapy**

   (1) *Phlebotomy.* Hematocrit should be reduced to 42% to 45% by removing 0.5 to 1 U of blood daily or every other day, with less frequent removal of smaller volumes in the elderly and in patients with cardiac disorders. Blood counts should be checked monthly, and hematocrit should be maintained below 45%. As iron deficiency develops, the need for phlebotomy decreases, and iron supplements are given only if symptoms develop (e.g., cheilosis, glossitis, weakness). Phlebotomy can **increase the risk of thrombosis** and does not affect splenomegaly, thrombocytosis, or signs and symptoms due to increased marrow turnover (hyperuricemia, pruritus, weight loss, fatigue).

   (2) *Myelosuppressive therapy.* Indicated with advanced age (>70), continued need for frequent phlebotomy, prior thromboses, symptoms due to splenomegaly, hypermetabolic state, and perhaps for platelet counts $>1 \times 10^6$ (an association between thrombocytosis and thrombosis is not established). Phlebotomies are also needed for several weeks until a response occurs. ^{32}P is convenient for elderly patients whose limited life expectancy offsets the risk of treatment-related leukemia. A single dose (2.3 mCi/m^2 IV, total dose <5 mCi/m^2) decreases the red cell mass in 2 to 3 months. A second dose may be required at 12 weeks, and unmaintained remissions last 6 to 18 months. Hydroxyurea (15–20 mg/kg/d PO continuously) or busulfan (4–6 mg/d PO until remission and then intermittently as needed) may be less leukemogenic than chlorambucil, but more studies are needed. Blood counts should be checked weekly or bimonthly, and dosages should be adjusted for thrombocytopenia or leukopenia, which may be protracted after busulfan. Rarely, prolonged use of busulfan can cause pulmonary fibrosis, hyperpigmentation, or a wasting syndrome.

   (3) *Recombinant interferon-α2b* (3×10^6 U/m^2 SC 3 times per week) can control erythrocytosis, thrombocytosis, splenomegaly and pruritus after several months of treatment. Side effects of malaise and fever may abate with continued therapy, but long-term sequelae remain to be defined.

   (4) *Allopurinol* (300 mg/d) for hyperuricemia; *cyproheptadine* (4 mg 3 to 4 times per day) or *cimetidine* (300 mg qid) for pruritus.

(5) ***Antiplatelet agents*** (aspirin, dipyridamole) may *not* prevent thrombosis and may increase the risk of gastrointestinal hemorrhage.

C. Iron Overload

1. **CLASSIFICATION.** Iron overload results from red cell transfusions or increased absorption of dietary iron due to idiopathic hemochromatosis (or both), thalassemia, chronic hemolytic anemias, myelodysplastic syndromes, and congenital dyserythropoietic anemias. Iron may be deposited in reticuloendothelial cells with little associated toxicity or in parenchymal cells with tissue damage resulting in cirrhosis, cardiomyopathy, diabetes mellitus, hypogonadism, and arthritis.

2. **DIAGNOSTIC TESTS.** Serum iron >160 μg/dL with transferrin saturations >60% (also occur with ineffective erythropoiesis, chronic hemolysis, and marrow hypoplasia without iron overload); serum ferritin >400 mg/dL (also increased by inflammation, cancer, and liver disease); urinary iron loss >2.2 mg/d after deferoxamine (10 mg/kg IM), but this test may be insensitive to early parenchymal iron overload. Liver biopsy with histologic and quantitative analyses of iron content is the best index of total body iron stores, iron distribution (parenchymal versus reticuloendothelial), and tissue damage (cirrhosis). Another diagnostic marker is a family history of anemia or signs and symptoms of iron overload.

3. **THERAPY.** Tea with meals decreases absorption; transfusions should be limited. Removal of iron by phlebotomy (1–2 U/wk until iron deficiency develops and then 3–4 U/y) in idiopathic hemosiderosis or by SC infusion of deferoxamine (1–4 g over 12 to 24 hours, with dose adjusted to achieve maximum urinary iron loss) in primary hematologic disorders prolongs survival and improves, stabilizes, or prevents cardiac dysfunction, cirrhosis, hyperpigmentation, and hypogonadism. Although vitamin C (100–200 mg/d PO) increases the effectiveness of deferoxamine, its use should be discouraged, as it may cause cardiac decompensation as iron is released from reticuloendothelial sites. Initially, serum ferritin, serum iron, and MCV are measured monthly and then two to three times per year after iron stores are depleted. HLA typing of patients with idiopathic hemochromatosis and their families permits identification of obligate homozygotes and carriers and appropriate genetic counseling.

Chanarin J. Investigation and management of megaloblastic anaemia. Clin Haematol 1976;5: 747–763.

Charache S, Terrin ML, Moore RD, et al. Effect of hydroxyurea on the frequency of painful crises in sickle cell anemia. N Engl J Med 1995;332:1317–1322.

Gordeuk VR, Bacon BR, Brittenham GM. Iron overload: causes and consequences. Ann Rev Nutr 1987;7:485–508.

Green R. Screening for vitamin B$_{12}$ deficiency. Ann Intern Med 1996;124:509–511.

Hillman RS, Finch CE. The Red Cell Manual, 5th ed. Philadelphia: FA Davis Co, 1985.

Silver RT. Interferon-α2b: a new treatment for polycythemia vera. Ann Intern Med 1993;119: 1091–1092.

Young MS, Barratt AJ. The treatment of severe acquired aplastic anemia. Blood 1995;33:67–77.

II. LEUKOCYTE DISORDERS

Malignant leukocyte disorders, including acute and chronic leukemias, lymphomas, and plasma cell dyscrasias, are discussed in Chapter 11.

A. Neutrophilia

Neutrophilia (neutrophil count >10,000/μL) occurs most commonly as a normal marrow response to inflammation or infection but may also occur in response to epinephrine or corticosteroids or as part of a myeloproliferative disorder. Neutrophilia per se produces no adverse effects, and therapy is directed toward the underlying disorder.

B. Neutropenia

Neutropenia (neutrophil count <1800/μL) may occur as an isolated finding or in association with anemia, thrombocytopenia, or both. It may be due to decreased marrow production (drug toxicity, intrinsic marrow disease, marrow infiltration, vitamin B_{12} or folate deficiency), increased neutrophil destruction (drug effect, overwhelming bacterial infection, immune neutropenia), or increased margination (inflammation, splenomegaly). **Unexplained isolated neutropenia** is most often drug induced, and all unnecessary drugs should be discontinued. The hematopoietic growth factors G-CSF and GM-CSF have been shown to shorten the period of chemotherapy-induced neutropenia. Treatment with G-CSF is effective in raising the neutrophil count and reducing the incidence of infection in most cases of acute or chronic neutropenia. Antibiotic management of infections in patients with neutropenia is discussed in Chapter 3. Severely neutropenic patients with documented bacterial or fungal infection are candidates for neutrophil transfusion therapy if they do not respond to appropriate antibiotic therapy within 24 to 48 hours.

III. DISORDERS OF HEMOSTASIS

A. Bleeding Disorders

Pertinent diagnostic information includes the type of bleeding, the nature of inciting events (spontaneous versus surgery or trauma), prior drug or transfusion therapy, the presence of any significant medical disorders, and family history. However, definitive diagnosis of a bleeding disorder depends on adequate laboratory data. Initial workup should include a **full coagulation screen.**

- *Platelet count.* The relationship between the platelet count and bleeding due to thrombocytopenia is discussed on page 397.
- *Bleeding time (BT),* normally 4 to 8 minutes, is a measure of in vivo platelet plug formation. With normal platelet function, BT = 30 – platelet count/4000. If BT exceeds the predicted value, platelet dysfunction is present. Abnormalities in platelet plug formation are usually clinically significant only if the BT is greater than 12 to 15 minutes.
- *Fibrinogen.* Clinically significant bleeding due to hypofibrinogenemia is not likely to occur unless the fibrinogen level is less than 80 to 100 mg/dL.

Values below 80 mg/dL will result in prolongation of the other clotting tests.
- *Thrombin time* will be prolonged in the presence of dysfibrinogenemia/ hypofibrinogenemia or fibrin degradation products. The test is most valuable as a sensitive indicator for the presence of heparin.
- *Prothrombin time (PT)* measures extrinsic pathway clotting and reflects levels of factor VII as well as the common pathway factors (X, V, II, fibrinogen). Clinically important factor deficiency usually prolongs the PT at least 4 to 6 seconds.
- *Partial thromboplastin time (PTT)* measures intrinsic pathway clotting and reflects levels of factors XII, XI, IX, and VIII as well as the common pathway factors (X, V, II, fibrinogen). Clinically important factor deficiencies usually prolong the PTT at least 8 to 12 seconds.
- *Fibrin degradation products* will generally be increased with significant fibrinolysis.

Depending on the results of the screening tests, specific coagulation factor assays and other special tests may be performed to further define the problem.

1. PLATELET DISORDERS
   a. **Thrombocytopenia** may be due to decreased production, increased destruction, or splenic sequestration. The peripheral blood smear should be examined to confirm the degree of thrombocytopenia, assess platelet morphology (large platelets suggest a high platelet turnover), and detect abnormalities in other cell lines. Examination of bone marrow megakaryocyte numbers provides an estimate of platelet production.

   In addition to treating any underlying disorders, general management includes **minimizing the chance of bleeding** by avoiding intramuscular injections, drugs that inhibit platelet function (e.g., aspirin), and activities that carry significant risk of trauma. Menses can be suppressed by hormonal therapy. In the absence of platelet dysfunction, spontaneous bleeding will not occur in most patients until the platelet count drops below 5000/µL. Bleeding may occur at higher levels (20,000 to 40,000/µL) in patients with platelet dysfunction (e.g., uremia, sepsis, exposure to drugs that impair platelet function). With trauma or surgery, counts as high as 50,000 to 100,000/µL may be needed for effective hemostasis. In the absence of significant bleeding, **platelet transfusions** should be reserved for patients with platelet counts under 5000 to 10,000/µL or for patients with counts below 50,000 to 100,000/µL who are about to undergo an invasive procedure.

   b. **Drug-induced thrombocytopenia** is common after cytotoxic drug therapy. It may also occur as an unanticipated reaction to other drugs on either a marrow suppressive or antibody-mediated basis. Unnecessary drugs should be discontinued. **Platelet transfusions** may be necessary but often are not effective in immune-mediated cases. Therapy with **corticosteroids** has not proved useful. **Plasma exchange** has been reported to be rapidly effective in some cases of quinine/quinidine-induced thrombocytopenia.

c. **Autoimmune thrombocytopenic purpura (AITP)** is an antibody-mediated disorder with decreased platelet survival and normal or increased numbers of megakaryocytes in the marrow. There may be large platelet forms and BT shorter than predicted by the platelet count. Increased amounts of IgG usually can be demonstrated on the platelet surface. The disorder may be primary or may be seen in association with systemic lupus erythematosus, non-Hodgkin's lymphoma, chronic lymphocytic leukemia, or HIV infection. Diagnosis depends on exclusion of other causes of thrombocytopenia. Prednisone 1 mg/kg should be given as initial therapy. Two thirds of patients will respond; the initial response usually occurs within 2 to 3 days but may take as long as 1 to 2 weeks. Once a maximum or normal platelet count is achieved, the drug dose should be tapered to ascertain the dose required to maintain an acceptable count. Approximately one third of responses will be durable. Splenectomy is indicated for patients in whom steroid therapy has failed or for those in whom the maintenance dose is unacceptably high. Seventy percent of patients will achieve a complete response with splenectomy. Splenectomy can usually be performed without excessive bleeding or the need for platelet transfusions, even in patients with severe thrombocytopenia. Most patients will respond to IV gamma globulin (1 g/kg/d for 2 days). The effect is short-lived, with severe thrombocytopenia usually recurring within 1 to 3 weeks. However, the transient improvement may be useful in getting the patient through an acute episode of bleeding or a surgical procedure. For patients in whom such therapy has failed, favorable results have been reported with danazol (an attenuated androgen), immunosuppressive agents (e.g., vincristine, vinblastine, azathioprine, cyclophosphamide), immunoabsorption with staphylococcal protein A columns, and administration of anti-D (in Rh-positive patients). Plasma exchange has not proved generally efficacious.

Platelet transfusions are normally reserved for patients with life-threatening hemorrhage, as the life span of the transfused cells is usually very short. However, platelet survival does vary, and administration of a trial platelet transfusion is reasonable for patients with significant bleeding or with severe thrombocytopenia if the diagnosis is uncertain.

d. **Thrombotic thrombocytopenic purpura (TTP)** is characterized pathologically by widespread deposition of platelet aggregates in the microvasculature and clinically by microangiopathic hemolytic anemia, thrombocytopenia, neurologic abnormalities, renal dysfunction, and fever. The syndrome is closely related to the hemolytic uremic syndrome and is often associated with infection by toxigenic strains of *Escherichia coli.* Untreated, TTP is often fatal. The principal therapeutic approach involves plasma exchange or plasma infusion. In severely affected patients, daily plasma exchange (1–1.5 plasma volumes) should be started immediately, with the replacement fluid being 50% to 100% plasma. Alternatively, if the cardiovascular status permits, 4–8 U of plasma may be infused initially followed by 3–4 U/d. The intensity of this therapy may be adjusted depending on the patient's response but should be continued at least 7 to 10 days before it is concluded that no effect is likely to occur. Less severely affected patients may be treated less aggressively, and some will respond to much less plasma. Prednisone (1–2 mg/kg/d) probably improves the response rate, and the dose can be tapered rapidly after maximal response is attained. Antiplatelet agents (aspirin 325–1300 mg/d with or without dipyridamole 400 mg/d) have been shown to be important in therapy in some cases and should probably be given and continued for 3 to 6 months if there is not significant bleeding. About 75% of cases will respond to this approach, with improvement in neurologic status and platelet count apparent after a few days. Therapy with vincristine, IV gamma globulin, or splenectomy may be effective in refractory cases. Platelet transfusions are usually not necessary in patients with TTP, and some reports have suggested that they may be detrimental.

e. **Posttransfusion purpura** is a rare disorder characterized by thrombocytopenia occurring about 1 week after transfusion in a patient who either has previously been pregnant or undergone transfusion. Platelet counts are usually less than 10,000/μL. Megakaryocytes are plentiful in the marrow, and high-titer platelet antibodies are demonstrable. Most commonly in patients negative for the platelet-specific antigen HPA-1a (Pl^{A1}), a previously made anti-HPA-1a antibody has been recalled (and possibly an autoantibody produced), resulting in the destruction of both autologous and transfused platelets. Untreated, thrombocytopenia may persist for weeks. High-dose prednisone (2–4 mg/kg/d), IV gamma globulin (0.4 g/kg/d for 2 to 5 days), or plasma exchange may improve the platelet count within a few days. Platelet transfusion is ineffective.

f. **Dilutional thrombocytopenia** may occur in massive transfusion. Platelet counts should be monitored in patients transfused with more than 1 blood volume, and platelet transfusion should be considered for clinically significant thrombocytopenia.

g. **Qualitative platelet abnormalities.** Acquired platelet function abnormalities occur with uremia, myeloproliferative disorders, paraproteinemias, disseminated intravascular coagulation, sepsis, and the use of drugs known to impair platelet function. Congenital platelet function abnormalities include von Willebrand disease and other more rare disorders. **The hallmark of platelet dysfunction is prolonged bleeding time** not explainable by the platelet count. Management of acquired platelet dysfunction involves treatment of the underlying disorder. The platelet defect in uremia is usually improved by dialysis. In both congenital and acquired disorders, platelet function may be transiently improved in some patients by cryoprecipitate (10–15 bags), deamino-D-arginine vasopressin (DDAVP [0.3 μg/kg]), or platelet transfusion. The patient should avoid drugs that impair platelet function.

h. **Thrombocytosis.** Extremely high platelet counts may be associated with abnormal bleeding or, less frequently, with venous or arterial thrombosis. These clinical manifestations are almost always limited to patients with myeloproliferative disorders and severe thrombocytosis (platelets $\geq 10^6/\mu L$). They do not occur in patients with secondary thrombocytosis. Therapy with myelosuppressive and antiplatelet agents is discussed in the section on essential thrombocythemia and polycythemia vera. If symptoms are life threatening, plateletpheresis will decrease the platelet count rapidly, but the effect is transient, and the count will rebound within a few days.

2. COAGULATION FACTOR ABNORMALITIES. The distinction between congenital and acquired coagulation factor abnormalities is usually apparent from the history, although the condition in some patients with mild congenital factor deficiencies may not become apparent until adulthood, often after a hemostatic challenge. In congenital disorders, the defect is usually the deficiency of a single coagulation factor; with acquired disorders there are usually multiple factor deficiencies.

   a. **Hemophilia.** Congenital deficiencies of factor VIII (hemophilia A) or factor IX (hemophilia B) are X-linked disorders. Patients with factor levels less than 1% of normal usually suffer frequent spontaneous hemorrhage. Spontaneous hemorrhage is unusual in patients with levels of 1% to 5%. With levels greater than 5%, bleeding may occur if patients are subjected to hemostatic challenge. Management involves factor replacement at the time of hemorrhage, patient and family education, genetic counseling, psychologic support, and inclusion of dentists and orthopedic surgeons on the health care team. Active but sensible exercise is encouraged to increase muscle tone and minimize the chance of bleeding. Patients should avoid aspirin-containing drugs as well as IM injections.

   The basic principle of therapy for bleeding episodes is that they be treated early—thus, the widespread use of home treatment. There must be a high level of suspicion that any unexplained symptom is an episode of bleeding. Pain usually occurs before any other evidence of bleeding, and treatment should not be withheld simply because there are no physical signs. Superficial cuts and bruises can usually be handled by local measures. If sutures are required, factor replacement should be provided. Initial factor levels of 30% to 40% should be attained with uncomplicated hemarthrosis, hematuria, and minor hematomas, with daily repetition of this dose until resolution. Surgery or major muscle hematomas require initial factor levels of 60% to 100%, with minimum levels of 40% to 50% maintained over the next 10 to 14 days. Factor levels should be monitored to ensure that the expected levels are being attained. Patients with head injury, even if only a hard blow, should be given factor replacement to initial levels of 50% to 60% even if there are no neurologic signs or symptoms. CT should be performed on any patient with neurologic abnormalities; if positive, a full surgical regimen of factor replacement is initiated. For oral surgical procedures or dental extractions, a single infusion of factors to bring the level to 50% to 100% is followed by administration of epsilon-aminocaproic acid (EACA) to inhibit clot lysis (see below).

   The component and dose required to achieve such factor levels depend on the particular factor involved and the patient's baseline level. For factor VIII, replacement is with either plasma-derived or recombinant factor VIII concentrate. The administration of 1 U/kg will result in an increase in plasma levels of 2%. Since the half-life of factor VIII is about 10 hours, the dose may have to be repeated every 12 hours. Factor IX replacement is achieved with factor IX concentrates. Because of the extravascular distribution of factor IX, the dose is twice that of factor VIII. The half-life of factor IX is approximately 24 hours. Thus, the repeated dose, if required, need be administered only every 24 hours. Although factor replacement is normally not indicated in the absence of bleeding, prophylactic replacement may be appropriate for frequent repeated hemorrhage.

EACA, a fibrinolytic inhibitor, is effective in achieving clot stabilization following dental or oral surgical procedures. The usual dose is 50 mg/kg every 6 hours for 7 to 10 days. Antifibrinolytic therapy is contraindicated in urinary bleeding.

DDAVP (0.3 µg/kg IV) mobilizes extravascular factor VIII and increases plasma levels by 2-fold to 3-fold. Its use in patients with mild hemophilia A who have acute bleeding or before scheduled minor surgery may eliminate the need for blood products. The effect is rapid, factor VIII levels being maximal within an hour and declining with the usual 10-hour to 12-hour half-life. Patients may be refractory to a second dose for 48 hours. Factor VIII levels should be monitored. DDAVP is not effective in hemophilia B.

Joint bleeding is a common manifestation of severe hemophilia. Treatment consists of early factor replacement and **joint immobilization** during the period of pain. Routine joint aspiration is not indicated but may be considered, if factor levels are adequate, for relief of severe pain and as a diagnostic procedure if infection is suspected. Chronic synovitis is best handled by prophylactic factor replacement and isometric exercises. Joint replacement can be accomplished with adequate factor replacement.

Approximately 10% to 15% of patients with severe hemophilia A develop antibodies to factor VIII. In most cases, the inhibitor titer will increase dramatically if factor VIII is given, making subsequent treatment difficult. Thus, management of mild bleeding episodes is limited to immobilization and analgesia. With more severe bleeding episodes, low-purity factor IX concentrates are often effective, presumably because of the presence of activated factors that bypass factor VIII in the coagulation sequence. Treatment with recombinant factor VII_a or porcine factor VIII may be effective. If the inhibitor concentration is low, large doses of factor VIII concentrate may be effective, but one may have only a few days before the titer increases to the point that further therapy is not possible. In desperate situations, inhibitor concentrations can be lowered with plasma exchange. Corticosteroids or cytotoxic agents have not proved useful. A state of immune tolerance may be induced in one half to two thirds of cases by daily infusion of factor VIII. After several months, the inhibitor titers fall and may disappear. Factor IX inhibitors develop in only 1% of patients with hemophilia B. Management is similar to that of patients with factor VIII inhibitors.

b. **Von Willebrand disease.** Von Willebrand disease (VWD) results from an inherited abnormality of von Willebrand factor (VWF). The most common form, type 1, is an autosomal dominant disorder characterized by a deficiency of all multimeric forms of the protein (15% to 60% of normal levels). Type 2 is characterized by selective deficiency of the larger VWF multimers, and type 3 is characterized by severe deficiency of all multimeric forms. VWF is necessary for the maintenance of factor VIII levels, which will be reduced in proportion to the level of total VWF protein. All forms of VWD are characterized by long BTs. Therapy is aimed at restoring the circulating level of VWF-factor VIII. For minor bleeding or for scheduled minor surgery, DDAVP (0.3 μg/kg) is effective in achieving adequate factor levels. This therapy may induce thrombocytopenia in some patients with the 2b subtype. For replacement of VWF-factor VIII, factor VIII concentrates that contain VWF should be used. Factor VIII levels necessary for hemostasis are those outlined for hemophilia A. After infusion, the BT correction lasts 4 to 6 hours, whereas correction of the factor VIII level is prolonged (24 to 48 hours). For surgery, component administration is needed preoperatively and at 12 and 24 hours postoperatively, and then at most once a day.

c. **Other factor deficiencies.** Deficiencies of other coagulation factors are inherited as autosomal recessive disorders and may also be associated with clinical bleeding. As with hemophilia, treatment of bleeding episodes is based on replacement of the factors to hemostatic levels (Table 10–5). With the exception of hypofibrinogenemia, which is treated with cryoprecipitate, replacement is with fresh frozen plasma.

d. **Vitamin K deficiency/antagonism.** Vitamin K deficiency may occur with malabsorption syndromes, biliary obstruction, poor diet in combination with broad-spectrum antibiotic therapy, therapy with certain third-generation cephalosporins, and high-dose aspirin therapy. Warfarin, a vitamin K antagonist, induces functional vitamin K deficiency. Screening test values include a normal fibrinogen level but prolonged PT and PTT, which correct to normal after mixture with normal plasma. Management depends on the urgency with

TABLE 10–5. Plasma Coagulation Factors

FACTOR	MINIMUM LEVEL NECESSARY FOR SURGERY (%)	NORMAL IN VIVO HALF-LIFE (h)
II	15	60
V	15–20	10
VII	10–15	5
VIII	25	10
IX	20–25	20
X	15–20	30
XI	10–25	70
XIII	5	230

which the hemostatic abnormality needs to be corrected. In patients with little or no bleeding, therapy with vitamin K_1 10–15 mg IV is sufficient and will correct the hemostatic abnormality within 24 to 72 hours if liver function is normal. Vitamin K deficiency can be reversed immediately with fresh frozen plasma, but this should be reserved for patients with significant bleeding or those about to undergo an invasive procedure. Low-purity factor IX concentrates should not be used to reverse vitamin K deficiency because of the risk of thrombosis due to the presence of activated clotting factors. In warfarin-treated patients, restoration to proper control may be achieved within a few days by adjusting the dose of either the anticoagulant or interacting drugs.

 e. **Liver disease.** Coagulation factor abnormalities in liver disease may be due to decreased factor synthesis, biliary obstruction with vitamin K deficiency, decreased clearance of fibrin degradation products, or dysfibrinogenemia. The PT and PTT are typically prolonged. For clinically significant abnormal laboratory values alone, therapy with vitamin K_1 (10 mg IV) is appropriate, but factor replacement is not required. If the patient is bleeding or is about to undergo an invasive procedure, coagulation factors should be provided, using fresh frozen plasma or, if the patient also needs red cells, whole blood. Because of the increased risk of thrombotic complications, low-purity factor IX concentrates should not be given to patients with liver disease. Factor replacement may be compromised in patients with ascites because the volume of distribution of the administered factors is greatly increased.

 f. **Defibrination syndromes.** Disseminated intravascular coagulation (DIC) is often associated with malignant disease, sepsis, tissue necrosis, shock, abruptio placentae, brain injury, and complement-mediated intravascular hemolysis. Diagnostically the most important laboratory findings are thrombocytopenia and hypofibrinogenemia. The PT and PTT are typically mildly to moderately prolonged. The thrombin time and BT may be prolonged because of the presence of fibrin degradation products. Clinical manifestations are most commonly bleeding and less commonly end-organ ischemia. Management of DIC is directed primarily toward correction of the underlying abnormality. Component replacement is usually appropriate only in patients who are bleeding or who require an invasive procedure. Most patients can be satisfactorily treated with a combination of **platelet transfusions** to keep the platelet count above 30,000 to 50,000/µL and **cryoprecipitate transfusion** to keep the fibrinogen above 80 to 100 mg/dL. Treatment with heparin is contraindicated unless the clinical manifestations are primarily tissue ischemia. Primary fibrinolysis occurs rarely except as a result of administration of fibrinolytic agents. It is manifested principally by hypofibrinogenemia. If treatment is necessary, hypofibrinogenemia may be reversed with cryoprecipitate.

 g. **Massive transfusion.** Patients who require large volumes of packed red blood cells may experience significant dilution of clotting factors. The extent of transfusion needed to produce a clinically important hemostatic abnormality depends on the baseline levels of the coagulation factors, but factor levels would be expected to be at 15% to 20% of the starting levels after the exchange of 2 blood volumes. Patients with laboratory evidence of clinically significant coagulation abnormalities may be treated with whole blood or with fresh frozen plasma. Dilutional thrombocytopenia will also occur under these circumstances and is nearly always of more clinical importance than dilution of the coagulation factors.

h. Circulating anticoagulants. Spontaneous inhibitors may develop to specific coagulation factors; the most common is directed toward factor VIII and may occur in association with rheumatologic, lymphoproliferative, and other disorders. Factor VIII inhibitors occurring in patients with hemophilia are discussed on page 401. The PTT is prolonged and does not correct on mixing with normal plasma. The diagnosis is confirmed by specific factor inhibitor assay. Management is similar to that in hemophiliacs with inhibitors, with three important differences: (1) spontaneous inhibitor titers usually do not rise in response to factor administration, so one can be more liberal in attempts to overwhelm the inhibitor with factor VIII infusion, (2) treatment with corticosteroids (prednisone 1 mg/kg/d) or cytotoxic agents (or both) is often effective, and (3) most spontaneous inhibitors do not cross-react with porcine factor VIII. Lupus inhibitors are immunoglobulins that interfere with clot generation in vitro. They occur in patients with such disorders as systemic lupus erythematosus, rheumatoid arthritis, drug reactions, and neoplasms, as well as in otherwise healthy individuals. These inhibitors are only rarely associated with a bleeding tendency; rather, they have been associated with an increased incidence of venous or arterial thrombosis and of spontaneous abortions. No specific therapy is indicated for the laboratory findings per se. If they are associated with thrombosis or frequent abortion, management includes anticoagulation therapy and immunosuppression with corticosteroids or cytotoxic agents.

3. **VASCULAR DISORDERS.** Purpura in the absence of identifiable hemostatic abnormalities can be seen in patients with vasculitis, scurvy, connective tissue disorders, Cushing's syndrome, Kaposi's sarcoma, cryoglobulinemia, and hyperglobulinemic purpura, as well as in patients with no obvious underlying disorder. Therapy is directed toward the underlying disorder.

B. Thrombotic Disorders

Thrombotic states of clinical importance include deep venous thrombosis, pulmonary embolus, and coronary or cerebral artery thrombosis or thromboembolism. These disorders are discussed in Chapters 4 and 7.

George JN, El-Harake MA, Raskob GE. Chronic idiopathic thrombocytopenic purpura. N Engl J Med 1994;331:1207–1211.

Lusher JM. Congenital coagulopathies and their management. In: Rossi EC, Simon TL, Moss GS, Gould SA, eds. Principles of Transfusion Medicine. Baltimore: Williams & Wilkins, 1996.

Thompson AR. Bleeding from acquired coagulation disorders and antithrombotic therapy. In: Rossi EC, Simon TL, Moss GS, Gould SA, eds. Principles of Transfusion Medicine. Baltimore: Williams & Wilkins, 1996.

IV. MYELOPROLIFERATIVE DISORDERS

A. Classification

Clonal stem cell disorders include **polycythemia vera, chronic myelogenous leukemia, paroxysmal nocturnal hemoglobinuria, agnogenic myeloid metaplasia with myelofibrosis,** and **essential thrombocythemia.**

B. Agnogenic Myeloid Metaplasia with Myelofibrosis

Agnogenic myeloid metaplasia with myelofibrosis is characterized by marrow fibrosis and extramedullary hematopoiesis leading to splenomegaly and anemia (often macrocytic) with granulocytosis, thrombocytosis, and teardrop-shaped red cells, nucleated red cells, large platelets, and immature granulocytes on the peripheral smear. Basophilia, eosinophilia, platelet dysfunction, hyperuricemia, and high serum lactic dehydrogenase levels are common. Leukocyte alkaline phosphatase may be high, normal, or low.

1. **DIAGNOSTIC TESTS.** Increased reticulin and collagen on bone marrow biopsy (but may be hypercellular or hypoplastic, and additional sampling may be needed), exclusion of folate and vitamin B_{12} deficiencies and disorders that cause secondary marrow fibrosis, such as other hematopoietic neoplasms (e.g., lymphomas, mastocytosis), solid tumors (e.g., prostate cancer), infections (e.g., tuberculosis), disorders with abnormal bone metabolism (e.g., renal osteodystrophy), rheumatologic diseases, and miscellaneous disorders (e.g., sarcoidosis, radiation therapy).

2. **THERAPY** includes transfusions (for symptomatic anemia), folate, allopurinol (for hyperuricemia). Androgens (p. 385) or pyridoxine (200–300 mg/d PO) may improve anemia. **Splenectomy** relieves local symptoms and improves cytopenias (but operative mortality is high and preoperative platelet transfusions may be needed for thrombocytopenia or platelet dysfunction). Splenic radiation relieves pain of splenic infarction and decreases spleen size in poor surgical candidates (but cytopenias may worsen from radiation of marrow included in the port). **Myelosuppressive agents** (e.g., busulfan 2–4 mg/d, 6-thioguanine 20–40 mg/d, ^{32}P) are given for splenomegaly or hypermetabolic symptoms (fever, fatigue, weight loss), but cytopenias may worsen. **1,25-Dihydroxyvitamin D$_3$** may improve anemia and thrombocytopenia, but hypercalcemia may occur. **Interferon** is minimally effective. **Bone marrow transplantation** may be useful in young patients with severe disease.

C. Essential Thrombocythemia

Essential thrombocythemia is characterized by thrombocytosis (platelets >600,000/mm^3 with giant forms on smear and atypical megakaryocytes in the marrow), bleeding, venous or arterial thromboses (less common), anemia, granulocytosis, and splenomegaly. Spurious elevations in serum potassium and acid phosphatase levels may occur. Diagnosis is made by bone marrow biopsy; platelet function tests, and BT (less consistently prolonged); exclude reactive thrombocytosis due to iron deficiency, acute hemorrhage, hemolysis, inflammation, or cancer (platelet function and morphology normal and pathologic bleeding or thrombosis does not occur); exclude other myeloproliferative disorders (e.g., polycythemia vera with complicating iron deficiency). **No treatment may be required** in patients less than 30 years old. **Myelosuppressive agents** in older patients (hydroxyurea 15–20 mg/kg/d PO, busulfan 4–6 mg/d PO) decrease platelet counts in 4 to 6 weeks. **Interferon-**α ($2–5 \times 10^6$ U/m^2 SC 3 times per week) may decrease the platelet count within 1 to 2 weeks. **Plateletpheresis, nitrogen mustard** (0.4 mg/kg IV), or hydroxyurea (30 mg/kg/d PO) is used for rapid reduction of platelet count in patients with acute bleeding or thrombosis. **Antiplatelet agents** (aspirin, dipyridamole, sulfinpyrazone) may help patients with digital ischemia or transient ischemic attacks, but risk of bleeding may be increased.

Gortelazzo S, Finazzi G, Ruggeri M, et al. Hydroxyurea for patients with essential thrombocythemia and a high risk of thrombosis. N Engl J Med 1995;332:1132–1136.
Tefferi A, Silverstein MN, Hoagland HC. Primary thrombocythemia. Semin Oncol 1995;22:334–340.

V. TRANSFUSION THERAPY

Modern transfusion therapy is based on the administration of specific components that are either collected directly from donors by apheresis techniques or separated from donated whole blood. Components can be divided into those containing red cells and those used to effect hemostasis.

A. Blood Components

1. COMPONENTS CONTAINING RED CELLS

   a. **Indications for transfusion.** A hematocrit value below which transfusions are universally required cannot be defined. The patient's age, underlying condition, symptoms, and the rate of change of the degree of anemia must be considered. Symptoms that may indicate a need for additional red cells include extreme fatigue, headache, dyspnea, angina, and palpitations. Patients rarely need transfusion if the hematocrit is over 30%. Patients who are otherwise healthy can often tolerate hematocrits of 15% to 20% without adverse effect. Patients with cardiorespiratory disease may develop symptoms when the hematocrit falls below 30%, but most patients do not do so until it falls below 25%. Each red cell unit can be expected to raise the hematocrit 3% to 4% in an adult recipient.

   In patients with acute hemorrhage, the immediate goal of maintaining intravascular volume can be achieved mostly, if not entirely, by administration of salt solutions or colloid preparations. Most patients without serious underlying disease can tolerate hemodilution to a hematocrit in the low 20s. Thus, it is probably reasonable to begin blood transfusion after loss of 30% to 40% of the blood volume, assuming the baseline hematocrit was normal.

   b. **Available products** include whole blood/modified whole blood, packed red blood cells, and other specialized red cell products. Whole blood/modified whole blood units contain approximately 200 mL red cells. If cryoprecipitate has been prepared from the unit, the suspending plasma will contain one half of the initial fibrinogen and

15% to 20% of the initial factor VIII, but other factors will be normal. With storage, factor VIII levels will fall to 30% of baseline in 2 to 3 days, factor V to 20% of baseline in 3 weeks, and other coagulation factors remain at baseline levels. There are no functional platelets or neutrophils. Packed red cells contain approximately 200 mL red cells suspended in a small amount of plasma or crystalloid solution (hct 70% to 80%). There is no significant amount of coagulation factors and no functional platelets or neutrophils. Leukocyte-poor blood is prepared by filtration and contains less than 5×10^6 leukocytes per unit. Indications for transfusion of leukocyte-poor blood include prevention of febrile transfusion reactions or transmission of CMV. Provision of leukocyte-poor blood products may also be useful in reduction of rates of platelet alloimmunization. Saline washed cells are indicated for patients with severe adverse reactions to plasma constituents and perhaps for patients with complement-mediated immune hemolytic anemia. Previously frozen deglycerolized red cells are suspended in a crystalloid solution and contain very few white cells and no coagulation factors.

Whole blood is appropriate for patients who require both intravascular volume and increased oxygen-carrying capacity (i.e., patients who are bleeding significantly). Hypovolemic patients may also be supported with packed red cells and colloid/crystalloid solutions, but if large volumes are required, supplementation with coagulation factors may be necessary. Patients who are not hypovolemic should be given packed red cells. Administration of whole blood to such patients may result in circulatory overload and also represents a waste of plasma components.

c. **Compatibility testing.** Patients should not be transfused with (1) red cells to which they have circulating antibodies, (2) red cells to which they are likely to form antibodies (Rh system), or (3) large amounts of plasma containing antibodies to the patient's red cells (small amounts of such plasma, as would be present in a unit of packed red cells, are usually not harmful). Although patients usually receive ABO group-specific components, appropriate substitutions are permissible (Table 10–6). A full crossmatch includes typing, testing the patient's serum for unexpected antibodies, and compat-

TABLE 10–6. **Blood Type Substitutions**

	PERMISSIBLE BLOOD TYPE SUBSTITUTIONS	
BLOOD TYPE	RED CELLS	PLASMA
O	None	A, B, AB
A	O	AB
B	O	AB
AB	A, B, O	None

ibility testing between the patient's serum and the donor's cells. If there is not time to complete compatibility testing, type-specific (ABO and Rh) blood or uncrossmatched O Rh-negative cells may be given.

   d. Administration of blood. Circulatory overload may occur if blood is given too quickly. Otherwise healthy patients with chronic anemia can be given packed red cells safely at a rate of 3–4 mL/kg/h. Patients with severe anemia or hypervolemia or both should not be given blood any more rapidly than 1 mL/kg/h. All blood products should be administered through a filter. Blood should not be mixed with any fluid except isotonic saline.

2. COMPONENTS FOR HEMOSTASIS

   a. Platelets. The indications for platelet transfusion are discussed on page 397. Platelet concentrates are prepared from units of whole blood or by apheresis techniques. A unit is defined as the number of platelets obtained from 1 unit of blood (approximately 0.7×10^{11} cells). Platelets obtained by apheresis usually contain the equivalent of about 6 units. Platelets are suspended in the donor's plasma and may be stored at room temperature for up to 5 days. Platelets should not be refrigerated. Transfusion of 1 unit of platelets will elevate the adult recipient's platelet count approximately 8000 to 10,000/µL. The usual adult dose is 4 to 8 units. Ideally, platelets should be ABO identical, but substitutions may be made. Rh-positive platelets should not be given to Rh-negative women of childbearing potential; if they are, Rh immune globulin should be administered. A platelet count should be obtained before and 1 hour after completion of the transfusion. In patients with sepsis, autoimmune platelet disorders, or platelet alloimmunization, the life span of transfused platelets may be so short that the posttransfusion platelet count is no different from the baseline. Management of alloimmunization depends on providing platelets from more closely HLA-matched donors. Other measures, such as IV IgG or plasma exchange, have not generally proved useful.

   b. Cryoprecipitate. Cryoprecipitate is prepared from single units of plasma by freeze/thaw techniques. Each bag contains approximately 100 factor VIII/VWF units, 250 mg fibrinogen, and 25% of the factor XIII in the original unit of blood. Cryoprecipitate is suspended in 10 to 20 mL (per bag) of either plasma or saline. Cryoprecipitate is indicated for documented deficiencies of fibrinogen. The adult dose is generally 10 to 20 bags.

   c. Factor VIII concentrates. Commercial factor VIII concentrates are prepared from large volumes of plasma and are supplied as a lyophilized powder. Modern manufacturing techniques have essentially eliminated the risk of viral transmission by these products. The dose is calculated on the basis of the patient's estimated blood volume, the increase in factor VIII level desired, and the assumption that 100% of the transfused factor will circulate. Transfusion of factor VIII concentrate is indicated for the treatment of patients with factor VIII deficiency. Only those preparations that contain von

Willebrand factor (VWF) should be used to treat von Willebrand disease.

d. **Factor IX concentrates.** These commercially prepared concentrates may be of high or low purity, the latter also being concentrates of factors II, X, and, variably, VII. Use of these preparations is generally limited to the treatment of patients with hemophilia B and of patients with factor VIII inhibitors. Doses for patients with hemophilia B are based on the level of factor IX desired and the assumption that 40% of the transfused dose will be retained in the plasma. Low-purity factor IX concentrates should be used with caution in patients with prior thrombosis or who have liver disease, as decreased clearance of activated factors may result in disseminated intravascular coagulation or thrombosis.

e. **Fresh frozen plasma.** A unit of fresh frozen plasma varies in volume from 200 to 350 mL and contains all of the coagulation factors in normal amounts. Transfusion of fresh frozen plasma is indicated for the treatment of documented factor deficiencies that cannot be treated more efficiently with other component preparations. Common indications include congenital factor deficiencies, liver disease, reversal of oral anticoagulation, and dilutional coagulopathy. Transfusion is usually indicated only in patients who are actually bleeding or are about to undergo an invasive procedure. In a 70-kg adult, factor levels will increase 2% to 3% per unit of plasma infused. Thus, reversal of oral anticoagulation will require approximately 4 units.

B. Transfusion Reactions

1. **HEMOLYTIC.** Intravascular hemolytic reactions are usually due to ABO incompatibility and are preventable. Most commonly, they result from clerical errors, mislabeled tubes, and improper identification of the recipient. Symptoms include chills, fever, chest pain, back pain, and nausea. If a hemolytic reaction is suspected, the transfusion should be stopped, the blood pressure carefully monitored, and the clerical work checked. Two to ten milliliters of the patient's blood should be centrifuged, and the plasma should be examined immediately. If a significant hemolytic reaction has occurred, the plasma will be red. If a reaction is confirmed by examination of the plasma, attempts should be made to maintain urine flow at >100 mL/h with diuretics (furosemide 20–80 mg IV) and sufficient IV fluids. Renal function and coagulation status should be monitored closely. A posttransfusion blood sample should be sent to the blood bank to determine the cause of the reaction. Delayed hemolytic transfusion reactions occur in patients who have been previously sensitized to a red cell antigen. The antibody, however, is undetectable at the time of transfusion. The transfusion itself is uneventful. An anamnestic response is triggered, and transfused red cells bearing the relevant antigen are destroyed. The patient's hematocrit suddenly drops 3 to 10 days after the transfusion. In addition, there may be fever, hemoglobinuria, and hyperbilirubinemia. The direct antiglobulin test may be positive if there are any remaining antigen-positive red cells. The indirect antiglobulin test will reveal a red cell alloantibody not present at the time of the transfusion. Since all

sensitized red cells may be rapidly destroyed, severe anemia may result, and additional transfusions using antigen-negative blood may be required.

2. FEBRILE TRANSFUSION REACTIONS are usually due to antibodies to white blood cells and are most often manifested by chills or fever or both beginning 30 minutes to 2 hours after the start of the transfusion. Since chills and fever can also be the only symptoms of a hemolytic transfusion reaction, it is important to rule out this possibility. Therapy with aspirin or acetaminophen is usually effective. The transfusion need not be discontinued if the reaction is mild, but slowing the infusion rate may be helpful. Patients with two consecutive febrile reactions should be provided with leukocyte-poor blood for subsequent transfusions. Febrile reactions to platelet transfusion may be due to cytokines that have accumulated in the suspending plasma during storage.

3. ALLERGIC TRANSFUSION REACTIONS are due to antibodies to plasma proteins. Urticaria is most common, although hypotension and bronchospasm can also occur. Serious reactions may result from antibodies to IgA, particularly in IgA-deficient patients. For mild cases, diphenhydramine 50 mg (either PO or IV) usually suffices. The transfusion may be slowed but should not be discontinued if urticaria is the only problem. For more severe reactions, the transfusion should be discontinued, and therapy with corticosteroids or epinephrine should be considered.

C. Other Adverse Effects of Transfusion

1. TRANSMISSION OF INFECTION. The per unit risk (1996) of transmission of hepatitis C and HIV by transfusion is approximately $1:10,000$ and $1:600,000$, respectively. CMV transmission to immunocompetent recipients may result in a mononucleosis-like syndrome. CMV transmission to profoundly immunosuppressed recipients, such as bone marrow transplant recipients, may result in serious infection. For such immunosuppressed patients not previously infected with CMV (i.e., negative for antibody to CMV), transmission of CMV by transfusion can be prevented by supplying blood products containing less than 5×10^6 leukocytes or blood products from donors who are also CMV seronegative.

2. ALLOIMMUNIZATION. Approximately 2% to 3% of transfusion recipients will develop red cell alloantibodies. Platelet alloimmunization occurs in 20% to 50% of patients receiving frequent transfusions.

3. GRAFT-VERSUS-HOST DISEASE. Graft-versus-host disease may occur if immunocompetent lymphoid cells are transfused into severely immunosuppressed recipients. Gamma irradiation (2500 rads) eliminates the possibility. All blood products provided for intrauterine transfusions, for neonatal exchange transfusions, and for transfusion in patients who have severe cellular immunodeficiency or Hodgkin's disease or who have undergone bone marrow transplantation should be irradiated. Irradiation of blood products is not necessary for patients with AIDS.

4. **CITRATE TOXICITY.** Blood for transfusion is collected in a citrate-based anticoagulant that prevents clotting by chelation of calcium. With extremely rapid transfusion of whole blood or plasma (500 to 1000 mL/10 min over a prolonged period), symptoms or signs of hypocalcemia may occur, and supplemental calcium (do not mix the calcium with the blood) should be considered.

Beauregard P, Blajchman MA. Hemolytic and pseudo-hemolytic transfusion reactions: an overview of the hemolytic transfusion reactions and the clinical conditions that mimic them. Transfus Med Rev 1994;8:184–199.

Rintels PB, Kenney RM, Crowley JP. Therapeutic support of the patient with thrombocytopenia. Hematol Oncol Clin North Am 1994;8:1131–1157.

11 11 11 11 11 11 11 11 11 11

ONCOLOGIC THERAPEUTICS

JULIE R. GRALOW
KAREN J. HUNT
STEPHEN H. PETERSDORF
ROBERT B. LIVINGSTON

11 11 11 11 11 11 11 11 11 11 11

Cancer currently afflicts an estimated 1,252,000 new patients annually and causes 547,000 deaths per year (Table 11–1), making it the second leading cause of death in the United States. Because epidemiologic studies have suggested that environmental risk factors are operative in the multifactorial pathogenesis of 80% to 90% of cancer cases, avoidance of carcinogenic factors (such as cigarette smoke, alcohol, and asbestos) is the most desirable method of reducing cancer morbidity and mortality. Unfortunately, intervention trials aimed at primary prevention of cancer have been limited in scope and efficacy, making therapy of established cancer an important medical priority. Three major types of treatment are used to treat neoplasms: surgery, radiation therapy, and systemic therapy (chemotherapy, hormone therapy, biotherapy). Surgery and radiation therapy are generally used in attempting to cure localized malignancies, whereas chemotherapy is used for disseminated neoplasms. Recently, the advantages of combined therapy have become evident, and an increasing number of tumors are now managed with combinations of these three therapeutic approaches (e.g., Ewing's sarcoma, ovarian carcinoma, osteosarcoma, some locally advanced breast and lung carcinoma). The rationale for such combination therapy comes from observations that surgery is most likely to fail locally at the edges of tumor resection (positive surgical margins), radiation therapy is most likely to fail in the center of tumors, and chemotherapy is most likely to fail in the presence of bulk disease.

Laboratory studies have validated clinical observations that small tumors are more likely to respond to chemotherapy than are large tumors. Small tumors generally have high growth fractions (i.e., most of the cells are actively proceeding through the cell cycle), whereas larger tumors have higher percentages of dormant cells resistant to cell cycle-active agents. Furthermore, smaller tumors are statistically less likely to contain cells that have acquired drug resistance by somatic mutation (estimated to occur every 10^6 cell divisions). Studies have shown that combination chemotherapy regimens with agents having different modes of action and exhibiting different forms of toxicity are more likely to be curative than single-agent therapy, as the chance of double resistance to two drugs is much less (10^{-12}) than the risk of single-drug resistance (10^{-6}). Maximally tolerated drug doses should be used because the fraction of cells killed is proportional to the dose employed. Single drugs, low doses, and long intervals between chemotherapy cycles encourage the development of resistant tumor cell clones.

Biologic response modifiers now play an established role in the treatment of certain cancers (e.g., IL-2 in renal carcinoma, interferon [IFN] as adjuvant therapy in melanoma, BCG as local therapy for bladder tumors). Other modifiers of biologic response include G-CSF (filgrastim) and GM-CSF (sargramostim), which stimulate the production of white blood cells. These

413

TABLE 11-1. **Estimated Relative Cancer Incidences and Deaths by Site and Sex (1995)***

SITE	RELATIVE INCIDENCES		CANCER DEATHS	
	MALE (%)	FEMALE (%)	MALE (%)	FEMALE (%)
Lung	14	13	33	24
Colorectal	10	12	9	11
Breast	<1	32	<1	18
Prostate	36	—	11	—
Leukemia/lymphoma	7	6	8	8
Pancreas	2	2	5	5
Ovary	—	5	—	6
Uterus	—	8	—	4
Urinary	8	4	5	3
Oral	3	2	2	1
Melanoma	3	3	2	1
Other	15	13	19	19

*Data from Wingo P, Tong T, Bolden S. Cancer statistics, 1995. Ca: A Cancer Journal for Clinicians 1995;45:8–17. Nonmelanoma skin cancer and carcinoma in situ have been excluded.

hematopoietic growth factors are used to aid in host recovery from severe chemotherapy-induced myelosuppression and may permit an increase in the dose intensity of standard chemotherapeutic agents.

II. CANCER CHEMOTHERAPY AND BIOTHERAPY

This brief introduction to the major chemotherapeutic agents currently in use presents standard doses for each drug given as a single agent. When given in combination, these doses may need to be modified. Expected side effects are summarized in Table 11–2. Before prescribing such agents, a physician should have a thorough pharmacologic understanding of these drugs beyond that which can be provided here.

A. Alkylating Agents

Alkylating agents are widely used cytotoxic chemotherapeutic agents having mutagenic and carcinogenic effects. Most alkylating agents form positively charged carbonium ions, which then attack the nucleophilic (electron-rich) sites on nucleic acids, resulting in a formation of covalent bond and subsequent cross-linking of DNA. Single-strand breaks occur primarily in the process of DNA repair and generally do not produce lethal damage. Most alkylating agents are cell cycle-phase nonspecific. Although the alkylating agents share a common mechanism of action, they do not display cross-resistance in experimental systems and are not uniformly effective against the same malignancies.

1. **CYCLOPHOSPHAMIDE (CYTOXAN)** requires activation by hepatic microsomal enzymes to the active moiety, phosphoramide mustard. A toxic metabolite, acrolein, may cause hemorrhagic cystitis. Cytoxan is well absorbed orally and is commonly administered in a daily, continuous

TABLE 11–2. Toxicities of Chemotherapeutic Agents

DRUG/ROUTE*	WBC†	PLATELETS‡	NAUSEA	OTHER GI	PULMONARY	RENAL	NEURO-LOGIC	ALOPECIA	VESICANTS§	OTHER
ALKYLATING AGENTS										
Cyclophosphamide (PO, IV)	3+	1+	2+	–	Fibrosis	Hemorrhagic cystitis	–	+	–	SIADH
Ifosfamide (IV)	2+	2+	1–2+	–	–	Hemorrhagic cystitis	+	+	–	–
Nitrogen mustard (IV, topical)	3+	3+	3+	–	–	–	–	+	+	–
Chlorambucil (PO)	2+	2+	1+	–	–	–	–	–	–	Leukemogenic
Busulfan (PO)	3+	3+	1+	–	Fibrosis	–	–	–	–	Skin toxicity
Melphalan (PO)	2+	2+	1+	–	–	–	–	–	–	Leukemogenic
Nitrosoureas (PO, IV)	3+	3+	2+	–	Fibrosis	1–2+ nephro-toxicity	–	–	–	Leukemogenic
Cisplatin (IV, IA, IP)	1+	1+	3+	–	–	3+ nephro-toxicity	2+	–	–	Ototoxic
Carboplatin (IV)	3+	3+	1+	–	–	–	–	–	–	–
ANTITUMOR ANTIBIOTICS										
Doxorubicin (IV)	3+	2+	2+	Mucositis	–	–	–	+	+	Cardiotoxic
Bleomycin (IV, IM, SC)	–	–	1+	–	Fibrosis	–	–	–	–	Skin, allergic reactions
Dactinomycin (IV)	3+	3+	2+	Mucositis, diarrhea	–	–	–	+	+	Radiation recall
Mitomycin C (IV)	3+	3+	2+	Mucositis	Fibrosis	Hemolytic-uremic syndrome	–	±	+	Cardiotoxic
Mitoxantrone (IV)	3+	2+	1+	Mucositis	–	–	–	–	+	Cardiotoxic

Toxicity severity: 1+, mild; 2+, moderate; 3+ marked. SIADH, syndrome of inappropriate antidiuretic hormone.
*Routes of administration: IV, intravenous; IM, intramuscular; IT, intrathecal; IP, intraperitoneal; IA, intraarterial; SC, subcutaneous; PO, oral.
†Likelihood of producing leukopenia.
‡Likelihood of producing thrombocytopenia.
§Vesicants cause extravasation ulcers.

Table continued on the following page

TABLE 11–2. Toxicities of Chemotherapeutic Agents (Continued)

DRUG/ROUTE*	WBC†	PLATELETS‡	NAUSEA	OTHER GI	PULMONARY	RENAL	NEURO-LOGIC	ALOPECIA	VESICANTS§	OTHER
PLANT ALKALOIDS										
Vincristine (IV)	1+	1+	−	−	−	−	3+	−	+	SIADH
Vinblastine (IV)	3+	3+	−	Mucositis	−	−	−	+	−	Myalgias
Etoposide (PO, IV)	2+	1+	1–2+	Mucositis	−	−	−	+	−	Hypotension, allergic reaction
Taxol (IV)	3+	1+	1+	Mucositis	−	−	2+	+	+	−
ANTIMETABOLITES										
Thioguanine (PO, IV)	2–3+	2–3+	1+	Stomatitis	−	−	−	−	−	Hepatotoxic
Mercaptopurine (PO)	2–3+	2–3+	1+	−	−	−	−	−	−	Hepatotoxic
Cytarabine (IV, SC, IT)	3+	3+	2+	Mucositis, pancreatitis	−	−	Ataxia	+	−	Hepatotoxic, conjunctivitis
Fluorouracil (IV)	1–2+	1+	1+	Stomatitis, diarrhea	−	−	Ataxia	−	−	Conjunctivitis, angina
Methotrexate (IV, IT, PO, IM)	2–3+	2–3+	1+	Stomatitis	Fibrosis	2+ nephrotoxicity	+	+	−	Hepatotoxic
MISCELLANEOUS										
DTIC (IV)	1+	1+	3+	−	−	−	−	−	+	Flu-like syndrome

Toxicity severity: 1+, mild; 2+, moderate; 3+ marked. SIADH, syndrome of inappropriate antidiuretic hormone.
*Routes of administration: IV, intravenous; IM, intramuscular; IT, intrathecal; IP, intraperitoneal; IA, intraarterial; SC, subcutaneous; PO, oral.
†Likelihood of producing leukopenia.
‡Likelihood of producing thrombocytopenia.
§Vesicants cause extravasation ulcers.

PO dose of 50–150 mg/m^2. The IV dose is 500–1000 mg/m^2 every 3 to 4 weeks. Hemorrhagic myopericarditis is the dose-limiting toxicity of cyclophosphamide when given at maximum doses (>120 mg/kg) in preparative regimens for bone marrow transplantation. This drug is active in the treatment of breast carcinoma, non-Hodgkin's lymphoma, small cell lung cancer, and ovarian carcinoma.

2. IFOSFAMIDE (IFEX) differs from Cytoxan only in the placement of one of its alkylating side chains. Hemorrhagic cystitis occurs commonly with this drug unless it is given with the uroprotectant mesna, which binds to acrolein in the urine. The standard dosage is 1.8–2.4 g/m^2 IV daily for 4 to 5 days every 3 to 4 weeks. Mesna is given IV at a dose 20% of the ifosfamide dose, immediately before, 4 hours, and 8 hours after ifosfamide. Ifosfamide is active in the treatment of soft tissue sarcomas and testicular carcinomas, as well as some lymphomas.

3. NITROGEN MUSTARD (MECHLORETHAMINE) is an analog of mustard gas and was the first chemotherapeutic drug to be tested clinically. The usual dosage is 8 mg/m^2 IV on day 1 and day 8 every 4 weeks. This drug has largely been replaced by cyclophosphamide, although it is still used in some regimens for Hodgkin's disease.

4. CHLORAMBUCIL (LEUKERAN) is well absorbed orally and may be given in a daily dose of 3–6 mg/m^2 or as a dose of 16 mg/m^2/d for 5 days every 4 weeks. Intermittent administration reduces the risks of irreversible bone marrow damage and secondary acute myelogenous leukemia that may occur with prolonged use. Chlorambucil is used in chronic lymphocytic leukemia.

5. BUSULFAN (MYLERAN) is well absorbed orally and given in a dose of 2–4 mg/m^2/d on an intermittent schedule. As with chlorambucil, myelosuppression may be prolonged and irreversible if excessive doses are used. This drug is used almost exclusively in the treatment of chronic myelogenous leukemia.

6. MELPHALAN (ALKERAN, L-PAM, PHENYLALANINE MUSTARD) is given orally or intravenously. The usual PO dosage is 8–10 mg/m^2 for 4 to 6 days every 4 to 6 weeks, adjusted to bone marrow tolerance. The IV dose is 16 mg/m^2, repeated every 2 weeks for four cycles, then monthly. Secondary leukemia may occur with prolonged oral use. It is administered most frequently to patients with multiple myeloma.

7. NITROSOUREAS. **Carmustine** (BCNU) and **lomustine** (CCNU) are highly lipid-soluble and cross the blood-brain barrier, producing CSF drug levels that are 30% to 50% of plasma levels. BCNU is given in a dose of 200–225 mg/m^2 IV, and CCNU is given as 100–150 mg/m^2 PO. Because these drugs produce delayed neutropenia and thrombocytopenia, they are administered every 6 to 8 weeks. BCNU is active in Hodgkin's disease, multiple myeloma, non-Hodgkin's lymphoma, brain tumors, and melanoma. CCNU is principally used in the treatment of brain tumors.

8. CIS-DIAMMINEDICHLOROPLATINUM (CISPLATIN, PLATINOL) is extensively protein bound, with a tissue half-life of 5 days. Twenty to seventy-five

percent is excreted in the urine within 24 hours of administration. The incidence of renal toxicity can be significantly reduced by vigorous saline hydration (e.g., 250 ml/h) for 4 hours before and after cisplatin administration. The standard dose is 100–120 mg/m^2 IV every 3 to 4 weeks or 20 mg/m^2/d for 5 days every 3 weeks. At high doses, the dose-limiting toxicities are peripheral sensory neuropathy and hearing loss. Cisplatin is active against testicular cancer, ovarian carcinoma, non-Hodgkin's lymphoma, non-small cell lung cancer, small cell lung cancer, and squamous cell carcinomas of the head and neck.

9. CARBOPLATIN (PARAPLATIN, CBDCA) is a nonnephrotoxic but myelosuppressive analog of cisplatin. Its administration does not require hydration. For patients with normal renal function, the standard dosage is 300–360 mg/m^2 IV every 4 weeks. Doses must be adjusted for renal dysfunction to prevent severe myelosuppression, particularly thrombocytopenia (J Clin Oncol 1989;7:1748).

B. Antitumor Antibiotics

1. ANTHRACYCLINES. **Doxorubicin (Adriamycin)** and **daunorubicin** are produced by species of *Streptomyces* and exert their cytotoxic effects by several different mechanisms, the most important of which may be interaction with the nuclear enzyme, topoisomerase II. Both of these antibiotics undergo extensive hepatic metabolism and biliary excretion. The usual dose of doxorubicin is 60–90 mg/m^2 via a short IV infusion or as a prolonged infusion over 96 hours every 3 weeks. It is also given as 15–20 mg/m^2 IV weekly. Daunorubicin is given in a dose of 30–60 mg/m^2 IV daily for 3 days. A 50% dose reduction is required in the presence of hepatic dysfunction (bilirubin > 2 mg/dL). These drugs probably should be withheld if the bilirubin is more than 5 mg/dL. Three forms of cardiac toxicity are produced by anthracyclines, the most important of which is a chronic dilated congestive cardiomyopathy, which is dose and schedule dependent. The risk is <10% with a total dose of doxorubicin < 450 mg/m^2. The incidence of congestive heart failure is significantly less if doxorubicin is administered either by continuous infusion or on a weekly schedule (Ann Intern Med 1983;99:745). At high total cumulative doses, cardiac function should be followed with serial left ventricular ejection fractions. Doxorubicin is active against a variety of malignancies, including non-Hodgkin's lymphoma, Hodgkin's disease, breast carcinoma, sarcomas, small cell lung cancer, ovarian cancer, and thyroid cancer. Daunorubicin is used primarily in the treatment of acute myelogenous and lymphocytic leukemias.

A third compound, **mitoxantrone (dihydroxyanthracenedione),** is closely related to the anthracyclines. It, too, appears to work through enzyme-mediated DNA cleavage. It is given IV at 12 mg/m^2/d for 3 days in the treatment of acute myelocytic leukemia (together with ARA-C), and at 12–14 mg/m^2 once every 3 weeks in breast cancer and non-Hodgkin's lymphoma. It causes minimal nausea/vomiting, usually no alopecia, and has a reduced potential for cardiotoxicity, all advantages over the anthracyclines. Reversible myelosuppression is dose-limiting and predictable. Its antitumor effect in breast cancer is inferior to that of Adriamycin, but it lends itself more readily to use in high-dose or transplantation regimens.

2. BLEOMYCIN is a mixture of small molecular weight glycoproteins produced by a species of *Streptomyces*. It induces single-stranded and double-stranded breaks in DNA through formation of superoxide and hydroxyl radicals. As almost all of the drug is excreted unchanged in the urine, doses should be reduced 50% to 75% for a creatinine clearance less than 40 mL/min. The usual dosage is 10–20 U/m^2 IV weekly or 15 U/m^2 by continuous infusion daily for 4 days. The most important toxicity is interstitial pneumonitis, most likely to occur in elderly patients with underlying pulmonary disease, previous pulmonary irradiation, and with cumulative doses of more than 400 U. Subsequent oxygen exposure may precipitate respiratory failure, and if patients who have received bleomycin require surgery, the Fio_2 should be kept as low as possible. Bleomycin is active against squamous cell carcinomas, non-Hodgkin's lymphomas, Hodgkin's disease, and testicular carcinomas.

3. DACTINOMYCIN (ACTINOMYCIN D) is a high molecular weight antibiotic isolated from a species of *Streptomyces* that intercalates between DNA strands blocking the DNA's ability to act as a template for both DNA and RNA synthesis. Dactinomycin is administered in doses of 2.5 mg/m^2 IV every 3 to 4 weeks in treatment of gestational choriocarcinoma, Wilms' tumor, and rhabdomyosarcoma.

4. MITOMYCIN (MUTAMYCIN) is a purple antibiotic isolated from a species of *Streptomyces*. The drug requires metabolic activation and produces damage to DNA either by alkylation or through generation of free radicals. The recommended dose is 10–20 mg/m^2 IV. Mitomycin produces prolonged, cumulative bone marrow suppression and should be administered every 6 to 8 weeks. This drug is used for gastrointestinal carcinomas, non-small cell lung cancer, and bladder carcinomas.

C. Plant Alkaloids

1. VINCA ALKALOIDS. The vinca alkaloids are derived from the ornamental shrub *Vinca rosea*. They bind to tubulin, inhibiting the assembly of microtubules and disrupting the mitotic apparatus. Spindle formation is the most sensitive to the action of these drugs, but they are not absolutely phase specific. Minute concentrations of these alkaloids kill sensitive cells. As vincristine and vinblastine undergo extensive hepatic metabolism, a dose reduction is advised in patients with bilirubin over 2 mg/dL.

   a. **Vincristine (Oncovin)** is given in doses of 1–1.4 mg/m^2 IV weekly. Most oncologists do not administer over 2 mg in a single dose. The dose should be reduced 50% if the bilirubin is over 2 mg/dL. The most important side effect is a peripheral neuropathy that usually resolves with time but may progress to muscle weakness. Loss of deep tendon reflexes is an indication to discontinue the drug. Oncovin is active in acute lymphocytic leukemia, non-Hodgkin's disease, and small cell lung cancer.

    b. Vinblastine (Velban) is given in doses of 4–8 mg/m² IV weekly. In contrast to vincristine, the dose-limiting toxicity of vinblastine is myelosuppression, although it may also cause peripheral neuropathy and constipation. Velban is used in the treatment of testicular cancer, Hodgkin's disease, breast carcinoma, and non-small cell lung cancer.

    c. Vinorelbine (Navelbine) is also administered weekly, usually at a dose of 25–30 mg/m². It is myelosuppressive like vinblastine but causes neurotoxicity much less frequently than either vincristine or vinblastine. It is used in the treatment of lung and breast cancer and will probably replace vinblastine for these disease indications.

2. ETOPOSIDE **(VP-16)** is a podophyllotoxin derived from the mandrake plant. It has no effect on microtubule assembly but acts through binding to the nuclear enzyme, topoisomerase II, which results in stabilization of DNA strand breaks that would otherwise be resealed. VP-16 is a schedule-dependent drug. The usual dose is 50–150 mg/m²/d for 3 to 5 days (total dose 300 mg/m²). Because the drug is excreted in the urine, the dose should be reduced in the presence of renal dysfunction. It is active against testicular carcinoma, lung cancer, non-Hodgkin's lymphoma, Hodgkin's disease, and Kaposi's sarcoma and may have activity in breast cancer. The drug is now available in an oral formulation. For this, the usual dose is 50 mg/m²/d for 14 to 21 days, repeated at monthly intervals.

3. TAXANES. These compounds also bind to the tubulin subunits that polymerize to form microtubular elements within the mitotic spindle. Unlike the vincas, which prevent polymerization, the taxanes inhibit depolymerization or takedown of the microtubules back to subunits. These compounds undergo extensive hepatic metabolism, and dose reductions are advised even in the presence of subtle liver function abnormality.

    a. Paclitaxel (Taxol) may be given as a 3-hour, 24-hour, or 96-hour infusion, at doses that vary from 135 to 225 mg/m² (lower doses are necessary for the more prolonged infusion). It produces myelosuppression, alopecia, stomatitis, and a sensory peripheral neuropathy that may become more severe with repeated dosing. Premedication with steroids and H₁ and H₂ blockers is necessary to prevent anaphylactic reactions. Treatment is usually repeated at 3-week intervals. The drug is active in breast, lung, and ovarian cancer and may be useful in head and neck cancer.

    b. Docetaxel (taxotere) is usually given as a short infusion every 3 weeks, at doses of 60–100 mg/m². In addition to the side effects of paclitaxel, it can cause accumulation of third-space fluid with repeated dosing, both as peripheral edema and as pleural effusion or ascites. In addition to the symptoms produced, these accumulations may be confused with progression of the underlying disease. Docetaxel may also produce a skin rash. It is active in breast cancer and in non-small cell lung cancer, with reported activity in the latter disease after failure on platinum-based regimens.

D. Antimetabolites

Antimetabolites act as fraudulent substrates for biochemical reactions, either inhibiting essential synthetic steps or becoming incorporated into molecules and interfering with cellular function or replication. They exert their major effect during the S phase of the cell cycle and, therefore, are most effective against actively replicating cells.

1. PURINE ANTAGONISTS. Thioguanine and mercaptopurine are analogs of the natural purines guanine and hypoxanthine, respectively. After activation, both drugs are capable of inhibiting multiple steps in purine synthesis and of incorporation into DNA.

   a. **Thioguanine (6-thioguanine, 6TG)** should be taken between meals to facilitate oral absorption. With a standard dose of 2 mg/kg/d, 6-TG is active in acute myelogenous and lymphocytic leukemias.

   b. **Mercaptopurine (6-mercaptopurine, 6-MP)** is administered in the maintenance phase of acute lymphocytic leukemia treatment at a dose of 2.5 mg/kg/d (adjusted to bone marrow tolerance). Allopurinol creates a metabolic block of 6-MP metabolism, and the dose of 6-MP needs to be reduced if allopurinol is given concurrently.

   c. **Adenosine analogs.** These include **fludarabine, pentostatin** (deoxycoformycin), and **cladribine** (2-CdA, 2-chlorodeoxyadenosine). Fludarabine inhibits DNA polymerase and is used to treat chronic lymphocytic leukemia and recurrent low-grade lymphomas, usually in doses of 20–40 mg/m^2/d IV for 5 days every 4 weeks. Its dose-limiting toxicity is myelosuppression, although nausea and drug-related fever as well as occasional, reversible neurotoxicity may occur. Pentostatin inhibits the catabolic enzyme adenosine deaminase (ADA), resulting in accumulation of deoxyadenosine triphosphate, which in turn suppresses ribonucleotide reductase and results in impaired DNA synthesis. Lymphocytes are particularly sensitive to ADA inhibition. Pentostatin is administered in a dose of 4 mg/m^2 IV every 2 weeks and produces nausea, some degree of neutropenia early, lethargy, and prolonged depletion of T cell function as side effects. Cladribine interferes with DNA synthesis and repair in both resting and proliferative lymphocytes and triggers programmed cell death (apoptosis). It is usually given at a dose of 0.1 mg/kg/d by continuous infusion for 5 to 7 days, and its dose-limiting toxicity is myelosuppression, with long-term suppression of CD4+ lymphocytes and opportunistic infections a potential consequence. It is active in chronic lymphocytic leukemia, hairy cell leukemia, and other low-grade lymphoid malignancies.

2. PYRIMIDINE ANTAGONISTS

   a. **Cytarabine (cytosine arabinoside, ARA-C)** is an analog of deoxycytidine that is converted to its active form, ara-cytidine triphosphate, by enzymes of the salvage pathway. It inhibits DNA polymerase and is an S phase-specific agent. ARA-C is administered as a continuous infusion in a dosage of 100–200 mg/m^2 IV q24h for 5 to 7 days. It is also given in higher doses as 3 g/m^2 IV q12h for 6 to 12 doses. Low-dose ARA-C (20 mg/m^2 IV or SC daily for 14 to 21 days) is used in treatment of myelodysplastic syndromes. The usual intrathecal dose is 50 mg/m^2. The duration of myelosuppression depends on the dose administered. Unique toxicities of high-dose ARA-C include cerebellar ataxia and pancreatitis. This drug is effective against acute myelogenous leukemia.

b. **Gemcitabine (Gemzar)** is also a cytidine analog, converted by kinase activity to an active triphosphate. It inhibits ribonucleotide reductase and DNA polymerase but is also incorporated into DNA, inhibits DNA repair, and is S phase specific. Its intracellular half-life is much prolonged compared with ARA-C, and its spectrum of anti-tumor activity involves solid tumors. The drug is active in pancre-atic, lung, and breast cancer. The usual dose is about 1 g/m^2/wk IV over 30 minutes for 3 weeks on a monthly schedule. Side effects include nausea/vomiting, generally modest myelosuppression, flu-like symptoms, and subclinical alterations in liver function.

c. **Fluorouracil (5-fluorouracil, 5-FU)** is an analog of uracil that has two distinct mechanisms of action after conversion to the nucleotide fluorouridine monophosphate (FUMP). Conversion to 5-FdUMP inhibits the enzyme thymidylate synthase and blocks DNA synthesis, probably accounting for most of its antitumor effects. The dosage and scheduling of 5-FU significantly alter its toxicity profile. The dose-limiting toxicity of IV bolus 5-FU (425 mg/m^2/d for 5 days, maximum of 800 mg/d) is hematologic. Continuous infusions of 5-FU (1000 mg/kg/d for 4 days or 200–300 mg/m^2/d for 4 to 6 weeks) produce significantly more GI side effects, particularly diarrhea and stomatitis, but very little myelosuppression. Another side effect of continuous infusion is palmar-plantar erythrodysesthesia (hand-foot syndrome). Patients with coronary atherosclerosis may experi-ence chest pain, ischemic ECG changes, and myocardial infarction when given 5-FU because of vasospasm of the coronary arteries. 5-FU or FUdR also has been infused via the hepatic artery to treat liver metastases, usually from colon cancer. Because there is extensive first-pass hepatic metabolism (especially for FUdR), only limited amounts of the drug administered in this manner reach the systemic circulation. 5-FU is used in treatment of breast cancer, colorectal carcinoma, gastric carcinoma, pancreatic cancer, and carcinomas of the head and neck.

3. **FOLATE ANTAGONISTS**

a. **Methotrexate (MTX),** a methylfolate derivative, inhibits dihydro-folate reductase, the enzyme that replenishes the intracellular pool of reduced folates to act as one-carbon donors for the synthesis of thymidine. To overcome potential resistance from either an altered dihydrofolate reductase or increased dihydrofolate reduc-tase levels resulting from gene amplification, MTX has been given in very high doses (1500 mg/m^2 or more), followed by leucovorin (N_3-formyltetrahydrofolate) rescue. The dose of leucovorin required depends on the dose of MTX administered and the measured plasma levels of MTX and may be as high as 100–200 mg/m^2 q6h for 48 hours or longer. These doses of MTX should be administered only by experienced physicians. The usual regimen of MTX IV or IM as a single agent is 30–60 mg/m^2 every 7 to 14 days. It is also administered intrathecally (12 mg). Because 90% of the drug is excreted by the kidneys, administration in the presence of renal dysfunction is potentially toxic. The risk of renal failure in patients receiving high doses can be lessened by vigorous hydration and alkalinization of the urine to increase the solubility of MTX. MTX accumulates in third-space fluids that act as a depot, slowly releasing the drug into the systemic circulation, which can produce unexpected toxicity. Hepatitis occurs sometimes in patients who are receiving low continuous oral doses but may also occur after single high doses. Liver biopsy is the only reliable method of determining the extent of liver damage. Intrathecal MTX can produce potentially permanent neurotoxicity consisting of motor weakness, cranial nerve palsies, coma, or seizures, as well as an acute arachnoiditis within 48 hours. MTX is active in acute lymphocytic leukemia, trophoblastic tumors, squamous cell carcinomas of the head and neck, breast cancer, and osteosarcoma.

4. HYDROXYUREA. Hydroxyurea inhibits ribonucleotide reductase, the enzyme responsible for the conversion of ribonucleotide diphosphates to the deoxyribonucleotide form. It is available commercially in an oral formulation as a 500 mg tablet. Common dosage schedules are 80 mg/kg as a single dose every 3 days or 20–30 mg/kg/d as a single dose, titrated to a desired level of white blood count suppression. The primary indication is treatment of chronic myelogenous leukemia. It is also sometimes used, in dosage of 1 g/m^2 q12h, to rapidly reduce potentially dangerous elevations of circulating blasts in patients with acute leukemia before initiation of conventional induction therapy. Side effects include myelosuppression, nausea/vomiting, and skin rash.

E. Miscellaneous Chemotherapy Agents

1. DACARBAZINE (DTIC, IMIDAZOLE CARBOXAMIDE-DIMETHYLTRIAZENO) is activated by hepatic microsomes producing an active methyl cation and exerts its cytotoxic action through methylation of DNA. The usual dosage is 250 mg/m^2/d IV for 4 days every 4 to 6 weeks. It is used in treatment of melanoma, soft tissue sarcomas, and Hodgkin's disease. The major side effect is nausea/vomiting, but myelosuppression that can be delayed and severe may be seen in about 20% of patients.

2. L-ASPARAGINASE is an enzyme that catalyzes the hydrolysis of asparagine. Most normal tissues are not affected by this reaction, as they contain asparagine synthetase, but in acute lymphocytic leukemia, the enzyme is often lacking, which makes asparagine an essential amino acid for the leukemia cells. Deprivation of this amino acid leads to cell death from an inability to complete protein synthesis. The dose commonly employed is 1000–20,000 IU/m^2/d or every other day for 10 to 20 doses, although single doses of 10,000–25,000 IU/m^2 produce prolonged blood levels and depletion of asparagine to zero for a week or more. It may be given IV or IM. Nausea, vomiting, fever, and chills are common acutely. Serious, potentially fatal toxicities include

hemorrhagic pancreatitis (seen in 15%) and cerebral dysfunction. L-Asparaginase does not cause myelosuppression and is, therefore, usually given in combination with other drugs to induce remission.

3. **PROCARBAZINE** is a drug that probably acts by methylation of DNA. It is available only in an oral formulation (50 mg capsule), and the usual dose is 100 $mg/m^2/d$ for 14 to 21 days. Its toxicities include nausea/ vomiting, myelosuppression, and neurotoxicity. Because it is also a monoamine oxidase inhibitor, alcohol or tyramine-rich foods and a number of drugs should be avoided during its administration. It is used primarily in the combination chemotherapy of Hodgkin's disease and primary brain tumors.

F. Biologic Response Modifiers

1. **BCG (THERACYS).** This is a freeze-dried suspension of an attenuated strain of *Mycobacterium bovis* that, when instilled intravesically, promotes a local inflammatory reaction in the urinary bladder, eliminating or reducing superficial cancerous lesions. Three vials, reconstituted and diluted in sterile saline, are given once weekly via Foley catheter for 6 weeks (induction), then by single instillations at 3, 6, 12, 18, and 24 months. The major complication in most patients is hemorrhagic cystitis, with associated dysuria, fever, and chills. However, systemic infection can develop from the organism (BCGosis), with persistent evidence of infection and even sepsis requiring therapy.

2. **INTERFERON.** Interferon-α (IFN-α) is used in the treatment of chronic myelogenous leukemia and renal cancer as an alternative to or after failure of cytotoxic agents. It is also shown to have effectiveness as an adjuvant therapy to prevent recurrence of malignant melanoma in high-risk patients. Dose and duration of therapy, which is given IM, SC, or IV, vary considerably, with dose-related fatigue and anorexia as the limiting toxicities on chronic administration. For adjuvant use in melanoma, the recommended schedule is 20 million U/m^2 IV, Monday through Friday for 4 weeks, then 10 million U/m^2 three times a week for 11 months.

3. **LEVAMISOLE.** This immunomodulator is taken in a dose of 50 mg PO tid for 3 days, repeated every 2 weeks for 1 year, in conjunction with 5-FU, for adjuvant therapy of colorectal cancer. Its use with 5-FU leads to reversible neurotoxicity in 5% of patients and laboratory evidence of mild liver dysfunction in 40%.

4. **INTERLEUKIN-2 (IL-2).** This glycoprotein is naturally produced by CD4+ T cells and produces its effects by binding to the IL-2 receptor expressed on lymphoid cells, resulting in clonal expansion of antigen-specific T cells, natural killer (NK) cells and monocytes or macrophages and upregulation of secretion of multiple other cytokines by mononuclear cells. It is clinically available as a recombinant preparation given parenterally. Doses and schedules in use vary widely, with both response and toxicity appearing to be dose related in renal carcinoma, the primary indication for its use at present. All patients develop chills, fever, and malaise. A vascular leak syndrome occurs at higher doses,

associated with weight gain, oliguria, tachycardia, and hypotension. Supraventricular arrhythmias may occur. Skin infiltration or rash with pruritus and gastrointestinal toxicity are also common. These side effects generally resolve rapidly on discontinuation of IL-2 therapy.

5. HEMATOPOIETIC GROWTH FACTORS. Those available at present include erythropoietin, which stimulates red cell production, granulocyte colony-stimulating factor (G-CSF), which stimulates white blood cell production, and granulocyte-macrophage colony-stimulating factor (GM-CSF), which has similar effects. Thrombopoietin, not yet commercially available, is in beginning clinical trials, but at present, no growth factor has been shown to ameliorate thrombocytopenia. Erythropoietin is usually given in a dose of 150 U/kg three times per week. G-CSF is given at 5 µg/kg/d, although higher doses are used to stimulate the circulation of more primitive hematopoietic progenitors for stem cell collection by apheresis. GM-CSF is given at 250 µg/m^2/d. All are administered SC. Erythropoietin is seldom associated with systemic side effects, but the granulocyte CSFs cause low-grade fever, myalgias, and a flu-like syndrome that rapidly resolves. These agents are used therapeutically when myelosuppression has already occurred and prophylactically when it is anticipated that a chemotherapy regimen will produce grade 4 toxicity, in order to shorten the duration of the neutropenic period. Erythropoietin is typically given when hematocrit falls below 28 to 30 and used to maintain hematocrit in the 30s. Both G-CSF and GM-CSF should be given until the total WBC reaches 5000 to 10,000, as premature discontinuation can result in repeated neutropenia.

G. High-Dose Therapy/Stem Cell Transplants: General Concepts

The basic principle of high-dose therapy in the treatment of cancer is that high chemotherapy concentrations may be able to overcome drug resistance. This appears to be particularly the case for the alkylating agents, which are at the core of such regimens, often combined with topoisomerase II-active drugs, which may potentiate effects of the alkylators by inhibiting DNA repair. Some high-dose regimens (e.g., cyclophosphamide, etoposide, cisplatin) do not require support with autologous hematopoietic stem cells, as they are not myeloablative. Other regimens (e.g., cyclophosphamide, BCNU, cisplatin, thiotepa, carboplatin) are essentially myeloablative and require stem cell support to prevent lethality. Formerly, the source of stem cells was bone marrow harvest. Today, the usual method of stem cell support involves administration of hematopoietic growth factors, such as G-CSF, with or without mobilizing chemotherapy to stimulate the transient circulation of stem cells in the peripheral blood, from which they are collected by apheresis using a celltrifuge and controlled-rate freezing. Autologous stem cell transplantation with peripheral blood stem cells (PBSC) leads to more rapid recovery of platelets and WBC counts, with a typical lag time of about 10 days after infusion, compared with 21 days or more for autologous bone marrow as a source. The acute toxicity shared by all programs that involve high-dose therapy and PBSC support is a period of effective aplasia that lasts about 2 weeks, during which support with antibiotics, given empirically in the setting of febrile neutropenia, and blood products is critical to the patient's survival. Other acute toxicities that are virtually universal in high-dose chemotherapy regimens include alopecia, stomatitis, nausea/vomiting, and anorexia, which is often prolonged and may necessitate the use of total parenteral nutrition for a period of weeks. Subacute and chronic toxicities are specific to the drugs employed in the regimen and certain risk features in the host and include interstitial pneumonitis (especially with BCNU), venous occlusive disease of the liver (all PBSC-requiring regimens), skin toxicity, and renal toxicity (especially with platinum and melphalan-containing regimens).

The current indications for high-dose therapy + PBSC include high-grade non-Hodgkin's lymphoma (relapsed) and acute myelocytic leukemia when an allogeneic donor is not available, usually in complete remission. High-dose therapy ± PBSC is commonly employed for stage IV breast cancer in remission and to complete the adjuvant therapy of high-risk primary breast cancer (stage II, ≥10 nodes, stage III). It is under investigation in myeloma, ovarian, and testicular cancer and certain other solid tumors.

Armitage JO, Antman KH. High-Dose Cancer Therapy: Pharmacology, Hematopoietins, Stem Cells. Baltimore, Williams & Wilkins, 1992.

Bensinger W, Appelbaum F, Rowley S, et al. Factors that influence collection and engraftment of autologous peripheral-blood stem cells. J Clin Oncol 1995;13:2547–2555.

Chabner BA, Longo DL. Cancer Chemotherapy and Biotherapy: Principles and Practice, 2nd ed. Philadelphia, Lippincott-Raven, 1996.

Norton L, Surbone A. Principles of chemotherapy: cytokinetics. In: Holland JF, Frei E III, Bast RC Jr, Kufe DW, Morton DL, Weichselbaum RR, eds. Cancer Medicine, 3rd ed. Philadelphia, Lea & Febiger, 1993, pp 598–617.

III. ONCOLOGIC EMERGENCIES

A. The Superior Vena Cava Syndrome

The superior vena cava syndrome (SVCS) occurs in 3% to 8% of patients with lung cancer or lymphoma because of extrinsic compression, thrombosis, or occlusion of the thin-walled SVC, resulting in impaired venous drainage of the head, thorax, and upper extremities. Malignancies are responsible for approximately 90% of cases of SVCS, with bronchogenic carcinoma (all types, but much more common with right-sided lesions) and lymphoma (especially diffuse large-cell) accounting for the majority of cases. The most common types of metastatic cancer that account for SVCS are breast cancer and testicular cancer. SVCS is also caused by thrombosis at the site of an indwelling vascular access device. The most common symptoms are dyspnea and swelling. Although SVCS has traditionally been called an "oncologic emergency," in the absence of tracheal obstruction, the effects of SVCS are unlikely to be life threatening. Delaying therapy for more than 1 week generally does not have a significant deleterious impact on the patient's survival (Cancer 1986;57:847–851). If SVCS is the initial presentation of the malignancy, efforts should be made to obtain a tissue diagnosis before initiation of treatment.

1. **THERAPY.** Traditional management of SVCS involves external beam radiation therapy with 400 cGy fractions for 3 to 4 days to the mediastinal mass, followed by continuation with 200 cGy fractions to a

total dose of 3000–4000 cGy for lymphomas and 4000–6000 cGy for lung cancer. Higher initial fractions will produce more rapid relief of symptoms. More than 75% of patients will respond to such management with symptomatic relief within 2 weeks of initiation of therapy. The degree of symptomatic relief correlates poorly with the magnitude of objective tumor response; dramatic resolution of symptoms commonly occurs without substantial reduction in tumor size. Failure of radiotherapy is most likely due to underlying thrombus. Supplemental oxygen, diuretics, and corticosteroids often are administered concurrently with radiation therapy.

Chemotherapy is as effective as radiotherapy in alleviating SVCS caused by small cell carcinoma of the lung or lymphoma. Chemotherapy is usually the treatment of choice, as these cancers generally require early institution of systemic therapy. When chemotherapy is to be the primary treatment, venous access should be obtained via lower extremity veins or a venous system that is not obstructed until SVC obstruction is relieved to prevent extravasation. Other approaches to the management of SVCS include thrombolytic therapy for pericatheter thrombosis, anticoagulation for similar indications if thrombolytic therapy is not indicated or after thrombolytic therapy, expandable wire stents when other modalities are ineffective or cannot be used, and, rarely, surgery.

2. **PROGNOSIS.** Although more than 80% of patients will obtain relief with the measures suggested, the median survival of patients with SVCS is only 5.5 months, with an overall 24% 1-year survival and a 9% 5-year survival. Survival depends highly on the histology of the underlying malignancy, with lymphoma patients enjoying a 41% 5-year survival compared with 5% for small cell lung cancer and 1% for non-small cell lung cancer patients. Recurrence of SVCS occurs in 10% to 20% of patients and is generally treated with symptomatic measures, chemotherapy, stenting, or surgery, as maximally tolerated radiation is usually administered at initial presentation.

Abner A. Approach to the patient who presents with superior vena cava obstruction. Chest 1993;103:394S–397S.
Armstrong BA, Perez CA, Simpson JR, et al. Role of irradiation in the management of superior vena cava syndrome. Int J Radiat Oncol Biol Phys 1987;13:531–539.
Escalante CP. Causes and management of superior vena cava syndrome. Oncology 1993;7:61–68.

B. Pericardial Tamponade

Neoplastic involvement of the heart is found in 3.4% of general autopsies and from 2% to 31% of patients dying of cancer. Two thirds of these patients have pericardial metastases, and of these, 29% become symptomatic, and 16% develop life-threatening cardiac tamponade. Lung cancer (37%), breast cancer (22%), hematologic malignancies (17%), sarcomas (4%), and melanoma (3%) are the most common causes of pericardial metastatic disease. Malignant pericardial effusion can be insidious in onset and is often difficult to diagnose. The most common symptom is dyspnea (more than 80% of patients). Other complaints are chest discomfort and orthopnea. Findings may include pulsus paradoxus, hypotension, jugular venous distention, and tachycardia. The presence of a pericardial rub is relatively uncommon.

TABLE 11–3. **Therapy of Malignant Pericardial Effusions**

THERAPY	RESPONSE RATE (%)	MAJOR COMPLICATION (%)
Tetracycline sclerosis	85	1–2
Indwelling pericardial catheter	76	1–2
Subxiphoid pericardiotomy	92	0–5
Thoracotomy with pleuropericardiotomy	86	0–8
Percutaneous balloon pericardiotomy	95	0

1. EMERGENCY MANAGEMENT. Acute pericardial tamponade is a medical emergency that mandates prompt withdrawal of pericardial fluid. Pericardiocentesis is effective in 97% of cases but may be associated with a 3% to 5% major complication rate (fatal dysrhythmias, right ventricular lacerations). Most of these untoward events can be avoided if pericardiocentesis is preceded by echocardiographic confirmation of location and size of pericardial fluid and performed in a catheterization laboratory under fluoroscopy with ECG or echocardiographic guidance. Pericardiocentesis should be avoided in patients with thrombocytopenia (platelets <50,000/mm^3), small effusions (<200 mL), or loculated effusions. Another approach is subxiphoid pericardiotomy, which can be substituted as a safe, rapid, and effective procedure. See Table 11–3 for a comparison of therapeutic interventions for malignant pericardial effusions. In situations in which immediate pericardiocentesis or subxiphoid pericardiotomy cannot be performed, IV infusion of fluids may be used temporarily to support cardiac output.

2. LONG-TERM MANAGEMENT. Although simple pericardiocentesis is generally effective in relieving acute symptoms and hemodynamic compromise, rapid reaccumulation of fluid generally leads to relapse within a few days unless more definitive measures are instituted.

   a. **Intrapericardial institution of sclerosing agents.** This is one of the most popular approaches for treatment of pericardial effusions due to solid tumors (e.g., lung cancer and breast cancer). An 18-gauge catheter is inserted into the pericardial space from a subxiphoid approach. The space is then aspirated dry, anesthetized with a small amount (10 mL) of 1% lidocaine (Xylocaine), and sclerosed with 500 to 1000 mg of tetracycline hydrochloride (dissolved in 20 mL of saline). Daily thereafter, the pericardial cavity is aspirated via the catheter, and if significant fluid is present (>25 mL), tetracycline is reinstilled. This technique is successful in resolving 81% to 91% of malignant effusions after an average of 2.8 instillations of tetracycline (Davis, 1984). Major complications are uncommon with this approach, although moderate pain (11%), fever (36%), and asymptomatic dysrhythmias (18%) may occur. Other agents that appear to be effective include bleomycin (which may be more readily available than tetracycline), 5-FU, thiotepa, bleomycin, cisplatin, quinacrine, and radioactive phosphorus (^{32}P).

b. **Surgery.** Operative relief of pericardial tamponade has historically involved the creation of a pleuropericardial window by an anterior thoracotomy approach. This technique is usually effective at achieving lasting relief of tamponade (94% of survivors) but is associated with significant morbidity and 8% operative mortality. Subxiphoid pericardiotomy has become a more popular means of providing pericardial decompression than the traditional pleuropericardial window. This procedure can be done under local anesthesia in 30 minutes, with negligible morbidity, no mortality, and virtually 100% efficacy. Pleuropericardial window can also be performed with a thoracoscopic approach, which is better tolerated. Radical pericardiectomy should be reserved for cases of constrictive pericarditis or those rare patients who have recurrent effusion after a pericardial window has been performed. A newer, less invasive approach is percutaneous balloon pericardiotomy. This is a well-tolerated procedure that can be performed in a cardiac catheterization laboratory with few complications. The success rate for this approach is 95%.

c. **Radiation therapy.** External beam radiation therapy (2500–3000 cGy in 150–200 cGy fractions over 3 to 4 weeks) is inferior to the aforementioned methods (efficacy rate 61% overall) and may be associated with constrictive pericarditis. It is most effective for hematologic malignancies (90% to 100% success rate) and breast cancer (69%).

d. **Systemic chemotherapy.** Chemotherapy often achieves rapid remission of hematologic malignancies and may successfully cure pericardial disease without the addition of local therapy in patients with leukemia or lymphoma.

3. **PROGNOSIS.** The survival of patients with malignant pericardial tamponade is generally dictated by the type of underlying malignancy. With relatively responsive tumors, such as lymphomas, survival is not affected by the presence of a pericardial effusion. However, for less responsive tumors, the presence of pericardial effusion indicates poor prognosis. Survival in most series varies from over a month to several years, with a median survival of less than a year.

Davis S, Rambotti P, Grignani F. Intrapericardial tetracycline sclerosis in the treatment of malignant pericardial effusion: an analysis of 33 cases. J Clin Oncol 1984;2:631–636.

Galli M, Politi A, Pedretti F, et al. Percutaneous balloon pericardiotomy for malignant pericardial tamponade. Chest 1995;108:1499–1501.

Rinkevich D, Borovik R, Bendett M, et al. Malignant pericardial tamponade. Med Pediatr Oncol 1990;18:287–291.

Vaitkus P, Herrmann HC, LeWinter MM. Treatment of malignant pericardial effusion. JAMA 1994;272:59–64.

Wilkes JD, Fidias P, Vaickus L, et al. Malignancy-related pericardial effusion. Cancer 1995; 76:1377–1387.

C. Pleural Effusion

Malignant pleural effusion is a common development in patients with advanced cancer. The occurrence of a malignant effusion is usually associated with median survival of less than 1 year. The pleural effusion results from either obstruction of mediastinal lymphatics by centrally located tumor (cytology negative) or pleural involvement with tumor by direct extension or seeding (cytology usually positive). Lung cancer is the most common cause of a malignant effusion in men and is second only to breast cancer as a cause in women. A pleural effusion may be asymptomatic when small but is usually associated with chest pain, cough, or dyspnea as it progresses. The best management of pleural effusions in patients with chemotherapy-responsive tumors (leukemia, lymphoma, small cell lung cancer) is systemic chemotherapy. For other tumors, thoracentesis is the most effective therapy. However, most effusions reaccumulate, and only in those rare circumstances in which effusions slowly recur is repeat thoracentesis appropriate. For most patients, pleurodesis or pleural sclerosis (usually with tetracycline, bleomycin, or talc) following chest tube drainage of the effusion is generally required. One randomized trial suggested that bleomycin was superior to tetracycline in effectiveness. Unfortunately, pleurodesis itself, regardless of the sclerosing agent employed, is often ineffective and may be associated with chronic pain as well as loculation of the pleural fluid. When an effusion is loculated, localization under ultrasonographic guidance is essential for safe thoracentesis.

For those patients who have recurrent effusion after pleurodesis, other approaches include pleurectomy and pleuroperitoneal shunt. Pleurectomy is the most efficacious approach but has rarely been used because of the requirement for major surgery in patients with short life expectancy. However, with new technologies, such as videoendoscopic thoracoscopy, pleurectomy and decortication may be performed with less morbidity.

Keller SM. Current and future therapy for malignant pleural effusion. Chest 1993;103:63S–67S.
Ruckdeschel JC. Management of malignant pleural effusion. Semin Oncol 1995;22:58–63.

D. Hypercalcemia of Malignancy

Neoplastic hypercalcemia occurs with an incidence of 150 cases per million people per year and is responsible for 20% to 25% of the cases of hypercalcemia diagnosed in the United States. The cancers that most commonly cause hypercalcemia are non-small cell lung cancer, breast cancer, multiple myeloma, non-Hodgkin's lymphoma, and renal cell carcinoma. Symptomatic hypercalcemia typically occurs when the calcium level is >12 mg/dL, depending on the level of serum albumin, which binds calcium, and on the rate of rise in calcium. Symptoms include nausea, constipation, mental status changes, abdominal pain, and polyuria. Coma, renal failure, and arrhythmias can occur with severe hypercalcemia (>14 mg/dL).

1. MANAGEMENT
    a. **Tumor cytoreduction.** The most successful long-term approach to the hypercalcemia of malignancy is the eradication of systemic tumor by surgery, radiation therapy, or chemotherapy. These definitive modalities should be used with the following palliative, temporizing measures.
    b. **Hydration and furosemide.** Initial management of all patients with malignant hypercalcemia should include vigorous hydration (e.g., 300 mL/h of normal saline) to correct volume depletion and to

promote urinary calcium excretion. Furosemide (20–40 mg IV) should be used to prevent volume overload and to augment urinary calcium wasting. Standard hydration therapy generally leads to a 2 to 3 mg/dL fall in the serum calcium level over 48 hours, but complete, sustained control is unusual.

c. **Mobilization.** Patients should be encouraged to remain ambulatory and physically active, as immobilization stimulates osteoclastic bone resorption.

d. **Diphosphonates (bisphosphonates).** The most potent agents for treating hypercalcemia are the diphosphonates: aminohydroxypropylidine diphosphonate (APD, pamidronate), ethane hydroxydiphosphonate (EHDP, etidronate), and dichloromethylene diphosphonate (Cl_2MDP, clodronate). These pyrophosphate analogs are incorporated into the hydroxyapatite of bone in areas of high bone turnover (e.g., metastatic lesions) and decrease the solubility of the crystals. All three compounds inhibit osteoclast function. Hypercalcemia improves in 70% to 100% of patients within 2 days from administration, with the serum calcium reaching its lowest level in 7 days. Pamidronate, the most potent of the available diphosphonates, is administered as a 60 mg IV infusion over 4 hours or 90 mg IV infusion over 24 hours. Pamidronate therapy also decreases pain and promotes healing of bone metastases. Etidronate is given at 7.5 mg/kg IV daily over 4 hours for 3 to 7 days. These agents are more effective if given after the patient is well hydrated. Toxicity associated with diphosphonate administration has consisted of mild fever (APD), phlebitis at the infusion site (APD), and mild gastrointestinal toxicity (mostly occurring with oral administration of these drugs). Osteomalacia can occur with long-term use of EHDP.

e. **Calcitonin.** Calcitonin is a potent inhibitor of osteoclastic bone resorption and also has a direct calciuretic effect at the level of the proximal tubule in the kidney. Commercial salmon calcitonin (4–12 IU/kg SC q8–12h) has the most rapid onset of action of all available agents, reducing elevated serum calcium levels within the first 24 hours in more than 80% of patients. In 2 to 3 days, however, osteoclasts escape from the effects of the hormone, and calcium levels begin to rise again. Interrupting therapy when escape occurs restores responsiveness to the drug after a few days. Concomitant use of corticosteroids (prednisone, 10 mg qid) delays the development of the calcitonin escape phenomenon for 4 to 9 days (Lancet 1985;21:907–910).

f. **Gallium nitrate.** An inhibitor of bone resorption, gallium nitrate acts by adsorbing to hydroxyapatite crystals rather than by osteoclast inhibition. A randomized trial demonstrated the superiority of gallium nitrate (200 mg/m^2 IV for 5 days by continuous infusion) over calcitonin (8 IU/kg IM q6h for 5 days) in achieving normocalcemia (75% versus 31%) and in duration of normocalcemia (>11 days versus 2 days). In a randomized study comparing it to etidronate, normalization of hypercalcemia occurred in more patients receiving gallium nitrate (82% versus 43%). Nephrotoxicity is the major adverse effect.

g. **Plicamycin (mithramycin).** This antineoplastic antibiotic inhibits osteoclast activity, reduces renal tubular calcium reabsorption, and lowers serum calcium levels. It is nearly always effective at a dosage of 25 µg/kg IV over 4 to 6 hours and usually has an onset of action in the first 24 hours and an effect that lasts 5 to 7 days. If no improvement in hypercalcemia is evident within 48 hours, a second dose of plicamycin should be given. Toxicity reported with plicamycin therapy includes hemorrhage due to thrombocytopenia, elevation of prothrombin time and transaminases, and renal failure. The platelet count, prothrombin time, liver transaminase levels, and creatinine level should be monitored during therapy.

h. **Corticosteroids.** Glucocorticoids (40–60 mg prednisone daily) are more likely to improve hypercalcemia in patients with multiple myeloma or other hematologic malignancies. Disadvantages of corticosteroid therapy for this condition include prolonged latency before clinical response occurs (5 to 10 days), immunosuppressive and catabolic side effects of steroids, and induction of skeletal demineralization by glucocorticoids.

i. **Phosphate therapy.** Oral phosphate therapy (250 mg PO qid of elemental phosphate) is safe and moderately effective in patients with hypophosphatemia. Careful dosage escalation (up to 2–3 g/d in divided doses) should be tried if no clinical response is observed after several days, although doses >2–3 g/d often cause intolerable diarrhea. Serum phosphate and creatinine levels should be monitored, and phosphate therapy should be discontinued if hyperphosphatemia or renal insufficiency develops.

2. **PROGNOSIS.** The survival of patients with hypercalcemia associated with malignancy is poor, with a median survival of 39 days despite achievement of normocalcemia. Death nearly always results from progressive disseminated disease. The only patients who survive longer than 6 months are those in whom systemic remissions can be achieved with radiation therapy, chemotherapy, or hormonal therapy.

Bilezikian JP. Management of acute hypercalcemia. N Engl J Med 1992;326:1196–1203.
Ralston SH, Gallacher SJ, Patel U, et al. Cancer-associated hypercalcemia: morbidity and mortality. Ann Intern Med 1990;112:499–504.
Ritch PS. Treatment of cancer-related hypercalcemia. Semin Oncol 1990;17(Suppl 5):26–33.

E. The Tumor Lysis Syndrome

Acute tumor lysis syndrome results from the rapid release of large quantities of intracellular potassium, phosphate, and nucleic acids from dying tumor cells, with resultant hyperkalemia, hyperphosphatemia, hypocalcemia, and hyperuricemia. The metabolic consequences include weakness, lethargy, paresthesias, muscular twitching, seizures, vomiting, ventricular dysrhythmias, and oliguric renal failure. Patients at risk for tumor lysis syndrome are those with bulky tumors that have high cell turnover rates and are sensitive to chemotherapeutic agents (especially Burkitt's and lymphoblastic lymphomas and acute leukemias). Most cases occur within 2 to 3 days of the initiation of chemotherapy.

1. **MANAGEMENT.** Prevention of tumor lysis syndrome is preferable to therapy. Patients at risk should be well hydrated (e.g., 3000 mL/m^2/d) for 24 hours before chemotherapy, and a brisk diuresis should be maintained with diuretics if necessary. Alkalinization of the urine (e.g., 50 mEq of sodium bicarbonate per liter of fluid) may inhibit deposition of uric acid crystals in the kidney (urine pH >7). Allopurinol (200–500 mg/m^2 PO or IV) is administered for 24 hours before therapy and for a week after therapy to inhibit the generation of uric acids from nucleic acids. Electrolytes, uric acid, and creatinine levels should be measured before chemotherapy and daily thereafter for several days in patients at high risk. If the syndrome evolves despite prophylactic measures, dialysis may be necessary to normalize metabolic parameters until renal function recovers.

F. Spinal Cord Compression

Epidural metastases cause spinal cord compression in 5% of patients with disseminated malignancies, or approximately 20,000 patients per year in the United States. The majority of cases of spinal cord compression in adults arise from metastatic breast, lung, prostate, and renal cell cancer and lymphoma. Compression usually results from epidural extension of metastatic tumor from an adjacent vertebra or from a pathologic vertebral compression fracture. In 95% of patients, the initial symptom of epidural spinal cord compression is progressive pain in an axial or radicular distribution. The pain of cord compression is often dysesthetic in nature, exacerbated by palpation or percussion over the spine and by recumbency. Weakness, sensory loss, and incontinence are later findings.

1. **MANAGEMENT.** Immediate intervention is mandatory in neoplastic spinal cord compression, as progression can be rapid, and lost neurologic functions are usually not regained. Emergency imaging of the spinal cord with MRI should be performed in patients suspected of having cord compression. Use of contrast enhancement with MRI increases the ability to detect leptomeningeal and intramedullary disease. Patients should undergo full spinal imaging before definitive therapy to exclude asymptomatic epidural disease at other levels that may later become symptomatic. Corticosteroid therapy should be instituted immediately on suspicion of spinal cord compression, but there is controversy about the optimal loading and maintenance doses. Dexamethasone is the most frequently used steroid, and commonly used doses include a loading dose of 10–100 mg IV followed by 4–24 mg qid. Radiation therapy is the definitive treatment for most patients, including those with slow progression (weeks to months), radiosensitive tumors (e.g., lymphomas), or contraindications to major surgery (e.g., terminal disease). Indications for surgical intervention with decompressive laminectomy include neurologic deterioration that develops during or following radiotherapy, radioresistant tumors, pathologic fracture causing cord compression by bone, instability of the spine, and an unknown primary tumor. Adjunctive postoperative radiation therapy has been shown to improve the final outcome compared with surgery alone.

TABLE 11-4. Treatment Outcome Following Neoplastic Spinal Cord Compression

PARAMETER	AMBULATORY POSTTHERAPY (%)
PRIMARY TUMOR TYPE	
Lymphoma	52
Multiple myeloma	50
Breast	33
Prostate	31
Lung	14
Kidney	10
PREOPERATIVE MOTOR STATUS	
Ambulatory	60
Paraparetic	35
Paraplegic	7

Modified from Bruckman JE, Bloomer WD. Semin Oncol 1978;5:135–140.

2. **PROGNOSIS.** Patients with neoplastic spinal cord compression generally have advanced cancer and short survival (16% to 20% 1-year survival). The results of treatment for spinal cord compression are best in patients who have minimal or no neurologic impairment and poorest in those with established paraplegia. About 60% to 70% of patients in the former category are able to walk after treatment, compared with 5% to 10% in the latter group. Treatment outcome according to tumor type and preoperative motor status is presented in Table 11–4.

Bates T. A review of local radiotherapy and cord compression. Int J Radiat Oncol Biol Phys 1992;23:217–221.

Boogerd W, van der Sande JJ. Diagnosis and treatment of spinal cord compression in malignant disease. Cancer Treat Rev 1993;19:129–150.

Byrne TN. Spinal cord compression from epidural metastases. N Engl J Med 1992;327:614–619.

Lozes G, Fawaz A, Devos P, et al. Operative treatment of thoraco-lumbar metastases, using methylmetacrylate and Kempf's rods for vertebral replacement and stabilization. Acta Neurochir 1987;84:118–123.

Zevallos M, Chan PYM, Munoz L, et al. Epidural spinal cord compression from metastatic tumor. Int J Radiat Oncol Biol Phys 1987;13:875–878.

G. The Serum Hyperviscosity Syndrome

Marked overproduction of monoclonal serum paraproteins resulting in elevation of the serum viscosity is seen in Waldenström's macroglobulinemia (85% to 90% of cases of hyperviscosity syndrome), multiple myeloma (5% to 10%), and lymphomas. Hyperviscosity syndrome is characterized by sludging and decreased perfusion of the microvasculature and vascular stasis, most commonly in the retinal, cerebral, cardiac, and peripheral vessels. Clinically, the syndrome is characterized by bleeding, visual signs and symptoms, and neurologic deficits. Diagnosis is confirmed by measuring the serum viscosity. Most patients begin to develop symptoms at serum viscosities >4 centipoise (normal 1.4 to 1.8). Untreated patients may progress to stroke, seizure, congestive heart failure, blindness, and significant hemorrhage.

1. **MANAGEMENT.** Plasmapheresis (plasma exchange of 3 to 4 L of plasma in 24 hours) is the therapy of choice for symptomatic hyperviscosity. Dehydration should be corrected, and rapid blood transfusion should be avoided, as these conditions will increase plasma viscosity and cause clinical deterioration. Concomitant antineoplastic therapy (with chlorambucil, melphalan, or cyclophosphamide and prednisone) must be administered to prevent recurrence of the syndrome, which generally relapses within 2 to 3 weeks unless tumor bulk is reduced. Maintenance plasmapheresis of 1 to 2 L at 1 to 2 week intervals may be necessary until definitive therapy is effective. Volume replacement is usually with fresh frozen plasma, since it replaces immunoglobulins and clotting factors. Hypocalcemia related to citrate anticoagulants may be observed.

2. **PROGNOSIS.** The prognosis for a symptomatic patient depends on that for the underlying disease. Plasma exchange is much more effective for IgM paraproteinemias because 80% of IgM is confined to the intravascular space. Removal of 1 L of plasma can reduce IgM levels by 15% to 20% and reduce relative viscosity by 50% to 100%. Reduction of IgG levels is much less satisfactory because of the large extravascular pool available for redistribution following plasmapheresis.

Crawford J, Cox EB, Cohen HJ. Evaluation of hyperviscosity in monoclonal gammopathies. Am J Med 1985;79:13–22.
Patterson WP, Caldwell CW, Doll DC. Hyperviscosity syndromes and coagulopathies. Semin Oncol 1990;17:210–216.

H. Hypercoagulable States Associated with Cancer

Thromboembolic events occur in 5% to 10% of patients with cancer and are manifested as deep venous thrombosis, arterial thrombosis, migratory thrombophlebitis, pulmonary embolism, and nonbacterial thrombotic endocarditis. Trousseau's syndrome is most commonly seen with metastatic mucinous adenocarcinomas of the GI tract (pancreas, stomach, colon, and gallbladder), lung, prostate, or ovary. Thromboses in cancer patients are often atypical (superficial, located in upper extremities) and refractory to conventional anticoagulation therapy. Patients with acute promyelocytic leukemia may have disseminated intravascular coagulation (DIC) that can initially worsen with induction chemotherapy as dying cells release procoagulant factors. Cancer can promote clotting through several mechanisms, including direct effects on platelets, endothelial cells, or other blood cells, inappropriate vascular coagulation and abnormal fibrinolysis due to release and activation of clotting factors and procoagulants, localized anatomic changes, such as tissue injury and venous obstruction, and patient immobilization.

1. **MANAGEMENT.** Therapy is directed at treating the acute event and reducing the risk for subsequent events. Thrombolytic agents (streptokinase, urokinase, plasminogen activators) are rarely used in cancer patients because of increased hemorrhagic risk factors found in this population (active bleeding, thrombocytopenia, CNS or pericardial metastases), but they may be necessary in the case of life-threatening thrombotic or embolic events. The anticoagulant drugs, heparin and

warfarin, prevent extension of established venous thrombosis and recurrent embolization by inhibiting blood coagulation. If anticoagulation is contraindicated or unsuccessful at preventing recurrent thromboses, vena caval interruption (with a Greenfield filter) to prevent the risk of pulmonary embolism from distal thromboses may be advisable. Surgical removal of the thrombolytic obstruction is indicated only when there is threatened gangrene of the limb because of extensive venous obstruction, acute circulatory collapse from massive pulmonary embolism, or in selected cases of chronic thromboembolic pulmonary hypertension with proximal pulmonary arterial obstruction. Acute thrombotic episodes are treated with IV heparin for 5 to 10 days (adjusted to maintain the aPTT 1.5 to 2 times control). Outpatient treatment with either adjusted-dose SC heparin (5,000–10,000 IU up to tid) or PO warfarin (maintaining an international normalized ratio [INR] of 2 to 3) is then given for at least 3 months or for the duration of time the patient is believed to be at risk. Warfarin alone frequently fails to prevent recurrent thromboses in Trousseau's syndrome, with SC heparin being required. Warfarin and heparin can produce a high incidence of potentially fatal hemorrhage in cancer patients, and the aPTT and PT must be closely monitored. Antiplatelet drugs are of questionable benefit for stopping the progression of thrombosis and for prophylaxis in patients with recurrent thrombosis. Results of clinical studies with new antithrombotic agents (including low molecular weight heparin) and the newer generation fibrinolytic agents may prove to be of benefit to the cancer patient with a hypercoaguable syndrome.

2. **PROGNOSIS.** Hypercoaguable states associated with cancer are often refractory to conventional anticoagulation therapy. Vital in the management of patients with Trousseau's syndrome is immediate and vigorous antitumor therapy. Thromboembolic events rank second to infections as a cause of death in patients with solid tumors. Pulmonary emboli have been found at autopsy in up to 50% of patients with disseminated cancer.

Bell WR, Starksen NF, Tong S, et al. Trousseau's syndrome: devastating coagulopathy in the absence of heparin. Am J Med 1985;79:423–430.

Levine M, Hirsh J. The diagnosis and treatment of thrombosis in the cancer patient. Semin Oncol 1990;17:160–171.

Rickles FR, Edwards RL. Activation of blood coagulation in cancer: Trousseau's syndrome revisited. Blood 1987;62:14–31.

Scates SM. Diagnosis and treatment of cancer-related thrombosis. Semin Thromb Hemost 1992;18:373–379.

IV. TREATMENT OF SPECIFIC DISEASE ENTITIES

A. Hematologic Malignancies

1. **ACUTE MYELOID LEUKEMIA.** Acute myeloid leukemia (AML) is characterized by a marked excess of nonlymphoid blast cells in the bone marrow (>30% of nucleated cells), usually in association with circulating blast cells. Seven subtypes have been defined, including myeloblastic (M1 and M2), promyelocytic (M3), myelomonocytic (M4), monocytic (M5), erythoblastic (M6), and megakaryocytic (M7). Treatment consider-

ations are similar for all of these subtypes except acute promyelocytic leukemia (M3).

a. **Chemotherapy**

(1) *Induction chemotherapy.* Newly diagnosed AML must be treated aggressively with myelosuppressive agents to achieve complete remission. Regimens including the anthracyclines idarubicin (12 mg/m^2/d IV for 3 days) or daunorubicin (30–60 mg/m^2/d IV for 3 days) along with cytosine arabinoside (100–200 mg/m^2 IV by continuous infusion for 7 days) induce complete remissions in 60% to 85% of patients.

Patients with acute promyelocytic leukemia (M3) may receive induction therapy with all-trans-retinoic acid (ATRA). This derivative of vitamin A induces differentiation of the promyelocytes to mature granulocytes without marrow aplasia and without risk of DIC, which is a complication of the treatment of M3 leukemia with standard chemotherapy. However, ATRA may cause pulmonary infiltrates and the retinoic acid syndrome, which produces an ARDS-like picture. Both chemotherapy and ATRA are equally effective at inducing remission, but overall survival is superior if patients are treated with ATRA at any time in their treatment course (induction, consolidation, or maintenance) (Proc Am Soc Hematol 1995; 85(10):488).

(2) *Consolidation chemotherapy.* Additional cycles of chemotherapy must be given after achievement of complete remission to prevent early relapse. A regimen similar to the original induction regimen is repeated as consolidation therapy 3 to 4 weeks after bone marrow recovery, provided that patients are ambulatory, afebrile, and off antibiotics and that their leukocyte count is >3000/mm^3 and their platelet count is >100,000/mm^3. Alternatively, multiple courses of high-dose cytarabine (HDAC; 3 g/m^2 IV over 1 to 2 hours q12h qod for six doses), have been shown to be the most effective consolidation regimen for patients under the age of 55 (N Engl J Med 1994;331:896–903). Patients receiving HDAC should be treated with topical corticosteroids to prevent painful conjunctivitis and must be monitored for early signs of cerebellar toxicity (e.g., nystagmus). Patients over the age of 55 should probably not receive this regimen because of a marked increase in cerebellar toxicity in this age group. The optimal number of cycles of consolidation chemotherapy with HDAC is four, which can achieve a long-term disease-free survival rate of 44%.

(3) *Maintenance chemotherapy.* Several trials have investigated the role of prolonged administration of low-dose chemotherapy for 1 to 2 years after consolidation therapy. Most studies show no benefit to maintenance therapy in AML, provided aggressive induction and consolidation therapy is given. Maintenance with ATRA may be helpful for patients with M3 leukemia.

(4) *Bone marrow transplantation.* Allogeneic bone marrow transplantation has been widely used in patients for whom a

suitable HLA-matched marrow donor is available. With histo-compatible transplants, long-term disease-free survival may be achieved in 50% to 60% of patients when transplantation is performed in first remission. This approach is generally recommended for patients with poor-risk AML who have an appropriate donor. Alternatively, recent studies of autologous transplantation (with and without purging of marrow stored in remission with 1-hydroperoxycyclophosphamide or mafosfamide) suggest that 40% to 50% of patients who have transplant in first remission may be cured with this approach. These results are similar to consolidation therapy with HDAC but inferior to allogeneic transplant (N Engl J Med 1995;332:217–223).

b. **Supportive care.** Patients usually must be hospitalized for 3 to 4 weeks with each cycle of chemotherapy. Central venous access, hyperalimentation, hydration, allopurinol, prolonged transfusional support, and empiric antibiotics for neutropenic fevers usually are required. Histocompatibility typing of patients and family members should be done to identify potential platelet and bone marrow donors. Patients with acute promyelocytic leukemia with DIC are often treated with low-dose heparin therapy (10–20 U/kg/h) during induction, although management with intensive blood product support is equally effective.

c. **Prognosis**

(1) *Conventional therapy.* Most AML trials report median remission durations of 12 to 13 months, median survivals of 20 to 24 months, and long-term disease-free survival rates of 15% to 25%. Patients with particular cytogenetic abnormalities t(8;21), t(15;17), and inv(16) have a better prognosis, particularly those patients who receive multiple cycles of HDAC, where 40% to 45% of patients may be long-term survivors.

(2) *Salvage chemotherapy.* Approximately 60% to 75% of patients with AML will experience leukemic relapse, and about half of these patients can be reinduced into a second complete remission. Unfortunately, virtually none of these patients will survive long term unless marrow transplantation is undertaken. Drugs commonly used in relapsed patients include HDAC and mitoxantrone plus etoposide (VP-16). Bone marrow transplantation may cure patients who recur with long-term disease-free survival rates of 25% to 30% in first relapse or second remission and 10% to 15% in end-stage refractory leukemia.

Linker CA. Treatment of acute leukemia in adults. Curr Opin Oncol 1992;4:53–65.

Mayer RJ, Davis RB, Schiffer CA, et al. Intensive post-remission chemotherapy in adults with acute myelogenous leukemia. N Engl J Med 1994;331:896–903.

Stone RM, Mayer RJ. Treatment of the newly diagnosed adult with de novo acute myeloid leukemia. Hematol Oncol Clin North Am 1993;4:47–64.

Tallman M, Andersen J, Schiffer C, et al. Phase III randomized study of all-trans-retinoic acid (ATRA) vs daunorubicin and cytosine arabinoside as induction therapy, and ATRA vs observation as maintenance therapy, for patients with previously untreated acute promyelocytic leukemia (APL). Proc Am Soc Hematol 1995;85(10):488.

Zittoun RA, Mandelli F, Willemze R, et al. Autologous or allogeneic bone marrow transplantation compared with intensive chemotherapy in acute myelogenous leukemia. N Engl J Med 1995;332:217–223.

2. ACUTE LYMPHOBLASTIC LEUKEMIA. Acute lymphoblastic leukemia (ALL) is the most common childhood malignancy (3.5 cases per 100,000 children). It peaks in incidence between 2 and 7 years of age. ALL is much less common in adults but still constitutes 20% of adult acute leukemias. Patients typically experience fatigue, malaise, epistaxis, fever, bone pain, lymphadenopathy, hepatosplenomegaly, and petechiae. Features that have been associated with an unfavorable outcome include age under 2 years or over 10, immunophenotype (B cell worse than T cell, which is worse than common ALL), elevated leukocyte count (>30,000/mm^3), delayed achievement of remission (>4 weeks), abnormal karyotype (especially translocations), male sex, hepatosplenomegaly, and the presence of CNS leukemia at diagnosis.

a. **Management.** Treatment of ALL can be divided into four phases: remission induction, consolidation, low-dose maintenance, and treatment of sanctuary sites (CNS and testicles). Treatment regimens are usually stratified in intensity, depending on the presence or absence of high-risk features.

(1) *Induction chemotherapy.* The standard remission induction regimen for childhood ALL includes vincristine (1.5–2 mg/m^2 IV qwk for 4 weeks), prednisone (40 mg/m^2 PO qd for 4 weeks), and L-asparaginase (6000 U/m^2 IM two to three times per week), following hydration, urine alkalinization, and allopurinol. High-risk childhood ALL and all cases of adult ALL should also be treated with an anthracycline (e.g., daunorubicin, 25–50 mg/m^2 IV on days 1 to 3) to improve remission rates and durations.

(2) *Consolidation chemotherapy.* After complete remission is achieved, chemotherapy must be continued, or most patients will have relapse within 1 to 2 months. There are a variety of consolidation regimens that are quite complex and require multiple courses of different chemotherapeutic agents. In children, consolidation may consist of high-dose methotrexate with 6-mercaptopurine, teniposide, L-asparaginase, and cytarabine. High-risk children and adults may require additional drugs, such as anthracyclines and cyclophosphamide, for several months after remission is attained and before institution of maintenance. Several regimens have been shown to improve survival (Blood 1991;78:2814–2822), but no single approach is generally accepted. Such patients should be referred to major cancer centers for entry into controlled clinical trials.

(3) *Maintenance therapy.* The use of maintenance therapy has been established in childhood ALL. Maintenance usually consists of 6-MP and methotrexate for 2 years. Similar regimens are used in adults. The addition of other agents has not been shown to be of benefit.

(4) ***Central nervous system prophylaxis.*** Before the advent of prophylactic measures, CNS leukemia occurred in 50% of childhood ALL cases. Conventional CNS prophylaxis with intrathecal MTX (6 mg in children <1 y; 8 mg, 1 to 2 y; 10 mg, 2 to 3 y; 12 mg, >3 y) for five doses (given every 3 to 4 days), in conjunction with cranial irradiation (2400 cGy), reduces the incidence of meningeal leukemia to 5% but is complicated by a substantial decrement in intellectual functioning. Therefore, less aggressive prophylactic measures are currently advocated for standard-risk children. Prolonged intrathecal chemotherapy without radiation (with MTX alone or combined with intrathecal cytarabine [30 mg/m^2] and intrathecal hydrocortisone [15 mg/m^2]), limitation of cranial irradiation to 1800 cGy, and use of systemic (instead of intrathecal) high-dose MTX have all been advocated for low-risk cases of ALL. Patients treated with intrathecal chemotherapy alone must receive intermittent doses over a prolonged period (1 to 2.5 years). Patients who are at high risk for CNS leukemia (infants, leukocyte counts >100,000/mm^3, T cell ALL, adults) should receive combined-modality prophylaxis. Patients with overt CNS leukemia at diagnosis should receive aggressive CNS treatment with cranial irradiation (24 to 28 Gy), weekly intrathecal MTX during induction chemotherapy (for 5 to 10 doses), and monthly intrathecal MTX for the first year of therapy.

(5) ***Systemic relapse***

    (a) ***Chemotherapy.*** Second remissions can be achieved in 70% to 90% of children and 50% of adults following leukemic relapse using the same chemotherapeutic regimens employed for initial remission induction. The chances of achieving a durable second remission are greatly increased in patients who have relapse after a disease-free interval of at least 18 months, especially if relapse occurs after cessation of maintenance chemotherapy. Second-line drugs that have been found to be active against disease recurrences refractory to standard regimens include mitoxantrone, HDAC, teniposide, and etoposide.

    (b) ***Bone marrow transplantation (BMT).*** The role of marrow transplantation for ALL is controversial. With improvements in combination chemotherapy, marrow transplantation is used in first remission only for high-risk cases (Philadelphia chromosome positive, null cell ALL, high WBC at presentation) because of the danger of submitting cured patients to potentially fatal treatment. Autologous transplant has not been shown to be superior to chemotherapy for patients in first remission. After relapse, however, the chances of achieving cure with conventional chemotherapy are greatly diminished. In children, several studies have suggested that allogeneic transplant is superior to chemotherapy in second remission. Few adults with

relapsed ALL can be cured with salvage chemotherapy, and BMT is generally recommended in this setting. Long-term disease-free survival can be achieved in 40% to 50% of high-risk patients undergoing allogeneic transplantation in first remission and in 20% to 40% undergoing transplantation in second remission.

b. **Prognosis.** The prognosis for children with ALL is generally excellent. More than 90% will achieve a remission, and 60% to 70% will be cured. In adults, 60% to 80% will obtain a remission, but cure rates appear to be only 25% to 35% for adults.

Barrett AJ, Horowitz MM, Pollock BH, et al. Bone marrow transplantation from HLA-identical siblings as compared with chemotherapy for children with acute lymphoblastic leukemia in a second remission. N Engl J Med 1994;331:1253–1258.

Cortes JE, Kantarjian HM. Acute lymphoblastic leukemia. Cancer 1995;76:2393–2417.

Horowitz M, Messerer D, Hoelzer D, et al. Chemotherapy compared with bone marrow transplantation for adults with acute lymphoblastic leukemia in first remission. Ann Intern Med 1991;115:13–18.

Linker CA. Treatment of acute leukemia in adults. Curr Opin Oncol 1992;4:53–65.

Linker CA, Levitt LJ, O'Donnell M, et al. Treatment of adult lymphoblastic leukemia with intensive cyclical chemotherapy: a follow-up report. Blood 1991;78:2814–2822.

3. CHRONIC MYELOGENOUS LEUKEMIA. Chronic myelogenous leukemia (CML) has an incidence of 1 per 100,000 and is responsible for 20% to 30% of cases of leukemia in Western countries. The disease typically occurs in middle age and is associated with an unequal reciprocal translocation (the Philadelphia chromosome), which transfers the c-abl oncogene from the 9th to the 22nd chromosome. Three phases of CML occur. An initial chronic phase, with a median duration of 42 months, is characterized by minimal symptomatology and sensitivity to low-dose chemotherapy. A transitional accelerated phase is characterized by progressive leukocytosis, anemia, basophilia, splenomegaly, fever, bone pain, new cytogenetic abnormalities, and increasing blast counts (usually >10%) despite escalating intensity of chemotherapy. A terminal blast crisis phase, with a median duration of 4 months, is associated with more than 30% blasts and promyelocytes in the marrow or blood and is generally refractory to therapy.

a. **Treatment**

(1) *Chronic phase.* Asymptomatic patients having white cell counts <50,000/mm^3 do not necessarily require treatment, as conventional therapy has not been shown to prolong survival or delay blast crisis. Patients who are symptomatic or who have progressive leukocytosis, anemia, thrombocytosis, or thrombocytopenia should be treated with either hydroxyurea (0.5–4 g PO qd), IFN-α (e.g., 2–5 million U SC or IM daily), or busulfan (initially 0.1–0.2 mg/kg/d). Hydroxyurea is rapid acting, nearly always effective, and has few side effects. IFN-α initially causes a flu-like syndrome in most patients, achieves hematologic remissions in 80% of cases, and is the only drug capable of inducing cytogenetic remissions (in 10% to 20% of cases). Busulfan is rarely used now because of its risk of pulmonary toxicity, its long half-life, and the availability of safer drugs. In at

least two randomized trials, IFN-α prolonged survival and delayed progression to blast crisis when compared with chemotherapy. Splenectomy should be employed only in patients with refractory hypersplenism. Leukapheresis is expensive and of evanescent benefit and is recommended only in patients who are pregnant or have leukostasis.

All patients under 60 with CML should have HLA typing done on family members for donor purposes in allogeneic bone marrow transplantation. Long-term disease-free survival can be expected in 50% to 65% of patients undergoing matched allogeneic transplantation when performed in the chronic phase. The best results are achieved when the transplant occurs within 1 year of diagnosis. No other therapy results in long-term cure. If the patient does not have an appropriately matched family donor, an unrelated donor search should be pursued, as results with unrelated donor transplants in the chronic phase are nearly as good as transplants from a matched family donor.

(2) *Accelerated phase.* Escalating doses of hydroxyurea are usually employed in the accelerated phase. Patients with refractory hypersplenism may benefit from splenectomy. Allogeneic bone marrow transplantation from a matched donor, the treatment of choice, results in the cure of 15% to 30%.

(3) *Blast crisis.* Myeloid blast crisis occurs in two thirds of cases of CML and is treated with regimens identical to those used in AML. Unfortunately, only 15% to 35% of patients will benefit from therapy, and few will be cured. One report suggests that plicamycin (mithramycin) plus hydroxyurea may be effective in returning patients with myeloid blast crisis to a second chronic phase (N Engl J Med 1986;315:1433–1438), but this study has not been confirmed. Lymphoid blast crisis occurs in a third of cases of CML and is characterized by lymphoid morphology and terminal deoxynucleotidyltransferase (Tdt) positivity of blast cells. Lymphoid crisis should be treated like ALL, with vincristine and prednisone, with or without L-asparaginase and daunorubicin. With such management, 50% to 60% of patients can be induced into a remission or second chronic phase, but overall survival is poor, with the reappearance of blast crisis within 2 to 3 months. Median survival for patients in blast crisis with conventional therapy is 10 weeks (27 weeks if a second chronic phase can be induced). Matched allogeneic marrow transplantation in blast crisis results in approximately 15% long-term disease-free survival and is the treatment of choice.

Clift RA, Buckner CD, Thomas ED, et al. Marrow transplantation for chronic myelogenous leukemia: a randomized study comparing cyclophosphamide and total body irradiation with busulfan and cyclophosphamide. Blood 1994;84:2036–2043.

Giralt S, Kantarjian H, Talpaz M. Treatment of chronic myelogenous leukemia. Semin Oncol 1995;22:396–404.

Tura S, Baccarani M, Zuffa E, et al. Interferon alpha-2a compared with conventional chemotherapy for the treatment of chronic myelogenous leukemia. N Engl J Med 1994;330:820–825.

4. CHRONIC LYMPHOCYTIC LEUKEMIA. Chronic lymphocytic leukemia (CLL) is the most common type of leukemia in the United States and Europe. It typically is seen in an elderly asymptomatic patient (median age 60 years) noted to have lymphocytosis on routine blood testing. Monoclonal B lymphocytosis (>5000/mm³ in blood, >40% in marrow), lymphadenopathy, hepatosplenomegaly, and hypogammaglobulinemia are typical. Most patients survive several years in relatively good health with minimal therapy before developing pancytopenia and succumbing to infectious complications. Numerous staging systems have been proposed to stratify the risk of death from CLL. One of the most commonly used is that suggested by Rai (Table 11–5). Other prognostic features include the degree of lymphocytosis (>40,000/mm³ is unfavorable) and the pattern of marrow infiltration, with a nodular or interstitial pattern being much more favorable than a diffuse involvement of the marrow.

a. **Therapy.** Asymptomatic stage 0–I patients should not receive therapy because survival is not improved with early drug administration. When patients develop systemic complaints (fever, sweats, fatigue), progressive lymphadenopathy or hepatosplenomegaly, progressive anemia or thrombocytopenia, or recurrent infections, oral chlorambucil (e.g., 0.1 mg/kg/d PO) with or without prednisone is usually started. Cyclophosphamide (2–3 mg/kg/d PO) may be substituted for chlorambucil in patients with marked thrombocytopenia, since the former has a less profound effect on platelet production. Pulse therapy with chlorambucil (0.7 mg/kg PO over 4 days every 3 to 4 weeks) or cyclophosphamide (20 mg/kg every 2 to 3 weeks) may be substituted for daily continuous therapy with equivalent efficacy and less hematologic toxicity. Patients with advanced disease (with significant anemia or thrombocytopenia) may benefit from early institution of combination chemotherapy (e.g., CHOP [cyclophosphamide, doxorubicin, vincristine, prednisone]). Newer agents that show considerable promise in CLL include fludarabine (response rate of 50% to 75%), 2-deoxycoformycin, and 2-chlorodeoxyadenosine. Fludarabine has been shown to be more effective than traditional alkylating agents, with 30% to 50% of patients obtaining a complete remission.

TABLE 11–5. **RAI Staging of CLL**

STAGE*	FEATURES	MEDIAN SURVIVAL (mo)
0	Lymphocytosis	<150
I	Lymphocytosis and lymphadenopathy	101
II	Lymphocytosis, lymphadenopathy, splenomegaly	71
III	Lymphocytosis, anemia (Hb <11g/dL)	19
IV	Lymphocytosis, thrombocytopenia (<100,000/dL)	19

*All stages have lymphocytosis (>15,000/mm³ and >40% in marrow). Cases are assigned stage according to their worst prognostic feature (e.g., lymphocytosis with severe anemia in stage III even if lymphadenopathy and hepatosplenomegaly are lacking).

Fludarabine is usually given at a dose of 25 mg/m^2/d for 5 consecutive days every 28 days for six cycles and may be considered as initial therapy, particularly for high-risk patients. Additional supportive care measures may include IV gamma globulin for patients with recurrent infections and splenectomy for severe refractory anemia or thrombocytopenia due to hypersplenism.

Faguet G. Chronic lymphocytic leukemia: an updated review. J Clin Oncol 1994;12:1974–1990.
Foon K. Chronic lymphoid leukemias: recent advances in biology and therapy. Stem Cells 1995;13:1–21.
Keating MJ, O'Brien S, Kantarjian HM, et al. Nucleoside analogs in the treatment of chronic lymphocytic leukemia. Leuk Lymphoma 1993;10:139–145.

5. **HAIRY CELL LEUKEMIA (HCL)** is a rare chronic leukemia that generally occurs in middle-aged males and is characterized by pancytopenia, splenomegaly, and recurrent infections. The malignant cell is derived from the B lymphocyte lineage and is characterized by numerous cytoplasmic projections (hairy cells) and by acid phosphatase activity that is tartrate resistant (TRAP positive). Conventional management has been splenectomy, which temporarily improves the peripheral blood counts in 90% of patients, but at least 50% of patients will eventually have progressive disease. Recently, many new agents have been introduced that have significant activity in this disease. Low-dose IFN-α (2–3 million units SC three times a week) will induce complete or partial response in 90% of patients. Pentostatin (2'-deoxycoformycin) at 4 mg/m^2 IV every other week demonstrates complete and partial response rates of over 80%, although this agent may be associated with rash, diarrhea, nausea, and vomiting. The most active agent appears to be 2-chlorodeoxyadenosine (2-CdA) at 0.1 mg/kg IV CI qd for 7 days, which produces complete or partial responses in more than 95% of patients. Very few patients relapse after 2-CdA, and those who do usually respond to a second course. Toxicity associated with 2-CdA is typically fever, neutropenia, and transient immune suppression.

Foon K. Chronic lymphoid leukemias: recent advances in biology and therapy. Stem Cells 1995;13:1–21.
Piro LD, Carrera CJ, Carson DA, et al. Lasting remissions in hairy cell leukemia induced by a single infusion of 2-chlorodeoxyadenosine. N Engl J Med 1990;322:1117–1121.

6. **MULTIPLE MYELOMA.** Multiple myeloma is a malignant plasma cell dyscrasia with an incidence of three or four cases per 100,000. It is characterized by marrow plasmacytosis (>10%), monoclonal gammopathy (serum M protein >3 g/dL), osteopenia, tissue plasmacytomas, and punched-out lytic bone lesions. Myeloma may also be associated with renal failure, hypercalcemia, and anemia. Patients are typically elderly (median age 62) and experience fatigue, bone pain, anemia, or infection.
   a. **Therapy.** Plasma cell dyscrasias may occur in several stages, including monoclonal gammopathy of unknown significance, smoldering myeloma, and multiple myeloma.
      (1) Monoclonal gammopathy of unknown significance (benign monoclonal gammopathy) is characterized by minimal gammopathy (M protein <3 g/dL in serum and negligible in urine), fewer than 5% marrow plasma cells, no bone lesions, and normal albumin and hematocrit values. No therapy is indicated for

these patients, but approximately 25% will progress to myeloma. Therefore, regular follow-up with serial serum protein electrophoreses is indicated.

(2) *Smoldering or indolent myeloma.* Patients with definite but mild myeloma (no anemia, bone lesions, or renal insufficiency) should be monitored with serial serum protein electrophoreses and should not receive treatment until symptoms develop or clear evidence of progression occurs.

(3) *Symptomatic or progressive myeloma.* Melphalan (0.25 mg/kg PO qd for 4 days every 6 weeks) and prednisone (1 mg/kg PO qd for 4 days every 6 weeks) have been standard therapy for myeloma for many years. These drugs induce objective regressions (75% decrement in M protein production) in 50% to 60% of patients (median survival of 2 to 3 years). A 25% reduction in melphalan dose is prudent for initiation of therapy in patients with modest renal insufficiency. Leukocyte and platelet counts should be checked every 3 weeks to guide dosage titration. A properly adjusted regimen induces modest midcycle cytopenias. At least three cycles of therapy should be administered before failure is declared. Therapy should be ended in responding patients when the M protein level reaches a plateau, as melphalan is leukemogenic. Cyclophosphamide (100 mg/m^2 IV every 3 to 4 weeks) produces response rates and survival durations comparable to those achieved with melphalan. The merits of multiagent combination chemotherapy in myeloma remain controversial. Combination therapy may be beneficial to patients with high tumor burdens and poor prognostic features in terms of rate of response, but a metaanalysis of 18 published trials shows no difference in overall survival. The role of IFN-α is controversial. Other treatment approaches for myeloma include radiation therapy for severe bone pain (90% response rate) and IV gamma globulin (300 mg/kg every 3 weeks) for recurrent infections, which may be useful in individual cases.

(4) *Refractory disease.* For patients who are refractory to alkylating agents, the salvage regimen of choice is VAD (vincristine, doxorubicin [Adriamycin], and dexamethasone), which produces a 65% to 70% response rate and a 22-month median survival in patients who respond. The most active drug in VAD is dexamethasone, and patients whose disease is primarily refractory to first-line chemotherapy fare as well with high-dose dexamethasone alone (27% response rate) as with VAD (32% response rate). Bone marrow transplantation is being employed with increasing frequency for the treatment of multiple myeloma. Patients may be cured with allogeneic transplant, with approximately 30% of patients being cured with HLA-matched donors, but there is a significant early mortality (20% to 30%) with this approach. Autologous transplants can be performed up to the age of 65 and may be associated with prolonged survival, although this approach is probably not curative.

Alexanian R, Dimopoulos MA, Delasalle K, et al. Primary dexamethasone treatment of multiple myeloma. Blood 1992;80:887–890.

Gregory WM, Richards MA, Malpas JS. Combination chemotherapy versus melphalan and prednisolone in the treatment of multiple myeloma: an overview of published trials. J Clin Oncol 1992;10:334–342.

Kyle RA. Newer approaches to the management of multiple myeloma. Cancer 1993;72:3489–3494.

7. **HODGKIN'S DISEASE.** There are approximately 7500 new cases of Hodgkin's disease diagnosed in the United States each year. The disease exhibits a bimodal age distribution, with peaks in young adulthood and in late middle age. Patients typically have painless lymphadenopathy, fatigue, night sweats, fever, or weight loss.

   a. **Staging.** The therapy of Hodgkin's disease depends on accurate staging as outlined by the Ann Arbor Classification.

   > Stage I: Single lymph node region or focal extralymphatic site
   > Stage II: Two or more sites on one side of the diaphragm
   > Stage III: Involved sites on both sides of the diaphragm
   > Stage IV: Disseminated involvement of an extralymphatic site

   Stages are substratified by the absence (A) or presence (B) of fever (>38°C), night sweats, or weight loss (>10% of body weight). A staging laparotomy is performed if its results will affect treatment planning (e.g., if the choice of radiation therapy or chemotherapy would be altered by the discovery of intraabdominal disease).

   b. **Management.** Several excellent therapeutic regimens with comparable curative potential are available for Hodgkin's disease. Management varies considerably from institution to institution, but the following recommendations are reasonably standard.

   (1) Initial therapy

   (a) Stages I and II. Conventional management of stages I and II involves subtotal nodal (mantle, paraaortic, and splenic fields) or total nodal (mantle plus inverted Y fields) irradiation (4000–4400 cGy in 200-cGy fractions), depending on disease location. This approach yields 10-year survivals of 95% and 93% and disease-free survival of 88% and 76% in stages IA and IIA, respectively. Patients with stages IB and IIB fare less well, with 77% overall survival and 69% disease-free survival at 10 years. Although several authorities have advised chemotherapy alone or chemotherapy plus radiation therapy for stages IB and IIB, the consensus is that chemotherapy with its toxicities should be reserved for the 30% of patients in whom radiation therapy fails. One subgroup for which the combined-modality approach is generally accepted, however, includes patients with large mediastinal masses (greater than one-third the thoracic diameter) because of unsatisfactory failure rates with radiation therapy alone.

   (b) Stage IIIA. Patients with disease limited to the spleen and upper abdominal lymph nodes (stage $IIIA_1$) fare better than those with involved lower abdominal nodes (stage $IIIA_2$), with reported 5-year survival rates of 94% and 65%, respectively, following radiotherapy alone. Radiation

therapy may be used for stage IIIA$_1$ disease, but combination chemotherapy is commonly used in this circumstance. The effectiveness of chemotherapy and avoiding the morbidity of exploratory laparotomy justify this approach.

(c) ***Stages IIIB and IV.*** Combination chemotherapy is essential for the management of patients with stage IIIB or stage IV disease. Several effective, curative regimens have been devised, including MOPP (mechlorethamine, 6 mg/m^2 on days 1 and 8; vincristine, 1.4 mg/m^2 IV on days 1 and 8; procarbazine, 100 mg/m^2 PO on days 1 to 14; and prednisone, 40 mg/m^2 PO on days 1 to 14), ABVD (Adriamycin, 25 mg/m^2 IV; bleomycin, 10 U/m^2 IV; vinblastine 6 mg/m^2 IV; and dacarbazine, 375 mg/m^2 IV on days 1 and 15), alternating MOPP/ABVD, MOPP/ABV hybrid therapy (half-cycles of MOPP and ABV each month), and BCVPP (carmustine [BCNU] cyclophosphamide, vinblastine, procarbazine, and prednisone). Chemotherapy is given for six to eight cycles (of 28 days each) or for two cycles beyond verification of complete remission (Table 11–6). MOPP was the initial regimen of choice, but ABVD appears to be equally efficacious and less leukemogenic and causes less male sterility. In randomized trials, the MOPP/ABV hybrid regimen, alternating MOPP/ABVD, and ABVD appear to be equivalent regimens. MOPP alone may be slightly inferior.

(2) ***Salvage therapy.*** Factors predictive of a favorable outcome for salvage therapy of relapsed Hodgkin's disease include a disease-free interval of over a year, absence of B symptoms, limited nodal sites of relapse, and treatment in first, as opposed to subsequent, relapse. For patients who relapse more than 1 year from completion of previous therapy, approaches to salvage therapy include radiation to recurrent lymph nodes,

---

TABLE 11–6. **Chemotherapy of Advanced Hodgkin's Disease**

REGIMEN	COMPLETE REMISSION RATE (%)	5-YEAR DISEASE-FREE SURVIVAL (%)	REFERENCE
MOPP*	60–84	40–70	J Clin Oncol 1986;4:1295
ABVD†	60–80	40–70	Cancer 1975;36:252–259
BCVPP	76	64	Ann Intern Med 1984;101:447
MOPP/ABVD*	91	67 (10 y)	J Clin Oncol 1996;14:1421
MOPP/ABV‡	89	69 (10 y)	J Clin Oncol 1996;14:1421

*Twelve cycles.
†Six cycles.
‡Eight cycles.
MOPP, mechlorethamine (Mustargen), vincristine (Oncovin), procarbazine, prednisone; ABVD, doxorubicin (Adriamycin), bleomycin, vinblastine, dacarbazine; BCVPP, carmustine (BCNU), cyclophosphamide, vinblastine, procarbazine, prednisone; ABV, doxorubicin (Adriamycin), bleomycin, vinblastine.

retreatment with the same chemotherapy, an alternate chemotherapy regimen, or high-dose therapy with autologous or allogeneic transplant. For patients who relapse within 1 year of completing therapy, the prognosis is poor, and the most effective salvage therapy is autologous or allogeneic bone marrow transplant.

(3) Side effects of therapy. Short-term toxicities of therapy include nausea, vomiting, alopecia, neuropathy, and radiation pneumonitis (5% to 20%). Longer-term sequelae include radiation-induced hypothyroidism (3% to 15%), pulmonary fibrosis, pericarditis, and sterility (80% to 100% of men and >80% of women over 25 years old after MOPP; 70% to 100% of men and 40% of women after total nodal irradiation). Most ominous is the occurrence of secondary malignancies. The magnitude of this risk has been estimated to be 17.6% at 15 years, including a 13.2% risk for solid tumors (lung and breast cancers, melanomas, and sarcomas), 3.3% for AML, and 1.6% for non-Hodgkin's lymphomas. Chemotherapy (especially mechlorethamine and procarbazine) is primarily responsible for the development of secondary leukemias, but both radiation therapy and chemotherapy contribute to secondary solid tumors. The risk of breast cancer in women is greatest in those women who receive mantle radiotherapy under age 20 to 25.

Anderson JE, Litzow MR, Appelbaum FR, et al. Allogeneic, syngeneic, and autologous marrow transplantation for Hodgkin's disease: the 21-year Seattle experience. J Clin Oncol 1993;11: 2342–2350.

DeVita VT, Hubbard SM. Hodgkin's disease. N Engl J Med 1993;328:560–565.

Mauch PM, Kalish LA, Marcus KC, et al. Second malignancies after treatment for laparotomy staged IA-IIIB Hodgkin's disease: long-term analysis of risk factors and outcome. Blood 1996;87:3625–3632.

Shulman LN, Mauch PM. Current role of radiotherapy on Hodgkin's and non-Hodgkin's lymphoma. Curr Opin Oncol 1995;7:421–425.

Viviani S, Bonadonna G, Santoro A, et al. Alternating vs hybrid MOPP and ABVD combinations in advanced Hodgkin's disease: ten year results. Blood 1996;14:1421–1430.

8. **NON-HODGKIN'S LYMPHOMAS.** Non-Hodgkin's lymphomas (NHL) are increasing in frequency, and more than 45,000 new cases are diagnosed in the United States annually. Features adversely affecting outcome include advanced stage, presence of B symptoms, aggressive histology, advanced age, bulky disease (>10 cm), elevated lactate dehydrogenase (LDH) levels, male sex, and elevated proliferative rate.

a. **Management.** Treatment of NHL depends primarily on the histology and, to a lesser extent, the stage of disease. In this chapter, NHL is subgrouped as outlined by the International Working Formulation and by the REAL classification (Table 11-7). Staging procedures are similar to those of Hodgkin's disease except that exploratory laparotomy is rarely employed.

(1) Indolent (low-grade) lymphomas. Stages I and II low-grade lymphomas should be treated with external beam radiation therapy with curative intent (>3500 cGy over 3 to 5 weeks). Stages III and IV indolent lymphomas are generally considered incurable with conventional management and are treated with

TABLE 11–7. **Classification of Non-Hodgkin's Lymphomas**

WORKING FORMULATION	REAL CLASSIFICATION
LOW GRADE	
Small lymphocytic (SL)	B-lymphocytic lymphoma
Follicular small cleaved cell (FSC)	Follicular center cell
Follicular mixed small and large cell (FMCL)	Follicular center cell, grade II
INTERMEDIATE GRADE	
Follicular large cell (FLC)	Follicular center lymphoma, grade III
Diffuse small cleaved cell (DSC)	Mantle cell
Diffuse mixed small and large cell lymphoma (DML)	Marginal zone
Diffuse large cell (DLCL)	Diffuse large B cell lymphoma
HIGH GRADE	
Diffuse large cell, immunoblastic	Diffuse large B cell lymphoma
Small noncleaved cell, Burkitt's and non-Burkitt's (SNCC)	Burkitt's lymphoma
Lymphoblastic (LB)	Precursor B-lymphoblastic lymphoma

palliative intent. Asymptomatic patients may be followed clinically with no intervention, provided normal organs are not impaired. A Stanford University study of 83 untreated patients revealed a 73% 10-year survival, a 23% spontaneous regression rate, and a necessity for eventual therapeutic intervention in 61% (after a median of 3 years). The overall survival is similar to that of patients treated at the time of diagnosis. Disseminated symptomatic disease can be treated with single alkylating agents (e.g., chlorambucil, 0.1 mg/kg/d PO qd or 0.7 mg/kg PO over 4 days every 3 to 4 weeks) with or without prednisone (1 mg/kg/d initially, followed by a taper over several weeks), with a response rate of about 70%. Relapsing or unresponsive disease can be managed with CVP (cyclophosphamide, 400 mg/m^2 IV on days 1 to 5; vincristine, 1.4 mg/m^2 IV on day 1; prednisone, 100 mg/m^2 PO on days 1 to 5, repeated every 21 to 28 days) or CHOP (cyclophosphamide, 750 mg/m^2 IV; doxorubicin [Adriamycin], 50 mg/m^2 IV; vincristine, 1.4 mg/m^2 on day 1; prednisone, 100 mg/m^2 PO on days 1 to 5). Newer agents, such as fludarabine, also appear to have activity against the indolent lymphomas.

Early intervention with C-MOPP (cyclophosphamide, vincristine, procarbazine, prednisone) or CHOP has been advocated for follicular, mixed small cleaved and large cell lymphomas on the basis of two studies showing prolonged disease-free survival when this histology is treated aggressively, but the role of aggressive chemotherapy for indolent lymphomas remains controversial.

(2) *Aggressive (intermediate and high-grade) lymphoma.* Stages I and II diffuse aggressive lymphomas (e.g., diffuse mixed lymphoma [DML], diffuse large cell lymphoma [DLCL]) are best

treated with combined-modality therapy (e.g., three cycles of a doxorubicin-based regimen [CHOP, ACOB] plus 3000 cGy involved-field radiation therapy). This approach yields a 95% to 99% complete remission rate and 84% to 96% disease-free survival at 2.5 years. Bulky stage II and stages III and IV aggressive lymphomas are best managed with CHOP or a similar regimen. The introduction of newer combinations, such as MACOP-B has not been shown to be of benefit. With this approach, 50% to 85% of stage III and IV patients can be expected to achieve complete remission, and 40% to 75% will enjoy long-term disease-free survival.

  b. Miscellaneous lymphomas

    (1) Cutaneous T cell lymphomas (CTCL). Patients with mycosis fungoides and other CTCLs usually have chronic skin plaques, tumors, and nodules, which may be associated with circulating cerebriform lymphocytes (Sézary cells), lymphadenopathy, and visceral involvement. Diagnosis is generally elusive for several years while the patient's skin disease is managed with emollients and steroid creams. Aggressive therapy of CTCL with total skin electron beam radiation therapy and chemotherapy can produce major responses in 90% of patients and may cure a minority of patients with early-stage (skin only) disease. For the majority of patients, early institution of aggressive therapy does not appear to improve disease-free survival. Therapies that may improve symptoms include photochemotherapy with retinoic acid in association with ultraviolet irradiation of lymphocytapheresed cells, topical nitrogen mustard, and psoralen and ultraviolet A (PUVA). Once lymph nodes and visceral organs are involved, CTCL is incurable with conventional therapy. Combination chemotherapy with CVP or CHOP will induce remissions in the majority of patients, but the remission durations are short.

    (2) Lymphoblastic lymphoma. This is typically a T cell disorder of young men, who have mediastinal masses. It responds poorly to conventional lymphoma regimens but is curable when treated with ALL-type regimens.

    (3) AIDS-related lymphomas. Patients with AIDS-related lymphomas have intermediate to high-grade disease, often in extranodal locations. The prognosis for these patients is generally poor. Although they may respond to standard lymphoma regimens, such as CHOP, patient tolerance is poor because of vulnerability to myelosuppression. The underlying disease, as well as the antiviral agents and antibiotics taken by patients infected with HIV, often produces a dysfunctional bone marrow that does not permit introduction of cytotoxic chemotherapy.

  c. Central nervous system disease. Patients with small noncleaved cell lymphomas, lymphoblastic lymphomas, T cell lymphomas, or large cell lymphomas with marrow, testicular, or sinus involvement are at high risk for spread to the CNS. Prophylactic therapy involves administration of intrathecal chemotherapy (e.g., intrathecal MTX), cranial irradiation (2400 cGy in 2.5 weeks), or treatment with drug regimens that penetrate the cerebrospinal fluid well (e.g., high-dose methotrexate or cytarabine). Therapy for documented CNS disease is more intensive and usually includes cranial irradiation (3600–4000 cGy) combined with intrathecal methotrexate (12 mg twice a week until the cerebrospinal fluid is clear, and then 12 mg intrathecally every 6 weeks for 1.5 years).

d. **Bone marrow transplantation for lymphomas.** Patients who have relapse following therapy with doxorubicin-based regimens are rarely curable with conventional chemotherapy. Consequently, high-dose chemotherapy in conjunction with syngeneic, allogeneic, or autologous bone marrow transplantation has become increasingly popular as salvage therapy for suitable candidates. Recent series from several institutions indicate that 11% to 60% of patients with relapsed lymphomas can be cured with marrow transplantation. The prognosis appears to be best for patients transplanted early after relapse with small tumor burdens (preferably after induction of a second remission). Patients with end-stage, resistant disease and large tumor burdens fare poorly with transplantation.

Armitage JO. Treatment of non-Hodgkin's lymphoma. N Engl J Med 1993;328:1023–1031.

Fisher RI, Gaynor ER, Dahlberg S, et al. Comparison of CHOP vs m-BACOD vs ProMACE-CytaBOM vs MACOP-B in patients with intermediate or high-grade non-Hodgkin's lymphoma. N Engl J Med 1993;328:1002–1006.

Longo DL, Young RC, Hubbard S, et al. Prolonged initial remission in patients with nodular mixed lymphoma. Ann Intern Med 1984;100:651–656.

Portlock CS. Management of the low-grade non-Hodgkin's lymphomas. Semin Oncol 1990;17: 51–59.

Sprano JA, Wiernik PH, Strack M, et al. Infusional cyclophosphamide, doxorubicin, and etoposide in human immunodeficiency virus- and human T-cell leukemia virus type I-related non-Hodgkin's lymphoma: a highly active regimen. Blood 1993;81:2810–2815.

Young RC, Longo DL, Glatstein E, et al. The treatment of indolent lymphomas: watchful waiting vs aggressive combined modality treatment. Semin Hematol 1988;25(Suppl 2):11–16.

B. Breast Cancer

In 1995, approximately 185,000 women and 1400 men were diagnosed with invasive breast cancer in the United States, and 46,000 people died of the disease. Carcinoma of the breast is the most common cancer in women in the United States and is second only to lung cancer as a cause of cancer death in women. The incidence of breast cancer has been increasing about 1% annually since the 1940s, but overall mortality has been relatively stable. The most dramatic increase has been seen in smaller primary breast tumors, partly because widespread use of screening mammography permits earlier detection. Risk factors associated with an increased risk of breast cancer include a personal and family history of breast cancer, endogenous endocrine factors (menstrual and pregnancy history), and exogenous endocrine factors (oral contraceptive and estrogen replacement therapy). It is estimated that approximately 5% of all women with breast cancer may have the recently identified germ line mutations in the BRCA1 and BRCA2 genes (Science 1994;266:66–71; Science 1994;265:2088–2090). Tamoxifen is being studied as a preventive agent in women at high risk for developing breast cancer, based on data from adjuvant studies showing a lower incidence of new contralateral primary breast tumors in patients treated with tamoxifen compared with untreated patients (Lancet 1992;339:1–15, 71–85). Fenretinide, a vitamin A derivative, is also being studied as a chemopreventive agent. Mammography is the most important screening modality for the early detection of breast cancer. It is estimated that the mortality from breast cancer in women over 50 can be reduced by 25% to 35% with regular screening mammography.

1. NONINVASIVE (IN SITU) DISEASE. With the increasing use of screening mammography, noninvasive (in situ) cancers are diagnosed more frequently and now represent 15% to 20% of all breast cancers. Ductal carcinoma in situ (DCIS) usually appears as microcalcifications on mammography or as a soft tissue abnormality. The traditional therapy is mastectomy. Experience with breast conservation surgery followed by radiotherapy suggests that it is a reasonable alternative to mastectomy in DCIS patients (Int J Radiat Oncol Biol Phys 1994;30:3–9; N Engl J Med 1993;328:1581–1586). The incidence of distant recurrence and death from the primary DCIS in treated patients is less than 2%. Lobular carcinoma in situ (LCIS) is usually an incidental finding when a biopsy is done for some other abnormality. It is considered a marker for the subsequent development of invasive disease rather than a premalignant lesion. LCIS is often widely distributed throughout the breast and is frequently bilateral. Secondary invasive cancers are as common in the contralateral breast as in the ipsilateral breast, and the incidence of invasive cancer developing in either breast over 25 years is 25%. The clinical management of the patient with LCIS is controversial. Patients may be given the option of close observation or bilateral mastectomy (Oncology 1994;8:45–49).

2. INVASIVE LOCOREGIONAL DISEASE. Invasive ductal carcinoma is the most common invasive cell type (70% to 80%). Invasive lobular carcinoma (10% to 15%) involves both breasts more frequently than other cell types and has a higher propensity to metastasize to meningeal and serosal surfaces. Inflammatory carcinoma of the breast, an aggressive presentation with high likelihood of systemic spread and recurrence, is a clinicopathologic entity characterized by diffuse induration and erythema of the skin, usually without an underlying palpable mass. This presentation is due to tumor embolization of the dermal lymphatics. Breast cancer is highly treatable with a combination of surgery, radiotherapy, chemotherapy, and hormonal therapy and is most often curable when detected in the early stages. Prognosis and selection of therapy are influenced by the age and menopausal status of the patient, stage of the disease, and pathologic characteristics of the primary tumor.

   a. **Primary surgery.** The optimal surgical procedure depends on the location and size of the lesion, appearance of the mammogram, breast size, patient age, and how the patient feels about preservation of the breast. Surgical options include mastectomy (with or without reconstruction) or conservative surgery (i.e., lumpectomy) plus radiotherapy. For appropriately selected patients, survival is equivalent in both mastectomy and conservative surgery approaches, as documented in prospective, randomized trials (N Engl J Med 1995;333:1456–1461; N Engl J Med 1995;332:907–911). An axillary lymph node dissection for histologic study should be performed in cases of invasive breast cancer, as approximately one third of patients with clinically negative nodes will have histologic involvement with tumor, which would make them candidates for additional systemic treatment. Some patients prefer breast reconstruction to lumpectomy plus radiotherapy, and when extensive resection is required, reconstruction may give a better cosmetic result. Reconstructive techniques include saline implants (often after use of a tissue expander), latissimus dorsi myocutaneous flap, transverse rectus abdominus myocutaneous flap (TRAM flap), and free flaps (usually obtained from the gluteus maximus muscle).

b. **Radiation therapy.** Several prospective, randomized trials demonstrate a higher in-breast recurrence rate with conservative surgery alone (43% at 9 years) compared with conservative surgery followed by radiation (12%) (N Engl J Med 1995;333:1456–1461). Radiotherapy following breast conservation surgery consists of external beam radiation to the entire breast, frequently including a boost to the tumor bed. Nodal irradiation is added in cases with significant nodal involvement with tumor (four or more positive nodes or extracapsular extension). Postmastectomy chest wall radiotherapy is not routinely indicated but should be considered in patients who are at high risk of local recurrence (positive surgical margins or four or more involved lymph nodes). Various chemotherapy-radiotherapy sequences have been advocated, and delaying radiotherapy for 4 to 6 months while adjuvant chemotherapy is administered is now common in many of the national adjuvant chemotherapy trials.

c. **Adjuvant systemic therapy.** Adjuvant systemic therapy can significantly reduce the risk of recurrence and death in patients with breast cancer. The challenge is to determine which patients have the highest risk of recurrence and, thus, are more likely to benefit from adjuvant therapy. The most important factor for long-term prognosis is the number of axillary lymph nodes involved with tumor (Cancer 1980;45:2917–2924). The presence of estrogen receptors (ER) and progesterone receptors (PR) on tumors is associated with a greater likelihood of responding to endocrine therapy and a greater likelihood of long-term survival even without endocrine therapy (Breast Cancer Res Treat 1993;28:9–20). Tumor size, histologic grading, tumor proliferation, and the status of oncogenes and tumor suppressor genes (including HER-2/neu and p53) can have prognostic significance as well (J Clin Oncol 1989;7:1239–1251; J Natl Cancer Inst 1992;84:845–855; J Clin Oncol 1992;10:1044–1048). The proportion of women with invasive breast carcinoma who are considered candidates for adjuvant systemic therapy has shifted considerably in the past several years as a result of metaanalyses showing statistically significant effects of chemotherapy and hormone therapy on breast cancer recurrence and mortality.

Node-negative breast cancer patients have a relatively low risk of recurrence, although up to 20% to 30% will die of metastatic disease with local treatment alone (Cancer 1989;63:181–187). It is important to characterize the subset of node-negative patients who are at high risk of relapse based on known prognostic factors and those who could benefit from adjuvant therapy. Some patients with small (<1 cm) node-negative tumors appear to be at low risk for relapse and may not require postoperative adjuvant hormonal therapy or chemotherapy. Adjuvant therapy has been shown to reduce the risk of relapse and improve overall survival in node-negative patients, with a reported 26% reduction in annual risk of recurrence at 10 years following the addition of chemotherapy or hormone therapy and an 18% reduction in mortality (Lancet 1992;339:1–15, 71–85).

Node-positive breast cancer patients have well-established benefit from the addition of adjuvant systemic therapy. In lymph node-positive patients, combination chemotherapy is the treatment recommendation for ER-negative breast cancer patients whether premenopausal or postmenopausal and ER-positive patients who are premenopausal. In postmenopausal, ER-positive patients, metaanalyses have found that hormone therapy with tamoxifen is equally beneficial as adjuvant chemotherapy. Combinations of chemotherapy and endocrine therapy have, in some studies, been shown to be superior to either alone in some subgroups of patients.

(1) *Adjuvant chemotherapy.* Numerous studies have shown that combination chemotherapy is superior to single-agent therapy in the adjuvant treatment of breast cancer (Lancet 1992;339: 1–15, 712–785). Adjuvant combination chemotherapy has been found to prolong the disease-free interval and survival for premenopausal and postmenopausal patients with both negative and positive nodes, with a 28% reduction in risk of recurrence and 16% reduction in mortality at 10 years. There is a trend toward greater efficacy in younger women. Commonly used combination chemotherapy regimens in breast cancer include CMF (cyclophosphamide, methotrexate, 5-FU), CAF (cyclophosphamide, doxorubicin [Adriamycin], 5-FU), CMFVP (cyclophosphamide, methotrexate, 5-FU, vincristine, prednisone), and AC (doxorubicin, cyclophosphamide) (Table 11–8). The standard duration of administration of such chemotherapy is generally 4 to 6 months. Retrospective analyses have indicated that the intensity of dose delivery may be important in the clinical outcome and that doses should not be reduced arbitrarily (J Clin Oncol 1989;7:1677–1684). Data from a small number of studies suggest that anthracycline-containing regimens (CAF, AC) may be associated with better disease-free survival in some circumstances, including tumors with four or more positive lymph nodes, estrogen receptor negativity, or HER-2/neu oncogene overexpression (Proc Am Soc Clin Oncol 1992;11:61; N Engl J Med 1994;330:1260–1266). In postmenopausal women, adjuvant chemotherapy has not been shown to be as effective as in the premenopausal setting, possibly because of underdosing. Recent studies with equal dose intensity in this group appear to show significant benefit.

TABLE 11–8. **Common Adjuvant Chemotherapy Regimens for Breast Cancer**

1. Intermittent CMF (Bonadonna)

Cyclophosphamide	100 mg/m^2/d PO days 1–14	Every 4 wk
Methotrexate	40 mg/m^2 IV days 1, 8	
5-FU	600 mg/m^2 IV days 1, 8	

2. Continuous CMFVP (Cooper)

Cyclophosphamide	60 mg/m^2/d PO	Continuously
Methotrexate	15 mg/m^2/wk IV	
5-FU	300 mg/m^2/wk IV	
Vincristine	1–2 mg/wk IV to total of 6–10 doses	
Prednisone	60 mg/d PO, taper to 10 mg/d then discontinue in 6 wk	

3. FAC (M.D. Anderson and variations)

5-FU	400–600 mg/m^2 IV	Every 3–4 wk for 6 cycles
Doxorubicin (Adriamycin)	40–60 mg/m^2 IV	
Cyclophosphamide	400–600 mg/m^2 IV	

4. AC (NSABP)

Doxorubicin (Adriamycin)	60 mg/m^2 IV day 1	Every 3 wk for 4 cycles
Cyclophosphamide	600 mg/m^2 IV day 1	

(2) *Adjuvant hormonal therapy.* Tamoxifen is the primary adjuvant hormonal therapy used in breast cancer. The benefit of tamoxifen in the adjuvant setting is clear. A metaanalysis of tamoxifen trials has shown a 25% reduction in recurrence and 17% reduction in mortality in node-positive breast cancer patients at 10 years (Lancet 1992;339:1–15; J Natl Cancer Inst Monograph 1992;11:105–116). The improvement in survival rate was only statistically significant in women over 50 years of age. In the United States, the standard tamoxifen dose is 10 mg PO bid (or 20 mg qd). The optimal duration of tamoxifen treatment in the adjuvant setting is being studied, but a recent interim analysis of one of these trials reports that 10 years of adjuvant tamoxifen was no better in terms of overall survival than 5 years. There is a small (threefold) increased risk of endometrial cancer related to the use of tamoxifen, which is <1% for all tamoxifen takers (J Clin Oncol 1993;11:485–490). Tamoxifen therapy in premenopausal women is associated with a rise in circulating estrogen levels and irregular menses. Ovarian ablation (through surgery, radiation, or hormone therapy) in premenopausal breast cancer patients has been shown to have a statistically significant improvement in both recurrence-free survival and overall survival in node-positive patients (Lancet 1992;339:1–15).

d. **Neoadjuvant chemotherapy.** Neoadjuvant chemotherapy given before definitive surgery and radiotherapy of the primary tumor is being used increasingly in the treatment of breast cancer. Tumors that are too large to be treated with breast conservation therapy might regress during chemotherapy and, therefore, require less extensive surgery. Because of their high risk of systemic disease, patients with locally advanced stage III disease or inflammatory breast cancer are commonly treated with a combined modality approach, with neoadjuvant chemotherapy followed by mastectomy and irradiation. Both local and distant control and cure rates are improved.

e. **Adjuvant high-dose chemotherapy.** The 5-year disease-free survival rate following systemic doxorubicin-based chemotherapy for patients with 10 or more positive lymph nodes is approximately 41% (Cancer 1992;69:448–452). Because of this high failure rate with conventional dose adjuvant therapy, several randomized trials are being conducted to investigate the addition of high-dose chemotherapy regimens (with or without stem cell support) to standard adjuvant chemotherapy in patients at high risk of recurrent disease. These approaches might be advantageous in terms of disease-free and overall survival (J Clin Oncol 1993;11:1132–1143). High-dose therapy is toxic, with treatment-related mortality rates of 5% to 15% and serious nonfatal complication rates in excess of 30% (J Clin Oncol 1992;10:1743–1747).

3. **METASTATIC DISEASE.** Metastatic breast cancer is often responsive to therapy, with durable complete remissions attainable in 10% to 20% of patients, although treatment is rarely curative at this stage of disease. Radiotherapy has a major role in the palliation of locally recurrent disease and symptoms, such as pain due to bone metastases. The estrogen receptor and progesterone receptor status of the tumor, the history of previous treatment, the site of recurrence, the disease-free interval, and patient age and menopausal status should be considered in selecting systemic therapy. The biologic markers CEA, CA 15-3, and CA 27.29 generally parallel the clinical course in metastatic disease and frequently are used along with imaging studies in assessing response to treatment.

a. **Chemotherapy.** Disease progression on hormonal treatment, hormone receptor-negative disease, a short disease-free interval (<2 years from adjuvant therapy), and visceral involvement (hepatic or lymphangitic lung disease) are all indications for chemotherapy in the treatment of metastatic breast cancer. Most responses to chemotherapy are incomplete, but 50% to 70% of patients will respond to an effective combination regimen for a median of 6 to 9 months. Survival from the start of treatment is 12 to 18 months on average and may be improved by programs of high-dose consolidative chemotherapy for patients who achieve remission. Of the available chemotherapeutic agents, doxorubicin is the most effective as a single drug. Cyclophosphamide, methotrexate, 5-FU, thiotepa, vinblastine, mitomycin, and mitoxantrone have shown activity in metastatic breast cancer as single agents. For patients with a recurrence after an anthracycline-containing regimen, paclitaxel and docetaxel have been FDA approved. Vinorelbine and etoposide have also demonstrated activity in patients who relapse after treatment with an anthracycline-containing regimen. The standard adjuvant regimens (CMF, CAF, AC) have been shown to have proven response rates in metastatic disease. In previously untreated patients, the overall response rate to CAF or CMF therapy ranges between 50% and 80%, and the complete response rate is between 10% and 25%.

b. **Hormone therapy.** If visceral disease is absent and ER or PR status is positive, hormone therapy is considered standard first-line therapy in metastatic breast cancer. If the tumor is negative for both ER and PR, the probability of response is less than 10%. For the majority of patients with positive hormone receptors, hormone manipulation alone offers a 60% chance of objective remission with minimal morbidity. In general, the endocrine therapies are equally effective in breast cancer, and the choice of agent is based on the relative toxicities. Hormone options for premenopausal patients include the antiestrogen tamoxifen or ovarian ablation (surgical or radiation ablation, chemical castration with LHRH agonists). Post-menopausal patients may benefit from tamoxifen, progesterone therapy with megestrol acetate (80 mg PO bid), or the addition of aromatase inhibitors (aminoglutethimide, arimedex). Androgen therapy and corticosteroids have also had some success but are generally not as effective in breast cancer as other hormone agents. Randomized trials have not shown an advantage for doses of tamoxifen >10 mg bid. The standard dose of the aromatase inhibitor aminoglutethimide is 250 mg qid, and because of its adrenal suppression, it must be given with hydrocortisone. Aromatase inhibitors have not been shown to be effective in women with intact ovaries. Some patients with an initial response to hormone therapy may have a response to withdrawal of the hormone lasting up to 10 months. Patients who respond to initial hormone therapy and then relapse should be considered for other forms of hormone therapy. Use of second-line hormone manipulation provides further useful response in 30% to 50%; second-line hormones almost never work if there was no initial response.

c. **High-dose chemotherapy.** For metastatic disease, very high dose chemotherapy (5 to 30 times higher than conventional doses) with or without stem cell support has been associated with a high response rate. To date, between 15% and 30% of women with metastatic breast cancer remain progression free after being treated with high-dose chemotherapy regimens, with the length of follow-up approaching 3 to 5 years in some studies (J Clin Oncol 1992;10: 102–110; J Clin Oncol 1992;10:1743–1747). In most high-dose chemotherapy protocols, an initial response is induced with standard-dose chemotherapy, and patients with stable or responsive disease then undergo high-dose chemotherapy (usually with a combination of alkylating agents). The results of these trials are difficult to compare with the results of conventional studies because patients whose disease progresses during the initial conventional dose phase of the study are dropped from the analysis.

Ayash LJ, Wheeler C, Fairclough D, et al. Prognostic factors for prolonged progression-free survival with high-dose chemotherapy with autologous stem-cell support for advanced breast cancer. J Clin Oncol 1995;13:2043–2049.

Cannon-Albright LA, Skolnick MH. The genetics of familial breast cancer. Semin Oncol 1996;23:1–5.

Early Breast Cancer Trialist's Collaborative Group. Systemic treatment of early breast cancer by hormonal, cytotoxic, or immune therapy: 133 randomized trials involving 31,000 recurrences and 24,000 deaths among 75,000 women. Lancet 1992;339:1–15.

Fisher B, Anderson S, Redmond CK, et al. Reanalysis and results after 12 years of follow-up in a randomized clinical trial comparing total mastectomy with lumpectomy with or without radiation in the treatment of breast cancer. N Engl J Med 1995;222(22):1456–1461.

Fisher B, Fisher ER, Redmond C, et al. Tumor nuclear grade, estrogen receptor, and progesterone receptor: their value alone or in combination as indicators of outcome following adjuvant therapy for breast cancer. Breast Ca Res Treat 1986;7(3):147–160.

Gale KE, Andersen JW, Tormey DC, et al. Hormonal treatment for metastatic breast cancer: an Eastern Cooperative Oncology Group phase III trial comparing aminoglutethimide to tamoxifen. Cancer 1994;73:354–361.

Goldhirsch A, Wood WC, Senn HJ, et al. Meeting highlights: International consensus panel on the treatment of primary breast cancer. J Natl Cancer Inst 1995;87:1441–1445.

Paik S, Hazan R, Fisher ER, et al. Pathologic findings from the National Surgical Breast and Bowel Project: prognostic significance of erbB-2 protein overexpression in primary breast cancer. J Clin Oncol 1990;8:103–112.

Wenger CR, Beardslee S, Owens MA, et al. DNA ploidy, S-phase, and steroid receptors in more than 127,000 breast cancer patients. Breast Ca Res Treat 1993;28:9–20.

C. Lung Cancer

In the United States, lung cancer is the second most common cancer (after skin cancer) and the most common cause of cancer death. In 1995, over 170,000 new cases were diagnosed and 150,000 people died from the disease. In 85% to 90% of cases, lung cancer is caused by cigarette smoking.

1. TREATMENT OF NON-SMALL CELL LUNG CANCER
   a. **Operable disease.** Non-small cell histologies (epidermoid or squamous, adenocarcinoma, and large cell) account for 75% of patients with lung cancer. Of these, approximately a third will be candidates for a surgical procedure with curative intent. When possible, the tumor and areas of known nodal involvement in continuity should be removed by a procedure less than pneumonectomy, as the outcome of treatment is not improved by more radical surgery and the patient is left with a worse pulmonary reserve. Lobectomy does, however, appear to be superior to wedge resection when possible. Operative mortality should be <3% from lobectomy and <8% from pneumonectomy. Some patients' tumors that are anatomically resectable will be medically inoperable and should be managed as described for localized inoperable disease. Stage I lung cancer is best treated by surgical resection alone, usually a lobectomy. Five-year disease-free survival is little influenced by cell type and (in properly staged patients) exceeds 60%. In stage II disease with hilar/lobar nodal involvement and in stage III resectable disease, the results of surgery are influenced by histologic type: epidermoid tumors have a better prognosis than large cell or adenocarcinomas because of the greater likelihood of hematogenous dissemination with the latter cell types. The 5-year disease-free survival for resected stages II and III is only 20% to 35% in the absence of gross

mediastinal nodal involvement. When the latter finding is present, most surgeons do not operate, since the mortality of pneumonectomy may be greater than the chance of cure. Whether to operate on patients with *microscopic,* not grossly apparent, involvement of mediastinal nodes is controversial.

b. Localized inoperable disease. This includes patients whose tumors are anatomically resectable but medically inoperable, as well as those who have stage III disease without distant metastasis. For these patients, radiation therapy has been the mainstay of treatment. Given 5000 to 6000 cGy over a period of 5 to 7 weeks, patients with inoperable disease confined to the lungs have a 2-year survival of about 15% (median 9 months), and those with evidence of extrapulmonary spread have a 2-year survival of 5% to 8% (median 6 months). A combination of chemotherapy and irradiation improves on the results of radiation therapy alone in localized inoperable disease (2-year survival of 25% to 40%). Another approach is to give chemotherapy, with or without irradiation, as initial treatment, followed by an attempt at surgical resection in patients for whom it becomes technically possible. Such combined modality therapy remains investigational and is best conducted in the context of a protocol.

c. Extensive inoperable disease. There is no standard therapy for these patients, who unfortunately make up 30% to 40% of the lung cancer population at the time of presentation. They have clinically detectable metastasis beyond the ipsilateral hemithorax and regional nodes. A definitive approach requires systemic chemotherapy. It is important to realize that palliation of selected symptoms (e.g., bone pain, hemoptysis, superior vena cava syndrome) may be more reliably achieved with appropriate irradiation, whereas other symptoms (obstructive atelectasis, hoarseness) rarely are improved by x-ray treatment. Chemotherapy for non-small cell lung cancer is in a state of evolution. Nonprotocol treatment is not indicated for patients who are less than fully ambulatory and is controversial for those who are fully ambulatory. The best treatment for the latter group is entry on a protocol study. If this is not possible, a reasonable approach is the administration of cisplatin and vinorelbine or carboplatin and taxol.

2. **TREATMENT OF SMALL CELL LUNG CANCER**
   a. Limited (unresectable) disease. In these patients (25% to 40% of the total), clinical staging fails to reveal evidence of spread beyond the ipsilateral hemithorax and regional nodes. It appears that concurrent chemotherapy and chest irradiation is superior to chemotherapy alone or the use of these modalities in sequence. Cisplatin and VP-16 with irradiation has become a standard form of induction chemotherapy. Whole brain irradiation is used by many centers as prophylaxis against relapse at that site in patients who achieve remission. At the completion of induction treatment, maintenance chemotherapy is no longer administered on a chronic basis. However, administration of pulsed intensive cycles of reinduction,

either with the initially employed program or with one made up of different non–cross-resistant drugs may be of value. With concurrent chemoradiotherapy, 40% of patients with limited disease will survive for 2 years and about 25% for 5 years, a major improvement over supportive care alone (median survival 12 weeks) or radiation therapy alone (median survival 6 months, and 2-year survival <5%).

b. Extensive disease. The majority of patients with small cell lung cancer have clinically evident spread to organs beyond the chest at the time of presentation, reflecting the aggressive growth and early hematogenous dissemination of this cell type. Standard therapy is the use of drugs in combination, with elective whole brain irradiation to prevent relapse in this pharmacologic sanctuary reserved for patients with a complete or near-complete response to chemotherapy. Using a program like CAV (cyclophosphamide, doxorubicin [Adriamycin], and vincristine) alternating with cisplatin/VP-16, the median survival is about 8 months, with almost no long-term survivors. About 60% will have tumor regression, but only 15% will achieve complete response.

Albain KS, Rusch VW, Crowley JJ, et al. Concurrent cisplatin/etoposide plus chest radiotherapy followed by surgery for stages IIIA (N2) and IIIB non-small cell lung cancer: mature results of Southwest Oncology Group phase II study 8805. J Clin Oncol 1995;13:1880–1892.

Aisner J. Extensive-disease small-cell lung cancer: the thrill of victory; the agony of defeat. J Clin Oncol 1996;14:658–665.

Dillman RO, Seagren SL, Propert KJ, et al. A randomized trial of induction chemotherapy plus high-dose radiation versus radiation alone in stage III non-small cell lung cancer. N Engl J Med 1990;323:940–945.

Holmes EC, Livingston R, Turrisi A. Neoplasms of the thorax. In: Holland J, Frei E, eds. Cancer Medicine, 3rd ed. Philadelphia: Lea & Febiger, 1993, pp 1285–1336.

Le Chevalier T, Brisgand D, Douillard J, et al. Randomized study of vinorelbine and cisplatin versus vindesine and cisplatin versus vinorelbine alone in advanced non-small cell lung cancer: results of a European multicenter trial including 612 patients. J Clin Oncol 1994;12:360–367.

McCracken JD, Janaki LM, Crowley JJ, et al. Concurrent chemotherapy radiotherapy for limited small cell lung carcinoma: a Southwest Oncology Group study. J Clin Oncol 1990;8:892–898.

D. Head and Neck Cancer

Head and neck cancers afflict approximately 40,000 Americans annually and occur three times as often in males as females. Each tumor site has a distinct natural history and epidemiology. Alcohol and tobacco abuse have additive carcinogenicity for squamous cell cancers, nickel exposure predisposes to sinus tumors, and Epstein-Barr virus infection, woodworking dust, and residence in southeastern China predispose to nasopharyngeal carcinomas. In general, tumors arising from the anterior head and neck region (lip or anterior tongue) are less aggressive than those arising posteriorly (nasopharynx, hypopharynx, or larynx). Prognosis also depends on tumor stage and differentiation as well as the presence of underlying medical conditions. The frequent occurrence of other medical problems, such as chronic obstructive pulmonary disease, coronary artery disease, and poor nutrition, places these patients at an increased risk for surgery and postoperative complications. As many as 15% to 30% will have a synchronous or metachronous primary tumor elsewhere in the aerodigestive tract. Isotretinoin (*cis*-retinoic acid) has been shown to prevent second primary cancers of the head and neck when given for 1 year after local treatment, decreasing the second primary rate from 24% to 4% (N Engl J Med 1990;323:795–801). Other drugs under investigation include beta-carotene and alpha-tocopherol, which are active in reversing leukoplakia.

1. LOCALIZED TUMORS. Either surgery or radiation therapy can be used as the sole treatment modality for small primary tumors (<2 cm). When tumors are larger, are resected with involved surgical margins, or are metastatic to regional nodes, radiation therapy is given after surgical resection. Adjunctive neck dissection or neck radiotherapy is performed when the risk of lymph node metastases is estimated to be over 15%. For patients with advanced (stage III or IV) laryngeal cancer, organ preservation with chemotherapy followed by radiation is an alternative to laryngectomy and postoperative radiation. A large, randomized study showed no statistical difference in 2-year survival rates of patients assigned to standard surgical therapy (total laryngectomy and postoperative radiation) or chemotherapy and radiation (three cycles of 5-FU and cisplatin, followed by radiation, providing there was at least a partial remission to chemotherapy). Sixty-four percent of the patients in the chemotherapy arm retained a functional larynx. Whether this treatment approach can be applied to cancers of other sites in the head and neck is under investigation.

2. LOCALLY ADVANCED TUMORS. Standard treatment for locally advanced unresectable cancers of the head and neck is radiation therapy, which cures less than 30% of such patients. Although cisplatin and 5-FU regimens produce remissions in 60% to 90% of previously untreated patients, randomized trials have failed to show a survival advantage to its use before or after local therapy. The concomitant use of radiation plus radiation-sensitizing chemotherapy (e.g., 5-FU and cisplatin) shows promise in improving response and disease-free survival compared with radiation therapy alone. Similarly, although radiation therapy has been the standard treatment for patients with nasopharyngeal cancer, recent reports indicate a better cure rate with the addition of concomitant chemotherapy.

3. METASTATIC OR UNRESECTABLE, RECURRENT DISEASE. Many chemotherapeutic agents have been shown to have activity against disseminated or locally recurrent head and neck cancer. Methotrexate produces tumor regressions in 20% to 30% of patients for a median of 4 to 6 months. Combination chemotherapy regimens (especially those containing cisplatin and 5-FU) yield higher response rates, but randomized trials have failed to demonstrate a survival advantage for the more aggressive chemotherapy regimens over methotrexate alone. Large tumor size, prior therapy, and poor performance status all adversely affect the response to chemotherapy.

4. SALIVARY GLAND CANCERS. Ninety percent of parotid tumors and 75% of submandibular tumors are benign and can be treated effectively with surgical resection with or without postoperative irradiation. The most common malignant salivary gland neoplasms are mucoepidermoid and adenoid cystic carcinomas. Prognosis of these tumors depends on the

tumor site, grade, stage, and effectiveness of local therapy. Surgical resection of the primary tumor and regional lymph nodes is the primary treatment modality, but adequate tumor margins are often difficult to obtain. Consequently, postoperative radiation therapy is commonly employed, especially for high-grade lesions. This approach is curative in 70% to 80% of patients. When metastases occur, they are most likely to involve the local region, lung, and bone. Neutron radiation achieves superior local control rates compared with photon radiation as treatment for unresectable salivary gland carcinomas but is available in only a limited number of treatment centers (Int J Radiat Oncol Biol Phys 1993;27:235–240). 5-FU and doxorubicin appear to be the most active chemotherapeutic agents for these tumors.

Department of Veterans Affairs Laryngeal Cancer Study Group. Induction chemotherapy plus radiation compared with surgery plus radiation in patients with advanced laryngeal cancer. N Engl J Med 1991;324:1685–1690.

Dimery IW, Legha SS, Shirinian M, et al. Fluorouracil, doxorubicin, cyclophosphamide, and cisplatin combination chemotherapy in advanced or recurrent salivary gland carcinoma. J Clin Oncol 1990;8:1056–1062.

Jacobs CD, Goffinet DR, Fee WE. Head and neck squamous cancers. Curr Probl Cancer 1990;14:1–72.

Snow JB. Surgical management of head and neck cancer. Semin Oncol 1988;15:20–28.

Vokes EE, Weichselbaum RR, Lippman SM, et al. Head and neck cancer. N Engl J Med 1993;328:184–194.

E. Gastrointestinal Malignancies

1. **ESOPHAGEAL CARCINOMA.** Esophageal cancer is diagnosed in approximately 12,000 Americans each year. Tobacco and alcohol abuse are strong risk factors for squamous cell carcinomas, which account for over half of all esophageal cancers. The incidence of adenocarcinoma of the gastroesophageal junction has been increasing at a rate of 5% to 10% per year. These cancers develop from dysplastic Barrett's epithelium, which results from chronic acid reflux. Prognosis depends on tumor size and differentiation, depth of invasion, lymph node involvement, and degree of weight loss and obstruction. Historically, surgery has been the primary therapeutic modality for patients with esophageal cancer. Aggressive preoperative correction of poor nutrition and improvements in surgical techniques have decreased the operative mortality to the range of 5% to 10%. Although the overall 5-year survival after esophagectomy remains low at 20%, patients with early stage cancers (without nodal involvement) have a significantly better prognosis. For patients with locally advanced, unresectable esophageal cancer, concomitant chemotherapy (cisplatin and 5-FU) plus radiation therapy is the optimal treatment. In a randomized comparison to radiation alone, 2-year survival was statistically superior in the combined modality arm (38% versus 10%). Concurrent chemotherapy and radiation have also been employed before surgical resection as neoadjuvant or induction therapy, achieving pathologically documented complete remission rates of 25% to 50%. It remains unclear if preoperative therapy improves survival over surgery alone or if surgery is necessary after concurrent chemotherapy and radiation. The major-

ity of patients fail, with distant metastases to the liver, lung, and bone. Chemotherapy for metastatic disease is palliative, producing response rates of 20% to 40% lasting a median of 4 to 6 months. Active agents include 5-FU, cisplatin, bleomycin, methotrexate, mitomycin, etoposide, paclitaxel, and vinorelbine. Methods of palliating dysphagia include esophageal dilatation, therapeutic laser endoscopy, placement of an intraluminal prosthesis, and radiation therapy.

Coia LR. Esophageal cancer: is esophagectomy necessary? Oncology 1989;3:101–110.

Forastiere AA, Orringer MB, Perez-Tamayo C, et al. Preoperative chemoradiation followed by transhiatal esophagectomy for carcinoma of the esophagus: final report. J Clin Oncol 1993;11:1118–1123.

Gill PG, Denham JW, Jamieson GG, et al. Patterns of treatment failure and prognostic factors associated with the treatment of esophageal carcinoma with chemotherapy and radiotherapy either as sole treatment or followed by surgery. J Clin Oncol 1992;10:1037–1043.

Herskovic A, Martz K, Al-Sarraf M, et al. Combined chemotherapy and radiotherapy compared with radiotherapy alone in patients with cancer of the esophagus. N Engl J Med 1992;326: 1593–1598.

2. **GASTRIC CANCER.** An estimated 23,000 people in the United States are diagnosed with gastric cancer each year, with an incidence that continues to decrease. Abdominal pain, anorexia, nausea, early satiety, and dysphagia are common presenting symptoms. Surgical excision remains the only curative treatment for stomach cancer, which is relatively insensitive to radiation and chemotherapy. Patients with large primary tumors, positive surgical margins, or positive regional nodes have improved local control with adjunctive intraoperative or postoperative radiation, without improvement in overall survival. 5-FU remains the most active drug for disseminated disease, producing tumor regressions in 20% of patients for 4 to 6 months. Combination chemotherapy regimens, which produce modestly higher response rates (25% to 50%), are more commonly employed: 5-FU and cisplatin, ELF (etoposide, leucovorin, 5-FU), FAMTX (5-FU, doxorubicin, methotrexate), FAM (5-FU, doxorubicin, mitomycin), and EAP (etoposide, doxorubicin, cisplatin), among others. No regimen has been unequivocally shown to provide superior survivals, although their toxicities vary considerably. Several have also been compared with 5-FU alone, with no statistical difference in survival.

Cullinan SA, Moertel CG, Wieand HS, et al. Controlled evaluation of three drug combination regimens versus fluorouracil alone for the therapy of advanced gastric cancer. J Clin Oncol 1994;12:412–416.

Fuchs CS, Mayer RJ. Gastric carcinoma. N Engl J Med 1995;333:32–41.

Hermans J, Bonenkamp JJ, Boon MC, et al. Adjuvant therapy after curative resection for gastric cancer: meta-analysis of randomized trials. J Clin Oncol 1993;11:1441–1447.

3. **COLORECTAL CANCER.** Colorectal adenocarcinoma is the second most common cause of cancer death in the United States. Potentially curative primary surgical resection (with lymph node sampling) is feasible in 75% of newly diagnosed patients. Approximately 65% of operated patients are cured by surgery, with the remainder developing metastatic disease, most commonly to the liver. Patients with tumor limited to the muscularis (stage I) have an 80% to 90% cure rate with surgery alone, and adjuvant therapy is not indicated for this group. Patients

with tumor involvement of regional lymph nodes (stage III) have a high risk for recurrence. One year of adjuvant chemotherapy with 5-FU and levamisole in such patients has been shown to reduce the risk of relapse substantially and improve the 3.5-year survival from 55% to 71%. Data on adjuvant 5-FU and leucovorin is equally promising. Studies using 6 to 12 months of this regimen in patients with stage II and III colon cancer have shown superior relapse-free and overall survivals over surgery alone. Whether adjuvant therapy benefits stage II patients (with tumor invasion into the subserosa or invasion of adjacent organs without lymph node metastasis) is unclear, although many investigators believe that stage II patients with other poor prognostic features (e.g., aneuploidy or perforation) should be considered for adjunctive therapy. Postoperative radiation therapy may be beneficial for selected patients whose primary tumor extends to adjacent viscera, the bladder, the uterus, or the pelvic side wall.

The prognosis of patients with disseminated disease (stage IV) is related to the extent of tumor replacement within the liver as well as to elevations of carcinoembryonic antigen (CEA) and LDH. Patients with a limited number of liver or lung metastases should be considered for surgical resection, which cures 20% to 40% of such patients. 5-FU is the most active drug for disseminated colorectal cancer, providing objective tumor reduction in 20% of patients. 5-FU can be biomodulated with a variety of agents, including leucovorin (folinic acid) and methotrexate. Several randomized studies showed that biomodulation of 5-FU with leucovorin improves the response and survival compared with 5-FU alone. However, a comparison of seven different methods of 5-FU administration showed that, with the exception of 5-FU and PALA (which was an inferior regimen), the others produced statistically similar response rates and survivals. Low-dose, continuous infusion 5-FU was the best-tolerated regimen in that study. Other active drugs include mitomycin and irinotecan.

Because the morbidity and mortality in colon cancer are due to hepatic metastases and as 95% of metastases derive their blood supply from the hepatic artery, regional therapy with hepatic arterial chemotherapy or hepatic artery occlusion has been tested. In randomized comparisons with intravenous chemotherapy, intraarterial chemotherapy achieves higher response rates but thus far has not been shown definitively to confer a survival advantage over intravenous therapy. One study, however, showed that quality of life was statistically better in patients receiving intraarterial chemotherapy (Lancet 1994;344: 1255–1260).

Adenocarcinoma of the rectum occurs in approximately 40,000 people in the United States each year. The surgical and chemotherapeutic considerations for rectal cancer are similar to those for colon cancer, except that rectal cancer patients have a higher risk of local recurrence after resection (30% to 50%). Accordingly, combined postoperative chemotherapy with infusion 5-FU and radiation therapy to the pelvis are recommended for patients with rectal tumors extending through the muscularis and deeper (stages II–III). Randomized studies have shown improved local control and survival compared with patients treated with either modality alone or with no adjuvant therapy. Preoperative chemotherapy and radiation can downstage locally advanced, unresectable rectal cancers. Although abdominoperineal resection has been the standard operation for distal rectal carcinomas, there may be a role for sphincter-sparing surgery combined with adjuvant chemoradiotherapy for small tumors.

Leichman CG, Fleming TR, Muggia FM, et al. Phase II study of fluorouracil and its modulation in advanced colorectal cancer: a Southwest Oncology Group study. J Clin Oncol 1995;13:1303–1311.

Minsky BD, Cohen AM, Kemeny N, et al. Enhancement of radiation-induced downstaging of rectal cancer by fluorouracil and high-dose leucovorin chemotherapy. J Clin Oncol 1992;10:79–84.

Minsky BD, Mies C, Rich TA, et al. Potentially curative surgery of colon cancer: patterns of failure and survival. J Clin Oncol 1988;6:106–118.

Moertel CG. Chemotherapy for colorectal cancer. N Engl J Med 1994;330:1136–1142.

NIH Consensus Conference. Adjuvant therapy for patients with colon and rectal cancer. JAMA 1990;264:1444–1450.

Nordlinger B, Guiguet M, Vaillant J-C, et al. Surgical resection of colorectal carcinoma metastases to the liver. Cancer 1996;77:1254–1262.

O'Connell MJ, Martenson JA, Wieand HS, et al. Improving adjuvant therapy for rectal cancer by combining protracted-infusion fluorouracil with radiation therapy after curative surgery. N Engl J Med 1994;331:502–507.

Patt YZ. Regional hepatic arterial chemotherapy for colorectal cancer metastatic to the liver: the controversy continues. J Clin Oncol 1993;11:815–819.

Willet CG, Tepper JE, Donnelly S, et al. Patterns of failure following local excision and local excision and postoperative radiotherapy for invasive rectal adenocarcinoma. J Clin Oncol 1989;7:1003–1008.

4. **ANAL CARCINOMA.** Epidermoid and cloacogenic carcinomas are responsible for 1% to 2% of large bowel cancers (approximately 1500 cases per year in the United States) and occur with increased frequency in HIV-infected patients, homosexual males, and patients with chronic anorectal irritation due to fissures, fistulas, hemorrhoids, or condylomata. Small (<2 cm) superficial tumors below the dentate line may be locally excised, with a cure rate of 45% to 88%. In the past, larger tumors were treated with abdominoperineal (AP) resection and inguinal node dissection, which provided a long-term disease-free survival of 55%. Within the past decade, however, it has been possible to cure more than 80% of patients with chemotherapy and irradiation. During radiation therapy, two cycles of chemotherapy, consisting of IV bolus mitomycin and a 4-day infusion of 5-FU, are administered. The drugs must be given concomitantly with radiation, as sequential administration is significantly less effective. Not only does this therapy spare the sphincter and avoid a permanent colostomy, but long-term survival also appears superior to that with AP resection. Chemotherapy agents that are active in the setting of disseminated disease include 5-FU, mitomycin, cisplatin, bleomycin, methotrexate, and doxorubicin.

Cummings BJ, Keane TJ, O'Sullivan B, et al. Epidermoid anal cancer: treatment by radiation alone or by radiation and 5-fluorouracil with or without mitomycin C. Int J Radiat Oncol Biol Phys 1991;21:1115–1125.

Hussain M, Al-Sarraf M. Anal carcinomas: new combined modality treatment approaches. Oncology 1988;2:42–48.

Leichman LP, Cummings BJ. Anal carcinoma. Curr Probl Cancer 1990;14:117–159.

5. **PANCREATIC CANCER.** Pancreatic cancer affects 27,000 Americans each year and has an annual mortality rate of 10.4 per 100,000. Overall 5-year survival for all patients diagnosed with this cancer is <5%. Because of the paucity of early symptoms, less than 20% of patients with pancreatic cancer present with resectable tumors. Pancreaticoduodectomy is the treatment of choice for the minority of patients with resectable disease. Improvements in perioperative management have decreased the operative mortality from 20% to <5%. Patients with tumors found to be unresectable at surgery should have a bypass procedure (e.g., gastroenterostomy and cholecystoenterostomy) as well as chemical splanchnicectomy with a neurolytic agent (e.g., 50% alcohol or 6% phenol) for palliation of pain. Intraoperative radiation therapy allows delivery of a large single fraction of radiation locally and may improve local tumor control. Because patients with unresectable or metastatic disease often have significant debilitation, patient selection for aggressive treatment is of utmost importance. Patients who are less than ambulatory (Karnofsky performance status <50%) are often best served by supportive care alone. Concomitant radiation and 5-FU palliate and improve survival of patients with locally advanced pancreatic cancer but can produce nausea, mucositis, and diarrhea. Chemotherapy agents that have activity against disseminated disease include 5-FU, gemcitabine, mitomycin, and streptozocin. Tumor regression occurs in <25% of patients and is of short duration.

Lillemoe KD. Current management of pancreatic cancer. Ann Surg 1995;221:133–148.
Warshaw Al, Fernandez-del Castillo C. Pancreatic carcinoma. N Engl J Med 1992;326:455–465.

6. **HEPATOCELLULAR CARCINOMA.** Hepatocellular carcinoma (HCC) is relatively uncommon in the United States, although it is a common cancer in other parts of the world. It is associated with cirrhosis in 50% to 80% of patients. HCC in association with cirrhosis is typically multifocal, rarely surgically resectable, and associated with a very poor prognosis (median survival 1 to 2 months). HCC in the noncirrhotic patient typically occurs as a single dominant mass, which when resectable is associated with a 25% to 30% 5-year survival. Hepatitis B and C infection appears to be a significant cause of HCC, particularly in patients with continuing antigenemia and in those who have chronic active hepatitis. Vaccination against the hepatitis B virus in regions where it is endemic should reduce the incidence of HCC in the future. Aflatoxin, a mycotoxin from *Aspergillus* fungi, has been implicated as a factor in the etiology of primary liver cancer in parts of the world where this toxin occurs in high levels in ingested foods. In the West, 80% to 90% of cases are related to ethanol-induced cirrhosis. The biologic marker α-fetoprotein (AFP) is useful in the diagnosis of this neoplasm and has been shown to be prognostically important, with the median survival of AFP-negative patients being significantly longer than that of AFP-positive patients (J Surg Oncol 1992;49:151–155). Prognosis depends on the degree of local tumor replacement and the extent of liver functional impairment. Surgery is the treatment of choice for the small number of patients with local disease. In a series of carefully selected patients, partial hepatectomy resulted in a 5-year survival of 10% (Surg Gynecol Obstet

1989;150:208–214). Because of the high proportion of patients who experience relapse following surgery for localized hepatic cancer, adjuvant approaches have been employed using regional arterial infusion of the liver or systemic therapy with chemotherapy. There are no data thus far that support improved survival with adjuvant approaches. For selected patients with localized unresectable hepatoma (particularly the fibrolamellar variant), liver transplantation may offer a potentially curative treatment option (Ann Surg 1991;214: 221–229; Transplant 1992;53:376–382). The results overall have been disappointing because of the high rate of recurrent malignant disease following transplantation. External beam radiotherapy and chemotherapy followed by radiolabeled antiferritin antibody produces objective response in up to 50% of patients with unresectable HCC (J Clin Oncol 1985;3:1573–1582). Antiestrogen therapy with tamoxifen may also be of some value for the treatment of unresectable HCC.

Farmer DG, Rosove MH, Sheked A, et al. Current treatment modalities for hepatocellular carcinoma. Ann Surg 1994;219:236–247.
Venook AP. Treatment of hepatocellular carcinoma: too many options? J Clin Oncol 1994;12:1323–1334.

F. Gynecologic Malignancies

1. **OVARIAN CANCER.** Ovarian carcinoma is the fourth leading cause of cancer death in women, with 26,000 new cases reported and more than 14,500 deaths in the United States in 1995. The strongest risk factor for developing ovarian cancer is a family history of the disease. Women who have a first-degree family relative with a diagnosis of ovarian cancer have an approximately five-fold increase in relative risk. Hereditary (as opposed to familial) ovarian cancer accounts for <5% of cases and is associated with increased breast cancer risk and the BRCA1 and BRCA2 genes (Science 1995;270:789–791; Nat Genet 1996;13:238–240). Epithelial neoplasms constitute 90% of all ovarian cancers, with sex cord stromal tumors and germ cell tumors comprising the remaining 10%. Ovarian cancer spreads via local shedding into the peritoneal cavity followed by implantation on the peritoneum, via local invasion of bowel and bladder, or via the lymphatics. Because ovarian cancer is often asymptomatic in its early stages, most patients have widespread disease (60% stage III–IV) at the time of diagnosis. Measurement of serum CA-125 is useful in the differential diagnosis of a pelvic mass, and it is elevated in 80% to 85% of patients with serious epithelial ovarian cancer. CA-125 is also useful in monitoring the results of therapy, and its rise and fall have been correlated with the clinical course of the disease.

   a. **Primary surgery.** In the absence of extraabdominal metastatic disease, definitive staging of ovarian cancer requires laparotomy. If disease appears to be limited to the ovaries or pelvis, it is essential at laparotomy to examine and biopsy the diaphragm, both paracolic gutters, the pelvic peritoneum, and periaortic and pelvic lymph nodes and to take cytologic washings of the entire peritoneal cavity. In addition, invasion of the bowel and bladder needs to be evaluated. Surgery alone (total abdominal hysterectomy, bilateral salpingo-oophorectomy, and omentectomy) is adequate treatment for well or moderately well differentiated stage IA and IB disease, and these patients have a 5-year survival of > 90%. In selected patients who have early stage, low-grade tumors who desire future childbearing, unilateral salpingo-oophorectomy may be considered. For higher grades and stages, addition of postoperative chemotherapy or radiation therapy can improve overall survival. For more advanced disease, the tumor is debulked to nodules <2 cm residual. There is considerable evidence that the volume of disease left at the completion of the primary surgical procedure is related to patient survival. Cytoreductive surgery is recommended to optimally treat all patients with ovarian carcinoma. Approximately 60% to 75% of tumors at the time of diagnosis can be satisfactorily debulked. This may require resection of large tumor masses and partial bowel resections, in addition to bilateral salpingo-oophorectomy, total abdominal hysterectomy, and omentectomy. The response rate to chemotherapy, the odds of a pathologically negative second-look operation, and eventual cure are directly related not only to optimal debulking but also to tumor stage and grade. The role of surgery in patients with extraabdominal disease remains to be established.

b. **Primary chemotherapy.** Ovarian cancer is highly chemosensitive, and the overall response rate for patients with advanced disease is 60% to 80%. Dose intensity is an important factor in achieving optimal results with chemotherapy in ovarian cancer. Cisplatin and carboplatin are the most active chemotherapeutic agents. Combination regimens based on cisplatin or carboplatin and cyclophosphamide given for six cycles produce overall objective response rates of 90%, with clinical and pathologic complete responses in the range of 40% to 60% and 25% to 30%, respectively. Recent studies have confirmed that carboplatin and cisplatin when combined with cyclophosphamide have comparable efficacy, but carboplatin has a more favorable therapeutic index (J Clin Oncol 1992;10:706–717; J Clin Oncol 1992;10:718–726). Therefore, carboplatin can be considered the drug of choice for primary therapy if the patient does not have decreased marrow reserve. The combination of cisplatin/taxol produced improved clinical response and median survival when compared with cisplatin/cyclophosphamide in suboptimally debulked stage III and IV patients (N Engl J Med 1996;334:1–6). Paclitaxel produces objective responses when used either as primary therapy or for recurrent disease, with response rates ranging from 21% to 48%. Retrospective studies have shown that complete response to chemotherapy depends on the volume of disease at the time of chemotherapy initiation. Patients with any residual mass larger than 2 cm in diameter postsurgery have a 10% likelihood of achieving a complete remission with chemotherapy. The objective response rates of advanced ovarian carcinoma to single alkylating agents (melphalan, chlorambucil, or cyclophosphamide) range from 15% to 65%. The vast majority of these responses are partial remissions, and the 2-year disease-free survival rate is less than 10%.

c. **Radiation therapy.** Radiation has not been used routinely in the United States as the primary therapy for patients with small-volume residual ovarian cancer, even though clinical trials have shown that whole abdominal radiation therapy is effective in such patients. Whole abdominal radiation, using either an open-field or moving-strip technique, can be delivered in doses of 3000 to 5500 cGy to the upper abdomen and pelvis, respectively. Whole abdominal radiation therapy is rarely curative in any patient with macroscopic residual disease. The complications include radiation enteritis and hepatic and renal damage. Intraperitoneal phosphorus-32 radiotherapy is less frequently used (only if residual tumor is <1 mm) and is associated with a significant number of late bowel complications.

d. **Second-look surgery.** The value of secondary cytoreductive surgery (a second-look operation) in patients with persistent or recurrent disease after chemotherapy is controversial. A postchemotherapy laparotomy is often performed because noninvasive studies have a high false-negative rate and approximately one half of the patients in clinical complete remission have disease documented at exploratory laparotomy. It is suggested that patients who have residual disease at second-look surgery may benefit from additional chemotherapy. A negative second-look laparotomy has limited prognostic value, however, as disease recurs in approximately one third of all patients with surgically confirmed complete remissions at laparotomy.

e. **Salvage therapy.** Chemotherapy is the primary form of therapy for ovarian cancer patients whose disease recurs after an initial response. If the interval between completion of chemotherapy and the development of recurrent disease is lengthy (i.e., a minimum of 5 to 12 months), patients may respond to repeat treatment with cisplatin or carboplatin, with a 25% to 56% response rate in combination with ifosfamide (J Clin Oncol 1991;9:389–393). For patients with platinum-refractory disease, treatment with paclitaxel should be considered. In addition, several other chemotherapeutic agents have demonstrated activity in platinum-refractory ovarian cancer, including ifosfamide (20% overall response rate), hexamethylmelamine (12% to 14% response rate), tamoxifen (20% response rate), 5-FU and leucovorin (10% to 17% response rate), and etoposide (6% to 26% response rate). Some reports suggest a potential role for intraperitoneal therapy in treating advanced ovarian carcinoma. Instillation of drugs, such as 5-FU, methotrexate, melphalan, doxorubicin, cytosine arabinoside, cisplatin, and IFN-α (Semin Oncol 1991;18:248–254), through a Tenckhoff catheter or Portacath implanted into the peritoneal cavity achieves local drug concentrations in the peritoneal fluid 10-fold to 1000-fold higher than the concentrations achieved with IV therapy. Surgically defined complete response occurs in about 30% of patients who have low volume disease (no nodule >0.5 cm) at the start of intraperitoneal therapy. Another experimental treatment modality includes high-dose chemotherapy with autologous stem cell transplantation.

f. Palliation. Intestinal obstruction is the inevitable outcome for most women who have persistent ovarian cancer. Surgical intervention can improve the quality of life with some type of palliative operation in 85% of obstructed patients, with a morbidity of 30% to 40% and a mortality of 12% to 16%. Palliation is rarely achieved when there are multiple areas of partial or complete obstruction, when the transit time is prolonged due to diffuse peritoneal carcinomatosis, or when anatomy requires a bypass that results in short bowel syndrome.

Advanced Ovarian Cancer Trialists Group. Chemotherapy in advanced ovarian carcinoma: an overview of randomized clinical trials. Br Med J 1991;303:884–893.

Cannistra SA. Cancer of the ovary. N Engl J Med 1993;329:1550–1559.

Claus EB, Schildkraut JM, Thompson WD, et al. The genetic attributable risk of breast and ovarian cancer. Cancer 1996;77:2318–2324.

Hoskins WJ, Bundy BN, Thigpan JT, et al. The influence of cytoreductive surgery on recurrence-free interval and survival in small-volume stage III epithelial ovarian cancer: a Gynecologic Oncology Group study. Gynecol Oncol 1992;47:159–166.

Neijt JP, ten Bokkel Huinink WW, van der Burg ME, et al. Long-term survival in ovarian cancer: mature data from the Netherlands Joint Study Group for ovarian cancer. Eur J Cancer 1991;27:1367–1372.

Redman JR, Petroni GE, Saigo PE, et al. Prognostic factors in advanced ovarian carcinoma. J Clin Oncol 1986;4:515–523.

2. ENDOMETRIAL CANCER. Cancer of the endometrium is the most common gynecologic malignancy in the United States and accounts for 13% of all cancers in women. It is a highly curable tumor. Only 7% of patients with endometrial cancer die from it, primarily because it is usually diagnosed early as a result of postmenopausal uterine bleeding. Endometrial carcinoma can develop in association with prolonged, unopposed estrogen exposure. An increased incidence of endometrial cancer has also been found in association with tamoxifen treatment of breast cancer. The pattern of spread of endometrial cancer is partially dependent on the degree of cellular differentiation. Well-differentiated tumors tend to limit their spread to the surface of the endometrium, and myometrial extension is uncommon. Myometrial invasion in poorly differentiated tumors is frequently associated with lymph node involvement and distant metastases. A hysterectomy is required in staging endometrial cancer to determine the degree of myometrial invasion. Patients with endometrial cancer who have localized disease usually can be cured by hysterectomy and bilateral salpingo-oophorectomy. Periaortic and selective pelvic node sampling are added if the tumor is poorly differentiated, involves the lower third of the corpus or the cervix, has vascular space or extensive myometrial space invasion, or has positive peritoneal cytology. Adjuvant radiation therapy is added when deep invasion of the myometrium is found, for positive lymph nodes, or with high-grade tumors. If disease is known to be advanced before surgery, preoperative intracavitary and external-beam radiation therapy followed by surgery may be indicated. Radiation may also be an effective palliative therapy in unresectable disease. Some patients have regional and distant metastases that, although occasionally responsive to standard hormone therapy, are rarely curable. Progestational agents (medroxyprogesterone, hydroxyprogesterone, megestrol) produce good antitumor responses in 15% to 30% of metastatic patients

(Semin Oncol 1994;21:100–106) and are being evaluated in the adjuvant setting. Responses to hormones are correlated with the presence and level of hormone receptors, with up to 75% of advanced patients with detectable progesterone receptors responding to progestins, compared with 7% without detectable progesterone receptors (Acta Oncol 1989;28:561–566). Tamoxifen will give a response rate of 20% in those who do not respond to standard progesterone therapy (Gynecol Oncol 1989;32:1–3). There is no standard chemotherapy regimen for patients with metastatic uterine cancer, although doxorubicin has activity in up to one third of patients, and platinum compounds are also active.

Moore TD, Phillips PH, Nerenstone SR, et al. Systemic treatment of advanced and recurrent endometrial carcinoma: current status and future directions. J Clin Oncol 1991;9:1071–1088.
Nori D, Hilaris BS, Tome M, et al. Combined surgery and radiation in endometrial carcinoma: an analysis of prognostic factors. Int J Radiat Oncol Biol Phys 1987;13:489–497.

3. CERVICAL CANCER. Cervical cancer accounts for 6% of all malignancies in women, with an estimated 16,000 new cases of invasive cancer of the cervix and 5000 deaths in the United States each year. In the past four decades, the incidence and mortality of invasive cervical cancer have declined in the United States by 75% as a result of early detection through the use of the Papanicolau (Pap) test. The Pap test allows detection of the disease at a preinvasive stage, and approximately 65,000 cases of cervical carcinoma in situ are found this way annually. Epidemiologic studies convincingly demonstrate that the major risk factor for the development of preinvasive or invasive carcinoma of the cervix is human papillomavirus (HPV) infection. HPV DNA typing may aid in identifying the HPV types (16, 18, 45, or 56) that are most strongly associated with premalignant squamous lesions of the cervix (Obstet Gynecol 1992;79:328–337). An increased risk of cervical carcinoma also results from immunosuppression. Human immunodeficiency virus (HIV)-infected women have more aggressive and advanced disease and a poorer prognosis (Cancer 1993;71:402–406).

Precursor lesions to invasive cervical cancer include cervical dysplasia and the in situ cervical intraepithelial neoplasia (CIN). Longitudinal studies have shown that in untreated patients with in situ cervical cancer, 30% to 70% will develop invasive cancer over 10 to 12 years. Methods to treat noninvasive ectocervical lesions include laser therapy, cold-knife conization, cryotherapy, and the loop electrosurgical excision procedure (LEEP). Total abdominal or vaginal hysterectomy is an accepted therapy for the postreproductive age group. For medically inoperable patients, a single intracavitary insertion with tandem and ovoids for 5000 milligram hours (8000 cGy vaginal surface dose) may be used. Properly treated, tumor control of noninvasive, in situ disease should be nearly 100%.

For early stage invasive disease, surgery (from cervical conization to radical hysterectomy and bilateral pelvic lymph node dissection, depending on the extent of disease) and radiation therapy are equally effective and can result in cure rates of 85% to 95%. Surgery may be preferable in younger patients to preserve ovarian function and avoid vaginal atrophy and stenosis. The presence of paraaortic and pelvic lymph node metastases results in lower survival rates, with 5-year survival rates of 92% for patients with negative lymph node involvement, 49% for those with involved pelvic nodes, and 10% for those with involved paraaortic nodes. Postoperative total pelvic radiation is recommended to decrease pelvic recurrence in patients with deep stromal invasion, lymphatic space involvement, large tumor size, and three or more positive nodes. For patients with obvious parametrial involvement, extension to the lower third of the vagina, or extension to the pelvic wall, the treatment option of choice is external-beam radiation with two or more intracavitary applications. The addition of hydroxyurea (80 mg/kg twice weekly during radiation) as a radiosensitizer may improve survival in this group (Am J Obstet Gynecol 1988;159:87–94). Clinical trials of adjuvant therapy, including combined radiation and chemotherapy (sequential or concurrent), neoadjuvant chemotherapy, altered radiation fractionation, and brachytherapy, are ongoing.

In metastatic cervical carcinoma, cisplatin has a 15% to 25% response rate (J Clin Oncol 1987;5:1791–1795), and ifosfamide has a 31% response rate (Cancer Chemother Pharmacol 1986;18:280–283). It has been reported that locally advanced squamous cell carcinoma of the cervix responded to therapy with 13-*cis*-retinoic acid and human IFN-α with a 50% response rate and 12% complete response rate (J Natl Cancer Inst 1992;84:241–245). A small, highly selected group of patients with locally recurrent disease may benefit from pelvic exenteration (Obstet Gynecol 1989;73:1027–1034).

Coia L, Won M, Lanciano R, et al. The Patterns of Care Outcome Study for cancer of the uterine cervix. Results of the Second National Practice Survey. Cancer 1990;66:2451–2456.
Dembo AJ, Balogh JM. Advances in radiotherapy in the gynecologic malignancies. Semin Surg Oncol 1990;6:323–327.
Lanciano RM, Wom M, Hanks GE. A reappraisal of the International Federation of Gynecology and Obstetrics staging system for cervical cancer: a study of patterns of care. Cancer 1992;69:482–487.

G. Genitourinary Malignancies

1. **RENAL CELL CARCINOMA.** Approximately 29,000 new cases of renal cell carcinoma were diagnosed in 1995 in the United States. Of renal cell cancers, 85% are adenocarcinomas, and these are divided into clear cell, granular, and sarcomatoid cell types. A unique aspect of renal cell carcinoma is the frequent occurrence of various paraneoplastic syndromes, including hypercalcemia, polycythemia, fever, cachexia, hypertension, and hepatic dysfunction. Renal cell carcinoma often can be cured if it is diagnosed and treated when still localized to the kidney and to the immediately surrounding tissue. Even when regional lymphatics or blood vessels are involved with tumor, a significant number of patients can achieve prolonged survival. Approximately 40% of patients diagnosed with renal cell carcinoma survive 5 years. Surgical treatment is the accepted, often curative therapy for early stages of this disease. Resection may be simple, radical (including removal of the kidney, adrenal gland, perirenal fat, and Gerota's fascia), or, in some selected cases, a partial nephrectomy. Lymphadenectomy is commonly

employed, but its effectiveness has not been definitively proved (Urology 1993;41:9–15). When present, intracaval tumor thrombi are resected during the operation. External-beam radiation has been given before or after nephrectomy without conclusive evidence that it improves survival compared with surgery alone, but it may be of benefit in patients with more extensive tumors. In patients who are not candidates for surgery, external-beam radiation therapy (Semin Surg Oncol 1988;4:100–102) or arterial embolization (Semin Surg Oncol 1988;4:124–128) can provide palliation. When distant metastases are present, disease-free survival is poor. Selected patients with solitary or limited numbers of metastases can achieve prolonged survival with surgical resection of the metastases (J Urol 1986;136:805–807). Systemic therapy has demonstrated only limited effectiveness, and responses to cytotoxic chemotherapy do not exceed 10% for any regimen (Semin Urol 1989;7:199–206). Renal cell carcinoma universally expresses p-glycoprotein, the protein associated with the multidrug-resistance (MDR) phenotype. Progestational agents (e.g., medroxyprogesterone) have been used in patients with renal cell carcinoma, but the frequency of response is low (J Urol 1987;138:1379–1381). Various biologic therapies, including intermediate doses of IFN-α (3–6 million U three times weekly) and IL-2 (with lymphokine-activated killer [LAK] cells in some trials), have been studied and may have response rates as high as 15% to 20% in appropriately selected patients (Semin Oncol 1988;15:30–34). Renal cell carcinoma is one of the few cancers in which well-documented cases of spontaneous tumor regression in the absence of therapy exist, but this occurs rarely.

Belldegrun A, Abi-Aad AS, Figlin RA, et al. Renal cell carcinoma: basic biology and current approaches to therapy. Semin Oncol 1991;18:96–101.

deKernion JB, Berry D. The diagnosis and treatment of renal cell carcinoma. Cancer 1980;45:1947–1956.

Sene AP, Hunt L, McMahon RF, et al. Renal carcinoma in patients undergoing nephrectomy: analysis of survival and prognostic factors. Br J Urol 1992;70:125–134.

Thrasher JB, Robertson JE, Paulson DF. Expanding indications for conservative renal surgery in renal cell carcinoma. Urology 1994;43:160–168.

2. **BLADDER CANCER.** Approximately 50,000 people in the United States develop bladder cancer each year. More than 90% of bladder carcinomas are transitional cell carcinomas derived from the uroepithelium. Clinical staging is determined by the depth of invasion of the bladder wall by tumor. Approximately 80% of patients with bladder cancer have disease involving the mucosa (including carcinoma in situ) or the submucosa. These patients are often curable, although the tendency for new tumor formation is up to 80% over 20 years, and progression to muscle-invasive disease occurs in 10% to 20% (J Urol 1995;153:1823–1827). Endoscopic transurethral resection (TUR) is the most common and conservative form of management. Intravesical chemotherapy with thiotepa, mitomycin, doxorubicin, or BCG is most often used in patients with multiple or recurrent tumors or as a prophylactic measure in high-risk patients after TUR. Intravesical IFN-α has also shown activity against superficial bladder cancer as both a primary and secondary treatment after failure of other agents (J Clin Oncol 1988;6:476–483).

Only 20% of patients with bladder cancer have disease invading bladder wall muscle. More aggressive forms of treatment are often required for more advanced stages of bladder cancer. Radical cystectomy with or without preoperative radiation, or external-beam radiation alone in nonsurgical candidates, may be employed. A partial cystectomy may be indicated in the few patients with small, solitary primary tumors located well away from the trigone and the bladder neck. Radical cystectomy includes removal of the bladder, perivesical tissues, prostate, and seminal vesicles in men and bladder, uterus, fallopian tubes, ovaries, anterior vaginal wall, and urethra in women and may or may not be accompanied by a pelvic lymph node dissection. Reconstructive techniques that fashion low-pressure storage reservoirs from the reconfigured small and large bowel eliminate the need for external drainage devices and, in some male patients, allow voiding per urethra (J Urol 1993;150:40–45). Multiple protocols are evaluating the potential of adjuvant chemotherapy administered before cystectomy, after cystectomy, or in conjunction with external-beam radiotherapy to improve local control, prevent distant metastases, or allow preservation of the bladder. The combination regimen M-VAC (methotrexate, vinblastine, doxorubicin, and cisplatin) produces a complete response in approximately 20% of patients treated before definitive surgery (Br J Urol 1989;64:250–256).

Currently, cure is not possible for the majority of patients with regional or distant metastases. Those with involvement of pelvic organs by direct extension or small volume metastases to pelvic lymph nodes can sometimes be cured by surgery, radiation, or a combination of modalities that include chemotherapy. The focus of care for many stage IV patients is on palliation of symptoms from a bladder tumor that is often massive. Urinary diversion may be indicated not only for palliation of urinary symptoms but also for preservation of renal function in candidates for chemotherapy. Recent combination chemotherapy regimens that include cisplatin, methotrexate, and vinblastine, with or without doxorubicin (CMV or M-VAC), are encouraging and have induced some pathologic complete responses in advanced patients (Cancer 1989;64:2448–2458). Gallium nitrate has shown some activity in patients who have recurrences following cisplatin-based chemotherapy (Semin Oncol 1991;18:585–595).

Hudson MA, Herr HW. Carcinoma in situ of the bladder. J Urol 1995;153:564–572.
Raghavan D, Huben R. Management of bladder cancer. Curr Probl Cancer 1995;119:1–64.
Richie JP. Surgery for invasive bladder cancer. Hematol Oncol Clin North Am 1992;6:129–145.
Skinner DG, Daniels JR, Russell CA, et al. The role of adjuvant chemotherapy following cystectomy for invasive bladder cancer: a prospective comparative trial. J Urol 1991;145:459–467.
Thrasher JB, Crawford ED. Current management of invasive and metastatic transitional cell carcinoma of the bladder. J Urol 1993;149:957–972.

3. **TESTICULAR CANCER.** Cancer of the testis affects 7000 males in the United States each year and accounts for 1% of malignancies in men. It is a highly treatable, often curable cancer that usually develops in young and middle-aged men. Of testicular tumors, 93% are of germ cell origin. Testicular cancers frequently occur at an early stage, are very sensitive

to chemotherapy, and are variably sensitive to radiotherapy. Optimal management depends on the histology and stage. Testicular carcinoma is broadly divided into seminoma and nonseminoma types for treatment planning, with seminomas being more sensitive to radiation therapy. Approximately 90% of nonseminomatous testicular cancers have an elevation of at least one tumor marker (α-fetoprotein [AFP] or the beta subunit of human chorionic gonadotropin [β-hCG]) at presentation. Persistent elevations after therapy indicate residual tumor. Elevation of β-hCG is found in approximately 10% of patients with pure seminoma, but seminomas do not secrete AFP. LDH, although not as specific, may occasionally be the only elevated serum marker and can, therefore, have clinical use. Tumors that have a mixture of both seminoma and nonseminoma components and tumors with a seminoma pathology but with elevated serum levels of AFP should be managed as nonseminoma. Transscrotal biopsy is always contraindicated when diagnostically evaluating a testicular mass because of the risk of local dissemination of tumor into the scrotum and the risk of inguinal lymph node involvement. Radical inguinal orchiectomy with initial high ligation of the spermatic cord is the procedure of choice.

a. **Nonseminomatous germ cell tumors.** The nonseminomatous tumors are a heterogeneous group that includes choriocarcinoma, teratoma, embryonal carcinoma, and yolk sac carcinoma. The majority of nonseminomas have more than one cell type, and the relative proportions of each cell type are specified. The natural history of nonseminomatous germ cell tumors tends to be less indolent and less predictable than that of seminomas, with a greater likelihood of dissemination via the blood to distant sites, sometimes bypassing the retroperitoneal lymph nodes. Risk of metastases is lowest for teratoma and highest for choriocarcinoma. It is important to note that even patients with widespread metastases at presentation, including those with brain metastases, may still be curable and should be treated with this intent. Evaluation of the retroperitoneal lymph nodes is an important part of treatment planning in adults with testicular cancer. Patients with negative scanning results have a 25% to 30% chance of having microscopic involvement of the lymph nodes. Patients with tumors localized to the testis have traditionally been treated by inguinal orchiectomy followed by (in adults) retroperitoneal lymph node dissection (RLND), with surgical cure rates of 80% to 90%. Recently, the necessity of lymphadenectomy with its risk of infertility has been questioned, and many experts advise orchiectomy alone followed by close observation with monthly serum markers, chest x-rays every 1 to 2 months, and CT scans of the chest and abdomen every 2 to 3 months for 2 years (Semin Oncol 1988;13:321–323; J Clin Oncol 1990; 8:4–8). Cisplatin-based chemotherapy is used to salvage the 25% to 30% of patients who have relapse during surveillance, and 90% to 100% of them are cured.

Patients with involvement of retroperitoneal lymph nodes are treated with inguinal orchiectomy and RLND with or without the addition of chemotherapy. Studies have demonstrated that adjuvant cisplatin-based chemotherapy can prevent a relapse in > 95% of stage II nonseminoma patients (N Engl J Med 1987;317:1433–1438). In patients with less than six positive lymph nodes at RLND, none of which are greater than 2 cm in diameter, and no evidence of extracapsular lymph node extension, the relapse rate without chemotherapy is only 10%, and most are curable with standard chemotherapy if they do relapse (J Clin Oncol 1991;9:1393–1396). Therefore, the option of surgery and careful follow-up, reserving chemotherapy for relapse, is reasonable in this subset. Patients whose tumor markers do not return to normal after RLND should be treated with chemotherapy. Three courses of BEP (bleomycin, etoposide, cisplatin) appear to be equivalent to four courses in patients with minimal or moderate extent of disease (J Clin Oncol 1989;7:387–391). Four courses of EP (etoposide, cisplatin) or PVB (cisplatin, vinblastine, bleomycin) produce similar survival outcomes (J Clin Oncol 1995;13:470–476; J Clin Oncol 1993;11:1300–1305). The BEP regimen appears to produce less neuromuscular toxicity and was more effective in patients with more advanced disease when compared directly with PVB (N Engl J Med 1987;316:1435–1440). For patients in whom presurgical staging reveals extensive retroperitoneal masses that are unresectable (generally >5 cm), radical inguinal orchiectomy followed by chemotherapy with delayed surgery for removal of residual retroperitoneal disease should be considered.

Germ cell tumors are unusual among solid tumors because cure is still possible after relapse or even after failure to achieve a complete remission with initial therapy. Durable complete remissions can be obtained in more than 70% of patients with disseminated disease with cisplatin-based chemotherapy regimens. In selected cases, surgery should be used after chemotherapy to remove residual masses to determine if viable tumor cells remain, since such a finding is an indication for further chemotherapy. Resection of these masses reveals necrosis and fibrosis in 40% of cases, adult teratoma in 40%, and residual nonseminomatous testicular cancer in 20%. Patients having necrosis or teratoma are usually cured with surgery alone, but those with remaining cancer should receive two additional cycles of chemotherapy. Patients who have brain metastases should be treated with chemotherapy and simultaneous whole brain radiation. Patients with refractory disease are treated with regimens containing ifosfamide, vinblastine, etoposide, cisplatin, or carboplatin. Salvage regimens can produce long-term complete responses in 20% to 45% of patients with disease that has persisted or recurred following other cisplatin-based regimens (Cancer 1990;66:2476–2481). High-dose chemotherapy with autologous stem cell transplantation has been used with some success in the setting of refractory disease (J Natl Cancer Inst 1993;85:1828–1835). One study suggested that maintenance daily oral etoposide may benefit patients who achieve a complete remission after salvage therapy (J Clin Oncol 1995;13:1167–1169). Overall, 95% to 100% of stage I–II and 80% of stage III nonseminomatous testicular cancers are cured with modern therapy.

b. **Seminomas.** Pure seminomas account for 30% to 40% of testicular germ cell tumors and are extremely sensitive to chemotherapy and radiation. The metastatic potential is low, and most patients present with early stage disease. Stage I–II seminomas are treated with radical inguinal orchiectomy and radiation to the retroperitoneum and ipsilateral inguinal lymph nodes, with cure rates of 97% in stage I and more than 80% in stage II. Because salvage treatment is so successful in seminoma and most early stage patients (up to 85%) are cured with orchiectomy alone, close surveillance is being reported as a viable option to radiation following orchiectomy to reduce short-term and long-term toxicity. For patients with bulky tumor masses, recurrence rates are high after surgery plus radiation, and therefore adjuvant chemotherapy with a cisplatin-based regimen should be considered to reduce recurrences (J Clin Oncol 1988;6:1856–1862). Chemotherapy is given with EP, BEP, or PVB combination regimens as described for nonseminomatous tumors. Disseminated seminoma is treated with cisplatin-based chemotherapy, with cure rates of 83% (Ann Intern Med 1988;108:513–518).

Einhorn LH. Complicated problems in testicular cancer. Semin Oncol 1988;15:9–15.

Fung CY, Garnick MB. Clinical stage I carcinoma of the testis: a review. J Clin Oncol 1988;6:734–750.

Mead GM, Stenning SP, Parkinson MC, et al. The second Medical Research Council study of prognostic factors in nonseminomatous germ cell tumors. J Clin Oncol 1992;10:85–94.

Motzer RJ, Bosl GJ. High-dose chemotherapy for resistant germ cell tumors: recent advances and future directions. J Natl Cancer Inst 1992;84:1703–1709.

Ozols RF, Ihde DC, Linehan WM, Young RC. Management of high risk patients with advanced testis cancer: National Cancer Institute Approach. Semin Oncol 1988;15:335–338.

Williams SD, Loehrer PJ, Nichols CR, et al. Disseminated testicular cancer: current chemotherapy strategies. Semin Oncol 1989;16:105–109.

4. **PROSTATE CANCER.** Carcinoma of the prostate is the most common cancer and the second most common cause of cancer death in men in the United States, with over 240,000 diagnoses and 40,000 deaths in 1995. Prostate cancer is predominantly a disease of older men, which frequently responds to treatment when widespread and may be cured when localized. The issue of screening asymptomatic men for prostate cancer with digital rectal examination, prostate-specific antigen (PSA), or ultrasound is controversial (JAMA 1994;272:773–780). A high false positive rate (and associated morbidity of workup), identification of tumors that do not threaten the patient's health or normal life expectancy, the high rate of metastatic disease in tumors detected by PSA screening alone, and the considerable cost are arguments against the widespread adoption of mass screening. Presenting complaints of prostate cancer include symptoms of urethral obstruction, hematuria, urinary tract infection, and bone pain. Ten percent of patients have localized tumors discovered incidentally after transurethral prostatectomy (stage A), 15% to 20% have palpable nodules (stage B), 40% have regional extension to periprostatic tissues (stage C), and 30% to 35% have metastases to lymph nodes (stage D1) or distant sites (stage D2).

Degree of tumor differentiation correlates with likelihood of metastases and death. Because of marked variability in tumor differentiation from one microscopic field to another, pathologists report the range of differentiation among the malignant cells present in the biopsy (Gleason's grade). The rate of tumor growth varies from very slow to moderately rapid, with some patients living 5 years or more even after cancer has metastasized to distant sites, particularly to bone. Since the median age at diagnosis is 72 years, many patients, especially those with localized tumor, may die of other illnesses without suffering significant disability from their cancer. Although under debate as a screening tool, PSA is a valuable organ-specific tumor marker with good sensitivity and high specificity for prostate tissue that is helpful in following response to therapy. After radical prostatectomy or radiation therapy, detectable PSA levels indicate local treatment failure or metastatic disease (J Clin Oncol 1992;10:1208–1217; Radiother Oncol 1992;23:236–240). Serum acid phosphatase is less specific than PSA in prostate cancer but can be a useful marker in following disease course.

a. **Localized tumors.** When cancer is confined to the prostate gland, the disease is frequently curable, and median survival in excess of 5 years can be anticipated. Well-differentiated, focal, asymptomatic tumors discovered incidentally after transurethral resection of the prostate (TURP) may be followed with observation alone, as only 2% will progress within 4 years. Patients with more extensive or poorly differentiated adenocarcinoma discovered at TURP or with palpable prostatic nodules may be treated with either radical prostatectomy, interstitial radiation, or external-beam radiation therapy, with comparable 10-year survival rates of 55% to 75%. Surgery is usually reserved for patients in good health who are under the age of 70. Prostatectomy can be performed by a perineal or retropubic approach. Complications of radical prostatectomy can include urinary incontinence, urethral stricture, and impotence. Newer nerve-sparing operations now preserve potency in up to 30% to 70% of men (J Urol 1993;150:905–907). Whether to subject all patients to a pelvic lymph node dissection is debatable (Br J Urol 1993;72:484–488). Pelvic lymph node dissection is not therapeutic but spares the patient with positive nodes the morbidity of prostatectomy or radiation, since radical prostatectomy is usually not performed if frozen section evaluation of pelvic nodes reveals metastases. In patients in whom the PSA is under 20 and the Gleason sum is low, a pelvic lymph node dissection is probably unnecessary. Laparoscopic pelvic lymph node dissection may accurately assess lymph node status while shortening the hospital stay and decreasing morbidity (J Urol 1993;150:898–901). Candidates for definitive radiotherapy must have a confirmed pathologic diagnosis of cancer that is clinically confined to the prostate or surrounding tissues or both. Impotence rates after radiation are low, with urinary incontinence rates of 5% to 10%. Interstitial implantation of radioisotopes, usually performed with pelvic lymphadenectomy, is under clinical investigation (J Clin Oncol 1996;14:304–315). Asymptomatic patients of advanced age or with concomitant illness may warrant careful observation without immediate active treatment. One population-based study with 15 years of follow-up has shown excellent survival without any treatment in patients with well or moderately well differentiated tumors clinically confined to the prostate (J Urol 1994;152:1753–1756).

b. **Regional disease.** Patients with locally advanced cancer are not usually curable, although median survival may be as long as 5 years. Patients with extracapsular extension of tumor to the seminal vesicles or regional lymph nodes are best treated with external-beam radiation therapy using a linear accelerator (Int J Radiat Oncol Biol Phys 1993;26:197–201). Definitive radiation therapy should be delayed until 4 to 6 weeks after TURP to reduce the incidence of urethral stricture. The 10-year survival with conventional radiotherapy techniques is 30% to 40% for stage C and 10% to 20% for stage D1. Trials have reported improved local control and survival with mixed-beam (neutron/photon) radiotherapy, compared with standard photon therapy (Am J Clin Oncol 1993;16:164–167). Fast neutron therapy also showed improved locoregional control compared with photon therapy, although no difference in overall survival was seen (Int J Radiat Oncol Biol Phys 1993;28:47–54). Control of urinary symptoms is an important consideration in treatment. This may often be accomplished by radiation therapy, radical surgery, TURP, or hormonal manipulation.

c. **Metastatic disease.** If prostate cancer has spread to distant organs, cure is rarely, if ever, possible. Median survival is usually 1 to 3 years, although indolent clinical courses lasting many years may be observed. The most common site of distant tumor spread in prostate cancer is the bone. Eighty-five percent of patients with disseminated prostate cancer experience tumor regression following a hormonal manipulation with bilateral orchiectomy, estrogens, androgen receptor antagonists, ketoconazole, aminoglutethimide, or luteinizing hormone-releasing hormone (LHRH) agonists. Responses to hormonal manipulation are rapid and effective for a median of 12 to 18 months. All treatments result in impotence; therefore, choice of therapy is dictated by other side effects. Benefits of bilateral orchiectomy include ease of the procedure, compliance, immediacy in lowering testosterone levels, and low cost. Disadvantages include psychologic effects, loss of libido, impotence, and hot flashes. The addition of an androgen receptor antagonist, such as flutamide or nilutamide, to surgical castration may produce superior objective response rates, bone pain relief, and freedom from progression, but it has not been shown to improve survival (Lancet 1995;346:265–269). Ketoconazole is an antifungal drug that in sufficiently high doses inhibits testicular and adrenal production of androgens. Doses of 400 mg tid can bring about a rapid symptomatic response. Administration of diethylstilbestrol (DES) at a dose of 3 mg/d will achieve castration levels of testosterone through inhibition of LHRH via a negative feedback loop. However, estrogen is seldom used today because of the risk of serious side effects, including myocardial infarction, cerebrovascular accident, and pulmonary embolism. LHRH agonists, such as leuprolide (Lupron), goserelin (Zoladex), and buserelin, will lower testosterone to castration levels (Semin Oncol 1988;15:366–370). Depot formulations now allow these agents to be given by injection every 1 to 3 months. The addition of androgen receptor antagonists to LHRH agonists can prevent tumor flare reactions at initiation of treatment and has been shown in some studies to improve progression-free survival (16.5 versus 13.9 months) and overall survival (35.6 versus 28.3 months) compared with leuprolide alone (N Engl J Med 1989;321:419–424).

In patients with progressive disease after an initial response to hormones, second-line hormone therapy is rarely effective. However, studies suggest that withdrawal of flutamide may induce a clinical response in some patients (J Clin Oncol 1993;11:1566–1572). Hormone-refractory patients are candidates for chemotherapy with cyclophosphamide, doxorubicin, methotrexate, cisplatin, 5-FU, or combinations of agents. Unfortunately, neither response rates nor duration of response have been convincingly improved with combination chemotherapy. One of the most active agents in prostate cancer is doxorubicin (J Urol 1984;132:1099–1102). More recent studies have investigated the drugs estramustine, vinblastine, and etoposide, which have been shown in small studies to produce response rates of 35% to 50% (J Clin Oncol 1992;10:1754–1761; J Clin Oncol 1994;12:2005–2012). Very rapid progression, particularly in patients with large local disease or hepatic metastases, should suggest differentiation into a small cell variant. This variant behaves like small cell lung cancer, and chemotherapy regimens, such as cisplatin and etoposide, can produce objective responses (J Urol 1992;147:935–937).

Painful bone metastases can be a major problem in prostate cancer, and palliative radiotherapy for bone pain can be very useful. Many strategies for palliation have been studied, including corticosteroids (J Clin Oncol 1989;7:590–597), bone-seeking radionuclides, such as strontium-89 (Cancer 1993;72:3433–3435), gallium nitrate, and bisphosphonates. Suramin, a synthetic polyanionic antiparasitic agent, has been shown to achieve significant palliation in patients with painful bony metastases unresponsive to other manipulations (Urol Clin North Am 1991;18:123–129).

Andriole GL. Serum prostate-specific antigen: the most useful tumor marker. J Clin Oncol 1992;10:1205–1207.

Austenfeld MS, Thompson IM, Middleton RG, et al. Meta-analysis of the literature: guideline development for prostate cancer treatment. J Urol 1994;152:1866–1869.

Chodak GW, Thisted RA, Gerber GS, et al. Results of conservative management of clinically localized prostate cancer. N Engl J Med 1994;330:242–248.

Duncan W, Warde P, Catton CN, et al. Carcinoma of the prostate: results of radical radiotherapy. Int J Radiat Oncol Biol Phys 1993;26:203–210.

Eisenberger MA. Chemotherapy for prostate cancer. J Natl Cancer Inst Monograph 1988;7: 151–163.

Garnick MB. Prostate cancer: screening, diagnosis and management. Ann Intern Med 1993;118: 804–818.

Grayhack JT, Keeler TC, Kozlowski JM. Carcinoma of the prostate: hormonal therapy. Cancer 1987;60:589–601.

Krahn MD, Mahoney JE, Eckman MH, et al. Screening for prostate cancer: a decision analytic review. JAMA 1994;272:773–780.

Lu-Yao GL, McLerran D, Wasson J, et al. An assessment of radical prostatectomy: time trends, geographic variation, and outcomes. JAMA 1996;269:2633–2636.

Raghaven D. Non-hormone chemotherapy for prostate cancer: principles of treatment and application to the testing of new drugs. Semin Oncol 1988;15:371–389.

H. Malignant Melanoma

The worldwide incidence of cutaneous melanoma continues to increase at a greater rate than that of any other cancer. In the United States, the incidence has doubled since 1980, and in 1995 an estimated 34,000 new cases were diagnosed. Patients who have had one malignant melanoma are at increased risk for developing another (5%, compared with approximately 1% lifetime risk in whites). Epidemiologic studies have linked sun exposure, especially in early life, to melanoma. There is also a genetic predisposition to malignant melanoma. Malignant melanoma arises from a benign pigmented nevus in 50% of cases. Early signs in the nevus that suggest malignant change include a darker or variable coloration, itching, or an increase in size. Prognosis is affected by clinical and histologic factors and by the anatomic location of the lesion. The depth of vertical invasion (Breslow's classification) or the anatomic level of local invasion (Clark's classification) or both of a primary melanoma are the most important prognostic factors determining the risk of recurrence or dissemination. Melanoma spreads by local extension through lymphatics and by hematogenous routes to distant sites. Melanomas that have not spread beyond the site at which they developed are highly curable.

1. PRIMARY SURGERY. Because surgical management of the primary lesion is the only treatment known to affect survival, proper local treatment is crucial. An important question in the management of primary cutaneous melanoma is the appropriate width of the margins of the excision. A diagnostic full-thickness skin biopsy with 1 to 2 mm margins should be performed for any lesion suspected of being a malignant melanoma. If pathology reveals a localized melanoma, surgical reexcision should be performed with margins proportional to the microstage of the primary lesion. For most thin (<1 mm), low-risk lesions, this means approximately 1 cm margins (Arch Surg 1993;126:438–441). For deeper lesions, surgical treatment includes wide local reexcision with 2 to 3 cm margins, with skin grafting or an appropriate flap if necessary (Ann Surg 1993;218:262–267). Using this technique, the local recurrence rate is about 7%.

2. REGIONAL LYMPH NODE DISSECTION. The role of prophylactic or elective lymph node dissection in the management of primary malignant melanoma is controversial. For melanomas <1 mm, the low incidence of nodal metastases does not justify the morbidity associated with lymph node dissection (J Clin Oncol 1988;6:163–172). For intermediate thickness lesions (1 to 4 mm), nonrandomized studies suggested a benefit from elective lymph node dissection (Cancer 1993;72:741–749). Prospective, randomized trials that included patients with all tumor thicknesses and clinically negative lymph nodes, however, have failed

to demonstrate improved survival for patients undergoing lymphadenectomy at the time of diagnosis compared with those undergoing delayed lymphadenectomy when clinically suspicious adenopathy appeared (Mayo Clin Proc 1988;61:697–705). A technique called sentinel lymph node mapping and resection may help in management decisions in intermediate and high-risk patients with clinically negative lymph nodes (Arch Surg 1992;127:392–399). The draining lymphatic vessels from high-risk primary melanoma are identified by injecting dyes, such as isosulfan blue. The sentinel (first) lymph node that takes up the dye is surgically removed and subjected to histologic analysis. If this node is not involved with melanoma, there is less than a 5% chance that any lymph nodes in the drainage site are pathologically involved. Patients with metastatic involvement of the regional lymph nodes are best treated with therapeutic lymphadenectomy. As many as 30% to 40% of these patients may continue to be disease free following such an approach.

3. **ADJUVANT THERAPY.** Patients at high risk of recurrence of melanoma after primary surgery include those who have clinically detectable nodes and have undergone therapeutic lymph node dissection, patients in whom microscopically positive nodes were found at elective lymph node dissection, and patients with deep (>4 mm) primary lesions. Studies conducted in this group of patients to date have shown that adjuvant therapy does not prolong overall or disease-free survival. The standard of care for patients with high-risk locoregional disease after definitive surgical treatment is still observation alone. However, because of the high rate of treatment failure in higher-stage patients, clinical trials continue to examine the addition of adjuvant chemotherapy, biologic therapy (IFN-α), and immunologically active agents (levamisole, BCG). Melphalan administered by isolated regional limb perfusion remains under study in the adjuvant setting (Cancer Invest 1992;10:277–284).

4. **METASTATIC DISEASE.** Malignant melanoma can metastasize to almost any organ in the body. The survival time for patients with metastatic disease ranges from 6 to 9 months when metastases are detected in multiple organ sites. The disease-free interval before development of metastatic disease may be up to 20 years. Malignant melanoma is the single most common tumor reported to spontaneously regress, although the incidence of spontaneous regressions is less than 1%.

    a. **Surgery.** Simple resections of melanoma recurrences should be done if the patient can be rendered free of disease without major morbidity. Isolated metastases to the lung, GI tract, bone, or occasionally the brain may be palliated by resection, with occasional long-term survival. The 5-year survival rate may be as high as 20% after resection of solitary pulmonary metastases.

    b. **Chemotherapy.** Advanced melanoma is refractory to most standard systemic therapy. Decarbazine (DTIC) is the single most active agent in the treatment of disseminated melanoma, with an overall objective response rate of approximately 20% (Cancer 1977;40:1010–1015). The results of a trial of DTIC plus tamoxifen suggest an additive effect (N Engl J Med 1991;327:516–523). Tumors that have responded to DTIC may subsequently respond to BCNU, nitroso-ureas, or cisplatin after progression. Taxol has been studied in melanoma in phase II clinical trials, with some complete responses reported (Cancer 1990;65:2478–2481). The nonsteroidal antiestrogen tamoxifen has only a 6% objective response rate as a single agent (N Engl J Med 1979;301:1241–1242) but has been shown to increase therapeutic responses when used in combination drug regimens. The combination of DTIC, cisplatin, BCNU, and tamoxifen has a reported response rate of 50% (Cancer 1989;63:1292). High doses of alkylating agents, such as melphalan and thiotepa, followed by autologous stem cell transplantation produce objective responses of up to 50%, but the responses generally last less than 6 months, and the treatment is associated with significant toxicity (N Engl J Med 1988;318:869–976). Regional limb perfusion with melphalan has been used to control regionally recurrent melanoma. Melphalan has been used in combination with interferon-γ (IFN-γ) and very high doses of tumor necrosis factor (TNF) in isolated perfusion of recurrent limb melanomas, with 90% of patients given 4 mg of TNF (5 to 10 times the maximally tolerated systemic dose) achieving a complete response lasting an average of more than 1 year (J Clin Oncol 1992;10:52–60).

c. **Biologic therapy and immunotherapy.** Several lines of evidence suggest that the immune response of the host alters the growth and dissemination of malignant melanoma. Well-documented cases of spontaneous regression of primary and metastatic lesions have been reported. Nonspecific immunotherapy, including BCG and *Corynebacterium parvum* treatments, has been used in the treatment of malignant melanoma for years, although it has had minimal impact on the natural history of the disease. DNA recombinant technology has allowed the production of cytokines and monoclonal antibodies, rekindling interest in biologic therapy and immuno-therapy. The combination of IL-2 and lymphocyte-activated killer (LAK) cells has produced objective responses in 20% to 30% of patients with advanced melanoma, including occasional complete responses (J Clin Oncol 1989;7:477–485). Bolus IL-2 alone has also been reported to produce a similar objective response rate and may be more effective than continuous infusion IL-2 schedules (J Clin Oncol 1991;9:641–648). Early reports of IL-2 given in association with tumor-infiltrating lymphocytes (TIL) derived from the patient's own melanoma suggest a higher response rate than with LAK cells (N Engl J Med 1988;319:1676). Fifteen percent of patients will have objective responses to IFN-α, although systemic toxicity limits its use in patients already debilitated by cancer (Semin Oncol 1989;16:34–44). Combinations of IL-2, IFN-α, cisplatin, DTIC, and tamoxifen have achieved complete responses in the 20% range (J Clin Oncol 1992;10:1919–1926). The toxicity of this combined ap-proach is considerable, with significant myelosuppression and a decline of performance status during therapy. Vaccine development for melanoma includes autologous melanoma cell preparations, allogeneic cell fraction preparations, and purified melanoma antigens. These melanoma vaccine strategies have occasionally produced tumor regression (J Clin Oncol 1990;8:1858–1867; Ann Surg 1992;216:463–482). Improved understanding of melanoma immunobiology, along with the isolation and cloning of specific melanoma tumor-associated antigens (P97 and MAGE), have stimulated the development of new melanoma vaccination treatment approaches.

Balch CM. The role of elective lymph node dissection in melanoma: rationale, results, and controversies. J Clin Oncol 1988;6:163–172.

Holstrom H. Surgical management of primary melanoma. Semin Surg Oncol 1992;8:366–369.

Kirkwood JM, Agarwala S. Systemic cytotoxic and biologic therapy of melanoma. PPO Updates 1993;7:1–16.

Koh HK. Cutaneous melanoma. N Engl J Med 1991;325:171–182.

Koh HK, Sober AJ, Day CL, et al. Prognosis of clinical stage I melanoma patients with positive elective regional node dissection. J Clin Oncol 1986;4:1238–1244.

I. Soft Tissue and Bone Sarcomas

Sarcomas are a heterogeneous group of tumors originating in mesenchymal tissues. In 1995, 8000 new cases were diagnosed in the United States, including 6000 cases of soft tissue sarcomas and 2000 cases of bone tumors. Genetic conditions associated with an increased risk for sarcoma include familial retinoblastoma, neutrofibromatosis, and the Li-Fraumeni syndrome. Multiple chromosomal aberrations have been identified in bone and soft tissue sarcomas (N Engl J Med 1991;324:436–442), including loss of the retinoblastoma tumor suppressor gene (13q14) in osteosarcoma and other soft tissue sarcomas and a t(11;22)(q24;q12) chromosomal translocation that is a characteristic abnormality of Ewing's sarcoma and peripheral neuroectodermal tumors (PNETs).

1. SOFT TISSUE SARCOMAS. Soft tissue sarcomas represent 0.7% of all adult malignancies. In children younger than 15 years of age, they represent 6.5% of all cancers and are the fifth leading cause of cancer death. There are approximately 70 different histologic types of soft tissue sarcomas. In adults, the most common types are malignant fibrous histiocytoma (MFH), liposarcoma, leiomyosarcoma, neurofibrosarcoma, angiosarcoma, alveolar soft part sarcoma, and epithelioid sarcoma. In adolescents and young adults, the most common soft tissue tumors are synovial cell sarcoma, epithelioid sarcoma, clear cell sarcoma, and PNET. Rhabdomyosarcoma represents 5% to 8% of all childhood cancers. Immunosuppressed patients develop soft tissue sarcomas, particularly Kaposi's sarcoma, with increased frequency. The most important predictor of the biologic aggressiveness of an individual tumor and its propensity to metastasize is the grade of the tumor. This difficult pathologic assessment is based on the frequency of mitoses and the degree of pretherapeutic necrosis, as well as on the cellularity and nuclear pleomorphism (Semin Oncol 1989;16:273). Grade I and, to some extent, grade II tumors are low grade and tend to recur locally rather than systemically. In general, they do not respond as well to chemotherapy as do the high-grade tumors (grade III), which are aggressive tumors with a high propensity for systemic dissemination. Sarcomas located in the extremities generally have a better prognosis than those not in the extremities. At the time of diagnosis, soft tissue

sarcomas are highly treatable, often curable tumors that are best treated by an experienced multimodality team.

a. **Primary surgery.** Soft tissue sarcomas commonly occur as asymptomatic, slowly enlarging, firm soft tissue masses anywhere in the body. The goal of treatment of local disease is local control followed by preservation of optimal function. The surgical margin achieved has a direct influence on the local recurrence rate. These tumors are frequently surrounded by a pseudocapsule containing viable tumor cells. Therefore, they should never be simply shelled out. The proper biopsy for all lesions >3 cm is a carefully placed small incisional biopsy, using a longitudinal incision on the extremities. After the diagnosis is established, primary resection of the sarcoma should be performed by wide excision including several centimeters of normal tissue in all directions as well as excision of previous biopsy sites. In general, it is not necessary to perform lymph node dissections. For patients with lesions amenable to a combined approach, that is, preoperative or postoperative radiation in conjunction with nonamputative excision, 5-year survival rates are roughly equivalent to those achieved in the past with more radical surgical procedures. Where conservative resection and radiation therapy are not feasible, amputation should be the primary recommendation to avoid high local recurrence rates. Retroperitoneal sarcoma poses a complex problem, as complete resection is not often possible because of anatomic constraints. In many cases, partial resection of a major organ is required, and even in a completely resected sarcoma, a recurrence rate of 50% to 70% is common.

b. **Neoadjuvant chemotherapy.** Preoperative or neoadjuvant chemotherapy provides a unique opportunity to pathologically assess the effectiveness of chemotherapy. Necrosis of more than 90% of the cells in the resected specimen has been shown to correlate with improved survival in patients with osteogenic sarcomas, and similar prognostic significance is assumed for soft tissue sarcomas. Preoperative chemotherapy may also facilitate surgery by shrinking tumors, potentially allowing limb salvage surgery rather than amputation. Preoperative regional (intraarterial) chemotherapy has been used in combination with reduced doses of radiation therapy and surgery in limb-sparing treatment (Proc Am Soc Clin Oncol 1990;9:309).

c. **Adjuvant chemotherapy.** Adjuvant chemotherapy is considered standard therapy for rhabdomyosarcomas and extraskeletal Ewing's sarcoma because of their high incidence of systemic micrometastasis and responsiveness to chemotherapy. The role of adjuvant chemotherapy in all other sarcomas remains controversial. Adjuvant therapy apparently does not improve disease-free survival or overall survival in patients with low-grade lesions. The most active agents for soft tissue sarcomas are ifosfamide (30% response rate), doxorubicin (26%), dactinomycin (17%), and dacarbazine (16%). Several trials have evaluated the role of adjuvant chemotherapy with doxorubicin either as a single agent or in combination with other drugs. The majority of studies accrued small numbers of patients and did not demonstrate either a metastasis-free or an overall survival benefit. A metaanalysis of these trials, however, suggested a small treatment benefit in favor of adjuvant chemotherapy (Br J Cancer 1995;72:469–475).

d. **Radiation therapy.** Preoperative and postoperative radiation therapy has been used in conjunction with surgery to improve local control of the tumor. If used postoperatively, a dose of 60–65 Gy is required to achieve local control (J Clin Oncol 1988;6:854–862). If radiation therapy is used preoperatively, the dose required is lower (i.e., 50–54 Gy), and the radiation field is usually smaller. The local control rate of inoperable soft tissue sarcoma treated with 6000–8000 cGy of conventional photon radiotherapy is only 10% to 12%. The use of neutrons (which have a higher linear energy transfer and are not dependent on oxygen for cell kill) increases the local control rate to 50% (Am J Clin Oncol 1986;9:397–400). Precisely shaped fields and immobilization are mandatory.

e. **Treatment of recurrent or metastatic disease.** The two most common types of disease recurrence are local recurrence and hematogenous spread that most commonly involves the lungs. Local recurrence should be treated with aggressive surgical resection or as a high-risk primary tumor, with preoperative chemotherapy followed by local therapy depending on the clinical situation. Eighty percent of local recurrences occur in the first 2 years, and all of them occur in the first 3 years (Cancer 1981;47:2391–2397). Patients with isolated local recurrences have a 5-year survival rate of 45% to 85% when treated with aggressive local therapy (Arch Surg 1992;127:548–554). Isolated pulmonary metastases represent the initial pattern of recurrence in 50% of patients who have relapse. Resection of pulmonary metastases is indicated for patients with favorable prognostic factors, including a tumor doubling time of longer than 40 days, a disease-free interval of more than 1 year, fewer than three nodules, unilateral disease, and MFH tumor histology (Cancer 1992;59:662–668).

For patients with less favorable prognostic factors or with widely disseminated disease, chemotherapy is the only available treatment option. Complete response rates range from 10% to 15%, and only one third of patients achieve long-term disease-free survival. The most active agents are ifosfamide and doxorubicin, with objective response rates of 15% to 35%. Trials have indicated better overall response rates with a combination of ifosfamide and doxorubicin (J Clin Oncol 1993;11:1276–1285). DTIC is another active drug, with an objective partial response rate of 15% to 20%. Combination regimens using DTIC appear to be mildly synergistic.

2. **BONE SARCOMAS.** Bone sarcomas account for 0.2% of all primary cancers in adults and 5% of childhood malignancies. Bone tumors metastasize almost exclusively by hematogenous spread. Osteosarcoma, the most common primary malignant bone tumor, is a high-grade spindle cell tumor with a high propensity for lung metastases. The introduction of

neoadjuvant chemotherapy has allowed conservative limb salvage surgery in 50% to 80% of patients, as well as offering early systemic therapy against micrometastases. The beneficial role of neoadjuvant and adjuvant chemotherapy in patients with osteosarcoma is well proven (N Engl J Med 1986;314:1600–1608). Active agents include doxorubicin, cisplatin, ifosfamide, high-dose methotrexate, and cyclophosphamide. Osteosarcoma tends to be markedly radioresistant. Chondrosarcoma is the second most common primary spindle cell tumor of bone, characterized by cartilaginous neoplastic tissue. Surgical removal is the treatment for chondrosarcoma; in general, chemotherapy is not effective. Radiation therapy may offer benefit in local control (Int J Radiat Oncol Biol Phys 1982;8:187–190). Ewing's sarcoma is a rare tumor that usually occurs in bone in the second decade of life. It is an undifferentiated, small, round cell tumor and is thought to be of neuroectodermal origin. Ewing's sarcoma is considered a systemic disease because even when a tumor is apparently localized, approximately 90% of cases include occult metastatic disease. Radiation therapy provides good local control of Ewing's sarcoma, and surgery is usually limited to diagnostic biopsy (Am J Surg Pathol 1986;10:54–62). The addition of chemotherapy can significantly improve disease-free survival, and adjuvant chemotherapy is now accepted as standard therapy for Ewing's sarcoma. The most active single agents include cyclophosphamide, doxorubicin, vincristine, dactinomycin, etoposide, and high-dose melphalan.

Antman KH, Eilber FR, Shiu MHJ. Soft tissue sarcomas: current trends in diagnosis and management. Curr Probl Cancer 1989;13:337–367.

Marcove RC, Sheth DS, Healy J, et al. Limb-sparing surgery for extremity sarcoma. Cancer Invest 1994;12:497–504.

Singer S, Antman K, Corson JM, et al. Long-term salvageability for patients with locally recurrent soft-tissue sarcomas. Arch Surg 1992;127:548–554.

Tierney JF, Mosseri V, Stewart LA, et al. Adjuvant chemotherapy for soft tissue sarcomas: review and meta-analysis of the published results of randomized clinical trials. Br J Cancer 1995;72:469–475.

J. Adult Central Nervous System Malignancies

Primary brain cancers represent 1% (18,000 cases) of all cancers and 2.4% (13,300 cases) of cancer deaths annually in the United States. Metastases to the brain from a primary tumor that is outside the central nervous system (CNS) are more common than primary tumors of the brain. The cellular classification for CNS malignancies includes glial tumors, or gliomas (astrocytomas, ependymomas, oligodendrogliomas, medulloblastoma), and nonglial tumors (pineal tumors, meningiomas, choroid plexus tumors, germ cell tumors, craniopharyngiomas). Astrocytomas, the most prevalent subtype of glioma, are subdivided into subcategories by grade, based on the degree of tumor anaplasia and the presence or absence of necrosis. Glioblastoma multiforme is the highest grade (grade IV, poorly differentiated, rapidly growing) of astrocytoma. Surgical removal of brain tumors is recommended for most types and in most locations and should be as complete as possible within the constraints of preservation of neurologic function. Radiotherapy has a major role in the treatment of most tumor types and can increase the cure rate and prolong disease-free survival.

Chemotherapy may prolong survival in some tumor types and has been reported to lengthen disease-free survival in patients with gliomas, medulloblastomas, and some germ cell tumors. Patients who have CNS tumors that are either infrequently curable or unresectable should be considered candidates for clinical trials that employ radiosensitizers, hyperthermia, or interstitial brachytherapy used in conjunction with external-beam radiotherapy to improve local control of the tumor or for studies that evaluate new drugs and biologic response modifiers.

Levin VA, Gutin PH, Leibel S. Neoplasms of the central nervous system. In: DeVita VT, Hellman S, Rosenberg SA, eds. Cancer: Principles and Practice of Oncology, 4th ed. Philadelphia: JB Lippincott Company, 1993, pp 1679–1737.

Shapiro WR. Therapy of adult malignant brain tumor: what have the clinical trials taught us? Semin Oncol 1986;13:38–45.

K. Cancer of Unknown Primary Site

In most patients diagnosed with cancer, the history and physical examination, chest x-ray, urinalysis, blood studies, and stool guaiac determination will reveal clues to the primary site. When these and other appropriate tests are unrevealing and the biopsied site is not believed to be the primary, the patient is said to have cancer of unknown primary (CUP). Two percent to 9% of patients with histologically diagnosed cancer have disseminated disease without evidence of the site of origin of the primary tumor. The most common presentations are abdominal masses or hepatomegaly (19% to 84%), lymphadenopathy (11% to 36%), and bone pain (6% to 28%). The primary site will eventually be identified in 25% to 30% of patients before death and at autopsy in another 60%. When the primary site is identified in patients with CUP, the most common primaries identified historically are lung cancer in presentations above the diaphragm and pancreatic cancer in presentations below the diaphragm (Semin Oncol 1977;4:53–58) (Table 11–9).

1. DIAGNOSTIC WORKUP. Patients with CUP are a heterogeneous group. As only 10% to 13% of patients with CUP have tumors responsive to current therapies, most patients will not benefit from an extensive diagnostic workup. General principles are to evaluate signs and symptoms and to do simple tests, with a focus on finding treatable malignancies. At a minimum, the workup should include a biopsy of the tumor for pathologic evaluation, a thorough history and complete physical examination (including head and neck, rectal, pelvic, and breast examinations), chest x-rays, a complete blood cell count, urinalysis, and examination of the stool for occult blood. The location of metastases often provides a valuable clue to the primary site. Isolated cervical adenopathy is most commonly caused by head and neck cancer. The presence of an abnormal axillary node most likely represents metastatic breast cancer in a woman, although lymphomas, lung cancer, and melanomas also present in this manner. Supraclavicular nodes are common metastatic sites for occult lung and breast cancers, whereas metastases to inguinal nodes implicate tumors arising in the leg, perineum, prostate, or gonads. Lung metastases are twice as common in primary sites ultimately found to be above the diaphragm.

TABLE 11–9. **Distribution of Primary Tumor Sites: Cancer of Unknown Primary (CUP) Versus General Incidence**

PRIMARY SITE	PRIMARY SITE EVENTUALLY IDENTIFIED IN CUP (%)	GENERAL RELATIVE INCIDENCE OF PRIMARY SITE (%)
ABOVE DIAPHRAGM		
Lung	17	14
Breast	3	15
Thyroid	5	1
BELOW DIAPHRAGM		
Pancreas	21	2
Liver	10	1.5
Colorectal	7	11
Gastric	10	2
Renal	3	2
Ovary	2	2
Prostate	3	19
Adrenal	2	<1
NOT CLASSIFIED	15	

Data from Nystrom JS, Weiner JM, Heffelfinger-Juttner J, et al. Metastatic and histologic presentations in unknown primary cancer. Semin Oncol 1977;4:53–58; Wingo P, Tong T, Bolden S. Cancer statistics, 1995. Ca: A Cancer Journal for Clinicians 1995;45:8–17.

Liver metastases are more common from primary disease below the diaphragm. The most useful diagnostic modality is pathologic evaluation of the biopsied cancer, using histologic, immunocytochemical, electron microscopic, hormone receptor, and gene rearrangement techniques. The histologic subtype of the tumor (adenocarcinoma, squamous cell carcinoma, poorly differentiated carcinoma, neuroendocrine differentiation) can be helpful in identifying the primary site and in making treatment decisions. Immunocytochemical stains of the tumor specimen that may be helpful in identifying the primary tumor site include cytokeratins (epithelial tumors), S-100 and HMB-45 (melanoma), leukocyte common antigen (lymphomas), chromogranin (neuroendocrine tumors), estrogen and progesterone receptors (breast cancer), AFP and hCG (germ cell tumors), and PSA (prostate cancer).

Specific chromosomal abnormalities have been identified in several types of lymphoma (N Engl J Med 1983;309:1593–1599). A few solid tumors are also associated with specific chromosomal abnormalities, including an isochromosome of the short arm of chromosome 12 in germ cell tumors (Proc Am Soc Clin Oncol 1989;8:131) and an 11:22 translocation in Ewing's sarcoma and peripheral neuroectodermal tumors (N Engl J Med 1983;309:497–498). Measurement of selected tumor markers in the serum (e.g., PSA, hCG, AFP) may also yield valuable information. Radiologic testing constituting an adequate evaluation for a primary site generally includes CT imaging of the chest, abdomen, and pelvis.

2. TREATMENT. The prognosis of CUP is generally poor, but there are subsets of patients who have a better outcome. As a group, median survival is ≤4 months, and <10% are alive at 5 years. If a primary tumor is identified, treatment is given accordingly. Cancers curable with local therapy (with or without systemic therapy) include head and neck, anal, and breast cancer. Cancers potentially curable with chemotherapy include germ cell tumors and lymphomas. Cancers responsive to systemic therapy include breast, prostate, thyroid, endometrial, ovarian, and neuroendocrine cancers. Adenocarcinomas are the most common type of CUP, and the overall prognosis within this subgroup is poor. Subgroups with a more favorable prognosis include

   a. **Squamous cell histology in the high cervical or midcervical lymph nodes.** This presentation is consistent with a head and neck primary. Regional therapy (radical neck dissection or cervical radiation) can give a 35% to 60% 3-year survival.

   b. **Squamous cell histology in the inguinal lymph nodes.** If treated as anal or vulvar/cervical/vaginal primary (inguinal node dissection with or without radiotherapy), there is potential for long-term survival.

   c. **Male extragonadal germ cell syndrome.** There is a subgroup of poorly differentiated carcinomas that behave as extragonadal germ cell tumors and are responsive to chemotherapy. Males younger than 30 with poorly differentiated carcinomas in the mediastinum, retroperitoneum, or lymph nodes may have extragonadal germ cell tumors even if hCG and AFP levels are not elevated. They should be treated with cisplatin plus etoposide (or vinblastine) with or without bleomycin (Ann Intern Med 1986;104:347–353). Responses can be obtained in 36% of such patients (including 22% complete responses), and 13% will achieve long-term disease-free survival.

   d. **Neuroendocrine carcinoma.** Poorly differentiated tumors with neuroendocrine features on electron microscopy or immunocytochemistry should be treated similarly to small cell carcinoma of the lung, and some types, like carcinoid tumors, may have a very indolent course. Cisplatin-based regimens can induce partial or complete remissions in 72% of such patients, and 10% to 20% can be cured (Ann Intern Med 1988;109:364–371).

   e. **Female peritoneal carcinomatosis.** Women with peritoneal adenocarcinomas should be treated as if they had an ovarian primary, with cytoreductive surgery and cisplatin chemotherapy. Approximately 40% will achieve a complete response, with a median survival of 23 months (Ann Intern Med 1989;111:213–217).

   f. **Female axillary adenocarcinoma.** This group should be treated for presumptive ipsilateral breast cancer with mastectomy, axillary dissection, radiation, and adjuvant chemotherapy or hormonal therapy. Disease-free survival is up to 70% at 5 years.

   Other subgroups of patients have a bleak prognosis. Empiric chemotherapy is commonly administered with various combinations of doxorubicin, mitomycin, 5-FU, and cyclophosphamide, but response rates are low (0% to 30%) and no survival benefit has been demonstrated for this approach. Radiation therapy should be used for palliation of painful metastases and prophylactically for prevention of pathologic fractures from long bone metastases.

Abbruzzese JL, Abbruzzese MC, Hess KR, et al. Unknown primary carcinoma: natural history and prognostic factors in 657 consecutive patients. J Clin Oncol 1994;12:1272–1280.

Hainsworth JD, Greco FA. Treatment of patients with cancer of an unknown primary site. N Engl J Med 1993;329:257–263.

Leonard RJ, Nystrom JS. Diagnostic evaluation of patients with carcinoma of unknown primary tumor site. Semin Oncol 1993;20:244–250.

12 12 12 12 12 12 12 12

ENDOCRINOLOGIC AND RELATED METABOLIC DISORDERS

NORMAN R. ROSENTHAL

12 12 12 12 12 12 12 12 12

The release of the anterior pituitary hormones thyroid-stimulating hormone (TSH), corticotropin (ACTH), luteinizing hormone (LH), follicle-stimulating hormone (FSH), prolactin, and growth hormone is regulated by releasing and inhibiting hormones produced in the hypothalamus and reaching the pituitary via the hypothalamic-pituitary portal venous system. The posterior pituitary stores oxytocin and vasopressin in preparation for release into the general circulation. The hypothalamus and pituitary form an integrated axis that maintains control over much of the endocrine system. Disorders of the hypothalamic-pituitary axis are usually clinically manifested either by syndromes of hormone excess or deficiency or by visual impairment from optic nerve compression. Treatment of pituitary tumors usually includes measures to correct hormone imbalance and reduce tumor mass. Expanding lesions in the pituitary typically cause pituitary hormones to drop out in a predictable sequence of growth hormone and gonadotropins early and ACTH and TSH late. Lesions originating in the pituitary do not cause antidiuretic hormone (ADH) deficiency (diabetes insipidus) unless the destructive process extends into the hypothalamus.

Deficiencies of ACTH, LH, FSH, and TSH are treated by replacing target organ hormones, that is, corticosteroids, sex steroids, and thyroid hormone. Glucocorticoid and thyroid hormone replacement are indicated in all patients with hypopituitarism, as untreated adrenal insufficiency and hypothyroidism are potentially life threatening. Replacement of sex steroids improves sexual function and well-being, defends bone mass, and is indicated in all but the very elderly. Diabetes insipidus, although not life threatening, causes bothersome polyuria and polydipsia, which can be easily treated. Treatment of growth hormone deficiency is necessary only in children and adolescents.

A. Hypopituitarism

1. **ACTH DEFICIENCY (ADRENAL INSUFFICIENCY). Prednisone,** 7.5 mg/d (5 mg in AM, 2.5 mg in PM), or **hydrocortisone,** 30 mg/d (20 mg in AM, 10 mg in PM), provides physiologic replacement of glucocorticoid for most patients. Adequacy of glucocorticoid replacement is indicated by restoration of the patient's sense of well-being, appetite, and weight. Excessive glucocorticoid replacement is indicated by the development of cushingoid features (e.g., rounded face, thin skin, hypertension). Orthostatic hypotension despite glucocorticoid replacement may signify a need for mineralocorticoid. **Fludrocortisone** (Florinef) is usually given as a single daily dose of 0.05–0.3 mg. Hypertension, hypokalemia, edema, and congestive heart failure are indications for a dose reduction.

At the first sign of illness (including minor infections such as gastroenteritis and febrile viral syndromes), patients should double their maintenance dose of glucocorticoid. If vomiting precludes the use of oral medication, arrangements must be made immediately for parenteral administration of corticosteroids. Patients should wear a bracelet or necklace identifying themselves as having hypopituitarism. An injectable form of glucocorticoid (dexamethasone phosphate, 4 mg) for self-injection should be available whenever the patient will be out of reach of medical care for more than a day. Patients with hypopituitarism require coverage with stress doses of glucocorticoids during serious illness or surgery.

2. HYPOTHYROIDISM. Treatment of hypothyroidism due to TSH deficiency consists of L-thyroxine in appropriate doses. The usual dose is 1.5–1.7 μg/kg body weight. The dose should be adjusted to maintain the patient's free thyroxine index in the midnormal range.

3. GONADOTROPIN DEFICIENCY IN MEN. In men, gonadotropin deficiency causes testosterone deficiency with accompanying impotence or infertility or both, whereas in boys, delayed puberty or short stature may be the result. Testosterone deficiency can also lead to loss of muscle tone and osteoporosis. This deficiency can be treated with a long-acting testosterone preparation, such as testosterone enanthate given by IM injection. The frequency of administration must be tailored to the individual, a typical regimen being 200 mg testosterone enanthate IM every 2 weeks. The frequency of injections should be adjusted to avoid periods of symptomatic hypogonadism. Another treatment option is the transdermal testosterone patch, a newly available delivery system, that can be applied to either the scrotum or chest and must be changed daily. Since testosterone can stimulate the prostate, careful examination of the prostate is performed to rule out cancer or benign hypertrophy before treatment is initiated.

4. GONADOTROPIN DEFICIENCY IN WOMEN. In women, gonadotropin deficiency may cause estrogen deficiency symptoms, including infertility, amenorrhea, vaginal mucosal atrophy, hot flashes, and breast atrophy. Treatment depends on whether or not fertility is being sought. If fertility is the goal of treatment, gonadotropins can be used in an attempt to induce ovulation. If fertility is not an issue, hypogonadism is treated with estrogens and, for women with an intact uterus, in combination with progestins.

B. Nonfunctioning Pituitary Adenoma

Clinically silent tumors, that is, microadenomas (<1 cm) that produce no neurologic symptoms or endocrine deficiencies, grow slowly, if at all. A reasonable approach to a patient with an incidentally discovered tumor who has normal pituitary function and visual fields is to withhold treatment unless serial measurements of visual fields or tumor size (measured by periodic MRI scanning) indicate tumor enlargement or if pituitary hormone deficiency develops. Treatment consists of surgery, external radiation, or both. Surgery is generally recommended for large tumors with suprasellar extension or optic nerve compression or both. External radiation is given after surgery if removal is incomplete or if the tumor recurs. External radiation as primary therapy is appropriate for intrasellar tumors that present no immediate threat to surrounding structures. Radiation usually consists of 4000–5000 cGy delivered over 4 to 6 weeks.

C. Hormone-Producing Pituitary Tumors

1. ACROMEGALY. This is a chronic disease associated with diminished life expectancy. Treatment designed to reduce growth hormone level produces improvement in cardiac function and hypertension. **Transsphenoidal adenomectomy** will initially normalize growth hormone concentration in up to 75% of cases, but in many, late relapse occurs. Thus, multimodality therapy should be considered. **External pituitary radiation** is reserved for patients who have residual disease after surgery. Since it takes years for radiation to effectively lower GH levels, medical therapy is given while awaiting the effects of radiation. Medical therapy consists of dopamine agonists and somatostatin analogs. **Bromocriptine** in doses up to 20 mg/d may be of use in the treatment of acromegaly. Although the majority of patients will describe a clinical improvement, only 20% to 50% will show significant biochemical response. **Octreotide,** usually given as 100 µg q8h by SC injection, will reduce GH levels in 80% to 90% of patients and is our most effective drug therapy. Although inconvenience and expense limit its use, it is generally well tolerated except for the uncommon occurrence of diarrhea and cholelithiasis. Longer-acting analogs, administered every 2 to 4 weeks, will be available in the near future.

2. CUSHING'S DISEASE. **Transsphenoidal adenomectomy** or **hypophysectomy** is the treatment of choice for most patients with Cushing's disease. In the hands of an experienced neurosurgeon, pituitary microsurgery is successful in nearly 80% of patients with a microadenoma. The outcome is less favorable for patients with a macroadenoma (tumors >1 cm in diameter), of whom less than 50% are cured with surgery. Preoperative localization of the pituitary tumor will usually reduce the extent of surgery and thus lessen the likelihood of hypopituitarism from extensive pituitary resection.

   Patients undergoing pituitary surgery require **glucocorticoid coverage** in stress doses, both intraoperatively and postoperatively. Glucocorticoid coverage is usually tapered to physiologic replacement doses over 5 to 7 days after surgery. After successful adenomectomy, glucocorticoid replacement therapy is often needed for 6 to 12 months as the remaining pituitary gradually recovers its homeostatic ability to produce ACTH. Pituitary radiation is most effective in children. The remission rate in children is 70% to 80%, but there is a lag between treatment and remission of 12 to 18 months. Remission rates in adults are lower; approximately 50% have a successful response a year after radiation therapy. Radiation may be useful as adjunctive therapy for patients not cured by surgery.

3. PROLACTIN-PRODUCING PITUITARY TUMORS. The most common functioning pituitary tumor is the **prolactinoma.** Women characteristically have amenorrhea, galactorrhea, or infertility or some combination of these. In men, erectile dysfunction and loss of libido can occur. Most prolactinomas are benign microadenomas (<1 cm), and less than 10% of microadenomas will grow over time. Macroadenomas (>1 cm) can cause mass-related symptoms. The decision to treat a prolactinoma depends on several factors, including tumor size, the patient's symptoms and age, and the option of fertility. Therapy for microadenomas is

directed at restoring gonadal function and reducing galactorrhea. Hyperprolactinemic women over childbearing age might not need treatment. Suprasellar extension and associated neurologic symptoms are common in macroadenomas, and strategies for therapeutic intervention must consider the growth potential of this tumor.

The treatment choices are surgery, radiation, or bromocriptine. Successful **transsphenoidal removal** of the microadenoma with preservation of normal pituitary function is achieved in up to 80% of selected patients. External **radiation therapy** will arrest tumor growth but does not generally normalize prolactin levels or restore menses. The treatment of choice is the dopamine agonist **bromocriptine.** Doses of 2.5–15 mg/d will rapidly suppress prolactin secretion, restoring menses in about 95%. Bromocriptine often produces nausea and lightheadedness and should be initiated gradually with a dose of 1.25 mg (½ tablet) at night with a snack, then 1.25 mg tid, gradually increasing the dose until the prolactin level is normalized or menses restored.

Large prolactinomas, even those with suprasellar extension, can be effectively treated with bromocriptine in 70% of patients. Surgical resection or debulking may also be necessary.

When the goal of treatment is to restore fertility, the potential effect of pregnancy on tumor growth must be considered in selecting therapy. Pregnancy is associated with pituitary enlargement due to expansion of pituitary lactotrophs. In a woman with a prolactinoma, expansion of the tumor or normal pituitary or both may compress the optic nerves, causing visual impairment. The risk appears to be quite small for microadenomas but is of greater concern for macroadenomas. Some authorities recommend surgical extirpation of macroadenomas if pregnancy is the goal of therapy. Although bromocriptine has been used successfully to restore fertility, it has not yet received FDA approval for this indication. If bromocriptine therapy is used to restore fertility, the drug should be discontinued once pregnancy is established.

D. Diabetes Insipidus

1. **GENERAL PRACTICES.** Diabetes insipidus (DI) results from a deficiency of, or resistance to, ADH. In the absence of ADH, urine volumes may exceed 6 L/d, making it difficult to maintain water balance by increased fluid intake. Approximately half of patients will have a neoplasm or infiltrative disease of the hypothalamus with the remainder labeled as having "idiopathic" DI.

2. **TREATMENT.** In patients with partial DI, a normal thirst mechanism and free access to water will usually allow maintenance of normal hydration. For those in whom the polyuria, polydipsia, and nocturia are troublesome, several agents are available.

   a. **DDAVP.** Desamino-D-arginine vasopressin (DDAVP), a synthetic analog of human ADH, is the drug of choice for most patients. It is administered by instillation into the posterior nasal cavity by a metered nasal spray. The dose is 10 µg per spray at a frequency based on duration of antidiuresis. For some patients, a single administration provides 24-hour antidiuresis, but for most, twice-daily dosing is necessary. For patients unable to use the nasal route, DDAVP can be given parenterally in a dose of 0.5–2 µg SC or IV. An oral form of DDAVP has been approved recently.

b. Pitressin. Pitressin tannate in oil given IM provides long-acting (24 to 72 hour) antidiuresis. Because of vasopressor effects, it may cause headache, increased blood pressure, exacerbation of angina, or uterine cramps. A single dose of 5–10 U will usually provide a 24 to 72 hour effect. Vigorous shaking of the vial is required to ensure that the active ingredient is adequately suspended.

c. Chlorpropamide. This potentiates the effect of ADH at the renal tubule and, in patients with partial DI, may provide satisfactory relief of symptoms. Chlorpropamide is given once a day in a dose of 100–500 mg. Hypoglycemia may occur, especially at higher doses.

Andreoli TE. The posterior pituitary. In: Wyngaarden JB, Smith LH, eds. Cecil's Textbook of Medicine, 17th ed. Philadelphia, WB Saunders; 1985, pp 1266–1272.

Davis DH, Laws ER, Ilstrup DM, et al. Results of surgical treatment for growth hormone-secreting pituitary adenomas. J Neurosurg 1993;79:70–75.

Frohman LA. The anterior pituitary. In: Wyngaarden JB, Smith LH, eds. Cecil's Textbook of Medicine. Philadelphia, WB Saunders; 1985, pp. 1251–1265.

Mampalan TJ. Transsphenoidal microsurgery for Cushing's disease: a report of 216 cases. Ann Intern Med 1988;109:487–493.

March CM, Kletzky OA, Davajan V, et al. Longitudinal evaluation of patients with untreated prolactin-secreting adenomas. Am J Obstet Gynecol 1981;139:835–843.

Melmed S. Acromegaly. N Engl J Med 1990;322:966–977.

Neuman CB, Melmed S, Snyder PJ, et al. Safety and efficacy of long-term octreotide therapy of acromegaly: results of a multicenter trial in 103 patients. J Clin Endocrinol Metab 1995;80: 2768–2775.

Orth DN. Cushing's syndrome. N Engl J Med 1995;332:791–799.

Schlechte J, Dolan K, Sherman B, et al. The natural history of untreated hyperprolactinemia: a prospective analysis. J Clin Endocrinol Metab 1989;68:412–418.

Vance ML. Hypopituitarism. N Engl J Med 1994;330:1651–1662.

II. THYROID DISORDERS

A. Hyperthyroidism

1. **GENERAL PRINCIPLES.** Several disorders of the thyroid can cause hyperthyroidism. In Graves' disease, toxic multinodular goiter, and toxic adenoma, overproduction of thyroid hormone occurs. Treatment is aimed at suppressing the overactive gland. The hyperthyroidism of thyroiditis results from uncontrolled release of hormone from the gland. Treatment of thyroiditis is directed toward ameliorating symptoms while waiting for the hyperthyroidism to subside. There are three means of treating an overactive thyroid: **thionamide medication, radioactive iodine, or thyroid surgery.** The thionamides (propylthiouracil and methimazole) are concentrated in the thyroid and interfere with the synthesis of thyroid hormone. Thionamides effectively lower hormone levels but usually do not cure the hyperthyroidism. Radioactive iodine (RAI) or surgery is usually required for definitive treatment. Since RAI accomplishes the same objective as surgery (i.e., ablating an overactive thyroid gland) without the risks of anesthesia and surgery, it is preferred for most patients. Thyroidectomy is usually reserved for pregnant patients (in whom RAI is contraindicated) who are allergic to

antithyroid medication or as definitive therapy for severely hyperthyroid patients not controlled by medication.

2. TREATMENT
   a. **Thionamides.** The thionamides **propylthiouracil** (PTU) and **methimazole** inhibit thyroxine synthesis by blocking the organification of iodide. In addition, PTU (but not methimazole) partially blocks the peripheral conversion of thyroxine (T_4) to the more metabolically active triiodothyronine (T_3). In patients with Graves' disease, thionamides can be used as lifelong therapy, but about 10% to 20% of patients will enter a long-term remission after 12 to 24 months of treatment. Patients with mild hyperthyroidism and small goiters are more likely to enter remission.

   The **starting dose of propylthiouracil is 100–200 mg tid or methimazole 10–30 mg as a single dose.** Thyroid function tests should be measured at an appropriate interval of time to determine the correct maintenance dose. Eventually, patients can usually be treated with twice-daily administration of PTU.

   Thionamides have several potential side effects. A maculopapular rash occurs in 1% to 2% of patients. Rarely, thionamides cause cholestasis, and PTU can cause vasculitis. The most serious adverse reaction of thionamides is **agranulocytosis,** a complication seen in approximately 0.1% of patients. Patients should be instructed to report fever, sore throat, or infection. In this situation, medication should be withheld until the patient's white blood cell count is known.

   b. **Radioactive iodine.** RAI is concentrated in the thyroid, where radiation causes injury to thyroid cells, rendering some or all incapable of continued hormone production. The result of radiation-induced injury to the thyroid is progressive atrophy and fibrosis, in many cases resulting in hypothyroidism. More than 50% of patients treated with RAI become hypothyroid within a year, and another 2% to 3% annually thereafter. At the commonly used doses of RAI (i.e., 5–10 mCi) 80% to 95% of patients are cured of hyperthyroidism with one dose, usually within 2 to 4 months. Patients advised to have RAI therapy are often concerned about the potential harmful effects of radiation. Several studies show no increase in incidence of malignancy or genetic defects in offspring of patients followed for decades after RAI therapy.

   c. **Beta-adrenergic blockers.** Several manifestations of hyperthyroidism appear to be due to increased sensitivity to circulating catecholamines. Beta-adrenergic blocking agents are effective in reducing palpitations, tremulousness, nervousness, and tachycardia. **Propranolol,** 40–200 mg/d in divided doses, or **atenolol,** 25–100 mg/d, will ameliorate these symptoms as other steps are taken to treat the underlying thyroid overactivity.

   d. **Oral cholecystographic agents.** Certain radiologic contrast agents used for gallbladder imaging inhibit the conversion of T_4 to the more active T_3, and the iodide contained in these agents also blocks all steps of thyroid hormonogenesis. Their rapid onset can be valuable when prompt control of hyperthyroidism is desired. Sodium ipodate

(Oragrafin) or iopanoic acid (Telepaque), 1 g/d or 3 g every 3 days, produce a dramatic fall in serum T_3 concentration within 48 hours. These agents contain iodide, and their use precludes RAI for a period of several weeks or months. If used in conjunction with a thionamide, these agents are usually given for the first 2 or 3 weeks of therapy while waiting for the thionamides to take effect.

e. **Overview.** RAI is preferred treatment for most patients with hyperthyroidism. Patients who are severely hyperthyroid can be treated initially with thionamides, since it usually takes 2 to 4 months to control hyperthyroidism with RAI. If thionamides are used in preparation for treatment with RAI, they should be discontinued for at least a week before RAI is given and, if necessary, resumed a week or more after. For patients who decline RAI, thionamide treatment is a reasonable alternative for long-term management. These patients can reconsider the choice of RAI therapy at any time or if they develop an untoward response to thionamides. Surgery is usually reserved for large multinodular goiters, pregnant patients who are not able to take thionamides, and patients who are not controlled by antithyroid medication.

3. **THYROIDITIS.** In subacute or silent thyroiditis there is generalized inflammation of the gland and leakage of stored thyroid hormone, usually enough to cause hyperthyroidism. Duration of hyperthyroidism is usually less than 3 months; the symptoms are usually mild. Transient hypothyroidism may follow subacute thyroiditis and may be severe enough to require treatment for 3 to 6 months, by which time thyroid function usually has returned to normal.

Treatment is directed toward relieving symptoms rather than suppressing thyroid function. **Beta-blocking agents** are useful for control of tachycardia, palpitations, nervousness, and tremor. **Aspirin,** 2–4 g/d, is usually effective in treating the pain of subacute thyroiditis. When aspirin fails to provide relief, a short course of prednisone (40 mg/d) is nearly always effective.

4. **SPECIAL CIRCUMSTANCES**
   a. **Ophthalmopathy.** The ophthalmopathy of Graves' disease is highly variable in severity and course. Minor symptoms of conjunctival irritation or periorbital edema are treated symptomatically with eyedrops and elevating the head of the bed. In the most severe cases, vision may be threatened by ulceration or infection of the cornea or by pressure on the optic nerve. Prednisone (80–120 mg/d) is usually the first measure used in the treatment of severe ophthalmopathy. In patients in whom steroids fail, external orbital radiation or orbital decompression may be indicated.
   b. **Pregnancy.** RAI is contraindicated in pregnant women because of potential harm to the fetal thyroid. PTU is used in preference to methimazole in pregnancy because more of the latter crosses the placenta and is associated with the minor congenital anomaly aplasia cutis. The dose of PTU should be carefully titrated to maintain thyroid hormone levels in the upper normal range. Monthly or more frequent testing of thyroid function is required to ensure that hormone levels are in the upper-normal range, thereby

TABLE 12-1. **Drugs Used in Treatment of Thyroid Storm**

DRUG	DOSAGE
Propylthiouracil (PTU)	200–400 mg q6h PO or by NG tube.
Iodide	PO: supersaturated potassium iodide (SSKI) 5 drops tid
	IV: Sodium iodide, 1 g IV infusion over 12 h
Propranolol*	PO: 20–120 mg q4–8h
	IV: 1 mg/min to a total dose of 2–10 mg q3–4h
Dexamethasone	2 mg PO, IM, or IV q6h
Sodium ipodate	1 g/d PO

*Diltiazem 120 mg PO q8h, or equivalent parenteral dosage, may be substituted in patients with asthma.

preventing fetal hypothyroidism as a complication of treatment. PTU may be used by breast-feeding mothers. Although present in breast milk, the amount of PTU passed to the infant is insignificant at doses of ≤300 mg/d.

c. **Thyroid storm.** This is a syndrome of multisystem malfunction and fever resulting from severe hyperthyroidism. In thyroid storm, the usual symptoms and signs of hyperthyroidism are grossly exaggerated, the patient seemingly burning up with unusable energy. The temperature is usually over 38°C. Supraventricular tachycardia or atrial fibrillation is usually present and may be associated with high-output cardiac failure. Nausea, vomiting, diarrhea, and jaundice are common GI manifestations. Mental status may be unaffected in the early stages, but agitation, delirium, and coma may occur later. General supportive measures include cooling blankets and acetaminophen for fever (aspirin is contraindicated because it displaces T_4 from thyroid-binding globulin, thereby increasing the proportion of free hormone), digitalis and diuretics for heart failure, anticoagulation with heparin or coumadin for atrial fibrillation, sedatives for the management of hyperkinesis and agitation, and specific drugs for hyperthyroidism (Table 12–1). These act by several independent mechanisms to lower the concentration or mitigate the effects of thyroid hormones and are usually used in combination for **rapid control** of thyroid storm.

B. Hypothyroidism

1. GENERAL PRINCIPLES. Defects in the thyroid, pituitary, or hypothalamus can produce hypothyroidism. The most common causes of hypothyroidism are Hashimoto's thyroiditis and previous surgery or radioiodine for treatment of hyperthyroidism. Hypothyroidism due to TSH deficiency occurs as a relatively late manifestation of destructive lesions of the pituitary.

2. TREATMENT. The treatment of hypothyroidism is straightforward and effective. L-thyroxine (T_4) (Synthroid, Levothroid) is the agent of choice. Because bioavailability may vary between manufacturers, the use of generic thyroxine is not recommended. The dosage of T_4 is **1.5–1.7 µg/kg/d. Thus, for a 75-kg patient, 100–125 µg is a reasonable**

starting dosage. A reduction of 25–50 μg might be necessary for elderly and chronically ill patients of comparable weight. Thyroid replacement therapy is best monitored by following the patient's TSH level, which should be maintained in the normal range. Treatment is begun with full replacement doses except for patients with coronary artery disease, who are usually started on lower dosages, 50 μg of L-thyroxine per day, because of the possibility of angina or cardiac arrhythmias. The dose can then be raised by 25–50 μg/d every 2 weeks.

3. SPECIAL CIRCUMSTANCES
   a. **Coronary artery disease and hypothyroidism.** The coexistence of coronary artery disease and hypothyroidism is a difficult therapeutic problem, as treatment of hypothyroidism increases myocardial oxygen demands. Angina may be exacerbated even with subtherapeutic doses of thyroxine. A trial of propranolol with small increments of thyroxine may allow gradual restoration of euthyroidism without provoking increased angina. In some cases, coronary artery bypass surgery may be required to allow return to a euthyroid state.
   b. **Myxedema coma.** Untreated, hypothyroidism can progress to myxedema coma, a state of deeply depressed metabolic activity characterized by hypothermia, bradycardia, hypoventilation, coma, and ultimately death. Measures to support circulation, ventilation, and temperature as well as thyroid hormone replacement comprise the essential foundation for treatment.
      (1) Hypotension. Severely myxedematous patients usually have diminished plasma volume requiring volume expansion with isotonic saline guided by central venous pressure monitoring. α-Adrenergic agents should be avoided.
      (2) Ventilation. Although respiratory failure may be insidious, emergency treatment may be necessary. Enlargement of the tongue, which may be associated with long-standing hypothyroidism, can lead to obstruction of the upper airway. Arterial blood gases indicating hypoventilation (i.e., a P_{CO_2} of more than 45 to 50 mm Hg) or upper airway obstruction by an enlarged tongue require immediate placement of an endotracheal tube and assisted ventilation.
      (3) Thyroid hormone replacement is urgent and takes precedence over concerns of precipitating cardiac arrhythmias or ischemia. Thyroid hormone should be given IV, **0.3–0.5 mg of L-thyroxine** initially, with subsequent daily doses of 0.05–0.2 mg IV until the patient is stable and capable of taking oral medication. Some improvement should be apparent within 6 to 12 hours.
      (4) Adrenocorticoid administration. Glucocorticoids should be administered (100 mg of hydrocortisone IV q8h) and tapered gradually over a period of 10 days to 2 weeks.

C. Palpable Abnormalities of the Thyroid
   1. SOLITARY THYROID NODULE. A palpable thyroid nodule is present in about 4% to 7% of the adult population. The low incidence (3% to 4%) of malignancy and relative benign behavior of most thyroid cancers

argues for a conservative approach to the evaluation of the solitary thyroid nodule. Features of the history and physical examination that might raise suspicion of malignancy include nodules in patients at the extremes of age, particularly males, prior neck radiation, family history of thyroid cancer, rapid tumor growth, lymphadenopathy, fixation to adjacent structures, and vocal cord paralysis. Surgery might be considered as the initial approach to patients with these high-risk features. For other patients, the most cost-effective, accurate, and direct means of differentiating malignant from benign nodules is by fine needle aspiration biopsy. Patients with benign cytology should be examined every 6 to 12 months for changes in size or shape of the nodule. Any increase in the size of the nodule should reopen the question of malignancy even if the biopsy result was negative. Recent evidence suggests that short-term exogenous thyroxine has no significant effect on the growth of thyroid nodules.

If the biopsy shows malignant cells, surgery is indicated. The usual procedure is a subtotal thyroidectomy, with resection of the involved lobe, isthmus, and most of the opposite lobe, being careful not to damage the parathyroids or recurrent laryngeal nerve. On the day after surgery, L-triiodothyronine (T_3, Cytomel) 25 mg tid is started. At 6 to 8 weeks after surgery, Cytomel is stopped; 2 weeks later, the patient is treated with 30–100 mCi of ^{131}I, which will ablate remaining thyroid tissue in 80% of patients. A follow-up RAI uptake and scan are done a year later, and patients with persistent RAI uptake are retreated with ^{131}I. Lifelong treatment with thyroid hormone replacement is mandatory.

2. NONTOXIC GOITER. A small, diffuse, nontoxic goiter in a young person may remain small and asymptomatic, may evolve into a multinodular goiter, or may become hypofunctional. Measurement of TSH can help to determine appropriate therapy, as even a slight elevation may contribute to gland growth or indicate mild thyroid insufficiency. In either case, thyroxine therapy may prevent the progression to clinical thyroid disease.

If the TSH is normal, a small (i.e., nonvisible) goiter may be simply followed with serial measurements of gland size. For a large or enlarging goiter, treatment with thyroxine and regular follow-up are recommended.

Blum M. Myxedema coma. Am J Med Sci 1972;264:432.

Gharib H, James EM, Charboneau JW, et al. Suppressive therapy with levothyroxine for solitary thyroid nodules: a double-blind controlled clinical study. N Engl J Med 1987;317:70–75.

Helfand M, Crapo LM. Monitoring therapy in patients taking levothyroxine. Ann Intern Med 1990;113:450–454.

Hennemann G, Krenning EP, Sankaranarayanan K. Place of radioactive iodine in treatment of thyrotoxicosis. Lancet 1986, pp. 1369–1371.

Ingbar SH. The thyroid gland. In: Wilson JD, Foster DW, eds. Williams Textbook of Endocrinology, 7th ed. Philadelphia: WB Saunders, 1985.

Larsen PR. The thyroid. In: Wyngaarden JB, Smith LH, eds. Cecil's Textbook of Medicine, 17th ed. Philadelphia: WB Saunders, 1985, pp 1275–1299.

Sawin CT, Surks MI, London M, et al. Oral thyroxine: variation in biologic action and tablet content. Ann Intern Med 1984;100:641.

III. ADRENAL DISEASE

A. Adrenal Insufficiency

1. GENERAL PRINCIPLES. Adrenal insufficiency may result from destruction of the adrenal cortex (Addison's disease), congenital enzyme deficiency (congenital adrenal hyperplasia), or pituitary disease with ACTH deficiency. The most common cause of adrenal insufficiency is suppression of the hypothalamic-pituitary-adrenal (HPA) axis by therapeutic glucocorticoids. Recovery from HPA suppression is slow, and patients remain at risk for adrenal insufficiency during periods of stress for as long as a year after discontinuing glucocorticoid therapy. Chronic adrenal insufficiency usually occurs insidiously, the usual symptoms being fatigue, anorexia with weight loss, hypotension, and hypoglycemia. In contrast, adrenal crisis is a dramatic, life-threatening condition characterized by prostration, hypotension, fever, and electrolyte disorders that, if untreated, can progress rapidly to shock and death.

2. TREATMENT

   a. **Chronic adrenal insufficiency.** Patients with primary adrenal insufficiency **(Addison's disease)** lack all three classes of adrenal corticosteroids: glucocorticoids, mineralocorticoids, and androgens. Prednisone, 7.5 mg/d (5 mg in AM, 2.5 mg in PM), or hydrocortisone, 30 mg/d (20 mg in AM, 10 mg in PM), provides physiologic replacement of glucocorticoid with adjustments for very large or small persons or in patients taking drugs that increase the metabolic clearance of glucocorticoids, such as phenytoin, barbiturates, and rifampin. The adequacy of glucocorticoid replacement is indicated by restoration of the patient's sense of well-being, appetite, and weight and resolution of hyperpigmentation. Hyponatremia suggests inadequate glucocorticoid replacement. Insomnia or cushingoid features may be signs of excess glucocorticoid dose. For mineralocorticoid replacement in patients with adrenal insufficiency (signaled by volume depletion or hyperkalemia or both), the synthetic mineralocorticoid fludrocortisone (Florinef) is usually given as a single daily dose of 0.05–0.3 mg. Hypertension, hypokalemia, edema, or congestive heart failure calls for a reduction in dosage. Changes in fludrocortisone dosage are usually made in increments of 0.05 mg/d.

   The primary goal in patients with adrenal insufficiency is the prevention of adrenal crisis. At the first sign of illness (including minor infections, such as gastroenteritis and febrile viral syndromes), patients should double their maintenance dose of steroid. If vomiting precludes the use of oral steroids, arrangements must be made immediately for parenteral administration of corticosteroids. Patients should wear a bracelet or necklace identifying them as having adrenal insufficiency. An injectable form of glucocorticoid, such as dexamethasone phosphate (4 mg), should be taken along whenever the patient is out of reach of medical attention.

   b. **Acute adrenal insufficiency (adrenal crisis).** Glucocorticoid requirements increase dramatically during stress. During events such as surgery, infection, or trauma, persons with adrenal or pituitary insufficiency are at risk of developing adrenal crisis. The diagnosis of adrenal crisis must be made on clinical grounds because treatment cannot wait for laboratory confirmation of the diagnosis. After a blood sample is taken (to measure serum cortisol and possibly ACTH levels later), treatment is started immediately.

Hydrocortisone, the steroid preparation of choice for acute adrenal insufficiency, is given 100 mg IV, followed by an infusion of 100 mg q8h. IV is continued for 48 hours, after which oral hydrocortisone can usually be substituted in a dose of 50 mg q8h for the next 2 days. Initial fluid replacement is 5% dextrose and isotonic saline (D_5NS), given at a rate of 250–500 mL/h for the first several hours, until the extracellular volume deficit is corrected. Patients with adrenal insufficiency may have a ≥10% deficit in extracellular volume and require 4 to 6 L of fluid in the first 24 hours. Serum sodium and potassium levels need to be monitored frequently during the early stages of treatment. If the serum potassium is greater than 6.9 mEq/L (or over 6.5 mEq/L in a patient with cardiac arrhythmia), 2 ampules (89 mEq total) of sodium bicarbonate should be added to each liter of IV $D_5\frac{1}{2}NS$ until the potassium drops to a safer level.

c. **Perioperative management.** Patients with known or suspected adrenal insufficiency (including those receiving exogenous steroids) require high doses of glucocorticoid to withstand the stress of anesthesia and surgery. Hydrocortisone 100 mg IV should be given in the morning of surgery, followed by hydrocortisone 100 mg IV q8h given over the day of surgery. In uncomplicated cases, the dosage may be reduced by 50% each day thereafter until maintenance dosage is achieved.

d. **Steroid treatment and withdrawal.** When glucocorticoids are used as pharmacologic agents in doses exceeding physiologic replacement, suppression of the HPA axis occurs. The degree is a function of the dose and duration of therapy. The correlation between the dose and duration of steroid therapy potential HPA axis suppression is shown in Table 12–2. The patient may remain at risk for adrenal insufficiency during periods of stress for months after steroids have

TABLE 12–2. **Relationship Between Dose and Duration of Prednisone Therapy and Adrenal Suppression**

DOSE	DURATION			
	1 wk	1 mo	6 mo	1 y
Replacement (<7.5 mg/d)	–	–	–	–
Alternate day (any dose)	–	–	–	–
10 mg/d*	–	–	±	+
15 mg/d*	–	±	+	++
>30 mg/d*	+	++	+++	+++

From Thygeson M. Glucocorticoid withdrawal. In: Metz R, Larson E, eds. Bluebook of Endocrinology. Philadelphia: WB Saunders, 1985.

*Single daily dose in the morning. Pluses and minuses indicated likelihood of adrenal suppression: – rare; ± some patients; + many patients; ++ most patients; +++ all patients.

been discontinued. In a patient who has previously received steroids, adrenal responsiveness to stress can be assessed by measuring cortisol before and after an infusion of synthetic ACTH (cosyntropin). A normal response (stimulated plasma cortisol >18 µg/dL 60 minutes after 250 µg cosyntropin IV) implies that steroid coverage during surgery is not necessary. An alternative and perhaps more practical approach is to simply provide steroid coverage for any patient who has received pharmacologic doses of steroids in the previous year.

When glucocorticoids are no longer required for the treatment of an illness, they should be discontinued. The major concern during and after steroid withdrawal is the development of acute adrenal insufficiency. The stress of an acute illness or injury may precipitate adrenal crisis in patients with adrenal suppression. If therapeutic steroids are to be discontinued, the main issue is whether to reduce the dose gradually. Tapering the dose of steroids does not protect patients from adrenal crisis or steroid withdrawal symptoms but does delay eventual recovery of the HPA axis. The rate at which steroids are withdrawn should be based on the dose of steroid necessary to maintain remission. Gradual reductions in dose are more useful in situations when the goal is to find the lowest dose required for optimal control of disease. Steroids should be reinstituted if the patient develops an intercurrent illness or signs of adrenal insufficiency, such as hypotension, fever, nausea, and vomiting.

B. Hyporeninemic Hypoaldosteronism

1. **GENERAL PRINCIPLES.** Isolated aldosterone deficiency is most often due to a deficiency or impaired function in renin, that is, hyporeninemic hypoaldosteronism. The typical patient with this condition is elderly and diabetic and has mild renal insufficiency with hyperkalemia, hyperchloremic acidosis, mild elevation of serum creatinine, and the absence of alternative explanations for hyperkalemia. Blood pressure may be high, normal, or low.

2. **TREATMENT.** When hyperkalemia is severe enough to need therapy, treatment depends on the patient's blood pressure. If the patient is hypertensive, a loop diuretic such as furosemide lowers blood pressure and tends to reverse the hyperkalemia. With normal or low blood pressure, fludrocortisone (Florinef) provides mineralocorticoid replacement, reversing the hyperkalemia and acidosis. The dose of fludrocortisone may need to be higher than for adrenal insufficiency, over 0.2 mg/d.

   Beta blockers, prostaglandin synthetase inhibitors, angiotensin-converting enzyme inhibitors, potassium-sparing diuretics, and potassium supplements may exacerbate hyperkalemia and should be avoided.

C. Adrenocortical Excess (Cushing's Syndrome)

1. **GENERAL PRINCIPLES.** Cushing's syndrome can result from pituitary overproduction of ACTH (Cushing's disease), a benign or malignant cortisol-producing adrenal tumor, or ectopic production of ACTH. Thus, the first step in Cushing's syndrome therapy is to identify its cause.

Restoring normal adrenal function in patients with Cushing's syndrome is not always possible, and in some cases, treatment may leave the patient with temporary or permanent cortisol deficiency.

2. **TREATMENT**

a. **Pituitary Cushing's syndrome (Cushing's disease).** See treatment of Cushing's disease under Hormone-Producing Pituitary Disorders.

b. **Adrenal neoplasm.** Surgical removal of a functional benign adrenocortical tumor will cure Cushing's syndrome. Postoperatively, patients have temporary adrenal insufficiency due to atrophy of the contralateral adrenal gland, and they should be treated for adrenal insufficiency after the overactive adrenal is removed. Glucocorticoid therapy can be tapered and withdrawn over a period of several months. Adrenal carcinomas are usually unresectable at the time of diagnosis. In these patients the adrenolytic agent o,p',DDD can retard tumor growth as well as lower cortisol production, although toxicity may limit its usefulness. The starting dosage is 250 mg qid, increased gradually to tolerance or 24 g daily, as required to induce and maintain remission. Hypoadrenalism may accompany the use of o,p',DDD, in which case corticosteroids are given concomitantly. Ketoconazole, metyrapone, and aminoglutethimide, drugs that block cortisol production, can also be used to lower the cortisol level in patients with adrenal carcinoma.

c. **Ectopic ACTH.** Ectopic ACTH production with Cushing's syndrome may occur in a number of tumors, most commonly oat cell carcinoma of the lung, bronchial carcinoid, and pancreatic islet cell tumors. The ideal treatment of Cushing's syndrome due to ectopic ACTH production is removal of the underlying malignancy. If the tumor is unresectable, drugs that block cortisol production can benefit the symptoms of Cushing's syndrome. Ketoconazole, the antifungal agent, also inhibits adrenal steroid synthesis and, in doses up to 1200 mg/d, may normalize serum cortisol levels. The drug is given PO in four divided doses, beginning at 600 mg/d. Elevated serum transaminase levels can occur and rarely an idiosyncratic hepatitis may develop. A second agent can be added if cortisol levels are not controlled on 1200 mg/d. Metyrapone, an inhibitor of 11β-hydroxylase, in doses of 250–500 mg tid, will normalize cortisol level in many patients. Aminoglutethimide blocks the conversion of cholesterol to Δ-5-pregnenolone and, in doses of 250–500 mg qid, can be used to suppress excess cortisol production. Both agents can produce adrenal insufficiency, and serial measurements of serum or urine cortisol levels should be used to determine dosage.

D. Pheochromocytoma

This is a tumor of the adrenal medulla or the extraadrenal chromaffin system, present in approximately 0.1% of patients with persistent diastolic hypertension. About 10% are bilateral or multiple, and nearly 10% are malignant. The medical treatment of pheochromocytoma involves preparing the patient for surgery. Careful preoperative medical management of blood pressure and volume status is essential to prevent complications. These patients are often hypertensive, vasoconstricted, and volume depleted.

Removal of the tumor without proper premedication can result in hypotension and shock. Use of adrenergic blocking agents before surgery reverses the effects of excessive catecholamines. α-Adrenergic blocking agents lower blood pressure and reexpand blood volume. **Oral phenoxybenzamine,** a long-acting alpha blocker, is preferred. The starting dose is 10 mg bid, increased by 10–20 mg/d to a maximum of 200 mg/d or until the blood pressure is stabilized. Even patients with normal blood pressure should be so treated before surgery to avoid sudden volume reexpansion when the tumor is removed. Extra saline may be needed to maintain normal upright blood pressure as the intravascular space expands. A 1 to 2 week period of adrenergic blockade is usually recommended before surgery. Propranolol, 10–40 mg q6h, may be added if tachycardia or atrial arrhythmias occur and should be given only after adequate α blockade has taken place.

For unresectable tumors, metyrosine (α-methyl-*para*-tyrosine), an inhibitor of tyrosine hydroxylase, can reduce catecholamine production by 50% to 80%. Metyrosine is administered PO in an initial dose of 250 mg qid, with daily increments of 250–500 mg. The maximal recommended dosage is 4 g daily.

Aron DC, Findling JW, Fitzgerald PA, et al. Cushing's syndrome: problems in management. Endocr Rev 1982;3:229–244.

Baxter JD. Adrenocortical hypofunction. In: Wyngaarden JB, Smith LH, eds. Cecil's Textbook of Medicine, 17th ed. Philadelphia: WB Saunders; 1985, pp 1425–1430.

Bayliss RIS. Adrenal cortex. Clin Endocrinol Metab 1980;9:477–486.

Boggan JE, Tyrrell JB, Wilson CB. Transsphenoidal microsurgical management: report of 100 cases of Cushing's disease. J Neurosurg 1983;59:195–200.

Bondy PK. Disorders of the adrenal cortex. In: Wilson JD, Foster DW, eds. Williams Textbook of Endocrinology, 7th ed. Philadelphia: WB Saunders; 1985.

Bravo EL, Gifford RW. Pheochromocytoma: diagnosis, localization and management. N Engl J Med 1984;311:1298–1303.

Schambelan M, Sebastian A. Hyporeninemic hypoaldosteronism. Adv Intern Med 1979;24: 385–405.

Schteingart DE. Cushing's syndrome. Endocrinol Metab Clin North Am 1989;18:311–330.

IV. HIRSUTISM

1. **GENERAL PRINCIPLES.** The definition of hirsutism, excessive androgen-dependent hair in women, is to some extent subjective and depends on both cultural standards of beauty and the patient's self-image. Mild to moderate hirsutism of gradual onset is rarely a sign of serious illness and usually is a cosmetic rather than a medical problem. If in addition to hirsutism there is evidence of masculinization or virilization, a serious disorder is present. Signs of virilization include temporal balding, thinning of scalp hair, deepening of the voice, male body habitus, and clitoromegaly. Treatment depends on the cause. Congenital adrenal hyperplasia is treated with physiologic doses of glucocorticoids. Ovarian or adrenal neoplasms are treated surgically.

2. **TREATMENT.** In most cases this should be limited to simple cosmetic measures, such as bleaching. Shaving, although unappealing to most women, is effective and does not increase the rate of hair growth. Depilatory waxes and creams can be effective but may cause skin sensitization. Electrolysis results in permanent removal of individual hair follicles but is expensive and uncomfortable and requires many

treatments to produce a noticeable effect. When hirsutism is severe, widespread, or psychologically distressing, medical therapy may be helpful.

a. **Spironolactone.** This interferes with testosterone synthesis and also competes with testosterone for cytosol and nuclear receptors in androgen-sensitive tissues, including hair follicles. Most patients with simple hirsutism have improvement, usually within 6 months, when treated with spironolactone in doses of 100–200 mg/d in divided doses. Side effects include menstrual irregularity and breast tenderness.

b. **Oral contraceptive agents (OCAs).** Ovarian androgen production is stimulated by LH, and estrogen and progesterone suppress it, thus producing a fall in ovarian androgen output. Oral contraceptive therapy is effective in only about 30% of patients. When contraception is desirable, OCAs are suitable agents for treatment of hirsutism, either alone or in combination with spironolactone. Of the progestins contained in the OCA, ethynodiol diacetate has less androgenic potential than norethindrone acetate.

c. **Dexamethasone.** Dexamethasone is the drug of choice for hirsutism of congenital adrenal hyperplasia (CAH). In addition to the typical case of CAH, which involves precocious puberty and virilization at an early age, a milder variant, late-onset 21-hydroxylase deficiency, may produce hirsutism that appears after puberty. In this condition, dexamethasone in a daily dose of 0.5 mg at bedtime has been uniformly successful. Dexamethasone at this dose does not generally depress the ACTH-adrenal response to stress. The effect of glucocorticoid suppression in simple hirsutism has generally been disappointing.

Biffignandi P, Massucchetti C, Molinatti GM. Female hirsutism: pathophysiological considerations and therapeutic implications. Endocrinol Rev 1984;5:498–509.

Ehrmann DA, Rosenfield RL. An endocrinologic approach to the patient with hirsutism. J Clin Endocrinol Metab 1990;71:1–4.

V. MENOPAUSE

1. **GENERAL PRINCIPLES.** The decline in estrogen levels that occurs at menopause can be associated with a number of effects, including hot flashes, emotional lability, atrophy of the urogenital tissues, and the long-term risk of osteoporosis and its consequences, vertebral compression fractures and hip fractures, as well as coronary artery disease. Estrogen replacement therapy can be used to relieve specific symptoms and to help preserve bone mass and urogenital tissue. If estrogens are given for treatment of hot flashes, therapy should be discontinued every 12 to 18 months to see if continued treatment is necessary. Atrophic vaginitis may require treatment for several years. To be maximally effective in treatment and prophylaxis of osteoporosis, estrogens should be started early after menopause and continued indefinitely. Whatever the indications for estrogens, the goals of treatment should be discussed with the patient and her preferences incorporated in the treatment plan. Past history of uterine or breast cancer and history of venous thromboembolic disease or gallbladder

disease are contraindications to estrogen use. The unopposed use of estrogens is associated with a 3-fold to 8-fold increase in incidence of uterine malignancy. Progestational agents antagonize the proliferative effect of estrogen on the endometrium and, when given in conjunction with estrogen, reduce the risk of endometrial carcinoma.

2. TREATMENT. Women who have had a hysterectomy should take estrogens daily, starting with a dose of 0.625 mg conjugated estrogen (Premarin). If hot flashes persist, the dose should be increased to 1.25 mg/d. For women with an intact uterus, a progestational drug, such as medroxyprogesterone (Provera), should be given in association with estrogen. One schedule of administration is to give estrogen cyclically 25 days per month, with progesterone (Provera 10 mg) given on days 15 to 25. Both hormones are withheld for the last 5 days of the month. On this regimen, most women will have withdrawal bleeding during the 5 days off hormones; bleeding at other times during the cycle is abnormal and if recurrent should be evaluated with an endometrial biopsy. An alternative to cyclic administration is to give estrogen and progesterone daily in combination (Premarin 0.625–1.25 mg and Provera 2.5–5 mg/d). This combination is preferred by most women, as it does not cause withdrawal bleeding and is easier to remember. Breakthrough bleeding can occur with the initiation of continuous therapy and is easily controlled by increasing the progestin dosage. The bone-sparing effect of estrogens occurs with doses of 0.625 mg conjugated estrogen (Premarin) or ≥25 µg ethinyl estradiol. Although estrogen by injection is effective, it offers no advantages over oral administration and is less cost effective. Symptoms of urogenital atrophy can be effectively treated with estrogen vaginal cream 1 g 2 to 3 times a week. Transdermal estrogen (Estraderm) requires only twice-a-week administration.

Gambrell RD Jr. The menopause: benefits and risks of estrogen-progesterone replacement therapy. Fertil Steril 1982;37:457–474.

Hammond CB, Maxson WS. Current status of estrogen therapy for the menopause. Fertil Steril 1982;37:5–25.

Prough SG, Aksel S, Wiebe RH, Sheperd J. Continuous estrogen/progestin therapy in menopause. Am J Obstet Gynecol 1987;157:1449–1453.

VI. CALCIUM DISORDERS

A. Hypercalcemia

1. GENERAL PRINCIPLES. Conditions that cause hypercalcemia vary in pathogenesis and treatment. Hypercalcemia, even when asymptomatic and found incidentally on routine blood testing, can be associated with long-term sequelae, such as kidney stones and osteoporosis. More severe hypercalcemia can cause lethargy, anorexia, constipation, and eventually death from obtundation or cardiac arrhythmia. The two most common causes of hypercalcemia are hyperparathyroidism and malignancy. Ideally, treatment of hypercalcemia is directed toward curing its underlying cause. Surgical removal of a parathyroid adenoma cures the hypercalcemia of hyperparathyroidism. A serum calcium concentration of greater than 14 mg/dL requires immediate therapy.

TABLE 12–3. **Emergency Treatment of Hypercalcemia**

Saline diuresis	Up to 6 L isotonic saline IV over 24 h with furosemide, 40–100 mg IV q2–4h as needed, to maintain a urine output of 200–300 mL/h (electrolytes and volume status must be monitored closely)
Mithramycin	25 µg/kg body weight by IV bolus or infusion; repeat q24–72h only as needed
Pamidronate	60–90 mg IV over 24 h
Glucocorticoids	Prednisone, 40–100 mg PO in divided doses, or hydrocortisone, 200–400 mg/d IV infusion
Calcitonin	25–50 U q6–8h SC, IM, IV (concomitant use of glucocorticoids may prolong effect of calcitonin)
Phosphate	Fleet's Phospha-soda (3.3 g sodium phosphate per 5 mL), 5 mL PO or PR tid or qid, to keep serum phosphate in normal range (use only if serum phosphate is low)
Dialysis	Hemodialysis or peritoneal dialysis with calcium-free dialysis fluid; first choice in hypercalcemia complicated by severe renal failure

2. TREATMENT. Several agents are generally used in combination for rapid lowering of serum calcium. (Table 12–3).

   a. **Forced saline diuresis.** Since many patients are volume depleted initially, normal saline should be infused until intravascular volume is normal. This is followed by a forced saline diuresis using furosemide to accelerate calcium excretion. Careful monitoring of electrolytes is mandatory, as potassium and magnesium depletion is likely to occur. In some patients, central venous pressure monitoring may be needed.

   b. **Mithramycin.** The cytotoxic antibiotic mithramycin is effective in treatment of hypercalcemia of any cause. A single dose of up to 25 µg/kg IV over 30 minutes will normalize serum calcium in 75% of hypercalcemic patients within 48 hours. This can persist for about a week. Subsequent doses of mithramycin should be withheld until and unless calcium begins to rise again, as the duration of calcium-lowering activity varies and depends partially on other steps taken to lower calcium. The toxic effects of mithramycin (thrombocytopenia, hepatic and renal toxicity) are rarely seen when only one or two doses are given.

   c. **Bisphosphonates.** As an inhibitor of bone resorption, **pamidronate** is first choice because of its efficacy and single dose convenience. An infusion of 60–90 mg IV over 24 hours will normalize calcium in 70% to 90% of patients. Its effect can persist for several weeks, and transient fevers and myalgias occur in 20% of patients. Etidronate disodium **(Didronel),** given IV at a dose of 7.5 mg/kg/d for 3 to 7 days will correct calcemia in about 60% of patients. In contrast to pamidronate, etidronate disodium can cause a significant rise in both phosphate and creatinine.

   d. **Glucocorticoids.** Glucocorticoids in pharmacologic doses increase urinary calcium excretion and decrease calcium absorption from the intestine. They are effective in treating hypercalcemia associated with myeloma, sarcoidosis, and occasionally breast cancer but have little effect on serum calcium in patients with primary hyperparathyroidism. Because their maximum calcium-lowering effect may not occur for several days, glucocorticoids should be used in conjunction with other modes of therapy for acute hypercalcemia.

e. **Calcitonin.** This inhibits release of calcium from bone and increases renal calcium excretion. By itself, calcitonin (4–8 IU/kg SC or IM q12h) is only mildly effective, and escape from its calcium-lowering effect is usually seen within the first hours or days of use. However, the concomitant use of glucocorticoids appears to block this escape phenomenon. The potential advantages of calcitonin are the rapid (although mild) therapeutic effect and lack of toxicity.

f. **Phosphates.** Oral phosphate will lower serum calcium and may be useful in the treatment of hypercalcemia associated with a low or normal serum phosphate. The deliberate induction of hyperphosphatemia by IV or high-dose oral phosphate has been advocated, but this protocol is not recommended because of the risks of hypocalcemia and metastatic calcification.

g. **Gallium nitrate.** Studies indicate that bone resorption is inhibited at doses of 200 mg/m^2/d IV for 5 days. Normalization of calcium occurs in 60% to 70% of patients, with mean duration of response noted at 7 days.

B. Hypocalcemia

1. GENERAL PRINCIPLES. Hypocalcemia may occur with either acute or chronic symptoms, depending on the level and rate of fall of serum calcium. Chronic mild hypocalcemia may lead to cataracts, calcification of the basal ganglia, and metastatic calcification of soft tissues. Tetany, seizures, and laryngospasm requiring immediate diagnosis and treatment may be the first manifestations of hypocalcemia. Acute hypocalcemia is most often seen in hospitalized patients after removal of or damage to the parathyroid glands during neck surgery. Hypocalcemia due to other causes is usually mild and typically involves chronic symptoms, such as fatigue, myalgias, muscle cramps, or cataracts.

2. TREATMENT
   a. **Chronic hypocalcemia.** Treatment usually requires a combination of supplemental calcium and vitamin D. The treatment regimen must be individualized and followed carefully. Correction of hypocalcemia of hypoparathyroidism usually requires vitamin D in doses of 50,000–150,000 U/d along with 0.5–2 g elemental calcium per day. Calcium and vitamin D in these doses frequently induce hypercalciuria and, with it, a risk of calcium stone formation. Drug dosage should be adjusted to maintain the serum calcium in the low-normal range while at the same time avoiding excessive urinary calcium excretion (24-hour urine calcium >4 mg/kg/d). A thiazide diuretic and restricted sodium diet can help to reduce urinary calcium losses. In renal insufficiency, 1,25(OH)$_2$ vitamin D (calcitriol, Rocaltrol), 0.5–2 μg/d, is preferred to vitamin D for the treatment of hypocalcemia. Serum calcium levels must be monitored frequently,

TABLE 12–4. **Sources of Calcium Supplementation**

SOURCE	ELEMENTAL CALCIUM (mg)	DAILY DOSAGE*
Calcium lactate (650 mg tablet)	85	18 tablets
Calcium gluconate (1 g tablet)	90	17 tablets
Calcium carbonate (Tums tablets)	200	7 tablets
Oyster shell calcium (Tums E-X tablets)	300	5 tablets
Os-cal 250 tablet	250	6 tablets
Os-cal 500 tablet	500	3 tablets
Milk (1 cup)	300	1¼ quarts

*No. of tablets needed to provide 1500 mg elemental calcium per day.

especially at the onset of treatment because of the danger of hypercalcemia.

b. **Acute hypocalcemia.** Tetany, laryngospasm, or seizures require immediate treatment with IV calcium **(10% calcium gluconate).** Initially, 10–30 mL are infused over 10 to 15 minutes. If the patient can swallow, oral calcium should be given in a dose of 200 mg q2h, increasing to 500 mg q2h if necessary. The calcium content of various calcium preparations is listed in Table 12–4. If the patient is unable to swallow or if tetany returns within 6 hours, administration of calcium by continuous IV infusion is indicated. 1 g of calcium (approximately 100 mL of 10% calcium gluconate) is added to 1 L of a 5% dextrose solution and infused at a rate sufficient to prevent tetany—usually between 30 and 100 mL/h. Serum magnesium should be measured because hypomagnesemia may inhibit both the release and action of parathyroid hormone. If the magnesium level is low (less than 0.8 mg/L), magnesium sulfate is given IV (1–2 g $MgSO_4$ as a 10% solution over 15 minutes) or by IM injection (1 g of 50% solution q4h) until the magnesium level has returned to normal. Once stabilized, the patient may, depending on the cause of hypocalcemia, need to be started on vitamin D in addition to calcium.

Arnaud CD. The parathyroid glands, hypercalcemia and hypocalcemia. In: Wyngaarden JB, Smith LH, eds. Cecil's Textbook of Medicine, 17th ed. Philadelphia: WB Saunders, 1985, pp 1425–1430.

Ryzen E, Martodarm RR, Traxel M, et al. Intravenous etidronate in the management of malignant hypercalcemia. Arch Intern Med 1985;145:449–452.

Schneider AB, Sherwood LM. Pathogenesis and management of hypoparathyroidism. Metabolism 1975;24:871.

Scholz DA, Purnell DC. Asymptomatic primary hyperparathyroidism: 10-year prospective study. Mayo Clin Proc 1981;56:473–478.

Singer FR, Fernandez M. Therapy of hypercalcemia and malignancy. Am J Med 1987;82:34–41.

Suki WN, Yium JJ, Von Minden M, et al. Acute treatment of hypercalcemia with furosemide. N Engl J Med 1970;283:836.

VII. METABOLIC BONE DISEASE

Pathologic loss of bone mineral density is most often due to osteoporosis or osteomalacia. These two disorders differ in both their pathogenesis and treatment. Osteoporosis, an age-related thinning of bone, is primarily a disease of postmenopausal women, 25% of whom will experience wrist, vertebral, or hip fracture after age 65. Osteomalacia, a defect in calcification of bone osteoid, is associated with low levels of circulating vitamin D. Conditions that interfere with intestinal absorption of vitamin D or hydroxylation of vitamin D in the liver or kidney may be associated with reduced levels of activated vitamin D and osteomalacia. Certain drugs may contribute to osteopenia. Glucocorticoids interfere with GI absorption of calcium and inhibit bone formation, and their extended use can be associated with the development of osteopenia. Phenytoin and the barbiturates interfere with the 25-hydroxylation of vitamin D in the liver, leading to osteomalacia in some patients.

A. Osteoporosis

1. NONPHARMACOLOGIC THERAPY. Risk factors for primary osteoporosis include sedentary lifestyle, excess alcohol consumption, and smoking. Eliminating these factors is the first step in treating postmenopausal osteoporosis. A regular exercise program is particularly helpful in maintaining bone mineral density. Elderly people should be encouraged to walk or swim regularly. Early restoration of mobility after a period of enforced bed rest should also be encouraged.

2. CALCIUM. Ensuring an adequate calcium intake is a basic requirement of any therapeutic regimen. The premenopausal female requires 1000 mg/d of calcium to maintain calcium balance, and the estrogen-deficient woman needs 1500 mg/d to meet this goal (Table 12–4).

3. ESTROGENS. Estrogens slow postmenopausal bone loss, and the bone-protecting effect of estrogen occurs with doses of 0.625 mg of conjugated estrogen (Premarin) or ≥25 μg of ethinyl estradiol. Estrogens are contraindicated in women with a history of breast or endometrial cancer, venous thromboembolic episodes, or gallbladder disease. Blood pressure should be monitored in women taking estrogens. Transdermal estrogen is preferable in women with elevated triclycerides so as to avoid the first-pass hepatic effect on lipid synthesis.

4. BISPHOSPHONATES. These drugs suppress bone resorption by limiting osteoclast access to resorptive areas and by inhibition of osteoclast cellular activity. When they are given as prescribed, bone mineralization is not impaired. Alendronate sodium **(Fosamax)** at 10 mg PO daily taken 30 minutes before breakfast is well tolerated, increases bone mass, and causes a 50% reduction in new vertebral fractures. This drug has supplanted previous use of intermittent, cyclical etidronate, and newer, more potent bisphosphonates are under investigation.

5. CALCITONIN. **Miacalcin,** a nasal spray calcitonin, in a dose of 200 U (one puff) daily, will decrease bone turnover and preserve bone mass in osteoporotic women. It is thus far difficult to draw conclusions about its effect on bone fracture rate, but a large study addressing this issue is near completion. Several studies have shown this drug to have analgesic effects, and it may prove beneficial for women with chronic back pain from fractures.

6. **OTHER AGENTS.** Studies have shown that daily **vitamin D 800 IU** (i.e., two multivitamins) plus calcium reduce hip fracture rate with no toxicity and should be offered to all postmenopausal women. Conventional sodium fluoride is not recommended, as it has not been shown to reduce fracture rate, but a slow-release formulation of fluoride is under consideration for approval by the FDA based on one new compelling study showing clinical efficacy. Promising new treatments not currently available include the antiestrogen raloxifene and intermittent, synthetic parathyroid hormone therapy.

7. **RECOMMENDATIONS.** Calcium supplements are virtually free of side effects and should be recommended to women of all ages as a means of reducing the risk of osteoporosis. In the absence of contraindications, estrogens should be prescribed for postmenopausal women with osteoporosis and those at increased risk because of race, body habitus, diet, family history, or lifestyle. In women who cannot or will not take estrogen, alendronate is a reasonable alternative for established osteoporosis but currently is not approved for the prevention of osteoporosis. Intranasal calcitonin can be used if the patient is intolerant of alendronate or as an analgesic for women with chronic back pain from osteoporotic bone fractures.

B. Osteomalacia

Osteomalacia responds dramatically to treatment with vitamin D. For patients with nutritional osteomalacia, oral vitamin D, 50,000 U once a week, is usually sufficient. For patients with more severe osteomalacia as evidenced by bone pain, extensive skeletal involvement, or markedly elevated alkaline phosphatase, initial treatment doses of vitamin D should be about 50,000 U/d. In patients with chronic renal failure, **calcitriol** (Rocaltrol, $1,25(OH)_2 D$) is used initially in a dose of 0.25 µg/d. Since calcitriol can induce hypercalcemia in just a few days, close monitoring (twice weekly) of the serum calcium concentration is indicated. A daily calcium intake of 1000 mg/d should accompany the vitamin D. Success in treating osteomalacia is indicated by a lessening of bone pain and normalization of serum calcium, phosphorus, and alkaline phosphatase. The dosage of vitamin D should be reduced when the 24-hour urine calcium approaches hypercalciuric levels, that is, over 4 mg/kg/d.

C. Drug-Induced Osteopenia

Phenytoin, barbiturates, and glucocorticoids can contribute to osteopenia—the anticonvulsants by interfering with the hydroxylation of vitamin D in the liver and glucocorticoids by inhibiting both intestinal absorption of calcium and new bone formation. If long-term treatment with these drugs is anticipated, steps to prevent bone loss should be considered, especially in older patients. Vitamin D, 50,000 IU 1 to 3 times weekly, in combination with calcium, 1–2 g/d, may retard the bone loss otherwise caused by these medications.

Liberman UA, Weiss SR, Brall J, et al. Effect of three years treatment with oral alendronate on fracture incidence in women with postmenopausal osteoporosis. N Engl J Med 1995;333:1437–1443.

Nordin BE, Heyburn PJ, Peacock M, et al. Osteoporosis and osteomalacia. Clin Endocrinol Metab 1980;9:177–205.

Overgaard K, Hansen MA, Jensen SB, et al. Effect of salcatonin given intranasally on bone mass and fracture rates in established osteoporosis: a dose-response study. Br Med J 1992;305: 556–561.

Pak CYC, Sakhaee K, Adams-Huet B, et al. Treatment of postmenopausal osteoporosis with slow release sodium fluoride. Ann Intern Med 1995;123:401–408.

Riggs BL, Hadgson SF, O'Fallon WM, et al. Effect of fluoride treatment on the fracture rate in postmenopausal women with osteoporosis. N Engl J Med 1990;322:802–809.

Riggs BL, Melton LJ. The prevention and treatment of osteoporosis. N Engl J Med 1992;327: 620–628.

Storm T, Thamsborg G, Steiniche T, et al. Effect of intermittent cyclical etidronate therapy on bone mass and fracture rate in women with postmenopausal osteoporosis. N Engl J Med 1990;322:1265–1271.

VIII. DIABETES MELLITUS

A. Diabetic Ketoacidosis

The basic defect in ketoacidosis is a severe deficiency of insulin with accelerated hepatic gluconeogenesis and ketogenesis, increased release of free fatty acids from adipose tissue, and decreased utilization of glucose. Hyperglycemia leads to osmotic diuresis, which produces volume and electrolyte depletion. Acidosis causes outmigration of intracellular potassium. The clinical indications of ketoacidosis include malaise, mental obtundation, nausea, and vomiting, which aggravate the volume and electrolyte depletion. Clinically, ketoacidosis is easily recognized (Table 12–5).

1. TREATMENT. This consists of (1) insulin in adequate dosage, (2) correction of fluid and electrolyte abnormalities, and (3) identification and treatment of any underlying or associated illnesses. The following measurements should be recorded on a bedside flow sheet: bedside **blood glucose test** every 1 to 2 hours and urine output measurement every 2 hours and serum pH or bicarbonate and potassium levels every 2 to 4 hours until the biochemical situation has stabilized.

2. INSULIN ADMINISTRATION. Various methods of insulin administration have been used successfully. The dose, frequency, and route of administration of insulin are probably less important than familiarity with a single protocol of proven effectiveness. Continuous IV infusion is widely used

TABLE 12–5. **Diagnosis of Diabetic Ketoacidosis**

SYMPTOMS	SIGNS	LABORATORY DATA
Polyuria, polydipsia	Tachycardia, postural	Hyperglycemia (blood
Postural dizziness	hypotension	glucose >300 mg/dL)
Anorexia, nausea, vomiting,	Drowsiness, stupor, or coma	Acidosis (pH <7.3 or serum
and abdominal pain	Kussmaul's breathing, odor	bicarbonate <15 mEq/L)
Dyspnea	of ketones on breath	Ketonemia (strongly positive
Malaise, drowsiness	Hypothermia	nitroprusside reaction in
	Facial flushing	serum diluted to half
		strength with water)

TABLE 12–6. **A Protocol for IV Insulin Administration**

1. An IV bolus of 10 U of regular insulin is given.
2. An infusion of 50 U of regular insulin in 500 mL of NS (i.e., 0.1 U of insulin per milliliter of NS) is started. The initial infusion rate is 60 mL (6 U of insulin)/h. The rate is maintained until the blood glucose level is recorded at or below 240 mg/dL. At that point, the insulin infusion rate is reduced to 30 mL (3 U)/h.
3. A separate infusion of NS is started simultaneously with the insulin infusion and administered at 500–1000 mL/h. When the blood glucose level falls below 240 mg/dL, the saline is replaced by D₅NS administered at a rate of approximately 150 mL/h.
4. With the dextrose solution running, the blood glucose level is monitored at intervals of 1 or 2 h, and the insulin infusion rate is adjusted up or down, usually 1 U/h, to maintain a blood glucose level between 100 and 240 mg/dL.
5. The course is maintained until the blood glucose level becomes stable between these limits and the patient is asymptomatic and eating normally. At that stage, the patient is given a dose of intermediate-acting insulin. If it is given in the morning, the customary daily dose is used, but if it is administered later in the day, the dose is reduced in proportion to that part of the day that has elapsed. The insulin infusion is discontinued 1–2 h after the intermediate-acting insulin is given. Booster doses of rapid-acting insulin are given at 6-h intervals, if necessary, to keep the blood glucose level below 240 mg/dL. The size of the booster doses is usually about one fourth of the usual daily dose of intermediate-acting insulin.
6. The patient is usually kept in the hospital another day or so for stabilization of the blood glucose level and observation on a maintenance insulin program.

because of its flexibility and effectiveness. We use the protocol given in Table 12–6 (dosages are for average-sized adults).

3. FLUID AND ELECTROLYTE REPLACEMENT. Patients with ketoacidosis show varying degrees of acidosis and depletion of saline, water, potassium, and phosphate. Fluid and electrolyte replacement must be individualized and guided by the results of monitoring. The degree of **volume depletion** is estimated clinically by assessing jugular vein pressure and by the degree of orthostatic hypotension. A drop in mean blood pressure of more than 20 mm Hg when the patient shifts from lying to standing indicates extracellular volume (ECV) depletion of at least 30%; in a patient weighing 70 kg, this would be 4.6 L ($70 \times 0.22 \times 0.30 = 4.6$ L).

Saline repletion is begun with NS. In the average adult patient, the initial infusion rate is 1000 mL for the first hour, then 500 mL/h until postural hypotension is corrected. At this point, 0.45% saline can be substituted for NS. As saline depletion is corrected, the infusion rate is reduced. Most adult patients with diabetic ketoacidosis require 4–5 L of fluid in the first 8 hours.

Bicarbonate therapy should be reserved for those patients with severe acidosis (a venous pH of less than 7.1). When bicarbonate is given, the initial IV solution should contain ½ NS with two ampules of sodium bicarbonate (each ampule contains 44.6 mEq bicarbonate) added per liter. Bicarbonate administration is discontinued when the serum pH reaches 7.1.

Serum **potassium** does not accurately reflect total body potassium in the presence of acidosis because of the transfer of potassium from the intracellular to the extracellular space. Most patients with ketoacidosis have profound deficits of total body potassium despite normal or even elevated serum potassium concentrations. On average, the potassium deficit in patients in diabetic ketoacidosis is approximately 5 mEq/kg of body weight (350 mEq in a 70-kg person). When the serum potassium level is elevated, potassium replacement is withheld until improvement in the acidosis brings about a fall in serum potassium into the normal range. Then, potassium chloride is added to the IV solution to deliver 10–20 mEq/h. This replacement dose is used from the beginning if the serum potassium level is normal initially. If the initial serum potassium level is low, the replacement rate should be 20–40 mEq/h. Potassium replacement must be done with caution in patients with renal failure or oliguria.

Diabetic ketoacidosis is also associated with depletion of **phosphate.** Theoretically, phosphate deficiency could delay recovery, but in practice, phosphate repletion has not been shown to be of benefit in the routine treatment of diabetic ketoacidosis.

4. IDENTIFICATION AND TREATMENT OF UNDERLYING ILLNESS. Patients develop diabetic ketoacidosis for a reason, although that reason often escapes identification. The precipitating factor may be an acute illness, such as urinary tract infection, bronchitis, pneumonia, gastroenteritis, myocardial infarction, or appendicitis. All patients should be evaluated for intercurrent illness, which, if detected, should be treated simultaneously with the ketoacidosis. Perhaps the most common cause of diabetic ketoacidosis is the failure to increase insulin dosage during the stress of minor illness.

B. Hyperglycemic, Hyperosmolar Coma

Hyperosmolar coma is less common than ketoacidosis but carries a greater risk of death. Most patients are elderly and have either no history of diabetes or mild diabetes controlled by diet or oral drugs. Hyperosmolar coma is rarely seen in patients with established insulin-dependent diabetes mellitus (Table 12–7). Focal neurologic defects and seizures are also common. Complications include vascular thrombosis, acute hepatocellular necrosis, and other sequelae of hypotension and circulatory collapse. The

---

TABLE 12–7. **Conditions that May Lead to Hyperosmolar Coma**

Drugs
  Glucocorticoids
  Phenytoin
  Thiazide diuretics
Volume loss
  Vomiting
  Diarrhea
High-glucose intake in a patient with diabetes
Renal failure
Other illnesses (infection, myocardial infarction) that increase insulin needs

overall mortality from hyperosmolar coma and the frequently present underlying illness may be as high as 50% in elderly patients.

Treatment is the same as that outlined for diabetic ketoacidosis, except for emphasis on correcting hyperosmolarity. Treatment is designed to correct volume depletion, hyperglycemia, potassium depletion, acidosis, and any precipitating illness. Establishing a well-designed flow chart and recording the amounts of insulin and IV fluids administered, as well as vital signs, fluid intake, urine output, blood glucose level, electrolytes, and creatinine concentration, are essential to proper management.

Fluid and electrolyte replacement must be tailored to the individual patient. Often the most immediate threat in hyperosmolar coma is shock from volume depletion. The degree of volume depletion is assessed by noting jugular vein distention and an orthostatic drop in blood pressure. If orthostatic hypotension is present, the ECV is decreased by at least 30% (4.6 L in a 70-kg patient). For signs of orthostatic hypotension, initial fluid therapy should be NS, 500–1000 mL/h, although faster rates may be necessary if hypotension is severe. Most patients with hyperosmolar coma require at least 5 L of saline within the first 12 hours.

After volume depletion has been corrected with NS, the infusion should be changed to 0.45% saline and continued at 500 mL/h to correct hyperosmolarity. The degree of hyperosmolarity (water depletion) may be estimated by the following formula.

$$\text{Plasma osmolarity} = 2(\text{Na} + \text{K}) + \frac{\text{glucose}}{18} + \frac{\text{blood urea nitrogen (BUN)}}{2.8}$$

(normal range: 280–300 mOsm/L)

Because most of these patients are elderly and often have diminished cardiac reserve, great care must be taken to avoid volume overload. Monitoring of central venous or pulmonary capillary wedge pressure is frequently indicated.

C. Medical and Surgical Illnesses Requiring Hospitalization

The physiologic reaction to acute illness involves release of humoral agents antagonistic to the action of insulin. Volume depletion may occur as a result of diaphoresis, anorexia, vomiting, diarrhea, or hyperglycemia-induced polyuria. These mechanisms lead to progressive hyperglycemia, ketosis, and volume depletion in patients with type I diabetes. The diabetes usually can be managed quite successfully with a straightforward protocol, the essentials of which are the following: (1) frequent monitoring of volume status and of glycemia and ketonuria (generally before meals and at bedtime if the patient is eating; every 6 hours in patients receiving IV nutrition), (2) supplemental rapid-acting insulin as indicated by the blood glucose readings, and (3) adequate intake of saline and carbohydrate.

    1. PATIENTS TREATED WITH INSULIN. The patient's usual daily insulin dose is given at the customary times. The blood glucose level is measured, and additional rapid-acting insulin is given whenever the glucose reading is ≥240 mg/dL. The dosage of supplemental rapid-acting insulin is typically one fourth of the usual total daily dosage of insulin. The goal is to maintain blood glucose concentration between 120 and 240 mg/dL.

Intake of at least 150 g of carbohydrate per 24 hours and enough saline to restore or maintain normal fluid volume is important. Patients with milder illnesses are usually able to take the requisite volume of fluid and allotment of carbohydrate by mouth.

2. PATIENTS WHOSE DIABETES IS MANAGED WITH DIET ALONE OR ORAL HYPOGLY-CEMIC AGENTS. For patients with non–insulin-dependent diabetes mellitus, the management is the same as that already described, except that no intermediate-acting insulin is given, at least initially. Rapid-acting insulin is used when the blood glucose level before meals or at bedtime is ≥240 mg/dL. Initial doses of 4, 6, or 8 U are generally effective for small-, medium-, or large-framed persons, respectively. These doses can be adjusted up or down by 2–4 U, depending on the initial therapeutic response. The dose should be adjusted to maintain the blood glucose level between 120 and 240 mg/dL.

3. PATIENTS TREATED ON CONTINUOUS SUBCUTANEOUS INSULIN INFUSION (INSULIN PUMP). Patients receiving insulin by an insulin pump can often be managed during illness in or out of hospital by increasing the insulin infusion rate. For blood glucose readings of ≥240 mg/dL, the basal rate is increased by 50%. In addition, boluses equal to the usual bolus given before dinner are administered at the 4-hour checkpoints whenever the blood glucose level is ≥240 mg/dL. The accelerated basal rate is maintained until a blood glucose reading of under 150 mg/dL is noted at a 4-hour blood glucose checkpoint.

4. BLOOD GLUCOSE MANAGEMENT DURING HYPERALIMENTATION. In the diabetic patient receiving parenteral hyperalimentation with concentrated glucose solutions, we recommend the addition of rapid-acting insulin to each liter of hyperalimentation fluid. A commonly chosen starting dose is 10 U/L. Substantially larger doses are often necessary, and amounts of 25–50 U/L sometimes are required to control hyperglycemia. Even higher doses may be needed. IV infusions of dextrose should be continued for several hours after discontinuation of hyperalimentation to prevent hypoglycemia as a result of residual insulin action.

5. MANAGEMENT OF DIABETES DURING SURGERY. The goals of diabetes management in the perioperative period are to avoid extremes of glycemia and to prevent ketosis. Blood glucose concentrations between 120 and 240 mg/dL are desirable but difficult to achieve, and in many cases, less stringent standards of between 100 and 300 mg/dL may have to be accepted.

On the morning of surgery, an IV infusion is started, using D_5 (usually in ½ NS), at 125 mg/h. The object of providing 150 g of glucose over 24 hours is to prevent excessive fat mobilization and ketone production and to protect against hypoglycemia. One half of the usual total daily dose of insulin is administered as intermediate-acting insulin (Lente or NPH). Each time the blood glucose level is ≥240 mg/dL, rapid-acting insulin is given in an amount equivalent to one fourth of the patient's usual total daily dose. This protocol is continued until the patient is able to eat, when the patient's usual insulin dose is restarted while continuing the supplemental regular dose for blood glucose concentrations of ≥240 mg/dL.

For the diabetic patient treated with oral agents or diet alone, an IV infusion is started using the same fluids and is administered at the same rate as described earlier. Blood glucose is measured every 6 hours, and rapid-acting insulin is given when the blood glucose level is ≥240 mg/dL. For the average-sized person, a dose of 6 U of rapid-acting insulin is usually adequate, but large patients or those undergoing very extensive surgery may require substantially larger doses. The oral antidiabetic agents are omitted the day of surgery and restarted only when the patient is eating again. The contingency doses of rapid-acting insulin at the 6-hour checkpoints should be continued until the blood glucose level is consistently below 240 mg/dL.

D. Iatrogenic Hypoglycemia

Patients who take insulin or an oral hypoglycemic medication can develop hypoglycemia causing confusion, stupor, coma, or convulsions. Patients with hypoglycemia and depressed levels of consciousness should not be given oral glucose because of the risk of aspiration. Glucagon, 1 mg IM, will usually correct hypoglycemia within 30 minutes by stimulating hepatic glycogenolysis. If qualified personnel are available, initial therapy in the obtunded or unconscious patient should be IV glucose, 50 mL, or 50% dextrose (D_{50}). All patients should be observed until they are fully alert and have eaten a snack or meal. Patients with hypoglycemia caused by insulin may then be sent home if they are fully capable of taking their usual meals and a bedtime snack.

Hypoglycemic coma caused by sulfonylureas may be profound and long lasting. Patients who take sulfonylureas and who have severe, symptomatic hypoglycemia should be hospitalized and kept under close observation, including frequent blood glucose monitoring, for at least 24 hours. If hypoglycemia recurs, an infusion of D_{10} should be maintained at a rate sufficient to maintain the blood glucose concentration between 100 and 200 mg/dL.

Some patients who have been profoundly hypoglycemic remain unconscious even after the blood glucose level has been restored to normal. In such patients, cerebral edema may be responsible for the persisting coma. Mannitol, 200 mL of a 20% solution given IV over 20 minutes, and dexamethasone, 10 mg IV, have been used with some apparent success in the treatment of persistent coma following hypoglycemia.

After treatment, the circumstances surrounding the episode of hypoglycemia must be reviewed with the patient, and measures to prevent recurrences must be implemented.

IX. HYPERLIPIDEMIAS

A. Hypercholesterolemia

Reducing hypercholesterolemia lowers the risk of coronary artery atherosclerosis. Two groups of experts, operating as a National Institutes of Health (NIH) Consensus Development Conference and the National Cholesterol Education Program, provided clinically useful recommendations for dealing with hypercholesterolemia.

Before deciding on a specific treatment program for the individual patient with hypercholesterolemia, the physician should follow these steps.

- Confirm the initial laboratory results. Variation in the levels of cholesterol and high-density lipoprotein cholesterol (HDLC) from both biologic and analytic causes is considerable.
- Search for specific and potentially remediable conditions that may be causing the hypercholesterolemia. Hypothyroidism, certain medications (especially thiazide diuretics and beta blockers), obstructive biliary disease, the nephrotic syndrome, diabetes, and dysproteinemia all may affect plasma cholesterol concentrations.
- Identify and eliminate other possible coronary artery disease risk factors, such as hypertension, cigarette smoking, sedentary lifestyle, and extreme obesity.
- Take into account the patient's age, attitude to therapy, response to previous therapy, if any, and presence of other conditions that may limit life expectancy in making treatment decisions.

The recommended treatment program is based on plasma cholesterol and low-density lipoprotein cholesterol (LDLC) concentrations. The total cholesterol level is used for initial case finding and for monitoring; LDLC is used for certain therapeutic decisions. LDLC is calculated by the equation given below but is only useful when the triglyceride level is less than 400.

$$LDLC = total\ cholesterol - (triglycerides \div 5 + HDLC)$$

Also taken into account in making treatment decisions are coronary artery disease risk factors, which, in addition to those already mentioned, include a family history of coronary artery disease, diabetes, and HDLC concentrations below 35 mg/dL (Fig. 12–1).

1. **DIET.** The foundation of treatment is a diet low in saturated fat and limited in cholesterol and, for overweight persons, restricted in calories. The American Heart Association has recommended that the total fat content of the diet should not exceed 30% and the saturated fat should not exceed 10% of caloric intake. Cholesterol should be limited to 300 mg/d. This is the so-called step 1 diet. If a more stringent diet is considered necessary, the step 2 diet limits the saturated fat to less than 7% of total calories and the cholesterol intake to less than 200 mg/d. Dietary therapy may be quite effective, especially in obese individuals and in patients with mixed hyperlipidemias (such as familial combined hyperlipidemia). Since the relationship between plasma cholesterol levels and atherosclerosis is less clear in patients in the seventh decade of age and beyond, it seems reasonable to be cautious about using medication in these older patients.

2. **MEDICATIONS FOR TREATING UNFAVORABLE PLASMA LIPID CONCENTRATIONS.** The primary objective of treating hypercholesterolemia is to reduce the patient's risk of atherosclerotic coronary artery disease. Therefore, raising HDLC may be at least as important as lowering total cholesterol and LDLC concentrations. Patients more suitable for treatment with the fibric acid derivatives are those with elevated triglyceride levels. The value in raising HDL levels may depend on initial lipid levels. The concomitant presence of hypercholesterolemia (unresponsive to diet)

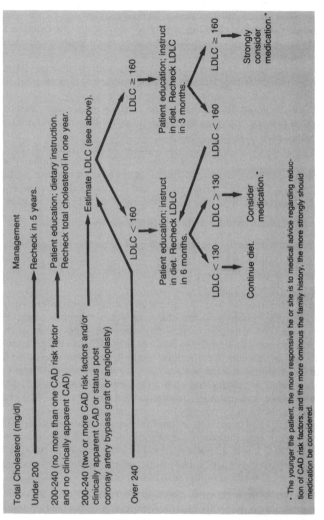

Total Cholesterol (mg/dl)   **Management**

Under 200   Recheck in 5 years.

200-240 (no more than one CAD risk factor   Patient education; dietary instruction.
and no clinically apparent CAD)   Recheck total cholesterol in one year.

200-240 (two or more CAD risk factors and/or   Estimate LDLC (see above).
clinically apparent CAD or status post
coronary artery bypass graft or angioplasty)

Over 240

LDLC < 160 → Estimate LDLC (see above).

LDLC ≥ 160 → Patient education; instruct in diet. Recheck LDLC in 6 months.

LDLC < 130 → Continue diet.

LDLC > 130 → Consider medication.*

LDLC < 160 → Patient education; instruct in diet. Recheck LDLC in 3 months.

LDLC ≥ 160 → Strongly consider medication.*

* The younger the patient, the more responsive he or she is to medical advice regarding reduction of CAD risk factors, and the more ominous the family history, the more strongly should medication be considered.

FIGURE 12-1. Therapeutic recommendations keyed to plasma cholesterol and LDLC concentrations.

would strengthen the indication for the addition of either niacin or HMG-CoA reductase inhibitors. Patients with more severely elevated plasma cholesterol concentrations might best be treated with agents that primarily reduce LDLC. Medications available are considered below.

a. **Fibric acid derivatives.** In a population of younger middle-aged men, treatment with **gemfibrozil** (600 mg bid) resulted in favorable changes in the levels of total cholesterol, LDLC, and HDLC of about 10%. Fatal and nonfatal coronary events were reduced by 34%, but there was no difference in overall mortality.

New third-generation (**clofibrate** having been the first and gemfibrozil the second generation) fibric acid derivatives, including **fenofibrate** and **bezafibrate,** may become available. The newer agents are more potent, are more effective in lowering LDLC, and still retain their capacity to raise HDLC levels. Fibric acid derivatives are almost always well tolerated, side effects being infrequent and generally mild. However, fibric acid derivatives can increase the risk of gallstones and potentiate warfarin.

b. **Compactin derivatives.** These agents competitively inhibit 3-hydroxy-3-methylglutaryl coenzyme A reductase, the rate-limiting step in cholesterol synthesis. The most studied of these agents to date is **lovastatin,** which markedly reduces plasma LDL concentrations both in familial and in less clearly categorized types of hypercholesterolemia. Lovastatin will reduce LDLC by 25% to 50% in a dose-dependent fashion as well as raise the HDLC by 10% to 15%. Newer inhibitors include **pravastatin, simvastatin,** and **fluvastatin.** Efficacy profiles indicate that lovastatin and pravastatin are equipotent, simvastatin is twice as potent, and fluvastatin is half as potent. If maximal LDLC reduction is desired, simvastatin is the most cost effective. These medications are all well tolerated and share similar risk profiles. Liver function changes occur in 1% to 2%, and myalgias, especially in conjunction with gemfibrozil, can occur. In familial hypercholesterolemia, the combination of lovastatin with a bile acid-sequestrating resin appears to be considerably more effective than either agent alone.

c. **Bile acid-sequestrating resins. Cholestyramine** and **colestipol** act by binding bile salts in the intestine, thereby preventing their enterohepatic recirculation. The need for increased synthesis of bile acids depletes hepatic cholesterol, their metabolic precursor, which in turn induces upregulation of hepatic B and E apoprotein receptors. This action has the effect of enhancing LDL clearance but also induces increased hepatic cholesterol synthesis, thereby tending to limit the efficacy of these agents. Therapy is usually started with a daily dose of two or three packets, each of which contains either 4 g of cholestyramine or 5 g of colestipol, stirred into water or juices. The dose is increased as indicated by serum cholesterol levels, to a maximal dosage of 24 or 30 g/d, in divided doses before meals. A pill form of colestipol is now available as 1 g tablets. These agents are expensive and unpleasant to take because of taste and insolubility. Many patients complain of bloating, constipation, or queasiness, and compliance is often suboptimal. At maximal doses, resins may reduce LDL by as much as 10% to 30%. Resins can be used in combination with other agents, such as compactin derivatives or nicotinic acid.

d. Nicotinic acid. Nicotinic acid inhibits very low-density lipoprotein (VLDL) production and, as a result, also decreases LDL production. The plasma cholesterol level may be reduced up to 25% by nicotinic acid, which is also the most potent agent for raising HDLC levels. Frequent undesirable side effects include flushing and pruritus (ameliorated by taking aspirin before each dose until tachyphylaxis eliminates the flushing) and upper GI discomfort. Aggravation of peptic ulcer disease, gout, and non–insulin-dependent diabetes mellitus may occur. The initial dosage is usually 250–500 mg/d, increased every week or two as tolerated, to a full therapeutic dosage of 2–7.5 g/d. Nicotinic acid can be used in combination with resins or HMG-CoA reductase inhibitors in the treatment of hypercholesterolemia.

B. Hypertriglyceridemia

1. **GENERAL CONSIDERATIONS.** The role of hypertriglyceridemia in atherogenesis is less certain. Several studies have failed to identify a relationship. However, members of some families with a high prevalence of hypertriglyceridemia seem to be susceptible to atherosclerosis.

   Hypertriglyceridemia often reflects the interaction of a genetic cause, such as familial hypertriglyceridemia or familial combined hyperlipidemia, and an acquired cause, such as poorly controlled diabetes mellitus, certain medications (estrogens, beta-blocking agents, thiazide diuretics, or glucocorticoids), alcohol consumption, obesity, hypothyroidism, or uremia. The combination of excessive endogenous triglycerides and hyperchylomicronemia may result in triglyceride concentrations of more than 1000 mg/dL or even 20 to 30 times that high. Patients with such high levels of triglycerides are in danger of developing the chylomicronemic syndrome, the manifestations of which include acute pancreatitis, nonspecific abdominal or, infrequently, chest pain, impairment of recent memory, hepatomegaly, and eruptive xanthomatosis.

2. **APPROACH TO TREATMENT.** Guidelines for treating hypertriglyceridemia are given below.
   - Always search for and treat conditions that may cause or aggravate hypertriglyceridemia. Oral estrogen therapy and alcohol consumption, even in very modest amounts, may greatly elevate triglyceride concentrations in susceptible individuals. Improving diabetes control, using alternative therapy in place of thiazides and beta-adrenergic blocking agents, changing oral estrogen to the transdermal patch system, dietary therapy for obesity, and elimination of alcohol may make specific treatment for hypertriglyceridemia unnecessary.
   - Patients with slightly to moderately elevated triglyceride levels (250 to 500 mg/dL) should be treated with dietary modification only.

- In patients with more severe hypertriglyceridemia (500 to 1000 mg/dL) who do not respond to diet alone and who have a family history of hypertriglyceridemia-associated atherosclerosis, the addition of medication to dietary therapy warrants consideration. In the absence of a family history of atherosclerosis, it is generally preferable not to use medication.
- Patients with severe hypertriglyceridemia (in excess of 1000 mg/dL) who do not respond to diet alone, including complete abstention from alcohol, should be treated with medication.

3. **THERAPEUTIC MODALITIES**

   a. **Diet.** The dietary treatment of hypertriglyceridemia is essentially the same as that for hypercholesterolemia. The essential feature is limitation of total fat and saturated fat and correction of obesity. Addition of fish oils rich in omega-3 fatty acids should be considered in patients not responding to standard dietary therapy.

   b. **Fibric acid derivatives.** Gemfibrozil (600 mg bid) is quite effective in lowering plasma triglyceride levels. In patients with familial hypertriglyceridemia or in those with family histories characterized by the combination of hypertriglyceridemia and atherogenesis, therapy using gemfibrozil along with either niacin or lovastatin may be preferable. Gemfibrozil may be lithogenic and can reduce the clearance of coumadin.

   c. **Nicotinic acid.** See relevant section under Hypercholesterolemia. As this drug can reduce elevations of both triglycerides and cholesterol, it is an excellent choice for treating familial combined hyperlipidemia disorders.

Brown G, Albers JJ, Fisher LD, et al. Regression of coronary artery disease as a result of intensive lipid-lowering therapy in men with high levels of apolipoprotein B. N Engl J Med 1990;323: 1289–1298.

Brown WB, ed. Fenofibrate, a third generation fibric acid derivative. Am J Med 1987;83(Suppl 5B):1–89.

Frick MH, Elo O, Haapa K, et al. Helsinki Heart Study: primary-prevention trial with gemfibrozil in middle-aged men with dyslipidemia. N Engl J Med 1987;317:1237–1245.

Grundy SM. Cholesterol and coronary heart disease. JAMA 1990;264:3053–3059.

Hegsted DM, Nicolosi RJ. Individual variation in serum cholesterol levels. Proc Natl Acad Sci USA 1987;84:6259.

Hoeg JM, Brewer HB. 3-Hydroxy-3-methyglutaryl-co-enzyme A reductase inhibitors in the treatment of hypercholesterolemia. JAMA 1987;258:3532–3536.

Vega GL, Grundy SM. Treatment of primary moderate hypercholesterolemia with lovastatin (mevinolin) and colestipol. JAMA 1987;257:33–38.

13 13 13 13 13 13 13 13

NUTRITIONAL THERAPEUTICS

A. HILLARY STEINHART
JEFFREY P. BAKER
ALLAN S. DETSKY

13 13 13 13 13 13 13 13 13

I. NORMAL NUTRITIONAL REQUIREMENTS

Normal dietary intake should provide a balanced supply of energy, protein, fluid and electrolytes, vitamins, minerals, and trace elements. Table 13–1 lists a summary of **recommended daily nutrient intakes** for people of both sexes and all ages. Individual variation in nutrient requirement does exist, depending on the person's level of activity, rate of growth, concomitant stress, or illness. This variation must be considered when tables such as these are used. Table 13–2 lists characteristics of therapeutic diets.

A. Energy

The average energy intake required to maintain body weight in adults is in the range of 25 to 35 kcal/kg/d. Energy expenditure can be measured by

TABLE 13–1. Average Daily Energy Requirements

AGE	SEX	AVERAGE WEIGHT (kg)	AVERAGE DAILY ENERGY REQUIREMENT (kcal/kg)	AVERAGE DAILY ENERGY REQUIREMENT (kcal/d)
Months				
0–2	Both	4.5	120–100*	500
3–5	Both	7.0	100–95	700
6–8	Both	8.5	95–97	800
9–11	Both	9.5	97–99	950
Years				
1	Both	11	101	1100
2–3	Both	14	94	1300
4–6	Both	18	100	1800
7–9	M	25	88	2200
	F	25	76	1900
10–12	M	34	73	2500
	F	36	61	2200
13–15	M	50	57	2800
	F	48	46	2200
16–18	M	62	51	3200
	F	53	40	2100
19–24	M	71	42	3000
	F	58	36	2100
25–49	M	74	36	2700
	F	59	32	1900
50–74	M	73	31	2300
	F	63	29	1800
75+	M	69	29	2000
	F	64	23	1500

*First and second figures are averages at the beginning and the end of the period.
Data from Canada Health and Welfare: Nutrition Recommendations. The Report of the Scientific Review Committee, 1990.

TABLE 13–2. Therapeutic Diets

TYPE	INDICATION(S)	MAIN FEATURES	COMMENTS
Diabetic	Diabetes—types I and II Gestational diabetes Impaired glucose tolerance	Increased CHO (50–55%) in form of soluble fiber Lower saturated fats Lower simple sugars	Timing of meals and snacks important (especially for patients on insulin) Weight loss for obese type II diabetics Diets based on food group substitutions
Lipid lowering	Prevention of coronary heart disease in moderate- to high-risk groups Blood cholesterol >75th percentile Blood triglyceride >90th percentile	20–30% of total calories as fat Cholesterol 100–300 mg/d Decrease or eliminate alcohol and sugars for hypertriglyceridemias Polyunsaturated/saturated fatty acid ratio >1	Degree of restriction depends on cholesterol and triglyceride levels and previous intake
Sodium restricted	Congestive heart failure Liver disease with ascites Salt-sensitive hypertension Renal disease with sodium retention Excess mineralocorticoid states	Degree of sodium restriction 22 mmol (500 mg)—very strict 44 mmol (1 g)—strict 87 mmol (2 g)—moderate 130–217 mmol (3–5 g)—no added salt	No salt added to foods Foods prepared and cooked without salt Low-sodium breads and butters may be required depending on restriction Dairy products and certain vegetables used in limited quantities
Controlled energy	Obesity (weight >20% above ideal)	Reduced caloric intake of nutritionally balanced foods Avoid diets of <4000 kJ (1000 kcal)/d	Gradual weight loss is best (1–2 lb per week) Physical activity important adjuvant Behavioral treatment often helpful
Renal	Renal insufficiency Chronic renal failure Acute renal failure	Energy, protein, fluid, electrolytes, vitamin and mineral intakes individualized depending on degree and type of renal impairment; use of dialysis and concomitant illnesses, such as diabetes, sepsis, hypertension	Moderate protein restriction may slow progression of renal failure (0.55–0.6 g/kg/d); increase protein for increased urinary protein losses; anorexia often a problem in chronic renal failure

Liver	Hepatic failure End-stage liver disease with encephalopathy	Protein restriction for encephalopathy (0–40 g/d) depending on stage	Plant protein sources may produce less encephalopathy
Portacaval shunt		Sodium (<2 g/d) and water (<1500 mL/d) restriction for ascites and hyponatremia	Hypoglycemia complicating hepatic failure generally requires IV glucose
Restricted lactose	Primary lactase deficiency Secondary lactase deficiency	Eliminate milk, milk products, and some processed foods; individual tolerance determined by adding foods containing small amounts of lactose; some yogurts, fermented cheeses, and lactose-reduced milks can be tolerated	May require calcium, riboflavin, vitamin D supplementation
Gluten-free	Celiac disease Dermatitis herpetiformis	Eliminate barley, wheat, rye, triticale, and usually oats, wheatstarch, and beer; may have secondary lactose deficiency early in course	Individual variation exists in sensitivity to oats, malt extracts, and derivatives
Antireflux	Gastroesophageal reflux disease ? Nonulcer dyspepsia	Avoid coffee, tea, alcohol, mints, cola, cocoa, chocolate, fat, onion, garlic; small, frequent meals; avoid lying down for 2–3 h after meals; weight loss in obesity	Drugs (NSAIDs, aspirin, anticholinergics) and smoking may be aggravating factors; individual tolerance to spicy foods and acidic fruit juices should be determined; elevate head of bed 4–6 inches on blocks
Postgastrectomy	Postoperative partial or total gastrectomy, vagotomy, and pyloroplasty Dumping syndrome	Small, frequent dry meals; separation of liquids and solids; low in simple carbohydrate with sufficient fat and protein	Can attempt gradual return to normal diet as tolerated; monitor weight, iron, folate and vitamin B_{12} status; watch for lactose intolerance and steatorrhea in some patients with diarrhea

means of indirect calorimetry. However, in most instances this is impractical and an easier alternative is to calculate the **basal energy expenditure** (BEE) by means of the Harris and Benedict equations for men and women.

$$\text{Men: BEE (kJ/d)} = 66.5 + 13.8W + 5H - 6.8A$$
$$\text{Women: BEE (kJ/d)} = 655 + 9.6W + 1.8H - 4.7A$$

where W is body weight (kg), H is height (cm), and A is age (y). The calculated BEE should be adjusted upward approximately 10% to account for the thermogenic effect of feeding (REE, resting energy expenditure). An adjustment also should be made for the degree of stress and activity. It

TABLE 13-3. **Recommended Daily Nutrient Intake Based on Age and Body Weight**

AGE	SEX	WEIGHT (kg)	PROTEIN (g)	THIA-MINE (mg)	RIBO-FLAVIN (mg)	NIACIN (NE[a])	n-3 PUFA[b] (g)	n-6 PUFA (g)	VIT A (RE[c])
Months									
0–4	Both	6	12[e]	0.3	0.3	4	0.5	3	400
5–12	Both	9	12	0.4	0.5	7	0.5	3	400
Years									
1	Both	11	19	0.5	0.6	8	0.6	4	400
2–3	Both	14	22	0.6	0.7	9	0.7	4	400
4–6	Both	18	26	0.7	0.9	13	1.0	6	500
7–9	M	25	30	0.9	1.1	16	1.2	7	700
	F	25	30	0.8	1.0	14	1.0	6	700
10–12	M	34	38	1.0	1.3	18	1.4	8	800
	F	36	40	0.9	1.1	16	1.1	7	800
13–15	M	50	50	1.1	1.4	20	1.4	9	900
	F	48	42	0.9	1.1	16	1.2	7	800
16–18	M	62	55	1.3	1.6	23	1.8	11	1000
	F	53	43	0.8	1.1	15	1.2	7	800
19–24	M	71	58	1.2	1.5	22	1.6	10	1000
	F	58	43	0.8	1.1	15	1.2	7	800
25–49	M	74	61	1.1	1.4	19	1.5	9	1000
	F	59	44	0.8	1.0	14	1.1	7	800
50–74	M	73	60	0.9	1.3	16	1.3	8	1000
	F	63	47	0.8[h]	1.0[h]	14[h]	1.1[h]	7[h]	800
75+	M	69	57	0.8	1.0	14	1.0	7	1000
	F	64	47	0.8[h]	1.0[h]	14[h]	1.1[h]	7[h]	800
Pregnancy (Additional)									
1st Trimester			5	0.1	0.1	0.1	0.05	0.3	100
2nd Trimester			20	0.1	0.3	0.2	0.16	0.9	100
3rd Trimester			24	0.1	0.3	0.2	0.16	0.9	100
Lactation (Additional)			20	0.2	0.4	0.3	0.25	1.5	400

[a]NE, niacin equivalents (1 NE = 1 mg niacin = 60 mg tryptophan).
[b]PUFA, polyunsaturated fatty acids.
[c]RE, retinol equivalents (1 RE = 1 µg (3.33 IU) retinol, 2 µg beta-carotene or 12 µg of other carotenoid provitamins).
[d]Smokers should increase vitamin C by 50%.
[e]Protein is assumed to be from breast milk and must be adjusted for infant formula.

appears that for patients on total parenteral nutrition, the maximum hypermetabolism secondary to stress is approximately 30%.

Nonprotein energy requirements can be provided in the form of either carbohydrate or fat. **Carbohydrate** provides 4 kcal/g, whereas fat provides 9 kcal/g. Current recommendations suggest reducing fat intake to <30% of total energy requirements, with one third of the fat in the form of saturated fats, one third as monounsaturated fats, and one third as polyunsaturated fats. A minimum amount of the essential n-3 and n-6 **polyunsaturated fatty acids** should be present in the diet (Table 13–3). **Cholesterol** should probably be restricted to less than 300 mg/d. Increasing the amount of

VIT D (µg)	VIT E (mg)	VIT C (mg[d])	FOLATE (µg)	VIT B$_{12}$ (µg)	CALCIUM (mg)	PHOS-PHORUS (mg)	MAGNE-SIUM (mg)	IRON (mg)	IODINE (µg)	ZINC (mg)
10	3	20	50	0.3	250[f]	150	20	0.3[g]	30	2[g]
10	3	20	50	0.3	400	200	32	7	40	3
10	3	20	65	0.3	500	300	40	6	55	4
5	4	20	80	0.4	550	350	50	6	65	4
5	5	25	90	0.5	600	400	65	8	85	5
2.5	7	25	125	0.8	700	500	100	8	110	7
2.5	6	25	125	0.8	700	500	100	8	95	7
2.5	8	25	170	1.0	900	700	130	8	125	9
5	7	25	180	1.0	1100	800	135	8	110	9
5	9	30	150	1.5	1100	900	185	10	160	12
5	7	30	145	1.5	1000	850	180	13	160	9
5	10	40	185	1.9	900	1000	230	10	160	12
2.5	7	30	160	1.9	700	850	200	12	160	9
2.5	10	40	210	2.0	800	1000	240	9	160	12
2.5	7	30	175	2.0	700	850	200	13	160	9
2.5	9	40	220	2.0	800	1000	250	9	160	12
2.5	6	30	175	2.0	700	850	200	13	160	9
5	7	40	220	2.0	800	1000	250	9	160	12
5	6	30	190	2.0	800	850	210	8	160	9
5	6	40	205	2.0	800	1000	230	9	160	12
5	5	30	190	2.0	800	850	210	8	160	9
2.5	2	0	300	1.0	500	200	15	0	25	6
2.5	2	10	300	1.0	500	200	45	5	25	6
2.5	2	10	300	1.0	500	200	45	10	25	6
2.5	3	25	100	0.5	500	200	65	0	50	6

[f]Infant formula with high phosphorus should contain 375 mg calcium.
[g]Breast milk is assumed to be the source of the mineral.
[h]Level below which intake should not fall.
Data from Canada Health and Welfare: Nutrition Recommendations. The Report of the Scientific Review Committee, 1990.

complex carbohydrates, such as starches and fibers, and decreasing the amount of simple sugars in the diet should be promoted.

B. Protein

Adequate daily protein intake for adults should be at least 0.6 g/kg, according to the World Health Organization. In North America, this amount is generally greatly exceeded. Requirements are higher for children, adolescents, and pregnant and lactating women. Although most of the population far exceed the recommended protein intake there exists a significant proportion—primarily children, the poor and socially disadvantaged, the elderly—who do not have adequate protein intake.

Foods high in protein include meats, poultry, fish, eggs, milk and milk products, nuts, seeds and some legumes, grains, and cereals. However, not all proteins are of equal quality. Some sources of protein, especially the vegetable sources, are lacking in one or more of the **essential amino acids.** These proteins are considered incomplete and must be taken with complementary sources of protein that provide the deficient essential amino acid(s). This is very important for people, such as vegetarians, whose major protein intake is from nonanimal sources.

C. Fluid and Electrolytes

Fluid intake should be 1500 to 2000 mL daily. There is no fixed requirement for dietary **sodium,** since normally functioning kidneys can adapt to either dietary sodium deficiency or excess. However, most sources advise avoidance of excessive sodium intake by keeping it in the range of 1.4 to 2 mmol (32 to 46 mg)/kg daily. Recommended daily intake for children is approximately 0.4 mmol (9 mg)/kg. **Potassium** is required for anabolic processes, such as protein synthesis and cellular glucose uptake. Recommended daily potassium intake is 0.75 mmol (29 mg)/kg for adults and 1.75 mmol (68 mg)/kg for children. Recommendations for fluid and electrolyte intake in normal subjects vary according to physical activity and environmental conditions, such as temperature and humidity.

D. Vitamins and Minerals

Recommended daily intakes of selected vitamins and minerals are listed in Table 13–3. These micronutrients are required for maintenance of normal metabolic processes. A lack of one is often associated with a specific deficiency syndrome. The food sources of the various vitamins and minerals and the signs and symptoms of the deficiency syndromes are listed elsewhere (see References).

E. Trace Elements

Trace elements are present in the diet in only extremely small amounts. Deficiency syndromes are rare but do occur. The importance of the trace elements is that these syndromes can occur if trace elements are not added to parenteral nutrition solutions given to patients who are not eating.

II. NUTRITIONAL ASSESSMENT

Before nutritional support is provided for the patient at risk of developing, or who has already developed, a nutrition-associated complication, the physician must first know whether nutritional support is required for this patient at the time. To determine this, it is first necessary to assess the patient's nutritional status. Assessment may range from a simple screening procedure based on data in the patient's history and physical examination to more elaborate laboratory techniques.

A. Diet History

This may be performed in a number of ways, such as observation of the patient's intake, determining food preferences and frequency of intake, keeping a 3 to 7-day record of food intake, or obtaining a 24-hour dietary recall. With these methods, one can determine if the patient's nutritional needs are being met based on standard requirements, with allowances made for the underlying disease(s) and stress.

B. Physical Examination

Physical examination can provide indicators of nutritional deficiencies. Some indicators of protein-calorie malnutrition are cachexia, muscle wasting, loss of subcutaneous fat, and edema or ascites. In addition, other signs of specific nutrient or vitamin deficiency syndromes may be detected.

C. Anthropometric Measurements

1. WEIGHT. There are a number of methods of expressing body weight to determine nutritional status. The current weight or **percentage of ideal body weight** based on height and body frame size, as outlined in the Metropolitan Life Insurance Company tables, can be used, but they do not make allowances for obese patients who have lost lean body mass although their total body weight may still be greater than ideal. This problem is avoided by the use of the **percentage of usual body weight** or by **recent weight change.** Weight loss of 20% to 25% of the usual body weight is associated with increased morbidity and mortality. However, when using these measurements, one must be aware that changes in body water, such as an increase in edema, can easily mask changes in muscle and fat content.

   The **body mass index** (BMI) is a simple way of expressing body weight in a standard manner. It is obtained by dividing the body weight (kg) by the square of the height (m). The resulting value correlates well with body fat. The normal range is 20 to 25 kg/m^2, with values below 18 indicating risk of nutrition-associated complications and values over 27 indicating risk of obesity-related complications. The BMI is difficult to interpret in the elderly, muscular athletes, and pregnant and lactating women. It should not be used in children or adolescents.

2. SUBCUTANEOUS FAT MEASUREMENTS. The use of calipers to measure **skinfold thickness** at various body sites—triceps, subscapular, suprailiac, anterior thigh, and umbilical—provides an indirect but reliable measurement of body fat stores. Standardized techniques performed by trained personnel using proper equipment must be ensured so that the results obtained are reliable. These measurements are not sufficiently sensitive to detect small or acute changes in body fat but can be used in monitoring chronic situations. Results can be compared with standard tables, and patients' percentiles can be determined. **Body fat**

depletion is indicated by a result below the 15th percentile. However, the results are limited by the fact that they do not account for differences in fat distribution, edema fluid, and hydration status.

3. SOMATIC PROTEIN MEASUREMENTS. Midarm muscle circumference (MAMC) is an indirect measure of muscle mass calculated based on the midarm circumference and the triceps skinfold thickness. Errors are due to failure to account for individual variation in skin compressibility and humerus diameter and for the incorrect assumption in the model that the arm and underlying muscle are cylindrical. The MAMC is not a reliable measure of acute changes in somatic proteins but, like subcutaneous fat measurements, can be used in monitoring chronic changes.

4. GROWTH CHARTS. The assessment of nutritional status in infants, children, and adolescents can be performed by means of following the growth patterns over time. Standard charts are available for plotting height, weight, or growth velocity. Deviations below the 5th percentile or a significant change in the growth pattern may indicate a nutritional deficiency, although numerous underlying disease processes can also alter growth without directly affecting nutritional status.

D. Biochemical Measurements

1. SOMATIC PROTEINS. These are indirect measures of the somatic protein compartment and include the **creatinine height index** and the **urinary excretion of 3-methylhistidine.** The creatinine height index involves three 24-hour urine collections to determine the creatinine excretion as an indicator of muscle protein stores. The results are compared with standard tables for creatinine excretion, and a percentage of ideal is determined. Creatinine excretion may be increased in patients with trauma or infection or in those who have undergone surgery. Excretion is decreased with increasing age, decreased GFR, and degenerative disease.

2. VISCERAL PROTEINS. A number of proteins that are synthesized in the liver can be measured in the serum (Table 13–4). These vary in their sensitivity and specificity for indicating malnutrition and in their circulating half-life in serum. Generally, the proteins with the shortest half-lives are the best indicators of acute or early changes in nutritional status.

E. Subjective Global Assessment (SGA)

The SGA is an easily derived measure based on data obtained from a screening history and physical examination (Table 13–5). These include patterns of weight change, dietary intake, gastrointestinal symptoms, functional capacity, the underlying disease process and its relation to nutritional needs, loss of subcutaneous fat, muscle wasting, edema, and ascites. The factors are weighted according to the examiner's subjective impression of their relative importance in that patient, and the patient is then given an overall rating of either well nourished (A), moderate or suspected malnutrition (B), or severe malnutrition (C).

TABLE 13-4. Nutritional Assessment: Visceral Proteins

PROTEIN	CONDITIONS CAUSING INCREASE	CONDITIONS CAUSING DECREASE	COMMENTS
Serum albumin	Dehydration	Malnutrition Maldigestion Malabsorption Protein-losing states Liver disease Congestive heart failure Cancer Acute stress Hypothyroidism Overhydration Prolonged bed rest	Serum half-life of 14–20 d Not sensitive to early deficiency or malnutrition Not specific for malnutrition
Transferrin	Iron deficiency Chronic blood loss Hypoxia Pregnancy	Malnutrition Iron overload Pernicious anemia Chronic infection Liver disease Protein-losing enteropathy	Normal range 2–2.6 g/L Serum half-life of 7–10 d Not sensitive to early deficiency or malnutrition
Thyroxine-binding prealbumin	Renal disease Hodgkin's disease	Malnutrition Liver disease Inflammatory bowel disease Hyperthyroidism Burns	Normal range 1.6–3 g/L Serum half-life of 2 days More sensitive to malnutrition than albumin or transferrin
Retinol-binding protein	Renal disease	Nephrotic syndrome Malnutrition Liver disease Acute metabolic stress Hyperthyroidism Cystic fibrosis	Normal range 0.3–0.8 g/L Serum half-life of 10–12 h Synthesized in the liver and catabolized in the kidney Very sensitive to early nutritional changes

TABLE 13–5. **Subjective Global Assessment (SGA)**

(Select appropriate category with a checkmark or enter numerical value where indicated by "#")

A. History

    1. Weight change

        Overall loss in past 6 months: amount = # _____ kg; % loss = # _____

        Change in past 2 weeks: _____ increase

                               _____ no change

                               _____ decrease

    2. Dietary intake change (relative to normal)

        _____ No change

        _____ Change _____ duration = # _____ weeks

                        _____ type: _____ suboptimal solid diet

                                      _____ full liquid diet

                                      _____ hypocaloric liquids

                                      _____ starvation

    3. Gastrointestinal symptoms (that persisted for >2 weeks)

        _____ none, _____ nausea, _____ vomiting, _____ diarrhea,

        _____ anorexia

    4. Functional capacity

        _____ No dysfunction (e.g., full capacity)

        _____ Dysfunction _____ duration = # _____ weeks

                        _____ type: _____ working suboptimally

                                        _____ ambulatory

                                      _____ bedridden

    5. Disease and its relation to nutritional requirements

        Primary diagnosis (specify) _____

        Metabolic demand (stress): _____ no stress   _____ low stress

                              _____ moderate stress _____ high stress

B. Physical (for each trait specify: 0 = normal, 1+ = mild, 2+ = moderate, 3+ = severe)

    # _____ loss of subcutaneous fat (triceps, chest)

    # _____ muscle wasting (quadriceps, deltoids)

    # _____ ankle edema

    # _____ sacral edema

    # _____ ascites

C. SGA rating (select one)

    _____ A = well nourished

    _____ B = moderately (or suspected of being) malnourished

    _____ C = severely malnourished

The SGA can be performed easily by properly trained physicians, house officers, dietitians, and nurses. It has been shown to be reliable among different observers to accurately predict the occurrence of nutrition-associated complications, such as infection, and it correlates well with more objective measures of nutritional status.

F. Prognostic Nutritional Index (PNI)

The PNI is a weighted index based on four objective measurements: **serum albumin, triceps skinfold thickness, serum transferrin, and delayed hypersensitivity reaction to three recall antigens.** This index can be determined in nontrauma surgical patients at the time of admission. It accurately predicts the risk of postoperative complications in this patient population.

$$PNI \ (\% \ risk \ of \ complications) =$$
$$158 - 16.6 \ (ALB) - 0.78 \ (TSF) - 0.2 \ (TFN) - 5.8 \ (DH)$$

where ALB is serum albumin (g/dL), TSF is triceps skinfold (mm), TFN is serum transferrin (mg/dL), and DH is maximal delayed hypersensitivity reaction to any of three antigens (0 = nonreactive, 1 = 5 mm reaction, 2 = greater than 5 mm reaction).

III. ENTERAL NUTRITION

When it has been determined that a patient has, or is at risk of developing, a nutrition-associated complication, a therapeutic approach must be selected. If the GI tract is functional, nutrition can often be provided orally or via tube feedings. Oral supplementation can be used if patients are able to take in enough by mouth to meet their needs. Consultation with a dietitian may be needed to design an adequate diet that is acceptable to the patient. In some cases, supplementation with one of the nutritionally complete commercially available formulas (e.g., Sustacal, Meritene, Ensure, Osmolite, Isocal) or with one of the specific supplements (e.g., potassium, magnesium, calcium, zinc, vitamins) will be indicated. If the patient is still unable to meet nutritional requirements, additional support—in the form of either enteral tube feedings or parenteral nutrition—is indicated.

A. Indications
- Patient has a functioning GI tract but is unable to meet nutritional requirements by means of oral feeding (anorexia, nausea, impaired swallowing, esophageal obstruction, major upper GI surgery, increased nutritional requirements, and so on.)
- Growth retardation in children with inflammatory bowel disease (feeds given nocturnally at home) and primary therapy of inflammatory bowel disease.
- Short bowel syndrome (more than 60 cm of functioning small intestine) or chronic partial bowel obstruction. Continuous pump infusion must be used in these situations.

B. Contraindications
- Any cause of a nonfunctioning GI tract (e.g., obstruction, perforation, ileus, some diarrheal states such as short bowel syndrome and severe active inflammatory bowel disease).
- High output fistula(s).
- Inability to obtain tube access to the GI tract.
- Refusal of patient or legal guardian.

C. Methods of Administration
  1. METHODS OF ACCESS TO THE GI TRACT
    a. Nasogastric (NG) tubes are soft, narrow-bore Silastic or polyurethane tubes with weighted tips placed in the gastric antrum, ideally.

Their position in the stomach should be confirmed fluoroscopically before initiation of feeding. These tubes have a tendency to clog and require frequent flushing. They are not suitable for high-viscosity formulas, such as the blenderized diets, but can be used for intermittent feeding.

b. Nasoenteral (NE) tubes. These are similar to but longer than the nasogastric tubes. They are placed in the distal duodenum or proximal jejunum under fluoroscopic control or guided by a gastroscope and are useful in patients with delayed gastric emptying, especially when complicated by reflux and aspiration. They require continuous infusion of formula as opposed to intermittent feedings.

c. Gastrostomy. These tubes can be inserted percutaneously under local anesthetic assisted by a gastroscope (PEG, percutaneous endoscopic gastrostomy) or under ultrasound or fluoroscopic guidance. They are considered to be the method of choice when long-term enteral feeding is required. They are useful when nasal irritation or necrosis occurs with NG or NE tubes and can be used for a blenderized diet. These tubes are easy to replace once the tract has matured. A smaller, mercury-tipped catheter can be passed through the gastrostomy tube down into the jejunum to avoid problems of impaired gastric emptying and reflux.

d. Jejunostomy is usually performed at the time of major upper GI surgery, such as a Whipple's procedure. It allows relatively early initiation of enteral feeding when the patient probably will not be able to eat for an extended period. It also avoids the problems of gastric retention and reflux or aspiration.

2. **METHODS OF FEEDING ADMINISTRATION**

a. Intermittent feeding. The total daily nutritional requirement is divided over four to eight separate feedings, aiming for a maximum volume of 300 mL per feeding. Each feeding is given over a minimum of 30 minutes, and the feeding tube is flushed and capped after completion. This technique allows greater patient freedom between feedings *but cannot be used for tubes in the duodenum or jejunum.*

b. Continuous infusion. Formula is continuously infused over all or part of the day depending on individual patient requirements and tolerance. Usually there is no need to initiate infusion with diluted formulas; rather, a slower infusion rate (10–50 mL/h) should be used, with gradual increase to the target rate as tolerated. Some patients, such as those with short bowels or those in the ICU, may be sensitive to variation in the infusion rate and will require administration by a pump to avoid diarrhea and metabolic complications of enteral feeding.

D. Enteral Formulas

There are numerous enteral formulas available for use. They can be divided into several broad categories: **blenderized, polymeric** (both milk-based and lactose-free), **elemental** (defined), **modular feedings,** and **formulas with altered amino acids.** For practical purposes, most clinicians need only be familiar with one or two formulas in each category (Table 13–6). Each nutritionally complete formula has a recommended daily volume. If this volume is not achieved, the patient is at risk of developing vitamin, mineral, or trace element deficiencies even though caloric intake may be adequate. Therefore, volumes should be continuously monitored and specific supplementation given accordingly.

E. Complications

1. MECHANICAL (TUBE) PROBLEMS
   a. **Improperly placed tube.** All NG and NE tubes should have their position confirmed radiographically before initiation of feedings. Percutaneous feeding tubes are placed under direct vision but can dislodge or migrate, especially during the first 10 days. This may result in pneumoperitoneum or leakage of gastric contents if the tract has not matured.
   b. **ENT irritation.** NG and NE tubes may cause local irritation to the nasal passageways, pharynx, and larynx. In extreme cases, this may result in necrosis and infection. When these complications arise, percutaneous tube insertion should be considered.
   c. **Tube clogging.** This problem occurs primarily with small-bore tubes but can happen with larger-bore tubes. To avoid tube clogging, use low-viscosity formulas, flush the tube with water or soda water after all feeds and medications, and use liquid suspensions of medications when available. Medications not available in suspension form should be crushed (except for slow-release or enteric-coated formulations).

2. GASTROINTESTINAL COMPLICATIONS
   a. **Gastric retention, gastroesophageal reflux, and aspiration.** Tubes that traverse the lower esophageal sphincter may cause an increase in gastroesophageal reflux and result in esophagitis, esophageal stricture formation, and pulmonary aspiration. These complications are less common with small-bore tubes and tubes placed in the jejunum. Gastric residual volumes should be checked when gastric feedings are used; if they are greater than 100 mL, corrective action should be taken. Prokinetic agents, such as metoclopramide, domperidone, or cisapride, can be used to avoid or treat gastric retention, but resistant cases may require percutaneous gastrostomy or jejunostomy. However, placement of a PEG may result in worsened gastric emptying, further aggravating reflux. This can be avoided by giving smaller feedings, keeping the head of the bed elevated, and passing a smaller-bore tube through the gastrostomy tube into the jejunum. Small bowel feeding tubes usually get around the problem of gastric retention but are not suitable for bolus feedings.
   b. **Nausea and vomiting.** This is often associated with gastric retention and reflux but may be due to bowel obstruction, ileus, or numerous central causes of nausea and vomiting.
   c. **Diarrhea.** Causes specific to enterally fed patients include an excessive rate or volume of feeding, use of hyperosmolar formulas,

TABLE 13-6. Enteral Formulas

CATEGORY	DESCRIPTION	INDICATIONS AND ADVANTAGES	DISADVANTAGES
Blenderized formulas (Compleat Formulas)	Purée of beef, vegetables, fruits, nonfat dry milk, sucrose, corn oil; variations can be prepared at home for less cost but content not standardized; provides approximately 1 kcal/mL	Requires functional GI tract; contains complex carbohydrate and fiber sources; variations can be prepared at home for less cost	High lactose content; may contain gluten; high viscosity; high osmolarity; commercial preparations are expensive
Milk-based polymeric formulas (Sustacal Powder, Sustagen, Meritene)	Whole proteins (caseinates, egg albumin, soy), carbohydrates (corn syrup, maltodextrins, disaccharides), fats (vegetable oils), vitamins, and minerals; nutritionally complete; most provide approx. 1 kcal/mL but Sustagen provides 1.6 kcal/mL	Requires functional GI tract; palatable for oral use; low viscosity; consistent standardized formulation	High lactose content; high osmolarity
Lactose-free polymeric formulas (Ensure, Ensure Plus, Enrich, Isocal, Osmolite, Isosource, Precision Isotonic, Portagen, Resource Liquid, Isotein, Sustacal Liquid, Sustacal HC, Sustacal with Fiber, Jevity)	Protein isolates (12–16%), oligosaccharides (50–55%), medium and long chain triglycerides (30%), vitamins and minerals; all nutritionally complete (approximately 1 kcal/mL) but Ensure Plus, Sustacal HC, and others have higher caloric density (1.5–2 kcal/mL); low residue (except Enrich, Jevity, and Sustacal with Fiber)	Requires a functional GI tract; palatable for oral use; low viscosity; consistent standardized formulation; tend to be lower osmolarity (300–400 mOsm/L) than lactose-containing formulas	Not palatable for all patients; may not be practical in patients with short bowel, partial bowel obstruction, fistulas (these often require elemental formulas)

540

Elemental (defined) formulas (Vivonex, Flexical, Vital, Travasorb, Peptamen Liquid, Criticare)	Nutrients in elemental or hydrolyzed form (amino acids and oligopeptides, glucose, and oligosaccharides); most calories provided by carbohydrates; very little fat as medium-chain or long-chain triglycerides (except Peptamen Liquid, which has 30% of calories as fat)	Indicated for short bowel (more than 60 cm functional bowel), malabsorption/maldigestion, partial bowel obstruction; requires minimal digestion; very low residue; low viscosity	Unpalatability restricts oral use; high osmolarity (from high concentration of simple sugars) results in higher incidence of GI intolerance and metabolic complications; low fat content results in potential risk of essential fatty acid deficiency
Modular feedings (Pro-Mix, Polycose, MCT oil)	Contain single nutrients (protein, carbohydrate or fat); vitamin/mineral supplemented	Can be combined with elemental or polymeric formulas to individualize a patient's nutritional prescription; useful for patients with special needs (liver disease, renal, cardiac, and respiratory failure)	Preparation of specialized formula is labor intensive; combination of formulas must be carefully planned to avoid deficiency states and metabolic complications

541

and bacterial contamination of the formula (especially if the hang time is more than 8 hours). Some evidence exists that patients with a low serum albumin (less than 27 g/L) have an increased incidence of diarrhea when they are enterally fed. These patients may require parenteral nutrition until their serum albumin is sufficiently high to allow enteral feeding. The use of concomitant medications—especially antibiotics—can be associated with diarrhea in enterally fed patients. Specific malabsorptive syndromes may also result in diarrhea (e.g., lactose intolerance, pancreatic insufficiency, celiac disease, inflammatory bowel disease).

d. **Constipation.** This is uncommon but can occur secondary to inadequate fluid or free water intake, the use of low-residue formulations, and the concomitant use of constipating agents. Water can be added to the daily feeding regimen, and a higher fiber formula (e.g., Enrich) can be used.

3. METABOLIC COMPLICATIONS

a. **Disturbances of water, sodium, potassium, phosphate, magnesium, and glucose balance.** Patients should be monitored periodically for occurrence of these imbalances. More frequent monitoring is indicated in very sick patients, in patients just starting enteral feeds, and in those experiencing high-volume diarrhea.

b. **Drug-nutrient interactions.** Enteral feeding may slow the absorption or alter the metabolism of some medications. The high vitamin K content of most formulas can make patients resistant to usual doses of coumadin.

c. **Essential fatty acid deficiency.** Patients on elemental formulas can theoretically develop this deficiency because of their low fat content. In practice, this rarely occurs.

IV. PARENTERAL NUTRITION

A. Indications

Indications for parenteral nutrition (PN) can be thought of as falling into one of three broad categories. Some patients may have more than one of these indications (e.g., patients with inflammatory bowel disease).

- Previously well-nourished patients who are unable to tolerate adequate oral intake or enteral feeding (for whatever reason) and will be unlikely to do so for at least 7 to 10 days
- Malnourished patients who are unable to tolerate oral or enteral feeds (e.g., short bowel syndrome with less than 60 cm small intestine remaining)
- Gastrointestinal disorders in which bowel rest is a primary mode of therapy (e.g., inflammatory bowel disease, enterocutaneous, and pancreatic fistulas)

B. Contraindications

- Adequate oral or enteral intake to meet nutritional requirements
- Lack of intravenous access (rare)
- Less than 5 to 7 days of PN likely required

- Terminal illness when aggressive management is not indicated
- Potential risks outweigh expected benefits
- Refusal of patient or legal guardian

C. Routes of Parenteral Nutrition

1. **PERIPHERAL PARENTERAL NUTRITION.** PN solutions are infused into a peripheral vein and must, therefore, not be of high osmolarity in order to minimize irritation and thrombosis. The concentration of dextrose and amino acids should not exceed 5%. The major source of nonprotein energy (80% to 85% of total nonprotein calories) is provided as lipid, which can be given in 10% or 20% concentrations because of its isotonicity. This method requires giving larger volumes of fluid to be nutritionally complete and should not be used for more than 7 days. If parenteral nutritional support is required for more than 7 days, the central route of PN administration should be used.

2. **CENTRAL PARENTERAL NUTRITION.** Solutions of high osmolarity are infused via a catheter placed into a central vein, usually the superior vena cava (SVC). The high blood volume flowing through the SVC allows the use of high-osmolarity solutions without irritative effects. Higher concentrations of dextrose (up to 25%) can be used as an energy source. This reduces the daily fluid volume required to meet nutritional requirements. Such fluid restriction is important in congestive heart failure, renal disease, and liver failure. In most cases, approximately 50% of the nonprotein energy is provided as dextrose and 50% as lipid. This ratio can be varied depending on the individual patient characteristics. For example, in patients with respiratory failure and CO_2 retention, it would be advantageous to use an energy source with a low respiratory quotient to minimize CO_2 production. This is achieved by increasing the relative percentage of calories provided by lipid.

D. Central Venous Catheter Insertion

The tip of the central venous catheter should be in the SVC. The catheter can be inserted via the subclavian vein or alternatively as a peripherally inserted central catheter (PICC) inserted into a peripheral vein in the arm and advanced under fluoroscopic control into the SVC. Central catheters should be inserted using strict sterile technique (gowns, masks, surgical scrubs, skin preparation) by an experienced operator.

The catheter once inserted and the position in the vein confirmed by return of blood, should be sutured in position with povidone-iodine ointment prophylaxis and a small gauze placed over the exit site and an Op-Site creating a watertight seal over the dressing. A chest x-ray, to verify position of the catheter tip in the SVC just above the right atrium, must be obtained before initiation of PN. For long-term PN, such as home PN, a Hickman catheter or Port-A-Cath is indicated.

E. The Parenteral Nutritional Prescription

Once it is decided to provide parenteral nutritional support for a patient, the daily fluid, protein, energy, electrolyte, mineral, trace element, and vitamin requirements for that patient should be determined. Since the requirements will vary according to the individual patient's previous nutritional status and underlying disease process, it is not possible to provide a standard prescription appropriate for all patients.

F. Parenteral Nutrition Solutions

Traditionally, parenteral nutrition has been provided as two separate solutions—one containing an amino acid and dextrose mixture to which electrolytes, trace elements, vitamins, and minerals were added and the second a lipid emulsion. The solutions are not mixed together before administration. Instead, the lipid emulsion is usually infused into the amino acid/dextrose administration tubing using a Y-connector. More recently, **total nutrient admixture (3-in-1)** systems have been gaining widespread use. Total nutrient admixture (TNA) allows increased flexibility in prescribing according to the individual nutrient needs of each patient. This may be particularly important in neonates, the elderly, critically ill patients, and patients with multisystem diseases or very specific metabolic or nutritional disorders. Although the mode of preparation of the parenteral nutrition solutions differs between TNA and the separate amino acid/dextrose and lipid systems, the principles of the nutrition prescription remain the same.

1. **AMINO ACIDS.** Balanced amino acid solutions are commercially available for use in the separate amino acid/dextrose and lipid systems. Concentrations of amino acids range from 3.5% to 10%. Amino acid solutions are also provided in premixed forms containing dextrose or electrolytes or both. Although this results in increased convenience of administration, it reduces individual flexibility. The osmolarity of amino acid solutions is approximately equal to the amino acid concentration multiplied by 100 (expressed in mOsm/L).

2. **DEXTROSE.** The range of dextrose concentrations used in the separate amino acid/dextrose and lipid systems ranges from 5% for peripheral PN to 25% for central PN. The osmolarity is approximately equal to the dextrose concentration multiplied by 50. Dextrose (as monohydrate) provides 3.4 nonprotein kcal/g. The use of dextrose as the exclusive source of nonprotein energy can result in the development of fatty liver. Generally, provision of 50% of the nonprotein energy in the form of dextrose is appropriate. In separate amino acid/dextrose and lipid systems, the dextrose is often provided by the hospital pharmacy in a single bag, mixed together with amino acids, electrolytes, vitamins, minerals, and trace elements.

3. **LIPID.** Lipid is provided in 10% and 20% emulsions. It provides a good source of nonprotein energy (1000 kcal/500 mL of 20% emulsion and 550 kcal/500 mL of 10% emulsion) and should be used in all patients except those with chylomicronemia. Both concentrations are isotonic and can be given via a peripheral vein without local irritation. It is also a useful source of nonprotein energy in patients with respiratory failure and CO_2 retention because of its low respiratory quotient as compared with dextrose. Generally, provision of 50% of the nonprotein energy in the form of lipids is appropriate. The lipid emulsions, when used in a separate amino acid/dextrose and lipid system, are usually infused via a Y-connector into the amino acid/dextrose administration tubing.

4. **TOTAL NUTRIENT ADMIXTURE.** In the TNA system, all of the macronutrients and the required additives are compounded together into a single bag that is able to hold up to 3 L. This solution contains a patient's daily nutritional prescription and can be administered continuously over 24 hours. This minimizes nursing time required for bag and tubing changes and minimizes the number of times that a central line is accessed. The TNA solution is stable within certain parameters of macronutrient composition and electrolyte and mineral additives. Because the prescription can be compounded in hospital pharmacies from high-concentration stock solutions of individual macronutrients, electrolytes, and minerals rather than premanufactured in specific ratios, the TNA system provides the highest degree of individualization of PN prescriptions. However, for practical purposes, it is advisable to have a number of standard amino acid/dextrose/lipid solutions that will meet the needs of the majority of patients within a single institution and to limit the use of individualized solutions to patients with very specific requirements that are not met by the standard solutions.

5. **ELECTROLYTES.** Sodium, potassium, calcium, magnesium, chloride, phosphate, and acetate are usually added to maintain electrolyte balance. PN solutions should be individually formulated by the addition or withholding of specific electrolytes as appropriate. Special attention needs to be paid to potassium, magnesium, phosphorus, and zinc, especially early in the course of PN, as these ions are taken up and used by cells as the patient becomes anabolic, thus resulting in low serum levels and potential complications. In addition, when malnourished patients are initially refed, they may have excessive sodium and water retention and the resulting risk of congestive heart failure. Thus, refeeding should be started gradually, avoiding large carbohydrate loads and carefully monitoring sodium and fluid balance.

6. **VITAMINS.** Standard multivitamin mixtures (e.g., Solu-Zyme, M.V.I.-1000, M.V.I.-12) should be added to PN solutions to provide water-soluble and fat-soluble vitamins and prevent deficiency states (Table 13–7). A water-soluble multivitamin preparation (e.g., Solu-Zyme) should be added 6 days per week, and the preparation containing both fat-soluble and water-soluble vitamins (M.V.I.-1000) should be added once weekly in most instances. Vitamin K_1, 10 mg, can be administered IM once weekly. There is some evidence that IV vitamin D is associated with hypercalcemia and pancreatitis in those receiving PN and should not be given in doses of more than 2500 IU/d.

7. **TRACE ELEMENTS.** See Table 13–8 for administration guidelines.

G. Monitoring

- Catheter exit site should be monitored daily and the dressing changed at least once a week. If there is evidence of infection at the exit site, swabs of the site are sent for culture. Infusion tubing is changed every 48 to 72 hours.
- Blood work should be done periodically following initiation of PN. Electrolytes, glucose, urea, and creatinine should be tested daily for the first 3 days and then three times weekly following that. Calcium,

TABLE 13–7. Vitamin Requirements on Parenteral Nutrition

VITAMIN	RECOMMENDED DAILY IV ADMINISTRATION	AMOUNT PROVIDED IN:		
		SOLU-ZYME (5 mL)	M.V.I.-1000 (10 mL)	M.V.I.-12 (10 mL)
A	2500 IU (= 750 µg retinol or 750 retinol equivalents)	—	10,000 IU	600 IU
D	? (see text)	—	1000 IU	40 IU
E	10 IU	—	10 IU	2 IU
K	10 mg/wk (IM)	—	—	—
B_1 (Thiamine)	5 mg	10 mg	45 mg	0.6 mg
B_2 (Riboflavin)	5 mg	10 mg	10 mg	0.72 mg
Niacinamide	50 mg	250 mg	100 mg	8 mg
B_6 (Pyridoxine)	5 mg	5 mg	12 mg	0.8 mg
B_{12} (Cobalamin)	12 µg	25 µg	—	1 µg
Pantothenic acid	15 mg	45 mg	26 mg	3 mg
Folic acid	600 µg	5 mg	—	80 µg
C (ascorbic acid)	300–500 mg	500 mg	1000 mg	20 mg
Biotin	60 µg	—	—	12 µg

TABLE 13–8. **Trace Element Requirements in TPN**

ELEMENT	RECOMMENDED DAILY IV ADMINISTRATION	COMMENT
Zinc	2.5–4 mg	Increase for GI losses (12 mg/L for small intestinal fluid or 17 mg/L for stool)
Iron (iron dextran)	1 mg	Increase to 2 mg/d in menstruating females; increase for other causes of blood loss; monitor iron stores periodically (especially in long-term PN)
Copper	0.5 mg	Increased GI losses in diarrheal illnesses; decreased excretion with impaired hepatic function (especially obstructive jaundice)
Chromium	10–20 μg	Deficiency associated with glucose intolerance
Selenium	40–120 μg	Deficiency associated with cardiomyopathy and muscle pain
Manganese	0.8 mg	Should not be given in obstructive jaundice
Iodine (potassium iodide)	120 μg	—

magnesium, phosphorus, AST, alkaline phosphatase, bilirubin, cholesterol, triglycerides, serum proteins, and complete blood count with differential count should be tested weekly. Monitoring of blood work should be more frequent in unstable patients or when specifically indicated.

- Urine is checked for glucose and ketones every 6 hours if patient has been hyperglycemic.
- Body weight is checked.
- Fluid intake and output are monitored.
- Nutritional status should be reassessed periodically to confirm that nutritional goals are being achieved.

H. Complications

1. **TECHNICAL**
   a. **Pneumothorax** occurs during catheter insertion. If small and not enlarging, it can be managed expectantly but sometimes requires insertion of a chest tube. If the catheter is properly within the SVC, it may be left in place.
   b. **Laceration of subclavian artery or vein.** Such injuries should be treated with local pressure and insertion of a chest tube if hemothorax occurs.
   c. **Injury to thoracic duct.** Remove the catheter and remove any resulting chylothorax by means of repeated thoracentesis until leakage of lymph stops.
   d. **Injury to brachial plexus**
   e. **Catheter embolization.** This occurs when a catheter placed through a metal cannula is withdrawn with the cannula still in the vein, shearing off the catheter.

f. **Air embolism.** This potentially fatal complication can occur during catheter insertion or later if the infusion tubing becomes disconnected from the catheter. The catheter should be immediately covered and the patient placed in the Trendelenburg position with the right side up.

g. **Venous thrombosis** around the tip of the catheter or in the SVC may be related to improper catheter position or to long-term usage. It is often associated with an underlying catheter infection and can sometimes be treated with streptokinase or urokinase to dissolve the fibrin clot and daily antibiotics but may require removal of the catheter. Urokinase is given as 7500 IU dissolved in 3 mL of normal saline, which is then injected into the catheter, up to a maximum of 2.5 mL. The catheter is capped for 3 hours and then flushed with 10 mL of normal saline containing 1000 U of heparin.

2. Septic. Catheter sepsis is an episode of sepsis that resolves after removal of the catheter. It is observed more commonly with the use of multilumen catheters and should be suspected when a patient receiving PN has a fever (even low grade), leukocytosis, or hyperglycemia. It is confirmed by a positive culture from blood or from the removed catheter tip. Not all episodes of sepsis occurring in patients on PN are catheter sepsis; efforts should be made to find other potential sources. An algorithm for managing the febrile PN patient is presented in Figure 13–1.

3. Metabolic
   a. **Hyperglycemia.** This is due to an excessively high rate of glucose administration or impaired glucose utilization or both. Impaired utilization is often associated with sepsis, trauma, stress, diabetes, liver disease, pancreatitis, and corticosteroid administration. Hyperglycemia can result in hyperosmolar nonketotic coma and dehydration when severe. The rate of dextrose infusion should be reduced and underlying conditions corrected when possible. If hyperglycemia persists, insulin therapy should be started. A constant IV insulin infusion allows close control of the blood glucose level, especially in the unstable patient.
   b. **Hypoglycemia.** This usually occurs when the infusion of dextrose is not constant throughout the day either because of mechanical infusion problems or when the dextrose infusion is suddenly stopped (usually when very high concentrations are used). Infusion pumps ensure constant rates of dextrose infusion. Avoid sudden discontinuation of dextrose infusion (e.g., for medications). When hypoglycemia occurs, constant infusion of the dextrose should be resumed immediately. Severe hypoglycemia should be treated with boluses of 50% dextrose.
   c. **Electrolyte disturbances.** Hypokalemia, hypophosphatemia, and hypomagnesemia are the most common electrolyte imbalances. They tend to occur early in the course of PN as these ions are taken up by cells during the process of protein synthesis. Additional supplementation of ions as necessary is adequate treatment.

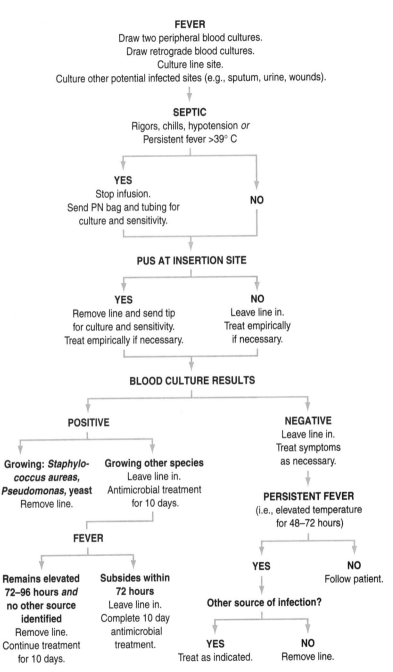

FEVER
Draw two peripheral blood cultures.
Draw retrograde blood cultures.
Culture line site.
Culture other potential infected sites (e.g., sputum, urine, wounds).

SEPTIC
Rigors, chills, hypotension *or*
Persistent fever >39° C

YES
Stop infusion.
Send PN bag and tubing for
culture and sensitivity.

NO

PUS AT INSERTION SITE

YES
Remove line and send tip
for culture and sensitivity.
Treat empirically if necessary.

NO
Leave line in.
Treat empirically
if necessary.

BLOOD CULTURE RESULTS

POSITIVE

NEGATIVE
Leave line in.
Treat symptoms
as necessary.

Growing: *Staphylo-
coccus aureas,
Pseudomonas,* yeast
Remove line.

Growing other species
Leave line in.
Antimicrobial treatment
for 10 days.

PERSISTENT FEVER
(i.e., elevated temperature
for 48–72 hours)

FEVER

YES

NO
Follow patient.

**Remains elevated
72–96 hours *and*
no other source
identified**
Remove line.
Continue treatment
for 10 days.

**Subsides within
72 hours**
Leave line in.
Complete 10 day
antimicrobial
treatment.

Other source of infection?

YES
Treat as indicated.

NO
Remove line.

FIGURE 13–1. Suggested algorithm for management of possible catheter sepsis in febrile PN patients.

    d. **Acid-base disturbances.** Hyperchloremic metabolic acidosis is the most common acid-base disturbance secondary to PN. It is due to the administration of excessive chloride or to the loss of bicarbonate through GI or renal routes. To treat, reduce chloride in the PN solution and substitute acetate (which is metabolized to bicarbonate). Treat sources of bicarbonate loss if possible.

    e. **Vitamin and trace element deficiencies.** These should be added to PN solutions on a daily basis as recommended, and appropriate adjustments should be made for individual patients.

    f. **Hyperlipidemia.** Hypertriglyceridemia is caused by excessive calorie administration (as either lipid or dextrose). Elevated cholesterol levels can be seen with very high rates of lipid infusion. Treatment is reduction of daily caloric or lipid intake or both.

    g. **Essential fatty acid deficiency.** This syndrome, characterized by dry, scaly skin and hair loss, is not seen in patients receiving lipid emulsion.

    h. **Pancreatitis.** Pancreatitis occurring in patients on PN may be due to hypertriglyceridemia or hypercalcemia. If it is due to hypercalcemia, vitamin D should be withdrawn from the PN solution.

    i. **Liver enzyme and liver function abnormalities.** Mild abnormalities of the serum alkaline phosphatase, AST, and ALT (less than two to three times normal) are common. These tend to be self-limited. Fatty infiltration of the liver is related to excessive calories being provided as dextrose. Cholestatic jaundice can also occur, but its cause is not clear. It may be related to underlying sepsis in the patient receiving PN. Fatty infiltration should be treated by reducing the caloric intake and replacing about 50% of dextrose with lipid emulsion. If cholestatic jaundice occurs, a search should be made for a source of sepsis.

V. HOME PARENTERAL NUTRITION

Occasionally, a patient will have an indication for parenteral nutrition that does not resolve over the course of a hospital stay. In these cases, PN is continued at home. The most common **indications** include short bowel syndrome, radiation enteritis, extensive Crohn's disease, and diffuse intestinal hypomotility. Home PN should be provided only by an experienced multidisciplinary group consisting of physicians, nurses, pharmacists, and dietitians. Not all patients who have an indication for home PN will be suitable for the program—usually because of poor social supports and inability or unwillingness to follow the strict aseptic techniques required. Patients should be trained in the techniques while in the hospital. This takes an average of 2 weeks depending on the complexity of the prescription and the patient's aptitude.

A. Infusion of PN Solutions

Infusion of PN solutions, usually via a Hickman catheter or Port-A-Cath placed in the SVC, is carried out overnight, thus allowing the patient to cap the catheter during the day to permit usual activities. The exact composition of the infusion solutions varies. For example, some patients with short bowel syndrome are able to eat and absorb sufficient calories and protein but require infusion of fluid and electrolytes to prevent imbalances due to excessive losses from their stomas. Such patients may also require once-weekly lipid infusions in order to avoid essential fatty acid deficiency. Although patients are receiving PN, they are also free to eat as tolerated, according to their underlying condition. Such intake should be accounted for when determining the PN prescription.

B. Complications

Complications of home PN are similar to those experienced with in-hospital PN. Line sepsis is a frequently occurring complication often treated with urokinase, as described, and 4 weeks of systemic antibiotics, thereby avoiding catheter removal. Stiffening and fracturing of the catheter are also more likely with prolonged PN. Certain metabolic complications, such as metabolic bone disease, iron deficiency, and trace element deficiencies, are more likely to develop when patients are receiving long-term home PN.

ASPEN Board of Directors. Guidelines for use of enteral nutrition in the adult patient. JPEN 1987;11:435–439.

ASPEN Board of Directors. Guidelines for use of total parenteral nutrition in the hospitalized adult patient. JPEN 1986;10:441–445.

ASPEN Board of Directors. Guidelines for use of home total parenteral nutrition. JPEN 1987;11:342–344.

Baker JP, Lemoyne M. Nutritional support in the critically ill patient: if, when, how and what. Crit Care Clin 1987;3:97–113.

Canada Health and Welfare. Nutrition Recommendations. The Report of the Scientific Review Committee, 1990.

Detsky AS, McLaughlin JR, Baker JP, et al. What is subjective global assessment of nutritional status? JPEN 1987;11:8–13.

FAO/WHO/UNU. Energy and protein requirements: report of a joint FAO/WHO/UNU Expert Consultation. Technical Report No. 724. Geneva, World Health Organization, 1985.

Ontario Dietetic Association–Ontario Hospital Association. Nutritional Care Manual, 6th ed., Don Mills, Ontario: Ontario Hospital Association; 1989.

Shils ME, Young VR, eds. Modern Nutrition in Health and Disease. Philadelphia: Lea & Febiger; 1988.

14 14 14 14 14 14 14 14

RHEUMATIC DISORDERS

GREGORY C. GARDNER
BRUCE C. GILLILAND

I. RHEUMATOID ARTHRITIS

Rheumatoid arthritis (RA) is a chronic inflammatory illness affecting predominantly peripheral joints in a symmetric distribution. The peak onset is the fourth through sixth decades of life, and women are affected three times more often than men. In the United States, 1% to 2% of the population is affected. The disease course is variable, with some patients having only mild joint swelling with long periods of remission, whereas others have a progressive destructive joint disease that seems unresponsive to any form of treatment. Prognostic factors that portend a poorer outcome include female gender, a positive rheumatoid factor, presence of rheumatoid nodules, higher number of joints involved, lower level of education, lower socioeconomic status, and carrying the HLA-DR4 antigen.

The clinical features of RA are presented in Tables 14–1 and 14–2. The 1987 criteria for diagnosis include morning stiffness lasting at least 1 hour, arthritis involving three or more joint areas, involvement of the hands, simultaneous involvement of joint areas on both sides of the body, rheumatoid nodules, positive rheumatoid factor, and radiographic changes characteristic of RA. At least four of these need to be present and symptoms need to be present for at least 6 weeks to diagnose RA.

Data appearing in the 1980s suggested that the usual pyramid approach to the treatment of RA was not preventing eventual functional incapacity of patients, and new treatment strategies are being developed. The newer approaches include more rapid institution of disease-modifying antirheumatic drugs (DMARDs), combination therapy with these agents, and a search for new medications, including biologic agents.

A. Treatment

The goal of treatment is to reduce or eliminate joint inflammation and thus prevent damage to the articular cartilage. By doing so, patient and joint function hopefully will be maintained. The treatment of RA must be thought of as a program and includes patient education, aerobic and joint-specific exercise programs, medications, and orthopedic surgery when necessary.

1. NONSTEROIDAL ANTI-INFLAMMATORY DRUGS (NSAIDs). NSAIDs constitute the mainstay of initial therapy for RA, especially in milder cases. Under the pyramid approach, patients would often be switched from one NSAID to another in hopes of finding the most effective agent. Currently, NSAIDs are thought of as adjunctive therapy to the DMARDs, and most rheumatologists would start one of the DMARDs at 12 weeks of persistent synovitis and use the NSAIDs primarily to help control pain.

    a. **Mechanism of action.** Aspirin and other NSAIDs help reduce inflammation and pain via two mechanisms. The first is by the ability of the NSAIDs to interfere with the conversion of arachidonic acid to inflammation and pain-producing prostaglandins by the enzyme cyclooxygenase (COX). This occurs at low to moderate dosing

TABLE 14–1. **Clinical Characteristics of Rheumatoid Arthritis**

Joint areas potentially involved: PIPs, MCPs, wrists, elbows, shoulders, hips, knees, ankles, MTPs, cervical spine
Joint pattern: Symmetric polyarthritis (peripheral joints predominantly)
Laboratory: Rheumatoid factor present in 80%; anemia; elevated ESR
Immunogenetics: HLA-DR4 present in over 70%

levels. It is now known that there are two forms of COX, COX-1 and COX-2. COX-1 is present in the GI tract and kidney and produces protective prostaglandins for those organs, and COX-2 is produced at sites of inflammation. Research is being directed at finding NSAIDs that target COX-2 specifically, which would avoid the loss of protective prostaglandins because of inhibition of COX-1. The second mechanism of NSAID action is their ability when given at higher dose to intercalate into the membrane of granulocytes and monocytes and interfere with the protein kinase C (PKC) activation pathway of these cells. This current understanding of the mechanism of actions explains why low doses help with pain but high doses are required to affect inflammation in any significant way.

   b. **Dosing.** Table 14–3 lists the current NSAIDs by their duration of action. An important principle to remember with dosing medications, including NSAIDs, is that it takes five half-lives to reach steady state and five half-lives to eliminate the drug from the body. Therefore, more patience is required when using an agent with a long half-life.

Salicylates have been a mainstay for the treatment of RA for many years. The plasma half-life is 3 to 6 hours, but salicylates exhibit dose-dependent characteristics, meaning that the higher the concentration, the longer the half-life. Salicylate levels can be measured, and the optimum level for anti-inflammatory activity is 20 to 30 mg/dL. Salicylates are started at 2 g/d in divided doses and gradually increased over 2 to 4 weeks to 4 g/d to achieve this level in the blood.

Other NSAIDs are generally started at a dose in the midrange and, remembering the five half-life rule, increased as needed to maximum dose if the response is inadequate.

TABLE 14–2. **Extraarticular Features of Rheumatoid Arthritis**

Ocular: Episcleritis, scleritis, scleromalacia
Pulmonary: Effusions, nodules, fibrosis
Cardiovascular: Small and medium-sized vessel vasculitis, aortitis (rare), pericarditis
Felty's syndrome: Neutropenia and splenomegaly
Sjögren's syndrome (secondary): Dry eyes and mouth (sicca)
Miscellaneous: Rheumatoid nodules

TABLE 14-3. Nonsteroidal Anti-inflammatory Drugs

DRUG	DAILY DOSE (mg) RANGE	SCHEDULE (DOSES PER DAY)	UNIT SIZE (mg)
Short-acting*			
Ibuprofen	1200-3200	3-6	300, 400, 600, 800
Fenoprofen	800-3200	3-4	200, 300, 600
Ketoprofen	150-300	3-4	25, 50, 75§
Indomethacin	50-200	2-4	25, 50†, 75‡
Tolmetin	600-2000	3-6	200, 400
Meclofenamate	200-400	4	50, 100
Diclofenac	100-200	2-4	25, 50, 75§
Intermediate-acting*			
Naproxen	500-1500	2	250, 375, 500§
Sulindac	300-400	2	150, 200
Diflunisal	500-1500	2	250, 500
Acetylsalicylic acid	1000-6000	3-4	325§
Etodolac	600-1200	2-3	300, 400
Oxaprozin	600-1200	1	600
Long-acting*			
Nabumetone	750-2000	1	500, 750
Piroxicam	20	1-2	10, 20
Phenylbutazone	300-400	1-4	100

*Drugs in the short-acting group have serum half-lives of about 1-4 h, in the intermediate-acting group about 10-20 h (dose dependent), and in the long-acting group about 45 h for piroxicam and 72 h for phenylbutazone.
†Also comes as a suppository.
‡Timed-release preparation.
§Standard size. Other unit sizes are available, depending on brand. Timed-release preparations are available.

c. **Adverse effects.** Table 14-4 outlines the variety of adverse effects of NSAIDs. The most important adverse effects are either GI or renal. NSAIDs may cause gastropathy by reducing levels of protective prostaglandins. Serious bleeding or even perforation may occur in the absence of prior symptoms. Misoprostol, a PGE-1 analog, has

TABLE 14-4. Adverse Reactions to Aspirin and NSAIDs

CNS: Headaches, cognitive dysfunction, psychosis, confusion, aseptic meningitis
Pulmonary: Exacerbation of asthma, pneumonitis
Gastrointestinal: Dyspepsia, nausea, ulceration, perforation, diarrhea, elevated transaminases, hypersensitivity hepatitis
Renal: Renal insufficiency, hyperkalemia, hypertension, interstitial nephritis, papillary necrosis
Hematologic: Impaired platelet function, aplastic anemia, agranulocytosis, thrombocytopenia
Cutaneous: Urticaria/angioedema, erythema multiforme, photosensitive eruptions, toxic epidermal necrolysis
Drug interactions: Increased blood levels of oral hypoglycemics, phenytoin, anticoagulants, lithium, methotrexate

been found to be effective in preventing NSAID-induced gastropathy. Etodolac and nabumetone may be more COX-2-specific agents and thus be less problematic. Another option in high-risk patients is the nonacetylated salicylates that have essentially no effect on prostaglandin production but remain effective anti-inflammatories at high dose.

Renal blood flow may be compromised by the NSAIDs, especially in patients with preexisting renal disease, congestive heart failure, cirrhosis, and hypovolemic states. Acetylated salicylates, such as aspirin, irreversibly bind to COX and interfere with platelet function during the life of the platelet. Other NSAIDs affect platelet function. The nonacetylated salicylates do not affect COX and have little direct effect on platelets and can be used in patients on anticoagulants.

Elderly patients are at particular risk for NSAID toxicity, and they should be used with caution in this group. All patients on long-term NSAIDs should be monitored. The current recommendations for monitoring are for a complete blood count, urinalysis, creatinine, potassium, and serum AST (glutamic oxaloacetic transaminase) at baseline, with follow-up at 1 to 3 months. These tests should then be done every 3 to 6 months while the patient is on the drug to monitor for toxicity.

2. **DISEASE-MODIFYING ANTIRHEUMATIC DRUGS.** DMARDs alter the manifestations of disease by suppressing the signs and symptoms of inflammation and by slowing radiographic evidence of joint space narrowing and juxtaarticular bone erosions. These agents may take 1 to 6 months before any clinical improvement is noted. The threshold for using these agents in patients with RA has declined over the last 20 years. The average time from diagnosis to institution of DMARDs has gone from an average of 2 years to less than 5 months, reflecting the concern about early intervention to prevent joint damage. Currently, the most frequently used DMARDs are hydroxychloroquine, sulfasalazine, and methotrexate.

Qualified generalist physicians may feel comfortable using either hydroxychloroquine, sulfasalazine, or methotrexate as a single agent in the treatment of RA. It is recommended that most RA patients be seen periodically by a rheumatologist to help in management, especially when combination therapy is deemed necessary or other DMARDs are being considered.

a. **Antimalarials.** Hydroxychloroquine and chloroquine are the two antimalarial agents in use for treating RA. Hydroxychloroquine is used more frequently because of concern about a greater risk of eye toxicity from chloroquine.

(1) *Mechanism of action.* Antimalarials affect immune activity, especially autoimmune activity, by interfering with the processing of antigen by antigen-presenting cells (APCs). These agents elevate the pH within the cells' vesicles, altering the way the antigen is degraded, bound to major histocompatability antigens, and presented to T cells. Both drugs are rapidly and

completely absorbed after oral administration and are concentrated in particular tissues, such as the retina, kidneys, bone marrow, and liver.

(2) ***Dosing.*** The ideal candidate for an antimalarial as a single agent is a patient with early, mild RA or with no evidence of bone erosions. Some clinical response may be noted by most patients at 8 to 12 weeks of therapy. The dosing is based on weight and is 6–6.5 mg/kg/d for hydroxychloroquine and 3.5–4 mg/kg/d for chloroquine. Standard dosages for adults are 200–400 mg/d of hydroxychloroquine and 125–250 mg/d of chloroquine. A recent metaanalysis of all DMARDs has shown that the antimalarials have one of the highest therapeutic-to-toxicity ratios, indicating that the efficacy is high and the toxicity is relatively low.

(3) ***Adverse reactions.*** Overall, only 8.5% of patients started on antimalarials stop these drugs because of adverse reactions. Most of these are GI related, with nausea, diarrhea, and abdominal pain most common. Rash is a less common cause for stopping. It typically is a full body, erythematous, maculopapular, pruritic rash that can be quite uncomfortable. With the dosing guidelines currently used, retinal toxicity, once the most feared adverse reaction, is fortunately quite rare. Nevertheless, it is important to obtain a baseline eye examination after the patient has demonstrated no acute toxicity from the drug (i.e., GI symptoms, rash) and repeat the eye examination at 6 to 12-month intervals. Other potential problems with the antimalarials include skin pigmentation, photosensitivity, and very rarely a neuromyopathy heralded by a decrement in the deep tendon reflexes.

(4) ***Monitoring requirements.*** Eye examinations should be performed every 6 to 12 months. It may be useful to document deep tendon reflexes initially and at regular intervals, as the loss of these reflexes may be a harbinger of neuromyopathy.

b. Sulfasalazine. Sulfasalazine was first used specifically for RA in the late 1930s. It did not attract much interest until the 1970s but has now emerged as a very useful agent for the treatment of RA.

(1) ***Mechanism of action.*** Sulfasalazine is a combination of sulfapyridine and 5-aminosalicylic acid (5-ASA). Sulfasalazine is cleaved by colonic bacteria in the intestine into sulfapyridine and 5-ASA. Sulfapyridine is absorbed and is the active component in treating RA, whereas 5-ASA remains in the GI tract, where it exerts an anti-inflammatory action in inflammatory bowel disease. The DMARD properties of sulfasalazine appear to occur from the ability of this agent to decrease the production of inflammatory cytokines, such as interleukin-1 (IL-1) and tumor necrosis factor (TNF). It also reduces the production of IgM rheumatoid factor.

(2) ***Dosing.*** Sulfasalazine generally comes in 500-mg tablets. The patient is started on 1000 mg in two divided doses, and the dose is increased over 1 to 2 weeks to 2000 mg/d. *Doses as high as*

3000–4000 mg/d may be used if there is a partial response to 2000 mg/d but only after 3 months of therapy at the 2000 mg/d level. With daily administration, steady-state levels in the blood are generally achieved in 4 to 5 days. The patient best suited for treatment with sulfasalazine is the patient with mild to moderate synovitis or one who has not responded to antimalarials. Improvement may begin in 3 to 6 weeks and continue for up to 24 months. Metanalysis of efficacy versus toxicity of sulfasalazine places it higher on the efficacy scale than antimalarials but with a higher potential toxicity.

(3) *Adverse reactions.* Short-term treatment trials place the discontinuation rate at 17% to 30%, but serious toxicity occurs in less than 5%. Most serious toxicity occurs during the first 3 months and is rare thereafter. The most serious adverse reaction is agranulocytosis, which occurs in 1.4% of treated patients and usually responds to drug withdrawal, although rare patients may need therapy with granulocyte-macrophage colony-stimulating factor (GM-CSF). The most common adverse reactions are nausea and diarrhea that responds to dose reduction but may require drug cessation. Other side effects include oral ulcers, hepatitis, thrombycytopenia, and CNS side effects (depression, headache).

(4) *Monitoring requirements.* Complete blood count (CBC) and transaminases every 2 weeks for 1 month, monthly for the next 5 months, then a CBC every 3 months thereafter.

c. **Methotrexate.** Methotrexate has emerged as one of the most useful agents for the treatment of RA.

(1) *Mechanism of action.* Although methotrexate at high doses inhibits folic acid metabolism, its activity at doses used in RA does not appear to depend on such activity. Indeed, the use of folic acid supplements appears to reduce the toxicity but not the efficacy of methotrexate. Recent data support the ability of methotrexate to promote the release and accumulation of adenosine, which in turn has significant effects on neutrophil function, including phagocytosis, release of toxic oxygen metabolites, and production of inflammatory cytokines. Methotrexate has a relatively rapid onset of activity (3 to 8 weeks), and when it is withdrawn, flare usually occurs within weeks, suggesting more of an anti-inflammatory activity than a true immune modulator.

(2) *Dosing.* Methotrexate can be administered orally, by subcutaneous or intramuscular injection, and intravenously. The oral absorption is approximately 75% of that given parenterally. Peak blood levels usually occur 1 to 2 hours after oral administration. Methotrexate comes in 2.5-mg tablets or in solution with a concentration at 25 mg/mL. The usual starting dose is 7.5 mg/wk PO in a single dose. This level is maintained for 4 to 6 weeks, and if there is no significant response, the dose is raised by 2.5 mg every 2 to 4 weeks to a maximum of 25 mg/wk. Most patients usually respond to 12.5 to 15 mg/wk, although some may require 20–25 mg/wk to achieve a therapeu-

tic response. As the dosage increases, many patients prefer to divide the therapy into two or three divided doses 12 hours apart. Some patients may respond better to parenteral administration of methotrexate, which can be tried if the response to oral dosing is insufficient. Patients can be taught to give the injections to themselves to reduce the cost. Patients with reduced renal function should receive methotrexate with extreme caution, if at all. NSAIDs or ASA should be used cautiously, since they can displace methotrexate from albumin, leading to elevated serum levels and potential enhanced toxicity.

The candidate for methotrexate is usually the RA patient with significant morning stiffness and synovitis or the patient who has not responded to either hydroxychloroquine or sulfasalazine. Methotrexate is currently the favored agent in the United States for treatment of RA because of its relatively rapid onset of action (3 to 8 weeks), high response rate (up to 75%), and high therapeutic index (efficacy versus toxicity).

(3) Adverse reactions. From 5% to 35% of patients stop methotrexate because of toxicity. The most common side effect of methotrexate is nausea and abdominal pain, which may necessitate drug withdrawal. Changing from oral to parenteral dosing may minimize GI toxicity. Also common are oral ulcers, which usually respond to administration of folic acid supplements, 1 mg/d. Serious hematologic toxicity may occur (leukopenia, anemia, thrombocytopenia) but also may be minimized by the use of folic acid. The most serious potential adverse reaction is hepatic toxicity. There was initially concern about the development of cirrhosis in patients on long-term methotrexate therapy, but prospective studies lasting up to 10 years have failed to demonstrate any major liver problems. Risk factors for hepatic toxicity include diabetes, obesity, previous liver injury, and alcohol use. Methotrexate should be used with caution in such individuals. Patients who refuse to stop using alcohol should not be given methotrexate. Methotrexate can have serious consequences on fetal development and should be given to women of childbearing age only with the understanding that precautions against pregnancy will be taken. A woman should be off methotrexate for at least one ovulatory cycle before conceiving. Other potential side effects include alopecia, which is usually mild, rash, pneumonitis, which may be quite severe, and very rarely, opportunistic infection.

(4) Monitoring requirements. CBC, transaminases, albumin, and creatinine at baseline, with CBC and transaminases every 4 weeks and creatinine and albumin every 3 months. A declining albumin may portend liver dysfunction even though the transaminases have been unimpressive. Some elevation of the transaminase level is common with initial therapy (two to three times normal) and usually normalizes with continued therapy or temporary dose reduction. Methotrexate should be stopped for pregnancy, serious leukopenia, persistent liver abnormalities, or pneumonitis. Patients should be advised to report a new

unexplained cough, as this may indicate methotrexate pneumonitis.

  d. **Gold compounds.** Gold compounds have been used since the 1930s for treatment of RA. Gold was once the most commonly used DMARD in RA but has fallen out of favor because of its toxicity. The RA patient for whom to consider gold treatment is one who has not responded to the preceding three agents either singly or in combination. Currently there are three compounds used: gold sodium thiomalate, gold thioglucose, both given by IM injection, and auranofin, an oral agent.

  (1) *Mechanism of action.* Even after over 60 years of use, the mechanism of action of the gold compounds is not well understood. The compounds inhibit the inflammatory activities of lymphocytes, monocytes, and, to a lesser degree, neutrophils.

  (2) *Dosing*

  (a) *Injectable compounds.* The initial dose should be 10 mg IM to preclude an idiosyncratic reaction, followed by 25 mg the next week, then 50 mg the third week. The 50-mg IM dose is then continued weekly until 1 g is reached. If there is no response at this point, gold should be stopped. Those patients with a good response can have the dose gradually decreased by giving 50 mg IM every 2 weeks for 2 months, 50 mg IM every 3 weeks for 2 months, and then 50 mg IM every month indefinitely.

  (b) *Oral agent.* The usual dose is 3 mg PO bid, with a maximum dose of 9 mg/d.

  (3) *Adverse reactions.* In a survey of 7000 patients on gold injections, adverse reactions occurred in 35%. The toxicity in decreasing order included skin reactions, stomatitis, postinjection flushing, and thrombocytopenia and leukopenia. Rare but potentially serious toxicity includes exfoliative dermatitis, aplastic anemia that may be fatal, and nephrotic syndrome. The presence of rash requires the cessation of gold therapy, but if the rash clears quickly, gold can be reinstituted at a lower dose, and the patient should be watched carefully. Any decrease in the cell counts on CBC is reason to stop gold treatment. A rechallenge may be cautiously attempted if the RA was well controlled on the gold. If protein in the urine reaches 300 mg in 24 hours, gold must be stopped and can be restarted cautiously when the urine clears. The oral agent auranofin has a propensity to cause significant diarrhea in up to one third of patients.

  (4) *Monitoring requirements.* Gold therapy requires rather intense monitoring. On the weekly schedule of gold injections, a CBC is done 1 week, alternating with a urinalysis the following week. It is generally advised that the laboratory work be done and reviewed before the injection. With auranofin, CBC and urinalysis are performed monthly.

  e. **Azathioprine.** Azathioprine is a cytotoxic agent and is generally not considered for initial DMARD therapy.

(1) Mechanism of action. Azathioprine is metabolized to 6-mercaptopurine (6-MP), and further metabolism of 6-MP produces compounds that interfere with the synthesis of adenine and guanine. Azathioprine acts by suppressing T cell function, decreasing immunoglobulin synthesis, and decreasing the secretion of IL-2.

(2) Dosing. The usual dose is 1–1.25 mg/kg/d, with a maximum dose of 2.5 mg/kg/d in unusual cases after at least 4 months of therapy on the lower dose. Rarely is an RA patient started initially on azathioprine. Its therapeutic ratio is lower than that of antimalarials, sulfasalazine, and methotrexate, and it is usually reserved for nonresponders or for use in combination regimens.

(3) Adverse reactions. Gastrointestinal toxicity (nausea, vomiting), oral ulcers, and rashes are relatively common but usually not serious and respond to either dose reduction or withdrawal. More significant is the hematologic toxicity, including leukopenia, anemia, and thrombocytopenia. Patients treated with azathioprine may experience a hypersensitivity reaction, with symptoms of fever, hypertension, arthralgias, and abnormal liver function tests. There is also a possible risk of increased lymphoproliferative malignancy in patients taking long-term azathioprine. Patients on allopurinol need only one-fourth the usual dose of azathioprine because of the inhibition of azathioprine metabolism caused by allopurinol. A combination of the two at the usual doses will result in significant azathioprine toxicity.

(4) Monitoring requirements. CBC and liver function tests every 2 weeks for the first 8 weeks, after which the monitoring may be reduced to every month if the patient is stable. The drug should be stopped for evidence of hepatitis or WBC less than 3000/mm^3.

f. **Cyclosporine.** Cyclosporine is not yet approved for use in RA but has been extensively studied in this disease. Recently, it has been shown to be beneficial in combination with methotrexate. There was statistically significant improvement in patients on methotrexate when cyclosporine was added to the regimens of those with only a partial response to methotrexate.

(1) Mechanism of action. Cyclosporine suppresses the immune response via its ability to inhibit the transcription of IL-2. Since IL-2 is critical in the activation of T cells in particular, the function of these cells is impaired. Other cytokines may also be affected.

(2) Dosing. The dosing is based on a per weight value, with the usual dose of cyclosporine in RA being 2.5–5 mg/kg/d. Levels above 5 mg/kg/d increase toxicity without any additional therapeutic value. Dosing should always start at the lower end of the range and be increased slowly according to response. This agent is poorly and variably absorbed orally, and excretion is principally via the biliary system. In general, cyclosporine

should be considered for the RA patients who are severely affected and not responding to less toxic agents. Cyclosporine should be used under the guidance of a rheumatologist.

(3) ***Adverse reactions.*** Gastrointestinal toxicity (nausea, diarrhea, vomiting, pain) is common, as are mild to moderate headaches, hypertrichosis, and gingival hyperplasia. The GI toxicity may respond to reducing the dose and then slowly increasing the dose back to a therapeutic range. The most serious toxicity is renal insufficiency and hypertension. Almost all individuals who take cyclosporine have an elevation in the creatinine by 25% or more. NSAID use may augment the risk of nephrotoxicity. Patients may require antihypertensives along with the cyclosporine to control blood pressure.

(4) ***Monitoring requirements.*** Blood pressure is taken weekly while instituting therapy and after increasing the dose. Serum creatinine is measured every 2 weeks for the first month, monthly for 6 months, and then at least every 3 months when stable.

g. Penicillamine. Because of its toxicity, this disease-modifying agent is used only after lack of response to other agents. The drug takes several weeks to months before clinical improvement. Penicillamine is started at 250 mg/d, and if there is no improvement after 3 months, the dose is increased to 500 mg/d for another 3 months. If there is no response, it is stopped. If the response is incomplete, the dose can be increased by 125 mg every 8 to 12 weeks to a maximum of 750 mg/d. If there is response at these higher doses, the dose is reduced slowly to 500 mg/d.

A CBC and urinalysis are done every 2 weeks for the first 6 weeks of therapy and then monthly.

(1) ***Adverse reactions.*** The side effects of penicillamine usually are encountered during the first 18 months of therapy. The most frequent is a rash, which when extensive requires stopping the drug. Patients also have an alteration or loss of taste perception. Aplastic anemia, leukopenia, and thrombocytopenia can develop. A white count of less than 3000/mm^3 or a platelet count below 100,000/mm^3 requires immediate discontinuation. Membranous glomerulonephropathy manifested by proteinuria and nephrotic syndrome can complicate penicillamine treatment. Urinary protein greater than 2 g/24 h requires discontinuing penicillamine. Patients with lesser degrees of proteinuria may be able to continue penicillamine at reduced dosage. Hematuria necessitates stopping the drug. When an autoimmune syndrome (myasthenia gravis, polymyositis, systemic lupus erythematosus, Sjögren's syndrome, Goodpasture's syndrome, or pemphigoid) develops in association with penicillamine, the drug should be discontinued.

3. GLUCOCORTICOIDS. Low doses of prednisone can be beneficial in patients with RA. The daily morning dose should not exceed 7.5 mg. Once there is response, prednisone is decreased by 1-mg decrements to achieve the lowest possible dose that will maintain clinical improvement. Other clinical situations in which low-dose glucocorticoids are beneficial: In a patient with active joint disease being started on a DMARD, low-dose prednisone will produce immediate clinical improvement and allow functioning during the time it takes the DMARD to become effective. Low-dose prednisone therapy also is justified in a patient whose continued functioning is necessary for maintaining a home or providing an income. Elderly patients with recent onset of RA often respond well to low-dose prednisone therapy alone.

Even with low-dose prednisone treatment, patients may be at risk for developing osteoporosis. Thus, these patients can be given supplemental calcium and vitamin D, and estrogens should be considered in postmenopausal women. Recent prospective data suggest that oral doses of glucocorticoids of 8 mg or less may not increase the risk of osteoporosis.

a. **Pulse intravenous methylprednisolone** therapy has been given to patients who are experiencing severe exacerbations. Methylprednisolone 1 g IV is given over 30 minutes. The patient's blood pressure should be carefully monitored during this infusion, as both hypotension and hypertension have been reported. IV therapy is usually given once a month for several months.

b. **Intraarticular glucocorticoids.** Intraarticular injection of glucocorticoids particularly helps the patient who has one or two swollen joints that have not responded to treatment. Joint injections are done under sterile conditions. The site of injection is anesthetized with 1% lidocaine; a small amount of lidocaine is also injected into the joint. The glucocorticoid preparations for intraarticular injection are in suspension and remain largely confined to the joint. The amount of steroid injected depends on joint size. The equivalent of 40 mg prednisone is recommended for injection of a knee, 10–20 mg for ankles, 5 mg for small joints of the hands or feet. In injection of the knee, 1–2 mL of 1% lidocaine can also be added. Care must be taken not to inject steroid into the soft tissue because this will cause atrophy of the overlying tissue. Joint pain several hours after injection due to chemical synovitis can be treated with an anti-inflammatory drug or analgesic.

4. OCCUPATIONAL AND PHYSICAL THERAPY. Occupational and physical therapy are important in RA. Patients should be instructed in joint protection and exercises to maintain strength and joint motion. Splinting of inflamed wrists relieves pain and permits continued use of the fingers. Splints are removed at least once a day so wrists can be exercised gently through a range of motion. Wrist splints worn at night often relieve symptoms of carpal tunnel syndrome. Diet instruction and sexual counseling are also important.

5. SURGERY. Synovectomy at selected sites may lead to improvement and prolongation of joint function. Synovectomy might be indicated in a knee with persistent synovitis of 6 months duration refractory to treatment. Synovectomy of the wrist and dorsal tendon sheath with resection of the ulnar styloid can reduce the risk of later extensor tendon rupture. Carpal tunnel release is indicated in patients with persistent symptoms or nerve conduction abnormalities of the median

nerve. Prostheses are now available for most joints, the most successful of which have been the hip and knee. Metatarsal head resection is indicated in patients with subluxation and pain not satisfactorily relieved by a metatarsal bar orthosis.

B. Extraarticular Manifestations of RA

1. **Vasculitis.** Patients with RA can develop symptomatic vasculitis, usually involving vessels ranging from small arteries to capillaries and venules. Manifestations include nailfold and volar pad infarcts of fingers, leg ulcers, mesenteric or coronary artery arteritis, and mononeuritis multiplex. Patients experiencing significant symptoms and organ damage require high doses of glucocorticoids: prednisone (60 mg/d) in divided doses initially, then gradually tapered to a single morning dose as dictated by clinical response. Cyclophosphamide 1–2 mg/kg/d may be given to patients who fail to respond initially to high doses of prednisone or require continued high doses of prednisone. Leg ulcers resulting from vasculitis present a difficult management problem requiring careful local care and elevation of the leg to minimize edema. Large skin ulcers may need skin grafts.

2. **Felty's syndrome,** characterized by RA, splenomegaly, and leukopenia, usually occurs in patients who have had RA for at least 10 years and in whom the titer of rheumatoid factor is high. Glucocorticoids may increase the neutrophil count but may not prevent infection. Both IM gold and methotrexate have been shown to improve neutropenia in patients with Felty's syndrome. The WBC count requires close monitoring in patients on those drugs. In most patients, splenectomy improves the neutrophil count and reduces the frequency of infection. Patients are given antipneumococcal vaccine (Pneumovax) before splenectomy.

3. **Sjögren's syndrome (secondary).** Patients who develop Sjögren's syndrome, manifested by dry eyes or mouth or both, are advised to use artificial tears or ointment regularly, especially at night, and to have regular dental care. Sjögren's syndrome in RA is usually not accompanied by the more severe system manifestations seen in the primary form of the disease.

Felson DT, Anderson JJ, Meenan RF. Use of short-term efficacy toxicity tradeoffs to select second-line drugs in rheumatoid arthritis. Arthritis Rheum 1992;35:1117–1125.

Gardner G, Furst DE. Disease-modifying antirheumatic drugs: potential effects in older patients. Drugs Aging 1995;7:420–437.

American College of Rheumatology Ad Hoc Committee on Clinical Guidelines. Guidelines for management of rheumatoid arthritis. Arthritis Rheum 1996;39:713–722.

American College of Rheumatology Ad Hoc Committee on Clinical Guidelines. Guidelines for monitoring drug therapy in rheumatoid arthritis. Arthritis Rheum 1996;39:723–731.

II. ANKYLOSING SPONDYLITIS

A. Clinical Characteristics

Ankylosing spondylitis (AS) is characterized by inflammation of the enthesis (areas of insertion of connective tissue into bone) that progresses to fibrosis and then ossification. Typically, AS begins with the insidious onset of

TABLE 14–5. Clinical Characteristics of Ankylosing Spondylitis

Joint areas potentially involved: Wrists, elbows, shoulders, hips, knees, ankles, spine, sacroiliac, sternoclavicular
Joint pattern: Symmetric sacroiliitis; progressive spinal involvement; asymmetric peripheral joint involvement in $^1/_3$; inflammation at insertion of Achilles tendon, plantar fascia, intercostal muscles
Laboratory: Anemia; elevated ESR
Immunogenetics: HLA-B27 in 90% of patients

bilateral sacroiliitis, with pain and stiffness occurring with inactivity and improving with movement. The pain is usually felt in the low back or buttock region and occasionally may radiate to the posterior thigh. In more severe cases, the entire spine may be involved and immobilized. Men are affected four times as often as women, and >90% of patients carry the HLA-B27 gene. The age of onset for most patients is 20 to 40 years. Other clinical features include peripheral arthritis usually of the large proximal joints, uveitis or iritis, and enthesitis of the plantar fascia or Achilles tendon. Patients with inflammatory bowel disease may develop AS but have a lower frequency of HLA-B27 than patients with AS alone (Tables 14–5 and 14–6).

B. Treatment

The goal of treatment is to reduce inflammation and stiffness to minimize spine deformity.

1. PHYSICAL THERAPY. The role of exercise to maintain spine range of motion cannot be overemphasized. Every patient with a recent diagnosis of AS should be sent to a physical therapist to be shown range of motion exercises and to discuss isometrics for the back and neck extensors. Posture should also be discussed. On each follow-up visit, the patient should be queried about compliance with these exercises.

2. NSAIDs. These agents have been the mainstay of therapy for AS and, by simply reducing stiffness and pain, may improve spine range of motion. The dose of NSAIDs for patients with AS is generally in the higher range. High doses interfere with WBC function (see NSAIDs in the rheumatoid arthritis section) and have a more profound effect on inflammation. The most effective NSAID is indomethacin, either 50 mg tid or 75 mg sustained-release bid. Naproxen and piroxicam as well as diclofenac are also effective in AS. Longer-acting agents are probably preferred for improved compliance in this age group. Remember to monitor these

TABLE 14–6. Extraarticular Manifestations of Ankylosing Spondylitis

Ocular: Episodes of acute uniocular iritis
Pulmonary: Fibrosis of upper lobes
Cardiovascular: Aortic insufficiency, conduction abnormalities
Neurologic: Cauda equina syndrome

TABLE 14–7. **Cytotoxic Drugs in Rheumatic Disorders**

DRUG	DOSE SCHEDULE	TOXIC SIDE EFFECTS
Azathioprine	Oral: 1–2 mg/kg/d	Marrow suppression, nausea, hepatitis, pancreatitis, oncogenesis, infection
Cyclophosphamide	Oral: 1–2 mg/kg/d IV: 0.5–1 g/m² of body surface area*	Marrow suppression, nausea and vomiting, infertility, hemorrhagic cystitis, bladder fibrosis, bladder carcinoma, infection, oncogenesis, pulmonary interstitial disease, alopecia
Chlorambucil	Oral: 0.1–0.2 mg/kg/d	Marrow suppression, nausea and vomiting, infertility, oncogenesis, hepatotoxicity
Methotrexate	Oral: 7.5–15 mg once a week† IV: 7.5–25 mg once a week	Marrow suppression, nausea and vomiting, diarrhea, stomatitis, cirrhosis, interstitial pulmonary disease

*Given at 1–3 mo intervals; see text.
†Given once a week in three divided doses, each separated by 12 h.

agents periodically for toxicity (see NSAID monitoring in the rheumatoid arthritis section).

3. **DMARDs.** Sulfasalazine has been studied for use in AS and is effective especially for the peripheral arthritis but may also be useful for inflammation of the spine. Sulfasalazine has been shown to reduce sedimentation rate and C-reactive protein and might, therefore, affect the long-term prognosis of the spine disease. Fewer data are available for methotrexate and azathioprine, but these agents have been effective in some patients. Dosing guidelines and monitoring are similar to those for RA (Table 14–7).

4. **CORTICOSTEROIDS.** Systemic corticosteroids are generally not useful in AS, but intraarticular corticosteroids may be used for treatment of the peripheral arthritis.

5. **SURGERY.** Surgery is occasionally needed for joint replacement of hips or shoulders. Patients with AS are prone to develop heterotopic ossification around the replaced joint, and this may be prevented by prophylactic low-dose radiation to the hip or shoulder or the use of postoperative indomethacin.

III. REITER'S SYNDROME

A. Clinical Characteristics (Table 14–8)

Reiter's syndrome (RS) is an inflammatory arthritis characterized by oligoarthritis (few joints), usually affecting the large joints of the lower extremities associated with either inflammatory eye disease (conjunctivitis, uveitis, iritis), recent urethritis, recent dysentery, or inflammatory low back pain. Over 80% of patients with RS are HLA-B27 positive. Patients frequently have enthesopathy similar to those patients with AS. Other features may include painless oral ulcers, hyperkeratotic rash on the palms or soles (or both) called keratoderma blennorrhagica, and a hyperkeratotic rash on the penis called circinate balanitis. When the digits are involved, they have the appearance of a sausage (dactylitis). Reiter's syndrome can follow an enteric infection with *Shigella, Salmonella,* or *Yersinia* or a genitourinary infection from *Chlamydia* or *Mycoplasma.*

B. Treatment

The main concerns when treating RS are peripheral joint inflammation, eye inflammation and enthesitis. Attacks of disease last 6 weeks to 6 months. Most patients have recurrent attacks, and some patients may have persistent disease that can be very difficult to control and require the institution of DMARD therapy.

1. **PHYSICAL THERAPY.** The emphasis of therapy for RS is on the peripheral joints rather than the spine. Significant spine disease is a late complication of more severe RS.

2. **NSAIDs.** As with AS, long-acting, high-potency NSAIDs in the high dosing range are useful for the joint inflammation and the enthesitis.

3. **DMARDs.** The same DMARDs used to treat AS can be used to treat RS. Dosing guidelines are the same as for RA (Table 14–7). Of note, RS and psoriatic arthritis may be more common in people infected with HIV, and risk factors for HIV should be ascertained, and appropriate testing should be done before using immunosuppressants, such as methotrexate or azathioprine.

4. **ANTIBIOTICS.** Some data support an initial 3 to 4 week treatment with antichlamydial antibiotics, such as doxycycline. This may shorten the initial episode and possibly prevent the development of a chronic disease state.

5. **CORTICOSTEROIDS.** As with AS, systemic corticosteroids are generally not helpful, but inflamed peripheral joints may respond well to injectable corticosteroids.

6. **MISCELLANEOUS.** Enthesitis involving the Achilles tendon and the plantar fascia can be particularly difficult to bring under control. Use of heel pads, arch supports, and soft tissue corticosteroid injection into the area of the plantar fascia may be of help. Injection of the Achilles tendon is not recommended.

TABLE 14–8. **Extraarticular Manifestations of Reiter's Syndrome**

Ocular: Conjunctivitis, uveitis
Urogenital: Urethritis, prostatitis, cervicitis
Mucocutaneous: Painless oral ulcers, circinate balanitis, keratoderma blennorrhagica on palms and soles, nail changes
Cardiovascular: Aortic insufficiency, conduction abnormalities

IV. PSORIATIC ARTHRITIS

A. Clinical Characteristics

Psoriatic arthritis is seen in 7% to 20% of people with psoriasis. Joint involvement may be either oligoarticular (affecting a few joints) or polyarticular, resembling RA. Psoriatic arthritis can also involve the spine, especially when the person carries the HLA-B27 gene. The affected digits typically take on a sausage appearance, similar to that with RS. Psoriatic arthritis can involve the DIP joints and is basically the only chronic inflammatory form of arthritis to do so. Another feature is nail pitting. The psoriatic rash may be limited to the scalp, navel, or intergluteal folds.

B. Treatment

1. **PHYSICAL THERAPY.** As for RA or other inflammatory forms of arthritis.

2. **NSAIDs.** Similar to other inflammatory forms of arthritis. NSAIDs should be the first medication used and may be the only agent necessary when only one or two joints are affected. One caveat is that some NSAIDs may exacerbate psoriasis. This should be considered when psoriasis gets worse with NSAID treatment.

3. **DMARDs.** In general, DMARDs used to treat RA, including gold compounds, can also be used to treat psoriatic arthritis. Doses are similar, and monitoring requirements are also the same. Methotrexate stands out as an agent that has been used to treat both the arthritis and the psoriasis. Antimalarials have been used successfully to treat psoriatic arthritis but have been implicated in worsening of the psoriasis in some patients.

4. **CORTICOSTEROIDS.** Oral corticosteroids frequently are helpful in psoriatic arthritis, as they are for RA. Some have cautioned that they may cause the development of pustular psoriasis. Intraarticular corticosteroids are useful for individual peripheral joint inflammation.

V. ARTHRITIS OF INFLAMMATORY BOWEL DISEASE

Ulcerative colitis and regional enteritis (Crohn's disease) may be associated with arthritis. Patients can have intermittent acute arthritis of peripheral joints or sacroiliitis and spondylitis. Back involvement is indistinguishable radiographically from primary ankylosing spondylitis. Bowel disease usually precedes ankylosing spondylitis. Peripheral joint disease involves episodes of acute arthritis in one or few joints, often the knee, that last a few weeks and then usually resolve completely without residual damage. Acute peripheral arthritis responds to a nonsteroidal drug or aspirin. These drugs also alleviate the pain of spondylitis. NSAIDs must be used cautiously because they have been reported to exacerbate the bowel disease. Sulfasalazine can serve a dual function in these patients, favorably affecting the inflammatory bowel disease as well as the arthritis.

Creemers MC, van Reil PL, Franssen MJ, van de Pitte LB, Gribnau FW. Second-line treatment in seronegative spondyloarthropathies. Semin Arthritis Rheum 1994;24:71–81.

VI. VASCULITIS

The vasculitides are a group of inflammatory disorders involving blood vessels, from capillaries and venules to large arteries. The disorders are classified according to the size of vessel primarily involved and the organ system(s) affected into four major groups: (1) hypersensitivity vasculitis, (2) polyarteritis and related disorders, (3) Wegener's granulomatosis, and (4) giant cell arteritis (temporal arteritis and Takayasu's disease).

A. Hypersensitivity Vasculitis

Hypersensitivity vasculitis (also called small-vessel vasculitis, allergic vasculitis, or leukocytoclastic vasculitis) affects capillaries, venules, and arterioles. Immune-mediated inflammation of small blood vessels can be induced by infection, collagen vascular disease, malignant disease, or drugs (Table 14–9).

Vasculitic skin lesions are palpable purpura (petechiae), vesicles, urticaria, erythema multiforme, or erythema nodosum, frequently appearing on the lower extremities below the knees. Other features include arthritis or arthralgias, myalgias, abdominal pain, GI bleeding, glomerulitis, pulmonary infiltrates, pleuritis, pericarditis, and peripheral neuropathy.

Henoch-Schönlein purpura (HSP) is a distinct form of hypersensitivity vasculitis that usually appears before the age of 20 but can occur at any age. HSP often occurs in the spring following an upper respiratory tract infection. The classic clinical triad of HSP is palpable purpura, arthritis, and abdominal pain. Patients may also experience gastrointestinal bleeding, proteinuria, hematuria, or renal insufficiency.

Mixed cryoglobulinemia is characterized by purpura, arthralgias, and glomerulonephritis. There is a high association of mixed cryoglobulinemia with hepatitis C, especially with type II mixed cryoglobulinemia (monoclonal IgM antibody and polyclonal IgG antigen). Hepatitis B may also be associated. Diffuse glomerulonephritis may progress to renal failure. In these patients, underlying chronic liver disease is usually present. Cold exposure may lead to infarction of ear lobes, tip of nose, or digits. In patients with mixed cryoglobulinemia associated with hepatitis C, treatment with interferon-α (IFN-α), 3 million U three times a week for 6 months, has led to reduction of skin lesions and improvement in liver function test and renal function. Unfortunately, the disease may exacerbate after discontinuing IFN-α. Other treatment regimens are under study.

TABLE 14–9. Differential Diagnosis of Hypersensitivity Vasculitis

Drugs
Bacterial endocarditis
Hypocomplementemic vasculitis
Henoch-Schönlein purpura
Mixed cryoglobulinemia
Connective tissue diseases
Malignant diseases

1. **THERAPY** is initially directed to removing or treating any responsible stimulus for the vasculitis. Infections, such as subacute bacterial endocarditis, are investigated and treated appropriately. A careful drug history should be obtained; however, usually the antigen or stimulus cannot be identified. **No treatment** of the vasculitis is necessary when it is mild and transient. In patients with more severe lesions, particularly those leading to skin ulceration or internal organ involvement such as glomerulonephritis, **prednisone** 40–60 mg/d is recommended. The dose is gradually tapered based on clinical response. Dapsone has also been effective in some patients. Prognosis is good in most cases of hypersensitivity or small-vessel vasculitis.

B. Polyarteritis Nodosa and Related Disorders

Polyarteritis nodosa (PAN) involves medium-sized arteries mainly in middle-aged patients. The vasculitis is segmental and has a predilection for branching points and bifurcations of arteries. Lesions are at different stages of development. Hepatitis B or hepatitis C is associated with the vasculitis in some patients. Symptoms are often nonspecific and include fever, malaise, myalgias, weakness, and weight loss. Tender nodules representing aneurysms can sometimes be palpated along the artery. Narrowing or occlusion of small arteries can cause digital gangrene or infarction of viscera, such as bowel or gallbladder. Kidney involvement can lead to hypertension and hematuria. Myocardial infarction and cerebrovascular accidents are other manifestations. of PAN; the lungs are spared. Vasculitis of the lung occurs in the disorder termed allergic angiitis and granulomatosis (Churg and Strauss). These patients usually have a history of asthma and peripheral blood eosinophilia.

A variant of PAN called microscopic polyarteritis affects predominantly small arteries. Organs involved tend to be kidney, lung, and skin. This form of polyarteritis is characterized by pauci-immune glomerulonephritis, pulmonary infiltrates and hemorrhage, and purpuric skin lesions. The antineutrophil cytoplasmic antibody (ANCA) test is positive for p-ANCA in many of these patients.

1. **TREATMENT.** This is started with **prednisone** 60 mg/d in divided doses, and **cyclophosphamide** 1–2 mg/kg/d is added. Once the patient's condition is stabilized, the dose of prednisone is gradually tapered to the lowest possible that will control symptoms. After the condition has been stable for several months, the dose of cyclophosphamide is cautiously reduced, and a close watch is kept for exacerbation. In some patients, the vasculitis is short-lived, whereas others may require treatment for months or longer. Although experience is limited, pulse cyclophosphamide treatment might be a reasonable alternative to daily cyclophosphamide and may reduce the risk of fibrosis and cancer of the bladder. Intervals between pulse treatment vary from 1 to 3 months, depending on the clinical response (see discussion of pulse cyclophosphamide treatment, Systemic Lupus Erythematosus, p. 259).

C. Wegener's Granulomatosis

This is characterized by necrotizing and granulomatous vasculitis involving the upper and lower respiratory tract and kidneys. A history of chronic sinusitis is frequent. Symptoms include cough (often productive of purulent sputum), hemoptysis, purulent nasal discharge, fever, myalgias and arthralgias, and weight loss. Hematuria, proteinuria, and a rising creatinine level indicate renal disease. Destruction of nasal cartilage produces saddle nose. Purpuric skin lesions can occur. The ANCA test is a useful diagnostic test and indicator of disease activity, but diagnosis is based on biopsy.

1. TREATMENT. Recognition of Wegener's granulomatosis is important, as untreated disease has a high mortality. Treatment is started with **prednisone,** 60 mg/d in divided doses, and **cyclophosphamide,** 2 mg/kg/d. Prednisone will reduce constitutional symptoms but is not sufficient treatment. The dose of prednisone is tapered to the lowest that controls constitutional symptoms. Cyclophosphamide is continued for several months, and the dose then can be tapered slowly. A reasonable alternative to daily cyclophosphamide might be pulse therapy given at intervals of 1 to 3 months, depending on the clinical response. Methotrexate has also been shown to be effective. Trimethoprim-sulfamethoxazole has been used in localized upper respiratory tract disease with some success and recently has been reported to prevent relapses in some patients after treatment with cyclophosphamide and prednisone.

D. Temporal Arteritis

Temporal arteritis, also referred to as cranial or giant cell arteritis, is granulomatous vasculitis affecting medium-sized arteries, primarily of the head. Headache is a common symptom, as are temporal artery and localized scalp tenderness. Patients may also experience decreased vision, diplopia, sudden blindness, vertigo, fever, malaise, weight loss, arthralgias, and jaw claudication. Temporal arteritis can involve symptoms of **polymyalgia rheumatica** (stiffness, aching pain, and soreness of the muscles of the shoulders, neck, and hip girdles). Patients often can give the exact time the symptoms started. The sedimentation rate is usually elevated above 50 mm/h and often higher (Westergren's method). When this diagnosis is considered, prednisone, 60 mg/d in divided doses, is immediately started, and a temporal artery biopsy is obtained within a few days. If it is negative, a biopsy is obtained from the other side. If this also is negative, a search should be made for other causes of these signs and symptoms.

1. TREATMENT. At least 40 mg prednisone per day is used for the first 4 to 6 weeks after diagnosis. If the patient is asymptomatic, very slow tapering of the prednisone dose is then started. Usually the patient will receive prednisone for an average of 2 years. Prednisone dosage is determined by signs and symptoms and not by the sedimentation rate. A modest elevation of sedimentation rate frequently occurs when prednisone is decreased and usually does not indicate a flare of disease. After the first several weeks of treatment, prednisone can be given as a single morning dose. Methotrexate has been used in the treatment of temporal arteritis to allow reduction of high doses of prednisone.

2. POLYMYALGIA RHEUMATICA. Patients may have polymyalgia rheumatica without clinical manifestations of temporal arteritis. For them, treatment with prednisone, 10–15 mg/d, is started. Dramatic improvement

usually occurs in 4 or 5 days or possibly a week. An excellent response to low doses of prednisone is typical of polymyalgia rheumatica. Low-dose prednisone is continued for several weeks and then is gradually tapered. Average duration of treatment is 1 to 2 years. Attempts should be made to find the lowest possible maintenance dose.

E. Takayasu's Arteritis

This is a disease of young adults (especially women) but can affect all ages. The disease usually involves the aorta and its major branches, with CNS ischemia, arm claudication, renal ischemia with hypertension, and mesenteric ischemia.

1. **TREATMENT.** Prednisone, 60 mg/d in divided doses, is started. The dose should be kept at ≥40 mg/d for at least 6 weeks, when slow tapering is begun. It is difficult to monitor treatment of this disorder because symptoms and signs are highly variable. The patient is observed for recurrent ischemic episodes. Vascular graft surgery is necessary in some patients to restore flow and prevent tissue infarction.

Agnello V, Romain PL. Mixed cryoglobulinemia secondary to hepatitis C virus infection. Rheum Dis Clin North Am 1996;22:1.

Conn DC, Hunder GG, O'Duffy JD. Vasculitis and related disorders. In: Kelley WN, et al., eds. Textbook of Rheumatology. Philadelphia: WB Saunders; 1993.

Gilliland BC. Vasculitis. Immunol Allergy Clin North Am 1993;13:335.

Guillevin L, et al. Prognostic factors in polyarteritis nodosa and Churg-Strauss syndrome. A prospective study in 342 patients. Medicine 1996;75:17.

Hoffman GS, et al. The treatment of Wegener's granulomatosis with glucocorticoids and methotrexate. Arthritis Rheum 1992;35:1322.

Hoffman GS, et al. Treatment of glucocorticoid-resistant or relapsing Takayasu arteritis with methotrexate. Arthritis Rheum 1994;37:578.

Mandell FB, Hoffman GS. Differentiating the vasculitides. Rheum Dis Clin North Am 1994;20:409.

Stegeman CA, Tervaert JWC, et al. Trimethoprim-sulfamethoxazole (co-trimoxazole) for the prevention of relapses of Wegener's granulomatosis. N Engl J Med 1996;335:16.

VII. OSTEOARTHRITIS

Osteoarthritis (OA) is the most common form of arthritis in the United States. The disease is characterized clinically by pain, restricted joint movement, and joint deformity. The disease affects predominantly middle-aged and older persons and increases with age. A number of conditions that alter cartilage or joint mechanics can lead to osteoarthritis. Injury to articular cartilage, torn meniscus, or ligamental instability can cause incongruity of joint surfaces and subsequently osteoarthritis. Classification of osteoarthritis is given in Table 14–10.

A. Clinical Characteristics

Commonly affected joints are hips, knees, lumbar and cervical spine, the distal and proximal interphalangeal joints of the hands, and the first carpal-metacarpal and first metatarsal-phalangeal joint. Pain usually begins insidiously and has a deep aching quality (sometimes poorly localized), initially brought on by activity and relieved by rest. It eventually becomes more constant and can be present at night. Pain, contractures, and deformity of joints limit physical activities. On physical examination, the

TABLE 14–10. Classification of Osteoarthritis

Primary: Localized, generalized (three or more joint areas affected), erosive (inflammatory form of OA of the hands)
Secondary: Trauma, congenital anomaly (Perthes' disease, congenital hip dysplasia), metabolic (CPPD, ochronosis, hemochromatosis, acromegaly, gout), postinflammatory arthritis (e.g., rheumatoid arthritis, infection), other (avascular necrosis, Charcot joint)

involved joint is swollen and tender and may be slightly warm and erythematous. The joint is enlarged because of both bony expansion and effusion. Crepitus may be felt on joint movement.

In primary osteoarthritis, routine laboratory tests, including the erythrocyte sedimentation rate, are normal. In secondary osteoarthritis, the laboratory reflects the underlying disease. X-rays initially are normal, but as the disease progresses, joint space narrowing, subchondral bone sclerosis, periarticular bone cysts, and osteophytes are observed.

B. Treatment

Therapy for OA should be thought of as a program intended to improve mobility and reduce pain to a more acceptable level.

1. **PHYSICAL THERAPY.** There are numerous studies that demonstrate the utility of range of motion, muscle strengthening, and aerobic conditioning. Aerobic activity especially may improve walk time and decrease pain scores and even depression levels. A visit or two to a physical therapist to discuss range of motion exercises, muscle strengthening, and joint protection and to develop an aerobic program is appropriate.

2. **ANALGESICS.** In a recent study comparing acetaminophen with ibuprofen for the treatment of OA, 4000 mg/d of acetaminophen was as helpful as 1200 and 2400 mg of ibuprofen. Patients with OA should be considered for acetaminophen therapy because of its relative safety and low cost. Some patients may also benefit from a small amount of a low-potency narcotic, such as propoxyphene or acetaminophen with codeine, to use when pain becomes more severe. Tramodol (Ultram) is a new analgesic that might be useful for some patients. The dose is one to two 50 mg tablets every 6 hours. It can cause dizziness, constipation, and nausea and can lower the seizure threshold in patients on antiseizure medications.

3. **NSAIDs.** These agents have been the mainstay of therapy for OA. Their potential for toxicity is greater in older persons with OA. Analgesic range doses (low dose) are usually sufficient in established OA when little inflammation is present. Many patients do well taking the NSAIDs as needed or before increased activity.

4. **CORTICOSTEROID INJECTIONS.** These can be quite helpful for treatment of symptomatic joints. Injections should be given no more than three or four times per year and no more than ten times total in any one joint. Pain relief may last weeks to months. Patients should be cautioned about being too active with a recently injected joint, since the joint may

574 I *14* RHEUMATIC DISORDERS

temporarily have reduced pain and proprioception. Loss of those protective mechanisms may allow OA to progress more rapidly.

5. SURGERY

   a. **Arthroscopy.** Arthroscopic surgery is warranted primarily for knee OA to remove loose bodies from the joint and trim torn menisci. Good candidates for arthroscopy usually have symptoms of locking or giveaway, have persistent joint effusions, and have mild OA on x-ray. Patients with more advanced OA of the knee generally are not candidates for arthroscopy.

   b. **Total joint arthroplasty.** One of the greatest advances in medicine in the last 40 years is the development of total joint arthroplasty. The appropriate candidate is the patient with moderate to severe OA who has not responded sufficiently to a medical therapy program, does not have significant underlying medical illness, is not content with a sedate lifestyle, and is willing to go through major surgery. Approximately 80% to 90% of patients who undergo total joint arthroplasty for OA, especially of the hip or knee, get excellent results.

Bradley JD, Brandt KD, Katz BP, Ralasinski LA, Ryan SI. Comparison of an anti-inflammatory dose of ibuprofen, an analgesic dose of ibuprofen and acetaminophen in the treatment of patients with osteoarthritis of the knee. N Engl J Med 1991;325:125–127.

Oddis CV. New perspectives on osteoarthritis. Am J Med 1996;100:10S–15S.

VIII. GOUT

Gout comprises a group of disorders that have in common clinical features caused by deposition of monosodium urate from supersaturated extravascular fluid. Gout is characterized by episodes of acute arthritis, by macroaggregates of monosodium urate (tophi) primarily in articular and surrounding tissue leading sometimes to crippling arthritis (chronic tophaceous gout), and by formation of urinary urate calculi. Any of these disorders can occur alone or in combination. Gout affects middle-aged and older men and is uncommon in women until after the menopause, when its frequency approaches that in men.

A. Causes of Hyperuricemia

The hallmark is hyperuricemia defined as a level 2 SD above the mean. The normal serum urate concentration in men is 5.1 mg ± 1 mg/dL and in women is 4 ± 1 mg/dL. Approximately 5% of normal persons are hyperuricemic, and only a few will develop gout. Hyperuricemia results from overproduction or underexcretion or both. The normal amount of urate excreted by the kidney in 24 hours is 600 mg. Approximately 90% of persons with primary gout have decreased renal clearance of urate, whereas about 10% are overproducers, excreting more than 1000 mg in 24 hours. This latter group is at greater risk of urinary calculi.

Hyperuricemia and gout are classified as secondary when they are associated with another disorder (renal failure, polycythemia, myeloproliferative and lymphoproliferative disorders, multiple myeloma, and a hereditary disorder, G-6-PD deficiency). Certain drugs and toxins decrease renal clearance of urate, including low-dose aspirin (less than 2 g/d), proximal loop diuretics (thiazide and furosemide), alcohol, and lead.

B. Clinical Characteristics

Acute gouty arthritis tends to affect distal joints in the lower extremities. The first metatarsal-phalangeal joint is most often involved, followed by tarsal joints, ankle, knee, and wrist. Urate-induced inflammation can also occur in bursae, in particular the olecranon and prepatellar. The onset of an attack is sudden. Untreated, the pain and swelling reach a peak in 24 to 36 hours and then subside over 3 to 10 days, usually without residual joint damage. Chronic tophaceous gout is characterized by aggregates of urate (tophi) in subchondral bone, cartilage, synovium, olecranon and other bursae, and soft tissue over the extensor surface of the upper forearm and over small joints of the hand, with insidious progressive joint destruction. Tophaceous gout becomes clinically apparent 10 or more years after the initial attack of gout.

C. Diagnosis

This is established definitively by identifying the characteristic rod-shaped or needle-shaped crystal either free in synovial fluid or in leukocytes under compensated polarized light.

D. Treatment

Goals are to (1) relieve pain and swelling of acute arthritis, (2) prevent future attacks of acute arthritis, (3) prevent or decrease the formation of tophi, and (4) prevent formation of urinary urate calculi.

1. ANTI-INFLAMMATORY DRUGS. Acute arthritis is treated with any one of several NSAIDs. The maximum daily dose schedule of NSAID is begun for 24 to 48 hours. Therapeutic blood levels are achieved faster with short-acting NSAIDs given in the recommended maximum daily dose. After 2 or 3 days, the dose is reduced to a midrange for the next 7 to 10 days. For example, indomethacin 50 mg is given q6h for 24 to 48 hours, followed by 25 mg qid for 7 to 10 days.

2. GLUCOCORTICOIDS. These are quite effective in treating acute gout and are a reasonable alternative in patients in whom large doses of NSAIDs are contraindicated. Treatment is started with 40 mg/d of prednisone, which can be given in a single dose. The dose is tapered by 5-mg decrements over the next 7 days. To prevent a poststeroid withdrawal flare of arthritis, a low dose of an NSAID (e.g., indomethacin 25 mg bid) or oral colchicine, 0.6 mg bid, is administered, beginning on the third day of treatment and continuing for 1 to 2 weeks after prednisone has been stopped.

3. INTRAARTICULAR GLUCOCORTICOIDS. In a situation in which systemic steroids or other medications are contraindicated, intraarticular steroids can be effective. The joint is first thoroughly aspirated when possible, then an intraarticular steroid preparation is injected. The injection dose for the knee is the equivalent of 40 mg of prednisone; for the ankle or wrist, 10–20 mg; and for the small joints of the hands and feet, 5 mg. Lidocaine 1% can be used to anesthetize the overlying skin

and soft tissue. However, this additional step may bring further discomfort and may not reduce the pain of injection. When possible, prophylactic colchicine therapy should be instituted to prevent rebound flare.

4. **COLCHICINE.** Oral colchicine has been replaced by other drugs in acute gout. However, in a patient experiencing several attacks of acute gout a year, low doses of oral colchicine (0.6 mg bid) will reduce the number and severity of episodes. An acute attack can be aborted by increasing colchicine to 0.6 mg/h for three to five doses when joint pain is first experienced. In patients with renal insufficiency or liver disease, the dose of colchicine should be reduced and WBC counts closely monitored. Colchicine blocks chemotaxis and phagocytosis by inhibiting the polymerization of microtubules.

   When a patient is unable to take anything by mouth, IV colchicine can be used to treat an acute attack; it does not cause the GI side effects of oral therapy. However, because of its potential severe toxicity and the availability of other therapies, IV colchicine is not recommended except in unusual circumstances. Colchicine 2 mg is diluted in 20 mL of saline and given over a 10-minute interval to reduce the possibility of severe thrombophlebitis. A secure IV line is important to prevent extravasation of colchicine, which can cause tissue necrosis. An additional 1 mg appropriately diluted can be given in 6 hours and in another 6 hours if required. Patients should not receive more than 4 mg IV for an attack of gout. IV colchicine should not be given to patients who have renal insufficiency, liver disease, or neutropenia. The dose should be reduced by one third to one half in elderly patients with decreased creatinine clearance. Colchicine toxicity includes marrow suppression, hepatocellular damage, myopathy, and neuropathy.

5. **HYPOURICEMIC THERAPY.** Drugs to decrease serum uric acid are indicated in patients who have tophaceous gout, frequent attacks of gout not controlled by prophylactic colchicine or NSAIDs, or recurrent urinary urate calculi. In addition, an antihyperuricemic drug is indicated in overproducers of uric acid, who are at risk of developing renal calculi. The 24-hour uric acid excretion in these patients is usually more than 1000 mg. Asymptomatic hyperuricemia or acute gout without apparent tophi does not usually require treatment with an antihyperuricemic drug, although some researchers disagree with this approach. Some recommend that uric acid be normalized in patients with nontophaceous gout. Renal disease due to parenchymal urate deposition is uncommon in patients with long-standing hyperuricemia. The antihyperuricemic drugs are probenecid, sulfinpyrazone, and allopurinol.

   a. **Uricosurics.** Probenecid and sulfinpyrazone are uricosuric agents. These drugs are preferably given to patients who are underexcreters of uric acid, have normal renal function, and have no renal calculi. When probenecid or sulfinpyrazone administration is started, **colchicine,** 0.6 mg bid, or low-dose NSAID is given to prevent flares of acute arthritis. Colchicine or an NSAID is continued for several months until the serum uric acid level is normal.

(1) ***Probenecid*** is started at 500 mg/d in two divided doses and increased by 500 mg/mo until serum uric acid is normalized. Most patients will respond to a dose between 1 and 3 g/d. The patient should be encouraged to increase fluid intake and to take the medication with meals. Probenecid should not be taken at bedtime when renal perfusion is low and the urine pH is acidic, conditions that foster the development of urate stones.

  (a) ***Adverse effects.*** Probenecid interferes with renal excretion of a number of drugs, raising their serum levels. These include NSAIDs, sulfonamides, sulfonylureas, methotrexate, penicillin, and ampicillin. Salicylates block the action of probenecid. Adverse reactions include rash, nausea, vomiting, and anaphylaxis.

(2) ***Sulfinpyrazone*** dosage is started at 100 mg/d in two divided doses. The dose is increased by 100 mg/wk until serum uric acid is normalized. Dosage can be increased to a maximum of 800 mg if necessary. The usual maintenance dose is around 400 mg/d in three or four divided doses.

  (a) ***Adverse effects.*** Sulfinpyrazone interferes with the excretion of sulfonamides and sulfonylureas and can potentiate the hypoglycemic effects of the latter. The drug also potentiates the action of Coumadin. Salicylates antagonize the uricosuric effect of sulfinpyrazone. Side effects include exacerbation of peptic ulcer disease and rash. Marrow suppression is rare. The drug also interferes with platelet aggregation.

b. Allopurinol is an antihyperuricemic drug that blocks the formation of uric acid by inhibition of xanthine oxidase. Since the drug is excreted in the urine, the dose of allopurinol should be reduced by at least 50% in those with significantly reduced renal function.

Allopurinol is the antihyperuricemic drug of choice in patients with widespread tophaceous gout and reduced renal function and in those with renal calculi. It should be used in patients with a history of stones who are overexcreters of urate, since they are at risk of developing more stones. Allopurinol should not be used to treat asymptomatic hyperuricemia. The starting dose of allopurinol is 100 mg/d and is increased by 100 mg/d until the serum uric acid concentration is less than 7 mg/dL. The dose can then be adjusted to the amount required to maintain a normal serum uric acid value. The maximum recommended daily dose is 800 mg/d. Most cases can be controlled with 300 mg/d.

  (1) ***Adverse effects.*** An important drug interaction of allopurinol is with the chemotherapeutic drug 6-mercaptopurine and its derivative azathioprine. Because these drugs are inactivated by xanthine oxidase, allopurinol will cause increased serum levels and potential toxicity. The dose of these chemotherapeutic drugs should be reduced by at least one third for a patient on allopurinol. Approximately 5% of patients on allopurinol will have a serious adverse reaction requiring discontinuation. The

most serious side effect is a life-threatening hypersensitivity reaction, with fever, rash, and hepatocellular injury. Types of rashes include pruritic maculopapular eruptions, erythema multiforme, toxic epidermal necrolysis, and generalized exfoliation. Patients with renal failure or who are receiving diuretics appear to be at greater risk of developing this serious drug reaction. Other side effects include nausea and diarrhea. An antihyperuricemic drug should not be started until after the acute gout attack resolves. These agents can prolong the attack by mobilizing urate from tissue sites to joint fluid. This same mechanism accounts for arthritis flares during the first several months of treatment. Patients with large tophaceous deposits may need to receive prophylactic doses of colchicine for a year or longer. In general, colchicine, 0.6 mg bid, or a low-dose NSAID should be given along with an antihyperuricemic drug until the uric acid level is normalized and tophi have resolved.

c. **Allopurinol with chemotherapy.** Allopurinol is also used to prevent acute uric acid nephropathy in patients undergoing chemotherapy for malignant disease. The patient should first be well hydrated and given a diuretic to increase urine flow and sodium bicarbonate to alkalinize the urine. Allopurinol, 8 mg/kg, is given in a single daily dose for 3 to 4 days. To prevent a gouty arthritis attack, colchicine, 0.6 mg bid, is also started; it is continued until allopurinol is stopped.

Emmerson BT. The management of gout. N Engl J Med 1996;334:445–451.
Levy M, Spino M, Read SC. Colchicine: a state of the art review. Pharmacotherapy 1991;11:196–211.

IX. CALCIUM PYROPHOSPHATE DIHYDRATE DEPOSITION DISEASE

Deposition of calcium pyrophosphate dihydrate (CPPD) crystals within articular hyaline cartilage and fibrocartilage can cause articular damage. Table 14–11 classifies CPPD crystal deposition disease.

A. Clinical Characteristics

Several different syndromes have been described in patients with CPPD crystal deposition disease.

1. PSEUDOGOUT is marked by episodes of acute arthritis, often as severe as urate gout, principally affecting the knees. Wrists, elbows, and even first-metatarsophalangeal joints also can be affected.

TABLE 14–11. Classification of CPPD Crystal Deposition Disease

Familial forms: Most autosomal dominant and associated with early osteoarthritic joint changes
Associated with metabolic disease: Hyperthyroidism, hemochromatosis, hemosiderosis, hypophosphatasia, hypomagnesemia, hypothyroidism
Idiopathic: Accounts for majority of cases

2. **PSEUDORHEUMATOID** is associated with polyarticular involvement, morning stiffness, synovial thickening, and in some cases, elevation of the sedimentation rate.

3. **PSEUDOOSTEOARTHRITIS** consists of degenerative changes in multiple joints, most often knees, wrists, metacarpophalangeal joints, hips, shoulders, ankles, and spine.

4. **PSEUDONEUROPATHIC** is a severe destructive joint disease, especially in the knees, and can be seen in the absence of a neurologic disorder.

5. **ASYMPTOMATIC CPPD.** Chondrocalcinosis, a radiographic sign of CPPD arthropathy, may be seen in the absence of symptoms.

B. Diagnosis

This is established by finding crystals either free in synovial fluid or in synovial fluid neutrophils. Crystals, appearing as small rods, cuboids, and rhomboids, can also be identified on synovial biopsy. They show weakly positive birefringence. X-rays show stippled or punctate deposits in articular cartilage and fibrocartilage. Calcifications can also be seen in tendons, ligaments, and joint capsules.

C. Treatment

Treatment is similar to that for acute gout. For prophylaxis, colchicine, 0.6 mg bid, or daily low doses of an NSAID will decrease the number and duration of attacks. Patients with chronic forms of disease are treated with an NSAID. Treatment of the underlying metabolic disorder does not affect the clinical expression of CPPD crystal deposition disease. Intraarticular injections of glucocorticoids are also quite effective in treating this disorder. Weightbearing joints should be injected only two or three times a year to prevent the possibility of accelerating joint damage.

X. HYDROXYAPATITE CRYSTAL DEPOSITION DISORDERS

Hydroxyapatite crystal deposition may lead to articular inflammation. The deposition of these crystals often occurs at sites of local tissue damage. Shedding of these crystals into the adjacent tissue results in phagocytosis by synovial lining cells and macrophages, followed by release of inflammatory mediators leading to tissue damage. Hydroxyapatite is a basic calcium phosphate that is partially carbonated. The crystals are 50 to 500 mm in length and form aggregates. They are detected by a calcium stain, alizarin red S. Definitive diagnosis requires special techniques such as electron diffraction or infra-red spectroscopy.

Hydroxyapatite crystal deposition occurs in periarticular tissues, especially around the shoulders. The supraspinatus tendon frequently is affected. Periarticular crystal deposition also occurs around the knees, hips, small joints. In a few patients, deposition of crystals may represent familial disease, but in most cases, crystal deposition is thought to occur as a result of metabolic abnormalities, exposure of crystal nucleating surfaces on collagen fibrils, and local tissue damage. In the majority of patients, the presence of hydroxyapatite crystals does not cause symptoms. The shedding of crystals into the surrounding tissue can result in acute inflammation involving bursae and tendons. Periarticular calcifications at the first metatarsal phalangeal joint can lead to acute inflammation, termed pseudopodagra. The periarticular calcifications subsequently disappear. Patients may experience acute shoulder pain and restriction of movement. Acute episodes resolve over days to weeks or, in some cases, even longer. During the acute attack, the calcific density may become indistinct and may disappear, only to reappear months to years later. An acute episode is usually treated with a NSAID using anti-inflammatory doses (see p. 553). Symptomatic relief also may occur with aspiration of the involved bursa, which may contain thick, chalklike fluid. Injection of corticosteroids may produce dramatic improvement, although there is concern that the corticosteroids may produce further calcification and tissue damage. Surgical removal of calcific deposits may be indicated in some patients for relief of symptoms. Patients undergoing chronic hemodialysis may also experience articular and periarticular inflammation. In patients with osteoarthritis, hydroxyapatite crystals are often found in cartilage and in synovium. The role of these crystals in osteoarthritis is unclear, and the treatment is that for osteoarthritis.

A unique destructive arthropathy of the shoulder has been associated with the presence of hydroxyapatite crystals. This syndrome affects mostly elderly women, leading to destruction of the rotator cuff and damage to the joint. The synovial fluid may contain fragments of cartilage and bone. The effusion is usually large and noninflammatory. Apatite crystals are present in the joint fluid. Some investigators have reported high levels of proteases, which may be released as a result of the hydroxyapatite crystals stimulating synovial cells to release proteases and other cytokines. The shoulder is most commonly involved, but the hip and knee can also be affected. Treatment is symptomatic, and a joint smoothing procedure or joint replacement could be considered in severe cases.

Halverson PB, McCarty DJ. Basic calcium phosphate (apatite, octacalcium phosphate, tricalcium phosphate) crystal deposition diseases. In: McCarty DJ, Koopman WJ, eds. Arthritis and Allied Conditions, 12th ed. Philadelphia, Lea & Febiger; 1993.

XI. SYSTEMIC LUPUS ERYTHEMATOSUS

SLE is an immune-mediated disorder that affects multiple organ systems. It strikes the young and old of both sexes. The female/male ratio is 9:1. The incidence is greater in African Americans than in whites.

The effects of estrogen on the immune system contribute to the high incidence of SLE in women during childbearing years. UV light, infections, and drugs are environmental factors that can trigger SLE. Abnormal immune regulation plays a critical role in SLE. Development of B cell hyperactivity results in hypergammaglobulinemia and autoantibodies, which are directed against antigens in the cytoplasm, nucleus, or the surface of cell membranes. Autoantibodies directed to cell membrane antigens cause hemolytic anemia, thrombocytopenia, or neutropenia. The serologic hallmark of SLE is antinuclear antibodies, in particular, antibodies to double-stranded DNA that are highly specific for SLE. Immune complexes are deposited in tissue, resulting in nephritis, arthritis, serositis, and vasculitis.

A. Clinical Characteristics

Table 14–12 lists the diagnostic criteria for SLE. Clinical expression and course are highly variable. Patients may have only one or a few features, such as rash, arthritis, or pleuritis, whereas others have multiple organ system involvement at presentation. Likewise, manifestations vary during the course, characterized by remissions and exacerbations. Fever, anorexia, weight loss, and fatigue occur frequently. Even after years of apparent inactivity, lupus can exacerbate and progress to death. Survival of SLE patients is 86% at 5 years and 76% at 10 years.

1. **MUSCULOSKELETAL.** The most frequent symptoms are arthritis and arthralgias. Arthritis is usually symmetric and nonerosive, involving small joints of hands and feet, wrists, knees, and ankles. Arthritis can be persistent or transient. Tenosynovitis can occur alone. Muscle pain and weakness can be due to inflammatory myositis or secondary to glucocorticoids, hydroxychloroquine, or hypokalemia.

2. **SKIN.** The most typical cutaneous manifestation of SLE is a butterfly erythematous facial rash over the malar areas and bridge of nose, which is often photosensitive and usually does not lead to scarring. SLE patients can also have lesions of **discoid lupus** that can cause severe disfiguring scars. Other skin manifestations include erythema multiforme, papulosquamous lesions, petechiae, vesicles, bullae, urticaria, angioedema, and panniculitis. Reversible or scarring alopecia can also occur. Small-vessel vasculitis can appear as palpable purpura, nailfold or volar fingerpad infarcts, erythema multiforme or nodosum, or livedo reticularis.

TABLE 14–12. Revised Diagnostic Criteria for Classification of Systemic Lupus Erythematosus

CRITERIA*	DEFINITION
Malar rash	Erythematous rash over malar eminences
Discoid rash	Erythematous patches with adherent keratotic scaling and follicular plugging
Photosensitivity	Rash as result of sun exposure
Oral ulcers	Oral or nasal ulceration
Arthritis	Nonerosive arthritis of 2 or more joints
Serositis	Pleuritis or pericarditis
Renal disorder	Persistent proteinuria >0.5 g/d or cellular casts
Neurologic disorder	Seizures or psychosis not associated with medications or metabolic derangement
Hematologic disorder	Hemolytic anemia or leukopenia (<4000/mm³) or lymphopenia (<1500/mm³) or thrombocytopenia (<100,000/mm³)
Immunologic disorder	Positive LE cell preparation or anti-DNA antibodies or anti-SM antibodies or false-positive VDRL
Antinuclear antibodies	

*For study purposes, a patient with 4 or more of these criteria simultaneously or serially is considered to have SLE.

From Tan EM, Cohen AS, Fries JF, et al. The 1982 revised criteria for the classification of systemic lupus erythematosus (SLE). Arthritis Rheum 1982;25:1271–1277.

3. **RENAL.** Clinically apparent renal disease occurs in more than half of SLE patients. Presenting signs of lupus nephritis are hematuria, proteinuria, and an active urine sediment consisting of red cell, white cell, and hyaline casts. Hypertension, nephrotic syndrome with either diffuse proliferative or membranous glomerulonephritis, and the complication of renal vein thrombosis also occur. Administration of an NSAID can worsen renal function.

   Lupus nephritis is classified pathologically into pure mesangial, focal segmental, diffuse proliferative, membranous, and advanced sclerosing glomerulonephritis. There may be overlap among these major histologic types. Of the first four types, diffuse proliferative glomerulonephritis carries the worst prognosis. Membranous glomerulonephritis can remain static for years. Histologic indices of activity and chronicity guide treatment decisions. Glomerular hypercellularity, fibrinoid necrosis, leukocyte exudation, hyaline thrombi, and interstitial inflammation are features of disease activity and usually respond to treatment. A high chronicity index based on glomerular sclerosis, fibrous crescents, tubular atrophy, and interstitial fibrosis portends irreversible disease, especially with azotemia.

4. **PULMONARY.** The most common pulmonary manifestation is pleurisy, occurring in more than half the patients. Pleural effusions are usually slight and show mononuclear cells. Patients can also develop acute lupus pneumonitis manifested by bilateral alveolar infiltrates. Infections should always be excluded because they account for most of the pulmonary infiltrates seen in SLE. Diffuse interstitial pneumonitis occasionally is observed. Pulmonary hypertension due to vascular involvement of pulmonary arteries is a serious complication of lupus and results in death in 1 to 2 years. Peripheral emboli resulting from peripheral thrombophlebitis also occur with greater frequency in lupus patients. Thrombophlebitis is associated with lupus anticoagulant or anticardiolipin antibodies.

5. **CARDIAC.** Pericarditis is the most commonly observed cardiac manifestation of SLE, occurring in about a third of patients. Fever, rub, tachycardia, and atrial fibrillation or flutter are clinical features. Tamponade is an uncommon complication. Patients can also develop myocarditis; Libman-Sacks endocarditis (nonbacterial verrucous vegetations) is usually asymptomatic and rarely diagnosed clinically. Coronary artery disease also occurs in SLE. Glucocorticoids, hypercholesterolemia, hypertension, and underlying coronary artery vasculitis are contributing factors.

6. **CENTRAL NERVOUS SYSTEM.** CNS disease covers a wide spectrum of manifestations ranging from subtle behavioral and cognitive abnormalities to strokes, seizures, and severe psychiatric disturbances. Other manifestations include aseptic meningitis, transverse myelitis, chorea, ataxia, and peripheral and cranial nerve neuropathies. Headache, often typical of migraine, is common in SLE. In patients with cerebrovascular accidents due to thrombosis there appears to be a relationship with the lupus anticoagulant or anticardiolipin antibodies.

7. **GASTROINTESTINAL.** Nausea and anorexia are common symptoms. Vasculitis of the bowel wall can cause abdominal pain, diarrhea, and melena, which can progress to bowel infarction or perforation. Acute pancreatitis can also occur as a feature of SLE or as a complication of glucocorticoid treatment.

8. **OCULAR.** Ocular manifestations are dryness (sicca syndrome), episcleritis, retinal artery vasculitis, and optic neuritis. Posterior capsule cataracts result from glucocorticoid treatment. Thrombotic glaucoma can occur in patients with anticardiolipin antibodies.

B. Treatment

An understanding of the disease by the patient and a good relationship among physician, patient, and family are essential. Patients should generally be seen by their physician about every 3 to 6 months to monitor the disease and adjust treatment. More frequent visits are needed during disease flares. Early recognition of disease flares or such complications as infections or drug reactions followed promptly by appropriate treatment can reduce morbidity and mortality. Patients should be told that estrogens used for birth control may increase the risk of lupus exacerbation. Fatigue is a common symptom in SLE. Patients should be encouraged to rest during the day and get a good night's sleep.

Since some patients experience flares of systemic disease or rash or both with exposure to ultraviolet (UV) light, they should be advised to stay out of the sun during peak hours (10 AM to 3 PM) of UV light, wear appropriate clothing, and use a high-grade sunscreen, which should be applied several times a day. Patients should also be warned about artificial sources of UV light.

The risk of infection is increased in SLE patients, especially those on glucocorticoids or cytotoxic drugs. Patients should be immunized with **pneumococcal** and **influenza vaccines,** the latter yearly. Prophylactic antibiotics are indicated in patients undergoing dental procedures and should also be considered in those having invasive diagnostic studies. Intrauterine devices carry an increased risk of infection.

1. **ARTHRITIS.** Arthritis is treated with a salicylate or NSAIDs. The dose is adjusted within the recommended range to control the symptoms. NSAID inhibition of prostaglandins within the kidney in lupus nephritis may worsen renal function. Occasionally, low-dose prednisone (5–10 mg/d) may be needed to control arthritis. For patients with persistent symptoms, hydroxychloroquine (200–400 mg/d) is useful.

2. **PERICARDITIS/PNEUMONITIS.** Pleurisy or pericarditis may respond to an NSAID but often requires glucocorticoids. The initial dose of prednisone is 20–40 mg/d. Symptoms usually respond in a few days, when dosage can be tapered by 5-mg decrements every 3 to 5 days, depending on the symptoms. A persistent pleural effusion should be aspirated to exclude other causes. Pericardial effusions can occasionally progress to tamponade, requiring pericentesis and instillation of glucocorticoids into the pericardium. Lupus pneumonitis also responds to the suggested doses of glucocorticoids after infection has been excluded.

3. **RASH.** Skin lesions may respond to topical fluorinated steroids. Fluorinated steroids, however, should not be used on the face because they will lead to thinning and atrophy of the skin. Hydroxychloroquine can be used for more extensive disease, especially in patients with discoid lesions and with subacute cutaneous SLE lesions. The initial dose is 400 mg/d. Once rash is under control, this can be reduced to 200 mg/d, and eventually to 200 mg qod. Because of the danger of retinal toxicity, the patient should have a careful baseline ophthalmologic examination, which should be repeated every 6 to 9 months. Prednisone, beginning at 40 mg in two or three divided doses, may be required when there is no response. The dose should be tapered as soon as possible to the lowest dose that will control the skin disease (see guidelines for steroid tapering under treatment of renal disease). Injection of glucocorticoids into the skin lesion can be quite effective but may lead to skin atrophy.

4. **RENAL DISEASE.** See Chapter 6 (pp. 258–259) for treatment of lupus nephritis.

5. **CEREBRITIS.** Both the diagnosis and treatment of CNS lupus are difficult. In patients with severe cognitive abnormalities and neuropsychiatric disturbances, prednisone can be tried in dosages ranging from 60 to 100 mg/d in two or three divided doses. When the patient improves, prednisone is given as a single morning dose, which is then tapered by 10-mg decrements at 5 to 7-day intervals until the dose is 40 mg and then by 5-mg decrements at 5 to 7-day intervals, depending on response. When the patient's symptoms cannot be controlled with prednisone 10 mg/d or less, alternative treatments should be considered.

   Patients already taking glucocorticoids may develop symptoms similar to those in CNS lupus. The distinction clinically between steroid psychosis and CNS lupus is difficult. When there is a question, the patient can be treated with high-dose prednisone (up to 100 mg/d) for 1 week. The prednisone dose is tapered slowly if the patient improves. If not, the symptom may be due to steroid psychosis, and prednisone should be tapered as quickly as possible. Haloperidol in doses of 1–4 mg bid or tid may help control psychiatric symptoms.

   Seizures can usually be controlled with phenytoin, 100 mg bid or tid. Prednisone, 60 mg/d in two divided doses, is also started; the dosage is then slowly tapered as previously described. It is difficult to know the end point of steroid therapy in this situation when seizures are the only evidence of activity. Patients with transverse myelitis and peripheral neuropathies can also be treated with prednisone.

   Strokes may be caused by vasculitis or possibly thrombosis secondary to a lupus anticoagulant or anticardiolipin. Patients should be treated with prednisone, 40–60 mg/d in two divided doses, which is tapered slowly. In a stroke patient who has a lupus antiphospholipid antibody, anticoagulation with heparin followed by Coumadin is probably indicated, assuming there is no evidence of bleeding. An alternate treatment is low-dose aspirin, 325 mg/d or qod.

6. **CYTOPENIA.** Hemolytic anemia and thrombocytopenia usually respond to **prednisone,** 40–60 mg in two or three divided doses. Occasionally, a patient may require 80–100 mg/d in divided doses. The initial dose is

continued until the platelet count or hematocrit has risen to a safe level. Prednisone dosage is then consolidated into a single morning dose, which is then tapered slowly. **Splenectomy** should be considered in thrombocytopenia or hemolytic anemia when cell counts cannot be controlled with glucocorticoids. When surgery is contraindicated, a patient with thrombocytopenia can be given **vincristine** or **vinblastine.** Danazol, 300–600 mg/d in divided doses, is also effective in some patients with thrombocytopenia or hemolytic anemia. IV gamma globulin, 40 mg/kg/d for 5 days, has been beneficial for some patients.

7. PULSE GLUCOCORTICOID TREATMENT. An alternative treatment to daily high doses of glucocorticoid in severe SLE is IV boluses of glucocorticoids. **Methylprednisolone** sodium succinate, 1 g IV, is given over a 30-minute period, and the dose is repeated on 3 consecutive days. Pulse therapy can be repeated in 3 months, depending on the patient's clinical status. After IV pulse therapy, the maintenance glucocorticoid dose is resumed; this can be further tapered on the basis of clinical parameters. Side effects include hypertension, hyperglycemia, and facial flushing. Rare complications are anaphylaxis, cardiac arrhythmias, and seizures.

C. SLE and Pregnancy

Recent data question the long-held notion that pregnancy exacerbates SLE. Nevertheless, it is clear that the incidence of adverse fetal outcomes is increased at least twofold in SLE. The most common problems are miscarriage, prematurity, and stillbirth. In the presence of lupus nephritis, the risk of fetal loss is even higher. The presence of anticardiolipin antibodies also seems to be a risk factor.

Since fetal survival is improved when lupus is under control, pregnancy should be planned at a time when the disease has been inactive for several months. In patients who have had recurrent spontaneous abortions and who have been shown to have antibodies to anticardiolipin, special steps should be taken. The pregnancy should be carefully monitored and treated as high risk. Early induction or cesarean section may be needed. Fetal survival has improved in some patients who were treated with prednisone and aspirin. Subcutaneous heparin also has been used. Glucocorticoids (prednisone, prednisolone, hydrocortisone) are metabolized by the placenta and do not affect the fetus. Dexamethasone should not be used during pregnancy. NSAIDs, antimalarials, and cytotoxic drugs should be avoided in patients contemplating pregnancy and during the pregnancy. Breast-feeding is considered safe in women who receive less than 30 mg/d of prednisone.

D. Drug-Induced Lupus

Several drugs can induce a lupuslike syndrome (Table 14–13). Procainamide is by far the most frequent cause of drug-induced lupus. The most common symptoms associated with drug-induced lupus are arthritis, arthralgias, pleurisy, and pericarditis. Renal and CNS disease are rare. Antinuclear antibodies (ANAs), most notably antihistone and anti–single-stranded DNA antibodies, are found in these patients. ANAs are also present in asymptomatic patients. Symptoms usually disappear a few weeks after stopping of the drug but occasionally will last for several months. The ANA test may remain

TABLE 14–13. **Drugs Associated with Lupuslike Syndrome**

MOST COMMONLY REPORTED	LESS COMMONLY REPORTED
Procainamide	Quinidine
Hydralazine	Practolol
Isoniazid	Penicillin
Hydantoin	Tetracyclines
	Sulfonamides
	Chlorpromazine
	D-Penicillamine
	Phenylbutazone
	Allopurinol
	Propylthiouracil

positive for months to years. Although symptoms usually disappear after stopping of the drug, patients may require salicylates or an NSAID. When symptoms are severe, glucocorticoids, 20–40 mg/d in two divided doses, are usually effective.

Hahn BH. Management of systemic lupus erythematosus. In: Kelley WN, et al., eds. Textbook of Rheumatology. Philadelphia: WB Saunders; 1993.
McCune WJ (Guest ed.). Systemic lupus erythematosus. Rheum Dis Clin North Am 1994;20:1.

XII. POLYMYOSITIS AND DERMATOMYOSITIS

Polymyositis (PM) and dermatomyositis (DM) are inflammatory disorders of unknown cause involving primarily proximal muscles of the upper and lower extremities. PM/DM occurs more often in women. The mean age of onset in adults is about 50 years. ANAs are frequently present, with anti-Jo-1, anti-PM/SCL, and anti-Mi appearing to have specificity for myositis. PM/DM occurs as a primary idiopathic disorder (type I and type II, respectively), in association with malignant disease (type III), in childhood (type IV), and in association with other collagen vascular diseases (type V). Inclusion, eosinophilic, and localized nodular myositis are classified as type VI.

A. Clinical Characteristics

PM or DM usually occurs as symmetric proximal muscle weakness causing difficulty in climbing stairs, rising from a couch, lifting heavy objects over the head, and combing the hair. Symptoms are often present for several months before the patient sees a physician. Some patients experience muscle pain and tenderness. Weakness of the muscles of the esophagus or pharynx produces dysphagia or dysphonia. Cardiac manifestations include cardiac arrhythmias, heart failure, and pericarditis. Interstitial fibrosis develops in about a third of patients. Patients are also at risk of aspiration pneumonitis. Raynaud's phenomenon, arthralgias, or arthritis may be experienced, as well as constitutional symptoms of malaise, weight loss, and fever.

In DM, rash can precede, coincide with, or follow the onset of muscle weakness. Typically, the patient develops an erythematous facial rash, often with a butterfly distribution, periorbital edema, and a dusky purple discoloration of the upper eyelids referred to as heliotrope. Scaly, purplish red papules develop over the dorsal surfaces of the interphalangeal joints, elbows, knees, and medial malleoli. Diagnostic tests for PM/DM are elevated muscle enzymes (CPK, aldolase, AST [SGOT]), myopathic changes on EMG (short-amplitude polyphasic potentials, fibrillations, irritability), and positive muscle biopsy (fiber necrosis, inflammatory infiltrate).

The course is highly variable. The cumulative survival rate is greater than 70% at 8 years.

B. Treatment

Initial treatment is with **prednisone,** 60–80 mg/d in three divided doses. After the first week, the dosage can be consolidated into a single morning dose. This dose is maintained until muscle enzyme values are normal. Improvement should occur within the first few weeks or month of treatment, at which time the dosage is tapered by 10-mg decrements every 5 to 7 days until it is 30 mg and then by 5-mg decrements at the same intervals. The patient's clinical state, muscle strength, and serum enzyme values are closely monitored and used as guidelines for reducing prednisone. Most cases respond to prednisone, and a low daily dose or alternate-day schedule can be used for maintenance. A cytotoxic agent should be added when myositis cannot be controlled with prednisone, ≤ 20 mg/d, after 2 to 3 months of starting prednisone. The most experience with cytotoxic drugs in PM/DM has been with azathioprine and methotrexate. The dose of **azathioprine** is 1.5–3 mg/kg/d. The initial dose of **methotrexate** is 7.5 mg/wk given in three divided doses 12 hours apart once a week. This dose can be gradually increased to 15 mg weekly. When a patient is unable to tolerate oral methotrexate because of GI upset, the drug can be given IM beginning with 10 mg once a week, which can be increased to 25 mg once a week depending on clinical response. Methotrexate should not be given to those with a creatinine value greater than 2 mg/dL or with liver disease. Concomitant aspirin or an NSAID, which are weak organic acids, can raise the blood level of methotrexate by interfering with its excretion and increase the risk of toxicity (see Rheumatoid Arthritis). When the rash in DM does not respond to prednisone, **hydroxychloroquine** can be used, beginning with a dose of 400 mg/d (see Rheumatoid Arthritis, pp. 556–557). For recalcitrant myositis, IVIG in a dose of 1–2 mg/kg/mo may be used. Cyclosporine also has been effective at a dose of 2.5–5 mg/kg/d. Both are expensive, and clinical experience is limited.

Steroid **myopathy** can complicate the clinical course of PM/DM and is likely when muscle weakness progresses in the face of normal muscle enzyme levels. The dose of prednisone is reduced to a level that will keep muscle enzymes normal. Steroid myopathy can also contribute to muscle weakness in a patient with active myositis, in which case, the dose of steroid is maintained and a cytotoxic drug (methotrexate) is added with the expectation that the dosage of prednisone can later be reduced.

During active disease, patients should regularly receive passive range-of-motion exercises to prevent contractures. Once the disease is under control, physical activity and muscle strengthening can gradually be increased.

Workman RL. Idiopathic inflammatory diseases of muscle. In: Weismann MH, Weinblatt ME, eds. Treatment of the Rheumatic Diseases. Philadelphia: WB Saunders; 1995, pp 201–216.

XIII. SYSTEMIC SCLEROSIS

Systemic sclerosis (scleroderma) is a chronic inflammatory disorder of unknown cause characterized by fibrosis of the skin and visceral organs, including the GI tract, lungs, heart, and kidney. The peak incidence of systemic sclerosis (SSc) is in the third to fifth decade; it is unusual in childhood and young men. Women are affected at least three times more often than men, especially during the childbearing age.

The degree and rate of skin and visceral involvement vary among patients. Two clinical subsets of SSc are recognized (Table 14–14). The first, referred to as diffuse cutaneous scleroderma, can have a rapid onset with early truncal involvement. These patients are at greater risk of developing pulmonary fibrosis and renal involvement within the first few years of their disease. In the other subset, limited cutaneous scleroderma, skin involvement is usually restricted to the distal extremities and face. Significant renal involvement is rare. The limited form of the disease is also referred to as CREST syndrome (calcinosis, Raynaud's phenomenon, esophageal dysmotility, sclerodactyly, telangiectasia). Although limited cutaneous disease is usually more benign, a few patients develop progressive pulmonary arterial hypertension, which is often fatal, or biliary cirrhosis. Although these two subsets are useful in predicting the course, some patients have overlapping features. In a few patients, systemic sclerosis may involve internal organs with little or no skin features, referred to as systemic sclerosis sine scleroderma.

A. Clinical Characteristics

1. **SKIN.** The first symptom of systemic sclerosis is usually Raynaud's phenomenon. The skin over the hands eventually becomes thickened,

TABLE 14–14. **Subsets of Systemic Sclerosis**

	DIFFUSE	LIMITED*
Skin involvement	Distal and proximal extremities, face, trunk	Distal to elbows, face
Raynaud's phenomenon	Onset within 1 year or at time of skin changes	May precede skin disease by years
Organ involvement	Pulmonary (interstitial fibrosis)	Gastrointestinal
	Renal (renovascular hypertensive crisis)	Pulmonary arterial hypertension after 10–15 y of disease in less than 10% of patients
	Gastrointestinal	Biliary cirrhosis
	Cardiac	
Nailfold capillaries	Dilatation and dropout	Dilatation without significant dropout
Antinuclear antibodies	Antitopoisomerase 1	Anticentromere

*Also referred to as CREST (calcinosis, Raynaud's phenomenon, esophageal dysmotility, sclerodactyly, telangiectasia).

From Gilliland BC. Systemic sclerosis (scleroderma). In: Fauci AS, et al. Harrison's Principles of Internal Medicine, 14th ed. New York: McGraw-Hill, 1996.

leathery, and tightly bound to underlying tissue. Digital ulcers, gangrene, and resorption of the distal phalanx may occur. Skin later becomes shiny, taut, and pigmented, with areas of hypopigmentation. Punctate telangiectases appear over the fingers, hands, face, mouth, lips, and tongue. Calcium deposits may appear in the volar pads of fingers and over extensor surfaces of the forearms, elbows, and knees. After many years, skin eventually softens in most patients but remains atrophic. Arthritis/arthralgias, joint contractures, fibrosis of tendon sheaths, and muscle atrophy may be present.

2. GASTROINTESTINAL. Systemic sclerosis affects the lower two thirds of the esophagus and lower esophageal sphincter. Patients complain of dysphagia, especially with solids. Reflux leads to esophagitis and strictures. Hypomotility of the small intestine produces bloating and abdominal pain, suggesting obstruction (pseudo-obstruction). **Bacterial overgrowth** in the atonic small bowel is responsible for causing malabsorption syndrome, manifested by steatorrhea, hypoalbuminemia, hypocalcemia, anemia, and weight loss. In the large bowel, wide-mouthed diverticula occur along the antimesenteric border of the transverse and descending colon. Hypomotility of the large bowel leads to obstipation.

3. PULMONARY. Pulmonary manifestations include interstitial pulmonary fibrosis, reduced diffusion capacity, and less commonly pleurisy. Pulmonary arterial hypertension also occurs and is seen mostly in patients with limited cutaneous involvement or CREST syndrome.

4. CARDIAC. Features of cardiac involvement are left ventricular dysfunction, heart failure due to myocardial fibrosis, pericarditis, and varying degrees of heart block and arrhythmia.

5. RENAL. Kidney disease is the most common cause of death in patients with systemic sclerosis. Scleroderma renal crisis most often occurs in patients with rapidly progressing diffuse cutaneous scleroderma and is usually manifested by malignant hypertension, proteinuria, and microscopic hematuria. If it is not treated, renal function rapidly deteriorates.

6. MISCELLANEOUS. Patients can also develop **hypothyroidism,** due to fibrosis of the thyroid gland or associated with Hashimoto's thyroiditis. **Biliary cirrhosis** is present in some patients with CREST syndrome. **Sjögren's syndrome,** with dry eyes and dry mouth, can also occur.

7. LABORATORY. Patients may have a hypoproliferative anemia secondary to chronic inflammation, and the ESR may be elevated. Patients may have hypergammaglobulinemia and a positive rheumatoid factor. ANAs are detected in 95% of patients using a cultured human laryngeal carcinoma cell line (HEp-2) substrate. Antitopoisomerase autoantibodies are found in approximately 40% of patients and are associated with diffuse cutaneous scleroderma, particularly in those at risk for developing pulmonary fibrosis. Anticentromere autoantibodies are found in 60% to 80% of SSc patients, predominantly those with limited cutaneous scleroderma. Antinucleolar and anti-RNP autoantibodies are also found in some SSc patients.

B. Treatment

Although no cure exists for systemic sclerosis, treatment of the involved organ system can be beneficial. The patient should be seen at least every 3 months or more often, depending on the severity of the illness and medications. Throughout their illness, patients will need repeated explanations and reassurances. Early recognition of scleroderma renal crisis can prevent potential renal damage.

1. PENICILLAMINE. Penicillamine is the most widely used drug for this disorder. Penicillamine has been shown to be immunosuppressive and to interfere with the molecular cross-linking of collagen. Retrospective studies show that patients on penicillamine have less skin thickening and reduced rate of new visceral organ involvement. To reduce adverse reactions, the dose is started low and increased slowly. The starting dose is 250 mg once a day, which is increased at 1 to 3-month intervals up to 1.5 g/d as tolerated. Because few patients can tolerate 1.5 g/d, a maintenance dose between 0.5 and 1 g/d is used for most. Doses of 500 mg or less can be given once a day. Higher amounts are given in two or three divided doses. The drug should be taken on an empty stomach. CBC and urinalysis are done monthly. See also p. 562.

2. RAYNAUD'S PHENOMENON. Patients are instructed to avoid frequent exposure to cold, to dress warmly, and to keep their body and face as well as their extremities warm. Vasodilators are used to treat Raynaud's phenomenon. These include reserpine, alpha-methyldopa, phenoxybenzamine, prazosin, and calcium channel blockers (nifedipine, diltiazem, and amlodipine). **Nifedipine** is recommended as the drug of choice in most patients. A sustained-release preparation has made nifedipine better tolerated. The usual dose of sustained-release preparation is 30 mg/d, but doses up to 60–90 mg/d may be required to control symptoms. Peripheral edema and tachycardia may be a problem with nifedipine in some patients. **Diltiazem,** 60 mg tid or qid, can be tried when the patient is unable to tolerate nifedipine. It may have less effect on relaxation of the lower esophageal sphincter than nifedipine has. **Amlodipine** is a long acting calcium channel blocker. The usual dose is 5 mg/d. Nitroglycerin paste applied to affected fingers and toes may also improve blood flow. Iloprost, a prostacycline analog, may decrease the severity of Raynaud's phenomenon and allow healing of digital ulcers. This drug is not yet available for general use. Pentoxifylline (Trental) improves blood flow through small vessels by increasing red cell deformability. Nitroglycerin paste applied to hands and feet is useful in some. Surgical sympathectomy can lead to transient improvement. Some patients benefit from learning **biofeedback** techniques for increasing skin temperature. Digital ulcers should be kept clean and protected from trauma by wearing of a finger guard. Antibiotics should be started at the first sign of infection.

3. ESOPHAGEAL DYSMOTILITY/REFLUX. Patients with esophageal reflux are advised to eat smaller meals, not to lie down for a few hours after a meal, to have the head of the bed elevated, and to avoid coffee, tea, and chocolate, which relax the lower esophageal sphincter. Antacids and H_2

blockers are also given. Omeprazole, a gastric acid (proton) pump inhibitor, is an effective drug in treating those patients with esophagitis, particularly those with erosive changes. Metoclopramide and cisapride, smooth muscle stimulators, increase gastrointestinal motility and increase lower esophageal sphincter tone. Esophageal dilation may be necessary in patients with strictures. Patients with malabsorption syndrome, often caused by bacterial overgrowth, improve with intermittent use of broad-spectrum antibiotics (tetracycline, metronidazole, or trimethoprim-sulfamethoxazole). In patients with constipation, stool softeners and mild laxatives are usually adequate.

4. MUSCULOSKELETAL. Polyarthritis is treated with an NSAID. The patient should do daily flexibility exercises to maintain range of motion. Patients with myositis usually respond to corticosteroids (prednisone 40 mg/d), slowly tapered based on the creatine kinase levels and muscle strength.

5. RENAL CRISIS. This is treated immediately with a potent antihypertensive agent. The angiotensin-converting enzyme (ACE) inhibitors (e.g., captopril, enalapril, lisinopril) are particularly effective in controlling blood pressure and improving renal function. This class of drug is the treatment of choice. Captopril, a short-acting ACE inhibitor, is generally easier to regulate for acute control of blood pressure. Other antihypertensives can be used to control blood pressure, including propanolol, clonidine, and minoxidil. Overdiuresis should be avoided, as it might decrease the effective plasma volume and renal blood flow. Patients with progressive renal failure should be prepared for the possibility of dialysis and renal transplantation.

6. PULMONARY HYPERTENSION/FIBROSIS. There is no long-term effective treatment for pulmonary arterial hypertension. Calcium channel blockers may provide transient improvement. Treatment for interstitial pulmonary fibrosis has largely been ineffective. Recently, cyclophosphamide has been reported in uncontrolled studies to be effective in treating interstitial pulmonary disease. The PO dose recommended is 1–2 mg/kg/d. Patients with lung involvement should receive Pneumovax and yearly influenza vaccinations. Home oxygen therapy may be necessary for patients with significant diffusion abnormality.

7. CARDIAC. Cardiac failure should be treated with diuretics with care not to overdiurese (see no. 5 above). Diuretics may decrease noninflammatory pericardial effusions.

C. Overlap Syndromes

Diagnostic criteria for more than one collagen vascular disease may be present. Overlap syndromes include systemic sclerosis and PM, SLE and RA, SLE and systemic sclerosis, and systemic sclerosis and RA. Myositis is also seen in conjunction with RA and SLE. Sjögren's syndrome may accompany almost any of the collagen vascular diseases. Mixed connective tissue disease (MCTD) defines a disorder with features of SLE, systemic sclerosis, polymyositis, and RA. In addition, patients also had in common high titers of antibodies to ribonucleoprotein (RNP). Clinical manifestations include

Raynaud's phenomenon, puffy hands, tight skin, esophageal dysmotility, rash, arthritis/arthralgias, pleurisy, pericarditis, aseptic meningitis, and myositis. These features appear sequentially over months and years. Eventually, about half of the cases of MCTD evolve into a clinical picture most consistent with systemic sclerosis, whereas others resemble SLE, RA, or Sjögren's syndrome or remain undifferentiated. The term "undifferentiated connective tissue disorder" has been suggested for cases that do not have diagnostic criteria for any one collagen vascular disease.

The inflammatory features of MCTD respond to corticosteroids, but treatment does not prevent this disorder from evolving into systemic sclerosis or other disorders. Inflammatory features of MCTD, such as pleurisy, pericarditis, or myositis, respond to **prednisone,** 40–60 mg/d. Mild disease can be managed with low doses of prednisone or an NSAID. Treatment of overlap syndrome is directed to the individual collagen vascular disease components.

D. Scleroderma-like Disorders

Repeated exposure to polyvinyl chloride (PVC) may lead to Raynaud's phenomenon, acroosteolysis, and scleroderma-like skin lesions. Hepatic fibrosis and angiosarcoma may also develop in workers exposed to PVC. In 1981, an illness developed in Spain after ingestion of adulterated cooking oil (rapeseed oil). This illness affected approximately 20,000 persons and was characterized by arthralgias and arthritis, interstitial pneumonitis, pulmonary hypertension, sicca syndrome, Raynaud's phenomenon, skin thickening, and resorption of distal digits.

In 1989, ingestion of a preparation of L-tryptophan caused an illness termed the eosinophilia myalgia syndrome. This syndrome consisted of severe myalgias, diffuse swelling of the extremities, polyneuropathy, pulmonary infiltrates, and cough. The extremity swelling progressed to thickening, with puckering of skin similar to that seen in eosinophilic fasciitis. In some patients, the disease progressed after discontinuation of the drug. Some patients died of pulmonary complications. Treatment consisted of high-dose prednisone, cytotoxic agents, plasmapheresis, and IVIG with variable results. L-Tryptophan has been removed from the market.

Scleroderma skin changes have been noted with the administration of pentazocine and bleomycin. With the latter drug, pulmonary fibrosis and gangrene of fingers have been seen. Recent studies have not shown a statistical association between silicone breast implants and the development of scleroderma or other defined connective tissue diseases.

E. Eosinophilic Fasciitis

This is characterized by rapid onset of pain, tenderness, and swelling of upper and lower extremities that develop after strenuous physical exercise in many patients. It affects both sexes equally. Onset is mostly between ages 30 and 65. Eosinophilic fasciitis is associated in a few patients with hematologic disorders, most often aplastic anemia and thrombocytopenia. The swelling progresses to brawny induration, followed subsequently by retraction of subcutaneous tissue leading to a cobblestone or puckered appearance. Biopsy specimen consisting of skin, fascia, and superficial muscles shows inflammation consisting of histiocytes, eosinophils, lymphocytes, and plasma cells involving the dermis and deep fascia. Patients also may experience polyarthralgias, arthritis, fever, fatigue, and weight loss. In some patients there is spontaneous improvement or improvement with glucocorticoids. Others go on to develop chronic fibrotic and atrophic skin changes and joint contractures, involving most often elbows, knees, ankles, wrists, and hands.

Treatment consists of **prednisone,** 40–60 mg/d, in divided doses and reduced gradually as previously described (see Systemic Lupus Erythematosus, Rash). Glucocorticoids should be given only for treatment of the acute inflammatory phase of disease and are of no benefit for chronic fibrotic cutaneous lesions. The response to prednisone is variable. Hydroxychloroquine, 400 mg/d, has also been effective in some cases.

Medsger TA Jr. Systemic sclerosis (scleroderma), localized forms of scleroderma and calcinosis. In: McCarty DJ, Koopman WJ, eds. Arthritis and Allied Conditions, 12th ed. Philadelphia: Lea & Febiger; 1993.

Steen VD. Renal involvement in systemic sclerosis. Clin Dermatol 1994;12:253.

Steen VD, et al. Therapy for severe interstitial lung disease in systemic sclerosis. A retrospective study. Arthritis Rheum 1994;37:1290.

15 15 15 15 15 15 15 15

DERMATOLOGIC DISEASES

MARK BERNHARDT
KENNETH A. ARNDT

15 15 15 15 15 15 15 15 15

I. GENERAL PRINCIPLES OF SKIN CARE

The two principal variables in dispensing topical medication—the medication itself and the vehicle—must both be appropriate for the condition under treatment. In general, **acute inflammation is best treated with aqueous, drying preparations, and chronic inflammation is treated with hydrophobic, more occlusive, lubricating compounds. Open wet dressings** cool and dry through evaporation. The resulting vasoconstriction decreases the augmented local blood flow present in inflammation. In addition, wet dressings cleanse the skin of exudates, crusts, and debris, help maintain drainage of infected areas, and decrease pain and pruritus. They are indicated in the therapy for acute inflammatory conditions, erosions, and ulcers. **Powders** promote drying by increasing the effective skin surface area. They are primarily used in intertriginous areas to reduce moisture, maceration, and friction. **Lotions** consist of suspensions of a powder in water. **Solutions** are lotions in which the active ingredients are dissolved, and consequently solutions are clear. **Tinctures** are alcoholic or hydroalcoholic solutions. As lotions and tinctures evaporate, they cool and dry; lotions leave a uniform film of medication on the skin. Sprays and aerosols act similarly. A **gel** is a transparent, semisolid emulsion that liquefies on contact with the skin, drying as a thin, greaseless, nonocclusive film. Lotions and gels are particularly useful for hairy areas. **Creams** are semisolid emulsions of oil in water. Although creams are often more cosmetically acceptable to patients, they may not be as effective for dry chronic dermatoses as **ointments,** which consist of an emulsion of water droplets suspended in oil or as an inert base, such as petrolatum.

An important consideration in topical therapy is dispensing the proper amount of medication. When inadequate amounts are prescribed, the patient may apply the medication too sparingly or less frequently than necessary. Table 15–1 gives conservative amounts needed for single or multiple applications of a cream, ointment, or lotion.

Arndt KA, LeBoit PE, Robinson JK, Wintroub BU, eds. Cutaneous Medicine and Surgery, An Integrated Program in Dermatology. Philadelphia: WB Saunders; 1996.

Champion RH, Burton JL, Ebling FJG, eds. Textbook of Dermatology, 5th ed. Oxford: Blackwell; 1992.

Fitzpatrick TB, Eisen AZ, Wolff K, Freedberg IM, Austen KF, eds. Dermatology in General Medicine, 4th ed. New York: McGraw-Hill; 1993.

Moschella SL, Hurley HJ, eds. Dermatology, 3rd ed. Philadelphia: WB Saunders; 1992.

II. DERMATITIS

Dermatitis is the most common inflammatory reaction pattern of the skin. The morphologic and histopathologic changes in all forms of dermatitis and eczema, terms that are used interchangeably, are similar. The earliest and mildest changes are erythema and edema. These may progress to vesiculation and oozing and then to crusting and scaling. Finally, if the process

TABLE 15–1. **Conservative Amounts of Topical Medications Needed for Single or Multiple Applications**

AREA TREATED	ONE APPLICATION (g)	TWICE DAILY FOR 1 wk (g)	THREE TIMES DAILY FOR 2 wk (g)
Hands, head, face, anogenital area	2	28	90
One arm, anterior or posterior trunk	3	42	120
One leg	4	56	180
Entire body	30–60	420–480	1.26–2.52 kg (42–84 oz)

TABLE 15–2. **Potency of Selected Topical Corticosteroids**

1 (most potent)	Betamethasone dipropionate ointment (optimized vehicle) (Diprolene)
	Clobetasol propionate ointment (Temovate)*
2	Fluocinonide cream, ointment, gel (Lidex)*
	Halcinonide cream (Halog)
3	Betamethasone valerate ointment (Valisone)*
	Fluticasone propionate (Cultivate)
4	Fluocinolone acetonide ointment (Synalar)*
	Hydrocortisone valerate ointment (Westcort)
5	Hydrocortisone butyrate cream (Locoid)
	Betamethasone dipropionate lotion (Diprosone)*
6	Desonide cream (Tridesilon; Desonide)
	Fluocinolone acetonide solution (Synalar)*
7 (least potent)	Hydrocortisone (Hytone)*

*Available as generic products. Studies to date have found that most generic topical corticosteroids are *not* biologically equivalent to the brand name products.

Modified from Cornell RC, Stoughton RB. Correlation of the vasoconstriction assay and clinical activity in psoriasis. Arch Dermatol 1985;121:63–67.

becomes chronic, the skin will be lichenified (thickened with accentuated skin markings), excoriated, and either hypopigmented or hyperpigmented. The factors that may initiate dermatitis are numerous, and its patterns dictate both the clinical classification and the therapy.

Atopic dermatitis is an intensely pruritic, chronic eruption. Although it may disappear with time, it is estimated that 30% to 80% of patients with atopic dermatitis will continue to have intermittent exacerbations throughout life, often when under physical or emotional stress. Approximately 70% of patients with atopic dermatitis have a family history of atopy, and about 50% of children with atopic dermatitis develop either rhinitis or asthma. **Lichen simplex chronicus** is a localized, chronic pruritic disorder resulting from repeated scratching and rubbing. Well-circumscribed lichenified plaques usually are located on ankles, anterior area of the tibia, and neck. Dry, keratotic papules and giant "scratch papules," or prurigo nodularis, are also a response to the repeated trauma of scratching. **Contact dermatitis** may be produced by primary irritants or allergic sensitizers. It is not the specific morphology that distinguishes contact dermatitis from other types of eczema but rather its distribution and configuration. This type of dermatitis is located in exposed or contact areas and typically has bizarre or artificial patterns characterized by sharp, straight margins, acute angles, and straight lines. **Hand dermatitis** is a common, chronic disorder that has as its most characteristic lesion myriads of small vesicles scattered on the sides of the fingers and, less often, throughout the palms. More severe changes include bulla formation and extreme inelasticity of the skin, with deep, painful fissures. **Nummular dermatitis** is characterized by round (coin shaped), eczematous plaques most commonly located on the dorsa of the hands and forearms, lower aspect of the legs, and buttocks.

A. General Principles

Topical corticosteroids are the primary agents in treatment. Effectiveness is related to the potency of the drug and its percutaneous penetration. Potency is most often assessed in vivo by the drug's ability to produce vasoconstriction on human skin, and results of this bioassay correlate well with clinical trials (Table 15–2). **Ointment** vehicles generally impart better biologic activity to the incorporated steroids than do creams or other vehicles. Occluding the treated area with nonporous plastic wraps dramatically raises the effectiveness of topical corticosteroids by increasing the hydration of the horny layer and the surface area of the skin, thereby both enhancing percutaneous absorption and inducing a reservoir of the medication in the stratum corneum. Folliculitis, miliaria, and maceration may occur from excessive occlusion.

Multiple **adverse effects** can be associated with use of topical corticosteroids. Burning, itching, and dryness are usually related to the vehicle: ointments are better tolerated when applied to inflamed skin than are creams or gels. Atrophy, telangiectasia, striae, and purpura may occur if potent preparations are applied over a week to a few months. The more potent the corticosteroid preparation, the more rapid and severe the adverse effects will be, especially if it is applied to those areas (face and intertriginous and anogenital areas) where there is greater absorption. Less common side effects include acneiform lesions, hypertrichosis, hypopigmentation, and ocular hypertension from application around the eyes. The greater absorption that occurs with occlusive techniques increases the risk of local steroid side effects as well as hypothalamic-pituitary-adrenal (HPA) axis suppression. It should be assumed that all patients undergoing substantial occlusive therapy have temporary suppression of the HPA axis. If used injudiciously, even without occlusion, the most potent formulations may induce mild hypercortisolism, HPA axis suppression, or rarely Cushing's syndrome. The use of topical corticosteroids is generally safe, however, if the appropriate strength is selected and used for a limited duration. Although the optimal frequency of corticosteroid application is unknown, there is probably no advantage to more than twice-daily usage. Repeated application of a topical corticosteroid may result in a diminished effect (tachyphylaxis). It is, therefore, best to treat effectively for days to 2 weeks and then have steroid-free intervals of 4 to 7 days or more.

All forms of dermatitis are intensely pruritic, and scratching may exacerbate atopic dermatitis and lichen simplex chronicus. Therapy with topical corticosteroids has some antipruritic effects, but specific measures aimed at reducing pruritus are also worthwhile. **Topical antipruritics** work either through decreasing the sensitivity of cutaneous nerve endings (e.g., phenol), through a counterirritant effect of substituting one sensation such as cooling for another, that is, itching (menthol), by surface anesthesia (**pramoxine,** Pramosone), or as a topical antihistamine (**doxepin hydrochloride,** Zonalon). Dermatitic skin will not always tolerate topical antipruritics, either because of a concomitant stinging or burning sensation or because of the greater chance of sensitization when potential allergens are applied to already inflamed skin. Often, a good emollient/moisturizer alone is the single best antipruritic therapy. **Oral antihistamines** often alleviate pruritus, allay anxiety, and allow sleep, even when itching is not directly related to histamine effects. The several chemical classes of antihistamines show only minor variations in their properties, and a side effect such as somnolence, which might preclude their use in one situation, may be advantageous in another. To be used most effectively, antihistamines should be gradually increased until either clinical remission occurs or side effects become bothersome (or intolerable).

B. Specific Treatments

1. ATOPIC DERMATITIS

a. Preventive measures. The environment should be kept at a constant temperature—comfortable, but not hot. Humidifiers will help alleviate skin dryness, especially during the winter; excess humidity should be avoided. Clothing worn next to the skin should be absorbent and nonirritating, laundered with bland soaps, and thoroughly rinsed. Overly frequent bathing, which promotes xerosis, must be eliminated. Baths are preferable to showers, and water temperature in either should be warm and not hot. Emollients or medications should be applied immediately after bathing to trap water in the skin and enhance absorption. Frequent application of bland lubricants soothes and physically protects the skin and is the most important single measure in atopic dermatitis therapy.

b. **Treatment of active dermatitis.** Compresses with aluminum acetate (Burow's) solution should be placed on exudative areas for 20 minutes four to six times a day. Alternatively the patient should be placed in a tub two or three times a day, to which an antipruritic colloid such as oatmeal (Aveeno, 1 cup to one-half tub of tepid water), has been added. Twice-daily application of a potent corticosteroid preparation will quickly quell inflammation and pruritus. If maintenance therapy is needed, it is advisable to use the least potent preparation (e.g., 1% hydrocortisone) that is effective. Tar compounds (Estar gel, T/Gel) are useful as adjunctive therapy in patients with chronic dermatitis (see Psoriasis below). They may be used alternately with corticosteroids or applied at the same time to the skin. Bath oil (Balnetar, four capfuls) is also helpful. Oral antihistamines should be used in an attempt to suppress pruritus. Hydroxyzine (Atarax, 10–25 mg PO q4–6h) is usually the best initial choice. Newer antihistamines, such as **cetirizine** (Zyrtec, 10 mg PO qd), a derivative of hydroxyzine, and **loratadine** (Claritin, 10 mg PO qd), are convenient alternatives when sedation is an intolerable side effect. Conversely, diphenhydramine (Benadryl 25 mg PO q4–6h) may be appropriate when some degree of sedation is desirable.

Acute flares of atopic dermatitis may be suppressed by a short course of prednisone (40–60 mg PO daily, tapered over a 10- to 14-day period) or a single IM injection (e.g., triamcinolone acetonide [Kenalog] 40 mg). Long-term administration of systemic corticosteroids plays no part in treatment of atopic dermatitis, and severe rebound flares may occur when either the corticosteroid dose is too low or the taper duration is too short. Photochemotherapy (psoralen-UVA [PUVA]) can induce remission in selected patients with recalcitrant chronic atopic dermatitis. Impetiginization should be managed with appropriate oral antibiotics. Treatment of *Staphylococcus aureus* infection (e.g., erythromycin, 250 mg PO q6h) may be helpful in selected patients.

2. LICHEN SIMPLEX CHRONICUS. Potent topical corticosteroids, usually applied under airtight occlusive dressings, are extremely effective. Intralesional injection of corticosteroids (e.g., triamcinolone acetonide [Kenalog] 2.5–10 mg/mL) is often the therapy of choice. Intralesional therapy has the potential risks of long-term potent topical corticosteroid use. Antihistamines may occasionally be of value, especially when administered immediately before bedtime.

3. CONTACT DERMATITIS
   a. **Preventive measures for primary irritant or hand dermatitis.** Exposure to household and work irritants, such as soaps, detergents, solvents, bleaches, ammonia, and moist vegetables and fruits, should be decreased. Without such avoidance, all other treatment is bound to be suboptimal. Patients need to receive frequent reinforcement in this rather tedious and difficult aspect of their care. Rings that occlude the underlying skin must be removed before any hand work is done. Waterless hand cleaners will remove stubborn soils and greases and are preferable to the use of other solvents. The skin

should be lubricated frequently with a bland cream or lotion. If possible, heavy-duty vinyl or plastic gloves should be worn during work. Thin, white cotton liners may be worn underneath the gloves to absorb sweat. Some allergens (e.g., nickel) and high concentrations of irritants (e.g., 10% potassium hydroxide) may penetrate rubber-based gloves. Furthermore, patients may occasionally become allergic to the rubber in lined rubber gloves. There are various barrier protective creams designed for use against aqueous compounds (Kerodex No. 71, SBS-44, and West No. 311), solvents (Kerodex No. 51, SBS-46, and West No. 411), or dusts (West No. 211). Barrier creams applied before work and during work breaks are moderately effective.

b. Preventive measures for allergic contact dermatitis. The patient should wash thoroughly as soon as possible after exposure to the allergen. Clothing or implements that may have become exposed should also be cleansed before being used again. Hyposensitization to allergic contact antigens, such as poison ivy and oak (and others), is of negligible, if any, benefit. Referral for patch testing may be necessary to identify specific allergens.

c. Treatment of acute dermatitis. Topical compresses or tub baths, such as those described for atopic dermatitis, are helpful for exudative, vesicular, or bullous lesions. After vesiculation subsides, topical corticosteroids will generally suffice for mild to moderate inflammation. For more severe cases, early aggressive treatment with systemic corticosteroids is indicated; prednisone, 60 mg PO daily, tapered over a 15 to 20-day course, should be used. Simultaneous use of topical corticosteroids may offer additional benefits. Some improvement in the rash and discomfort is usually observed within 48 hours after therapy is initiated. If inadequate amounts of systemic steroids are given for too short a time, a rebound reaction with generalized exacerbation may occur. Acute reactions to a strong irritant should be treated with forceful and prolonged irrigation by water. Acid burns should not be rinsed with alkali, and vice versa; doing so causes an exothermic reaction and further tissue damage. Industrial toxicity texts should be consulted concerning specific therapy for offending chemicals. Oral antihistamines should be administered as needed.

d. Treatment of chronic contact or hand dermatitis. The affected area should be soaked for 5 minutes in water, and then a hydrophobic emollient (e.g., petrolatum) or a potent topical corticosteroid ointment should be applied immediately. Tar preparations may be useful. The affected area should be soaked in a solution of two capfuls of Balnetar or other tar compound in tepid water for 15 minutes and then rinsed; a topical steroid ointment should be applied immediately. Phototherapy is frequently helpful in chronic hand dermatitis.

4. **NUMMULAR DERMATITIS.** Nummular dermatitis is treated by the general measures described for dermatitis, pp. 597 and 598. In addition,

iodochlorhydroxyquin (Vioform), which has mild antibacterial and antifungal effects, may help, especially when used in combination with a tar or a corticosteroid preparation or both. As is true with any dermatitis, bacterial superinfection may occur and should be treated with appropriate topical and systemic antibiotics.

Cowan MA. Nummular eczema: a review, follow-up and analysis of 325 cases. Acta Derm Venerol 1961;41:453–460.
Epstein E. Hand dermatitis: practical management and current concepts. J Am Acad Dermatol 1984;10:395–424.
Hanifin JM. Atopic dermatitis: new therapeutic considerations. J Am Acad Dermatol 1991;24: 1097–1101.
Jorizzo JL, Gatti S, Smith EB. Prurigo: a clinical review. J Am Acad Dermatol 1981;4:723–728.
Tan PL, Barnett GL, Flowers FP, et al. Current topical corticosteroid preparations. J Am Acad Dermatol 1986;14:79–93.

III. PSORIASIS

Psoriasis is a chronic, proliferative epidermal disease that affects 2 to 8 million people in the United States. Age of onset is most often in the third decade, although psoriasis may appear at any time from infancy to old age. A family history is found in 30% of patients, and a polygenic mode of inheritance appears most likely. The pathogenesis of psoriasis remains unclear but is multifactorial, involving keratinocytic and immunologic (T cell) abnormalities. Recent evidence suggests that there is an aberration throughout the skin of psoriasis patients that is modified to disease expression by certain stimuli (e.g., infection, trauma, drugs, inflammation). The psoriatic lesion is an erythematous, sharply circumscribed plaque covered by loosely adherent, silvery (micaceous) scales. Any area of the body may be involved, but lesions tend to occur most often on the elbows, knees, scalp, genitalia, and intergluteal cleft. In most patients, the disease remains localized as discrete plaques, although generalized involvement may develop.

A. General Principles

1. **PHOTOTHERAPY.** This is the treatment of choice for most cases of moderate to severe psoriasis, with involvement of more than 25% body surface area. It should be administered only by a qualified dermatologist. The ultraviolet (UV) spectrum is subdivided into three bands: UVC (200 to 290 nm), UVB (290 to 320 nm), and UVA (320 to 400 nm). UVC radiation has virtually no medical applications except as used in germicidal lamps. UVB radiation is responsible for most of the therapeutic effects of sunlight. Although exposure to sunlight is certainly less expensive and more pleasant than acquiring UV light in medical surroundings, inherent difficulties in its control and monitoring dictate that UVB phototherapy be administered via an artificial source in phototherapy booths. Numerous protocols involving repeated exposure to UVB light alone or with prior application of tar compounds (the Goeckerman regimen) have demonstrated effectiveness. The disadvantages of UVA and UVB phototherapy derive from the known deleterious effects of UV radiation on the skin. Long-term exposure has been related

to actinic keratoses, basal cell carcinoma, squamous cell carcinoma, and atypical melanocytic lesions, including melanoma, and has been demonstrated to promote the epidermal and dermal changes popularly ascribed to "aging." Since UVB light is that portion of the solar spectrum that is most responsible for sunburning (erythemogenic), patients for whom phototherapy is being considered should be properly advised and periodically observed for atypical keratinocytic or melanocytic lesions. UVA light is most frequently administered in combination with a photoactive drug, psoralen, to reduce the increased epidermal turnover characteristic of psoriasis. Psoralen-UVA (PUVA) photochemotherapy, as well as more conventional UVB light treatment, has numerous cutaneous and even systemic immunologic effects. In photochemotherapy, the psoralen is administered PO 2 hours before exposure to UVA light, but patients remain photosensitive for up to 24 hours. Phototoxicity, both acute and cumulative, is an even greater concern for PUVA than for UVB therapy.

2. **TAR COMPOUNDS.** If phototherapy is one of the more recent advances in the treatment of psoriasis, tar compounds must be considered one of the oldest. The ability of coal tars to inhibit epidermal DNA synthesis might account for their effectiveness in treating psoriasis. Coal tars are carcinogenic for the skin of experimental animals and are photosensitizing. The risk of developing skin cancer from the therapeutic use of coal tars with or without phototherapy, however, appears to be low. Coal tars are available in a wide range of vehicles, including creams, ointments, gels, shampoos, and bath preparations. Tar sensitizes the skin to long-wave ultraviolet light, and caution is in order to avoid phototoxicity. Patient acceptance is often limited by the distinctive odor and propensity for staining of the tar preparations.

B. Specific Treatments

Potent topical corticosteroids applied twice daily are very effective. Ointments are preferable, except for use on the scalp, where a gel or liquid vehicle is easier to use and more acceptable cosmetically. Overnight occlusion with plastic wrap, body suit, or shower cap may facilitate the initial response but should be discontinued once the lesions subside. Injection of corticosteroids (e.g., triamcinolone acetonide [Kenalog] 2.5–5 mg/mL) beneath individual plaques will cause involution within 7 to 10 days and is particularly helpful in patients with just a few lesions. Coal tar therapy may be used alone or in conjunction with topical corticosteroids. **Calcipotriene** (Dovonex ointment, bid), a vitamin D analog, inhibits cell proliferation and induces cellular differentiation. Its effectiveness in psoriasis is comparable with that of potent topical corticosteroids without the complications of the latter. The potential side effects from calcipotriene consist of local irritation and the (mainly theoretical) potential for hypercalcemia with long-term, widespread use. **Anthralin** (Drithocreme, Lasan), a synthetic derivative of a substance originally extracted from the *Andira araroba* tree of Brazil, reduces epidermal mitotic activity, perhaps through interference with mitochondrial DNA. Anthralin preparations may be irritating and will stain both skin and clothing. Initially, the lowest strength (0.1%) should be applied for 4 to 6 h/d, and both the concentration of the anthralin and the duration for which it is applied should gradually be increased until a therapeutic effect is seen. Alternatively, the higher concentrations (0.5–1%) may be used for shorter periods (10 minutes to 1 h/d). **Salicylic acid** acts like a keratolytic and thus helps remove adherent scales from psoriatic lesions. This removal in turn promotes the penetration and efficacy of other modalities, including corticosteroids, tars, and phototherapy. Keralyt Gel (6% salicylic acid, 60% propylene glycol, and 20% ethyl alcohol) is particularly useful when applied under occlusion to hydrated skin overnight.

Phototherapy is the treatment of choice for widespread or recalcitrant psoriasis. Antimetabolites (hydroxyurea, methotrexate) and immunomodulating drugs (cyclosporine) should be reserved for patients with serious disease unresponsive to other treatments in whom economic or social consequences justify the side effects. The same considerations apply to the use of etretinate (Tegison), a synthetic retinoid particularly useful in the most severe erythrodermic and pustular variants of psoriasis. All of these forms of therapy are generally administered by dermatologists familiar with their use.

Berth-Jones J, Hutchinson PE. Vitamin D analogues and psoriasis. Br J Dermatol 1992;127:71–78.
Simpson KR, Lowe NJ. Trends in topical psoriasis therapy. Int J Dermatol 1994;33:333–336.
Thune P, Brolund L. Short- and long-contact therapy using a new dithranol formulation in individually adjusted dosages in the management of psoriasis. Acta Derm Venereol Suppl (Stockh) 1992;172:28–29.

IV. ACNE

The clinical spectrum of acne lesions ranges from mild and purely comedonal (whiteheads and blackheads) to more moderate inflammatory (papules and pustules) to severe cystic (cysts and nodules). Therapy for acne not only must be appropriate for the predominant clinical type and severity of disease but must also take into consideration any aggravating (e.g., androgen excess) or complicating (e.g., gram-negative folliculitis) factors. The diverse agents that have been successfully used for acne reflect its multifactorial nature.

A. Mild Involvement (Few to Many Comedones, Few or No Inflammatory Lesions)

Tretinoin (Retin-A) is the most effective comedolytic agent. Its irritant effect sometimes limits its usefulness, although this can be minimized by proper application and a gradual increase in the potency of the formulation until the therapeutic effect is achieved. Therapy should be started with either the 0.01% gel or the 0.025% cream. If no improvement is seen after 12 weeks, a higher concentration (0.025% gel, 0.05% cream) is used. A small amount should be applied once daily, or initially, on alternate days, to all affected areas, avoiding the periorbital and perioral areas. The skin should be thoroughly dry before application; if the patient has washed, at least 15 minutes should pass before tretinoin is administered. Some patients will sunburn more easily, and excessive sun exposure must be avoided when using this product. Sunscreens ≥SPF 15 must be used with regularity.

Bacteriostatics are thought to improve acne by decreasing the formulation of harmful by-products as well as the actual number of *Propionibacterium acnes* bacteria. There are numerous gel-based benzoyl peroxide products (Desquam-X, Benzagel, and Persa-Gel). The lower concentration (2.5%) is usually better tolerated and is often as effective as the higher (5% to 10%) ones. Benzoyl peroxide washes are also useful adjuvants in any acne treatment regimen. These agents should be applied twice daily; if excessive erythema and dryness develop, the concentration and frequency of application should be decreased, or an alternative therapy should be adopted. Topical antibiotics are most effective for papular and pustular lesions. Clindamycin and erythromycin appear to be the most effective and easiest to use. All topical antibiotics are applied twice daily. Clindamycin phosphate (Cleocin T) is available in solution, lotion, or gel form. Erythromycin base is available as a solution (Staticin, A/T/S), pledgets (Erycette), gel (Emgel), or combined with benzoyl peroxide (Benzamycin). Combined tretinoin-benzoyl peroxide therapy is very effective for comedonal and papular acne. These agents must be applied at different times, not simultaneously, because mixing the highly unsaturated tretinoin with the reactive oxidant benzoyl peroxide inactivates both. The irritant response to this regimen limits its use. The latest addition to the anti-acne armamentarium is **azelaic acid** cream (Azelex). Applied bid, it is effective in mild to moderate acne, exhibiting both comedolytic and anti-inflammatory activity.

B. Moderate Involvement (Numerous Inflammatory Lesions or Cysts)

Topical therapy should be initiated, as suggested above. Oral antibiotics work through reduction of the normal cutaneous flora (particularly *P. acnes*) and direct anti-inflammatory effects. The results of antibiotic therapy cannot be adequately assessed for at least 6 to 8 weeks. If antibiotic is given for long periods, every attempt must be made to decrease to the lowest effective dose. Numerous oral antibiotics are useful. The choice of a particular drug is empiric and should take into consideration cost, convenience, and effect of previous treatments. **Tetracycline** (250 mg PO qid or 500 mg bid) is usually the drug of choice. It is inexpensive and, except for GI irritation and candidal vaginitis, relatively free of side effects. Erythromycin (250 mg PO qid) is usually the next drug of choice. Minocycline is quite effective, although its higher cost precludes use as a first-line therapy. Transient dizziness and nausea are usually avoidable if treatment is initiated with a dosage of 50 mg PO bid, increasing to a maximum of 100 mg PO bid, as needed. Doxycycline (50–100 mg bid) may also be effective, but its ability to photosensitize limits its use in sunny climates. Ampicillin (250 mg PO qid) is useful in certain patients, particularly pregnant women, in whom the use of tetracycline or minocycline must be avoided. An occasional complication of long-term broad-spectrum antibiotic therapy is gram-negative folliculitis. Patients will notice the sudden appearance of numerous pustules or inflammatory cysts infected with *Proteus, Pseudomonas,* or *Klebsiella* species. Any sudden change in clinical severity or morphology warrants gram stain and bacterial culture.

C. Severe Involvement Unresponsive to Other Therapy

Estrogens (administered as anovulatory agents) may help young women with severe acne. Most or all of the estrogen effect is the result of inhibition of adrenal androgen production. Thus, combination oral contraceptives should contain a nonandrogenic progestin, such as ethynodiol diacetate (Demulen). Estrogen therapy is rarely indicated before age 16, after which time there will be no problem with growth retardation. **Prednisone** (5–7.5 mg PO every evening) is helpful in female patients with severe acne unresponsive to conventional therapy who suffer from overproduction of androgens by the adrenal glands. **Spironolactone** (100–200 mg/d PO), an aldosterone antagonist with antiandrogenic side effects, is an alternative for women with androgen excess who cannot use oral contraceptives or corticosteroids.

Patients with severe cystic acne unresponsive to high-dose antibiotic therapy should be considered for treatment with **isotretinoin** (Accutane), a drug that inhibits sebaceous gland function and alters the inflammatory response. Isotretinoin is administered on a basis of 0.5–1 mg/kg/d for 5 months. Aside from its known teratogenic effects, most of the other side effects of isotretinoin are transient and mild, including cheilitis, xerosis, alopecia, and hypertriglyceridemia. Although patients may experience a temporary flare in cystic lesions when therapy is initiated, this does not affect ultimate response. Asymptomatic vertebral hyperostoses are a recognized side effect of isotretinoin therapy that may not become apparent for 6 to 12 months after treatment. The therapy of choice for cystic lesions and acne abscesses is intralesional injection of small amounts of corticosteroid preparations (e.g., triamcinolone acetonide [Kenalog] 2.5 mg/mL). Most lesions will flatten and disappear within 48 hours after injection.

Dicken CH. Retinoids: a review. J Am Acad Dermatol 1984;11:541–552.
Stern RS, Pass TM, Komaroff AL. Topical versus systemic agent treatment for papulopustular acne. Arch Dermatol 1984;120:1571–1578.

V. SKIN INFECTIONS

A. Superficial Fungal Infections

1. **CANDIDIASIS.** *Candida albicans* is a frequent cause of paronychial, intertriginous, oral, and vulvovaginal infections. Diagnosis can be easily confirmed by microscopic examination using potassium hydroxide or by culture. There are four classes of agents most commonly used for topical treatment of candidal infections: haloprogin (Halotex); the synthetic imidazole compounds, miconazole (Monistat-Derm), clotrimazole (Lotrimin, Mycelex), ketoconazole (Nizoral), and econazole (Spectazole); ciclopirox olamine (Loprox); and the polyene antibiotic nystatin. The imidazoles are at least as effective as nystatin for treating cutaneous candidiasis and in cream form may be superior to nystatin in the treatment of candidal vulvovaginitis. Ciclopirox is probably as efficacious as the imidazoles. Creams may be used for most cutaneous and vulvovaginal infections, although patients with the latter might prefer vaginal suppositories. Systemic therapy is indicated when

dealing with either oropharyngeal or stubborn vaginal candidiasis. Although older therapies, such as nystatin suspension or clotrimazole troches, remain useful, especially when cost is a main consideration, newer treatments, such as **fluconazole** (Diflucan, 150 mg PO one time only for vulvovaginitis; 200 mg PO, then 100 mg PO qd for oropharyngeal involvement), are safe, rapidly effective, and convenient alternatives. Paronychial and oral infections require more frequent applications, as often as five times a day, because the medication does not remain in contact with the skin or mucous membranes. Vulvovaginitis and other cutaneous candidal infections will respond to once-daily or twice-daily dosage, depending on the drug and dosage form.

Orally administered nystatin (500,000 U tid or qid) is useful when recurrent or resistant infections in the perianal, vulvar, or diaper areas are due to reinfection from gut organisms. Candidal paronychia can be managed with amphotericin B lotion, alcoholic solutions of 1% gentian violet, or 2% to 4% thymol in absolute alcohol. Although esthetically unappealing, gentian violet solution is particularly useful in severe, recalcitrant oral infections. Predisposing factors, particularly excessive moisture and maceration, must be eliminated.

DeVillez RL, Lewis CW. Candidiasis seminar. Cutis 1977;19:69–83.

2. **DERMATOPHYTE INFECTIONS.** The anatomic site, not the specific species of dermatophyte fungi, determines the appropriate treatment. Infections of the body and groin and superficial involvement of the beard area, palms, and soles can be managed by topical measures. Oral therapy is indicated when such measures fail, as well as when scalp and nails are affected. The synthetic imidazoles, haloprogin, tolnaftate, and the allylamine derivatives naftifine (Naftin) and terbinafine (Lamisil) will clear most superficial dermatophyte infections within 1 to 4 weeks. Econazole, ketoconazole, and the newer imidazoles, sulconazole (Exelderm) and oxiconazole (Oxistat), are used once daily except for tinea pedis, where a twice-a-day dosage is more effective. The other antimycotics are applied twice a day. Therapy should be continued for 4 weeks to decrease the relapse rate. A keratolytic agent, such as Keralyt or Epilyt gel (see Psoriasis), should be used for thick, hyperkeratotic involvement, as on the palms or soles. Open wet dressings (see Dermatitis) should be applied to acute vesicular lesions.

Azole and allylanine antifungals have supplanted griseofulvin as the treatment of choice in most dermatophyte infections. **Ketoconazole** (Nizoral, 200 mg PO qd), fluconazole (Diflucan, 125 mg PO qd), and **itraconazole** (Sporanox, 200 mg bid for 7 days, for tinea pedis; 100 mg for 30 days for tinea capitis; 200 mg qd for 12 weeks for onychomycosis) are all effective with minimal side effects other than the potential for hepatotoxicity. When used in a pulsed-dose fashion (200 mg PO bid for 1 week per month), itraconazole is the treatment of choice for onychomycosis. A 3-month course is sufficient to treat most infections of the fingernails; an additional month of therapy is usually necessary to adequately treat toenails. The absorption of these medications can be influenced by dietary and other factors. For example, ketoconazole is best absorbed when taken in the morning, and its absorption will be impaired by any antacids. Antacids will also interfere with the absorption of itraconazole, which to be absorbed must be taken with either a fatty meal or carbonated beverage. The drugs of choice are itraconazole and terbinafine (Lamisil) (250 mg for 2 weeks for tinea corporis and tinea cruris; 2 to 4 weeks for tinea capitis; 6 and 12 weeks for finger and toenail infections, respectively).

Elewski BE, Hazen PG. The superficial mycoses and the dermatophytes. J Am Acad Dermatol 1989;21:655–673.
Jacobs PH. Treatment of fungal skin infections: state of the art. J Am Acad Dermatol 1990;23:549–551.

3. **TINEA VERSICOLOR.** This asymptomatic eruption is caused by the lipophilic yeastlike organism *Pityrosporum orbiculare,* the pathogenic form of the normal skin resident *Pityrosporum ovale.* A peculiar aspect of tinea versicolor is its propensity to cause either hypopigmented or hyperpigmented lesions, which are highly confluent, round, finely scaled, thin plaques most often located on the upper torso. Most treatments will remove any evidence of active infection (i.e., scaling) within several days, but the pigmentary changes may take several months to resolve. In general, treatments should be used for 2 weeks, at which time a repeat application of a potassium hydroxide preparation will yield negative results if therapy has been successful. The synthetic imidazoles, ciclopirox, haloprogin, and tolnaftate, applied once or twice a day, are all effective. Selenium sulfide suspension (Exsel, Selsun) is applied once daily to the affected areas, allowed to dry, and then washed off after 5 minutes. Zinc pyrithione-containing shampoos (Head & Shoulders, Zincon) are applied in a similar fashion. Tinver lotion (25% sodium hyposulfite, 1% salicylic acid, and 10% alcohol) is applied twice a day. Tretinoin (Retin-A) cream (0.05% bid; see Acne) not only will cure tinea versicolor but also will promote more rapid fading of hyperpigmented lesions. Ketoconazole (a single 400-mg dose or 200 mg for 5 to 10 days), fluconazole (a single 400-mg dose), and itraconazole (200 mg qd for 7 days) are all effective both mycologically (negative results on potassium hydroxide test) and clinically (prompt fading of the lesions). Griseofulvin is ineffective against tinea versicolor.

Borelli D, Jacobs PH, Nall L. Tinea versicolor: epidemiologic, clinical, and therapeutic aspects. J Am Acad Dermatol 1991;25:300–305.

B. Herpesvirus Infections

1. **HERPES SIMPLEX.** Cutaneous herpes simplex infections take two distinct forms: (1) the painful and disabling primary infection of previously uninfected individuals and (2) the common, bothersome recurrent form, colloquially known as cold sores or fever blisters. Herpes simplex infections may be particularly severe and widespread in patients with certain skin disorders (e.g., atopic dermatitis) or immunodeficiencies. Infection by herpes simplex or varicella-zoster virus can be readily confirmed by cytologic examination of a scraping obtained from the base of a vesicular lesion and by culture. A Tzanck preparation will reveal characteristic multinucleated giant keratinocytes.

Acyclovir (Zovirax), a purine nucleoside analog, revolutionized the treatment of herpesvirus infections. Its safety and specificity depend on two factors: (1) a viral enzyme, thymidine kinase, is necessary for conversion of the drug to its active form, and (2) once activated, acyclovir inhibits a virus-specific DNA polymerase required for viral replication. Treatment promptly aborts new lesion formation, reduces viral titers, promotes healing, and ameliorates pain. IV acyclovir (5 mg/kg q8h) also prevents reactivation of herpes simplex in seropositive, immunocompromised patients undergoing chemotherapy or transplantation. Oral acyclovir (200 mg five times daily for 10 days) promotes resolution of primary herpes simplex infections, if begun within 3 days of onset. Although treatment of the primary episode will not per se affect the frequency or severity of future recurrences, if given continuously (400 mg PO bid) to patients with frequent recurrences (more than six per year), it will significantly reduce or even prevent outbreaks. Topical acyclovir (5% ointment applied q3h) has a modest effect on primary genital herpes simplex infections if begun within 72 hours of onset. Clinical studies have failed to show any benefit from its use in nongenital or recurrent episodes. Aside from transient renal dysfunction when IV acyclovir is administered too rapidly, acyclovir appears remarkably free of side effects. The greatest concern is that its overuse will promote the emergence of resistant viral strains. Thymidine kinase-deficient mutants have been recognized but seem to be less pathogenic to humans. Two new antiviral medications, **valacyclovir** (Valtrex, 500 mg PO bid) and **famciclovir** (Famvir, 125 mg PO bid) have a more convenient dosing schedule, and appear to be just as safe and effective as acyclovir in the treatment of recurrent genital herpes simplex. Open wet compresses (10 minutes tid or qid) or sitz baths are indicated for acute vesicular outbreaks. Mouthwashes (benzalkonium chloride [Zephiran] 1 : 1000 or tetracycline suspension 250 mg/60 ml of water) are cleansing and soothing in primary herpetic gingivostomatitis. Topical antibacterials (see Impetigo) should be applied to cutaneous herpes infections to prevent bacterial superinfection. Herpes simplex infection is one of the few instances in which use of topical anesthetics is effective and justifiable. Dyclonine hydrochloride (Dyclone), elixir of diphenhydramine hydrochloride (Benadryl elixir), or viscous lidocaine (Xylocaine) may be used for oral lesions, and benzocaine aerosol (Americaine) or pramoxine hydrochloride (Tronothane) ointment may be used for the anogenital area. They can be applied as frequently as necessary.

2. VARICELLA. Many patients with varicella require only symptomatic therapy. A drying antipruritic lotion (calamine alone or with 0.25% menthol or 1% phenol or both) should be applied. Phenol should not be used in pregnant women. Administration of oral antihistamines may decrease pruritus (see Dermatitis). Acyclovir (800 mg PO qid for 5 days) reduces the duration and severity of varicella but does not affect the incidence of complications (e.g., secondary bacterial infection, pneumonitis, meningoencephalitis). Results are best if therapy is started within the first 24 hours of development of vesicles. Severe varicella,

especially in the immunocompromised patient, is best treated with IV acyclovir, as is disseminated herpes zoster. High-risk susceptible patients (e.g., those with lymphoma or leukemia or immunodeficiency; the newborn child of a mother with varicella) under 15 years of age who have had close exposure to varicella or zoster should be passively immunized with varicella zoster immunoglobulin (VZIG). This immunization will moderate or even abort clinical infection if administered within 72 hours of exposure but is of no value in established infections.

3. **HERPES ZOSTER.** The more general measures described for herpes simplex and varicella are also applicable to herpes zoster. Acyclovir (800 mg PO five times a day for 7 to 10 days), valacyclovir (1 g PO tid for 7 days), and famciclovir (500 mg PO tid for 7 days) all alleviate the discomfort and shorten the course of localized zoster. The last has also been shown to reduce the chance of postherpetic neuralgia. The maximal benefit from any of these medications is seen if treatment is initiated within 48 hours of onset. IV acyclovir can prevent or abort dissemination in the immunocompromised patient.

Balfour HH Jr, Kelly JM, Suarez CS, et al. Acyclovir treatment of varicella in otherwise healthy children. J Pediatr 1990;116:633–639.
Feder HM. Treatment of adult chicken pox with oral acyclovir. Arch Intern Med 1990;150: 2061–2065.
McKendrick MW, McGill JI, White JE, et al. Oral acyclovir in acute herpes zoster. Br Med J 1986;293:1529–1532.
Wheeler CE Jr. Antiviral drugs and vaccines for herpes simplex and herpes zoster. J Am Acad Dermatol 1988;18:161–238.

C. Impetigo

Nonbullous impetigo, once regarded as solely streptococcal in origin, is now recognized as a manifestation of infection with either streptococci or *Staphylococcus aureus*. It occurs most often on the face or other exposed areas. It is highly contagious among infants and children but less so in older persons. Untreated impetigo usually resolves in about 10 days. The overall incidence of postpyodermal acute glomerulonephritis is 2% or less. Bullous staphylococcal impetigo is also seen primarily in children and is caused by group II type 71 staphylococci. These organisms produce a toxin that induces a superficial intraepidermal blister. The classic streptococcal impetigo lesion begins as a small erythematous macule that rapidly develops into a fragile vesicle. The vesicle then breaks, leaving a red, oozing erosion surmounted by a "stuck-on," thick golden crust. Bullous impetigo lesions appear as flaccid blisters, initially clear and then cloudy, that have a thin varnishlike crust when they rupture.

Mupirocin (Bactroban, applied tid) is the first topical antibiotic as effective as oral medication in the treatment of impetigo caused by either *Staphylococcus* or *Streptococcus*. Widespread involvement warrants systemic therapy.

Bullous staphylococcal impetigo should be treated with a semisynthetic penicillin (e.g., dicloxacillin, 250 mg PO qid) or erythromycin or a cephalosporin drug if the organisms are sensitive to this drug. Streptococcal impetigo should be treated with one IM injection of benzathine penicillin

(1.2 million U). An alternative therapy is 10 days of erythromycin (250 mg PO qid) or phenoxymethyl penicillin (250 mg PO qid).

Lesions should be soaked three or four times a day in warm tap water, saline, or a soap solution to remove the crusts. In addition, it is advisable to have both the patient and the family bathe once or twice daily with a bactericidal (e.g., povidone-iodine [Betadine]) or bacteriostatic solution (e.g., pHisoDerm, chlorhexidine gluconate [Hibiclens]). Avoid sharing personal toiletries. Nasal carriers may be sources of reinfection and should be treated with twice-daily applications of mupirocin to the anterior nares. A topical antibiotic ointment (e.g., povidone-iodine [Betadine], polymyxin B-bacitracin [Polysporin]) should be applied to the base of lesions after the crust has been removed.

Dahl MV. Strategies for the management of recurrent furunculosis. South Med J 1987;80:352–356.
Mertz PM, Marshall DA, Eaglstein WH, et al. Topical mupirocin treatment of impetigo is equal to oral erythromycin therapy. Arch Dermatol 1989;125:1069–1073.

D. Scabies

Scabies is caused by infestation with the mite *Sarcoptes scabiei*. Principally acquired through close personal contact, it may be transmitted by clothing, linens, or towels. The widespread, intensely pruritic eruption of scabies represents the host's immune response to the parasite. The mite itself can be found in inconspicuous linear papules (burrows) most often located on the interdigital spaces, wrists, elbows, nipples, umbilicus, lower abdomen, genitalia, and intergluteal cleft. Microscopic examination of a thin epidermal-shave biopsy specimen of such a lesion will demonstrate the mite, its eggs, or mite feces (scybala). Permethrin 5% cream (Elimite) is the treatment of choice for scabies. It is applied at bedtime to the entire body from the neck down. Medication should be left on for 8 to 12 hours before being washed off. At that time, clothing, towels, and linens should be laundered. A second application of permethrin 1 week later is necessary only if there is evidence of residual active mites. Lindane (Kwell, Gamene) when used in the same manner as permethrin is also effective. Lindane should be avoided in pregnant and nursing women, young children, and infants. Crotamiton (Eurax) cream, applied twice and left on during a 48-hour period, is an alternative that is more antipruritic but less scabicidal than lindane. A single PO dose of ivermectin (150–200 µg/kg) has been found to be an effective treatment in healthy and HIV-infected patients.

Persistent itching in treated patients may be due to continued infestation, residual hypersensitivity reaction to the mite, or irritation from overzealous use of lindane. If hypersensitivity is the reason, treatment with topical corticosteroids or a short, tapering course of oral corticosteroids will bring relief. Occasionally, persistent, intensely pruritic nodules remain after successful scabietic therapy. These nodules respond to intralesional corticosteroids.

Haustein U-F, Hlawa B. Treatment of scabies with permethrin versus lindane and benzoyl benzoate. Acta Dermvenerol 1989;69:348–351.
Meinking TL, Taplin D, Hermida JL, et al. The treatment of scabies with ivermectin. N Engl J Med 1995;333:26–30.
Orkin M, Maibach HI. Scabies therapy—1993. Semin Dermatol 1993;12:22–25.

E. Warts

Warts are intraepidermal tumors of the skin caused by infection with the human papillomavirus (HPV). Numerous types of HPV have been defined. In general, there is no absolute correlation between infection by a given HPV type and any particular lesional morphology, although certain HPV types characteristically affect special target areas. Warts may be found in persons of any age but are most common in those between the ages of 12 and 16. They may spread by contact or autoinoculation; anogenital warts (condylomata acuminata) are particularly contagious. HPV types 16 and 18 in condylomata acuminata likely increase the risk of cervical and anorectal carcinoma. Electrodesiccation, curettage, cryosurgery, and laser surgery are effective treatments that require additional training and equipment.

Keratolytics, such as 5% to 20% salicylic acid and 5% to 20% lactic acid in flexible collodion (Duofilm, Occlusal), may produce good results for most types of warts except the mosaic plantar variety. Keratolytic agents act by mechanically removing infected cells and by provoking an inflammatory reaction that elicits a virus-specific immune response. Keratolytic agents are used as follows.

- The area should be washed thoroughly with soap and water.
- The surface of the wart should be rubbed gently with a mild abrasive, such as an emery board, pumice stone, or callous file.
- The keratolytic should be applied to the wart with a toothpick or orangewood stick.
- The keratolytic should be allowed to dry.

This regimen is repeated nightly until a response is seen, undue irritation develops, or it is obvious that the warts are resistant. (This may take as long as 12 weeks to ascertain.)

Cantharidin is a mitochondrial poison that causes an intraepidermal blister. The lesion is painted with the solution, allowed to dry, and then covered with a nonporous occlusive tape (e.g., Blenderm). The tape is removed in 24 hours, following which a blister, often hemorrhagic, develops. Any residual wart evident at a 1 to 2 week follow-up can be retreated. **Podophyllum** resin (podophyllin), a cytotoxic agent that arrests mitosis in metaphase, is used primarily for treatment of condylomata acuminata. Care must be taken to avoid applying the medication to normal skin. When therapy is initiated, the podophyllin is washed off 1 to 4 hours after application to avoid undue inflammation and discomfort. If no response is seen at 1-week follow-up, the length of time the medication is left on is progressively increased, up to 24 hours. Podophyllin may cause systemic neurotoxic effects if absorbed. It is, therefore, inadvisable to apply it in large amounts on mucous membranes or to use it during pregnancy because of its possible cytotoxic effect on the fetus. **Podofilox** (Condylox) is a derivative of podophyllin developed for patient self-treatment. It is applied bid for 3 days of the week with no treatment on the subsequent 4 days. When podofilox is effective, results should be seen within 4 weeks of treatment. Like podophyllin, podofilox can be quite irritating when applied to normal skin.

Intralesional injection of interferon-α (Intron-A) may be considered for patients with recalcitrant condylomata acuminata, but the discomfort, side effects, and cost of this therapy severely limit its utility.

Relatively painless treatments include painting lesions with trichloroace-
tic acid, dichloroacetic acid, or monochloroacetic acid (often applied under
occlusion with 40% salicylic acid plaster) or localized submersion under
heated water (50°C for 30–60 s for one to four treatments) baths.

Androphy EJ. Human papillomavirus. Arch Dermatol 1989;125:683–685.
Cobb MW. Human papillomavirus infection. J Am Acad Dermatol 1990;22:547–566.
Greene I. Therapy for genital warts. Dermatol Clin 1992;10:253–267.

VI. PRURITUS

Itching is the cardinal symptom of most dermatologic diseases. It may be
localized or generalized, paroxysmal or unremitting. Itching and pain are
transmitted along similar, if not identical, peripheral neural pathways, and
itching does not occur in an area insensitive to pain. Histamine is the classic
but not the only mediator of pruritus, since most itchy conditions are not
accompanied by other signs of histamine release (i.e., wheal and flare), nor
are antihistamines always effective in reducing itch. Various proteases,
peptides, and prostaglandins potentiate histamine's effect without being
directly pruritogenic. Kallikrein, substance P, and serotonin may also be
primary mediators. The patient with itching and no rash poses a particularly
challenging diagnostic and therapeutic dilemma. Excessively dry skin
(asteatosis, xerosis) can be quite pruritic. Pruritus accompanied by no skin
changes other than those produced by scratching itself may also be
secondary to numerous systemic diseases (Table 15–3). Especially when no
definitive cure of the underlying illness may be offered, specific therapy
aimed at reducing such pruritus is most welcome.

A. Xerosis

Dry skin is a common condition, especially among the elderly. When severe
enough to provoke inflammation, it is also known as asteatotic eczema.
Environmental factors are important: repeated exposure to solvents, soaps,
and disinfectants will remove lipid from the skin, increasing transepidermal
water loss up to 75 times the normal amount. Decreased relative humidity
and cold, dry winds will literally pull water from the skin. Factors that
decrease the relative humidity include increased ambient temperature and
ventilating with cold, dry air.

TABLE 15–3. Systemic Diseases Associated with Pruritus

Uremia
Obstructive biliary disease (e.g., primary biliary cirrhosis)
Myeloproliferative disorders (e.g., polycythemia vera, Hodgkin's disease)
Iron deficiency
Endocrine disorders (e.g., thyrotoxicosis)
Visceral malignancies
Neurologic disorders (e.g., brain abscess)

Modified from Denman ST. A review of pruritus. J Am Acad Dermatol 1986;14:375–392.

1. **PREVENTIVE MEASURES.** Room temperatures must be kept as low as comfortable. Use of humidifiers (built-in or portable) should be encouraged. Bathing should be restricted to once every 1 to 2 days, and warm, not hot, bath water should be used. Bath oils may be used, but these can make the tub dangerously slick and are of limited therapeutic benefit. Excessive exposure to soaps, solvents, or other drying agents must be avoided. A mild soap, such as Dove, should be used. Finally, emollients should be applied frequently. These agents are most effectively applied when the skin is already moist (i.e., immediately after bathing). When choosing an emollient, one should sacrifice esthetics for efficacy because thicker, less appealing preparations (e.g., Eucerin, petrolatum) are more effective than lighter lotions (e.g., Alpha-Keri, Lubriderm).

2. **TREATMENT OF EXISTING DRYNESS.** The primary means of correcting dryness is to add water to the skin first and then apply a hydrophobic substance to keep it there. Emollients are only moderately effective at actually moisturizing the skin, despite advertising claims to the contrary. When used alone, hydrophobic emollients hydrate the skin simply by preventing the normal transepidermal water loss. Maximal hydration is achieved by the use of 40% to 60% propylene glycol in water applied under plastic occlusion overnight. Keralyt gel is a salicylic acid and propylene glycol formulation that is extremely effective at hydrating and simultaneously removing scaling. Creams containing urea or lactic acid or both (e.g., Carmol, Lac-Hydrin, and U-Lactin) are particularly helpful. Topical corticosteroid ointments used with occlusive dressings are the most effective and rapid therapy for symptomatic xerosis and associated eczematous changes.

B. Uremic Pruritus

Renal failure is the most prevalent of all systemic diseases associated with pruritus. Pruritus has become a much more common problem for uremic patients, although it remains unclear whether this is due to dialysis itself or is simply a product of patients' greater longevity. Of patients on hemodialysis, 80% to 90% at some time experience significant pruritus, 42% find that their itching is most severe during or immediately after dialysis treatments. The cause is unknown. Efforts aimed at correcting calcium and phosphorus abnormalities common in chronic renal failure will often, although not invariably, alleviate pruritus. Increased levels of magnesium and vitamin A within the skin have also been postulated to contribute to itching. The dry skin to which uremic patients are prone may further aggravate their itching.

1. **SPECIFIC TREATMENTS.** UVB phototherapy is almost always effective, with a decrease in itching usually seen after eight suberythemogenic daily doses. Parathyroidectomy may result in dramatic relief of itching within 24 to 48 hours in patients with secondary hyperparathyroidism. The response is not invariable, and if patients become hypercalcemic postoperatively, the pruritus can recur. Activated charcoal (6 g/d PO for 8 weeks) may be effective; it will nonspecifically bind other orally administered drugs. Finally, cholestyramine (5 g PO bid) may alleviate not only hepatic but also uremic pruritus (see below).

C. Cholestatic Pruritus

Pruritus occurs in 25% of patients with cholestatic liver disease but is rarely seen in hepatitis without biliary obstruction. Although purified bile salts applied to the skin are pruritogenic and lowering the serum bile concentration usually ameliorates cholestatic pruritus, no convincing evidence has been found that total or individual levels of bile salts, either circulating or within the skin, correlate with the presence or absence of itching.

1. **SPECIFIC TREATMENTS.** Cholestyramine (Questran 4 g PO qd–tid), an ion exchange resin, is frequently effective, although its antipruritic effect seems separate from its ability to normalize bile salt levels. Cholestyramine is a powder that is mixed with water or another fluid before ingesting. Ursodeoxycholic acid (Actigall 300 mg bid) is beneficial in alleviating cholestatic pruritus. Colestipol (Colestid) is another ion-exchange resin that may be substituted in patients who find cholestyramine too constipating. Like charcoal, ion-exchange resins may bind other orally administered drugs. Oral vitamin K supplements (10 mg a week) should be given concurrently. Phenobarbital (3–4 mg/kg/d PO) can reduce cholestatic pruritus, although the mechanism by which it does so remains unknown. Phenobarbital is sedating and may interfere with the metabolism of many drugs. UVB phototherapy is often helpful in treating cholestatic pruritus. Rifampin (150 mg PO bid or tid) is also effective in some patients with cholestatic pruritus. The presumed mode of action is rifampin's inhibition of intrahepatic bile acid uptake or stimulation of microsomal enzymes that detoxify nonbile salt pruritogens or both. Newer agents include nalmefene and ondansetron, which may help in refractory cases.

D. Hematologic Pruritus

Of patients with polycythemia vera, 14% to 52% have pruritus. Although elevated plasma and urine histamine levels, correlating with an increased number of basophils, have been found in two thirds of patients with polycythemia vera, antihistamines are usually ineffective at controlling their pruritus. Iron deficiency, with or without anemia, may also be associated with pruritus. Pruritus is frequently seen in Hodgkin's disease, often before the correct diagnosis is evident; severe, generalized pruritus may indicate a more serious prognosis.

1. **SPECIFIC TREATMENTS.** Cimetidine, a histamine$_2$ (H$_2$) blocker (300 mg PO qid), or cyproheptadine, an antihistamine and antiserotonin agent (4 mg PO qid), may reduce the pruritus of polycythemia vera, although double-blind studies have not confirmed their effectiveness. **Recombinant interferon-**α (3 million U IM three times a week) has been reported to dramatically reduce the severity of polycythemia vera-associated pruritus. The high cost and frequent side effects of this therapy limit its usefulness. Iron replacement will abolish pruritus due to iron deficiency, often before any measurable change in the hematologic status.

E. General Treatment Measures

Antihistamines are usually ineffective for pruritus caused by systemic illness. Coexisting conditions that may aggravate the pruritus—particularly xerosis, as is frequently observed in chronic renal failure—should be appropriately managed. Dietary manipulation may occasionally be helpful; low-protein diets have been successful for uremic pruritus, whereas diets rich in polyunsaturated fatty acids may help relieve cholestatic pruritus.

Finelli C, Gugliotta L, Gamberi B, Vianelli N, et al. Relief of intractable pruritus in polycythemia vera with recombinant interferon alfa. Am J Hematol 1993;43:316–318.

Gregorio GV, Ball CS, Mowat AP, Mieli-Verangi G. Effect of rifampicin in the treatment of pruritus in hepatic cholestasis. Arch Dis Child 1993;69:141–143.

Kantor GR. Evaluation and treatment of generalized pruritus. Cleve Clin J Med 1990;57:521–526.

16 16 16 16 16 16 16 16

NEUROLOGIC DISEASES

PHILLIP D. SWANSON

The number of neurologic conditions managed with medical therapy may surprise those who view diseases of the nervous system as poorly amenable to treatment. Although many therapeutic measures are not curative, a rather extensive therapeutic armamentarium is available to manage neurologic disorders.

I. SEIZURE DISORDERS

Epileptic seizures are commonly encountered in medical practice. The physician must be able to treat seizures immediately and manage patients on a long-term basis. Seizure management requires understanding of both seizure classification and anticonvulsant drugs.

A. Classification

Seizures are grouped into two principal categories: (1) primary generalized and (2) partial (Table 16–1). Three problems may lead to confusion with this classification. First, the category of primary generalized seizures includes both absences (petit mal seizures) and grand mal or other seizures associated with convulsive movements. Second, partial seizures may become secondarily generalized. Third, absence seizures and complex partial (psychomotor, temporal lobe) seizures may not be readily distinguishable on descriptive clinical grounds, in which case an incorrect anticonvulsant choice is likely to be made.

B. Treatment

1. **WHEN TO TREAT A SEIZURE.** Certain clinical situations associated with seizures can be managed **without** anticonvulsant drugs, including uncomplicated febrile seizures and seizures due to withdrawal from alcohol or sedative/hypnotic drugs. Even in children with multiple febrile seizures, or febrile seizures that are prolonged or are partial at the onset, prophylactic medication (usually phenobarbital) is no longer recommended. Drug and alcohol withdrawal seizures are not treated prophylactically because of difficulties in following these patients and because seizures should not recur if substance abuse is terminated. A common management problem is whether to treat a person who has had a single seizure of unknown cause. Estimated risk of recurrence is 31% to 71% within the first 3 years. Some physicians may prefer to wait until a second seizure occurs before instituting long-term anticonvulsant therapy. Prophylactic therapy (usually with phenytoin) has been used for patients with open head injuries or documented contusions. A randomized study showed that phenytoin reduced seizure frequency only during the first week after a severe head injury. Thus, the drug may be safely discontinued after the first week if no seizures have occurred. If a seizure has taken place, medication is continued for 6 months to a year. For concussion without evidence of contusion, anticonvulsants are not recommended.

TABLE 16–1. **International Classification of Epileptic Seizures**

I. Partial seizures (seizures beginning locally)
  A. Simple partial seizures (consciousness not impaired)
    1. With motor symptoms
    2. With somatosensory or special sensory symptoms
    3. With autonomic symptoms
    4. With psychic symptoms
  B. Complex partial seizures (with impairment of consciousness)
    1. Beginning as simple partial seizures and progressing to impairment of consciousness
      a. With no other features
      b. With features as in A.1–4
      c. With automatisms
    2. With impairment of consciousness at onset
      a. With no other features
      b. With features as in A.1–4
      c. With automatisms
  C. Partial seizures secondarily generalized
II. Generalized seizures (bilaterally symmetric and without local onset)
  A. 1. Absence seizures
    2. Atypical absence seizures
  B. Myoclonic seizures
  C. Clonic seizures
  D. Tonic seizures
  E. Tonic-clonic seizures
  F. Atonic seizures
III. Unclassified epileptic seizures (inadequate or incomplete data)

Abstracted from Commission on Classification and Terminology of the International League Against Epilepsy. Proposal for revised clinical and electroencephalographic classification of epileptic seizures. Epilepsia 1981;22:489–501. This classification was approved by the International League Against Epilepsy in September 1981.

2. **INITIAL ANTICONVULSANT.** The guiding principle is to select the least toxic agent most likely to control the type of seizure being treated. To minimize toxicity, many agents are started at a dose lower than the expected final one. In general, at a fixed dose, 5 drug half-lives are needed to achieve a steady state. In the pediatric age group, the dosage is based on the patient's weight. Tables 16–2 and 16–3 list characteristics of many of the available anticonvulsant drugs.

  a. **Absence attacks.** Ethosuximide (Zarontin) is the first drug used. Valproic acid (Depakote or Depakene) is also effective in this type of seizure. With the latter drug, hepatic function should be assessed periodically. Hepatotoxicity has almost always occurred within 6 months of beginning of therapy.

  b. **Primary generalized convulsions.** Phenytoin (Dilantin), valproic acid, phenobarbital, or carbamazepine (Tegretol) may be selected. In **juvenile myoclonic epilepsy,** seizures characteristically occur in the morning after arising. Myoclonic jerks without loss of consciousness or preceding a convulsion are common. Divalproex sodium (Depakote) is the antiepileptic agent of choice. Potential side effects

TABLE 16–2. Comparison of Selected Anticonvulsants Commonly Used for Treatment of Seizures

DRUG	USUAL TOTAL DAILY DOSE FOR ADULTS (mg)	TARGET PLASMA LEVEL (µg/ml)	PLASMA HALF-LIFE IN ADULTS (h)	COMMON SIDE EFFECTS	APPROXIMATE $ COST OF 100 TABLETS OR CAPSULES	COMMENTS
Phenytoin (Dilantin)	300–400	10–20	24–72	Gingival hyperplasia, ataxia, fetal malformations	22 (100 mg)	
Phenobarbital (Luminal)	90–300	10–40	90–120	Drowsiness	4 (30 mg)	
Carbamazepine (Tegretol)	600–1200	6–12	10–20	Dizziness, leukopenia	12 (250 mg)	Blood counts necessary
Ethosuximide (Zarontin)	750–2000	40–100	30–50	Nausea	30 (250 mg)	Agent of choice for absence (petit mal) seizures
Primidone (Mysoline)	500–1500	5–15 (phenobarbital, major metabolite)	7–14	Sedation	5 (250 mg)	Do not use with phenobarbital
Valproic acid (Depakote)	1000–3000	50–100	10–12	GI disturbances, sedation	45 (250 mg)	Can raise serum level of phenobarbital
Gabapentin (Neurontin)	2400–3600	N/A	5–7	Fatigue, somnolence	85 (300 mg)	Not metabolized; half-life is renal function dependent
Lamotrigine (Lamictal)	100–150 (on VPA) 300–500 (not on VPA)	N/A	12–61	Rash, abnormal cognition, dizziness	150 (25 or 100 mg)	Slow titration reduce side effect risk

Data from Swanson PD. Anticonvulsant therapy. Postgrad Med 1979;65:147–154; Bleck TP. Convulsive disorders: the use of anticonvulsant drugs. Clin Neurophysiol 1990;13:198–209; and Graves N. Guide to antiepileptic agents. Pharmacy Practice News, Retail Pharmacy News 1995;22(2):14–17.

TABLE 16-3. **Selected Anticonvulsants with Limited Application**

DRUG	COMMENTS
Mephenytoin (Mesantoin)	Useful for generalized and partial seizures; bone marrow suppression possible
Mephobarbital (Mebaral)	No advantage over phenobarbital
Methsuximide (Celontin)	Ancillary drug for generalized or partial seizures
Clonazepam (Klonopin)	Used for myoclonic seizures; high incidence of drowsiness and ataxia
Phenacemide (Phenurone)	Uncommonly used because of side effects of aplastic anemia, liver damage, and psychiatric disturbances
Clorazepate (Tranxene)	Longer acting than diazepam
ACTH	Used for infantile spasms
Lorazepam (Ativan)	Because of short half-life, usefulness limited to status epilepticus
Diazepam (Valium)	Used IV for status epilepticus
Felbamate (Felbatol)	Used for partial and generalized seizures including Lennox-Gastaut syndrome; risk of aplastic anemia limits usefulness

Adapted from Swanson PD. Anticonvulsant therapy. Postgrad Med 1979;65:147–154.

must be considered when choosing a drug, especially in women of childbearing age. Although anticonvulsant effects on the fetus remain controversial, certain results must be discussed with the patient: (1) severe midline defects such as meningomyelocele have been reported in children born of mothers taking valproic acid or carbamazepine, (2) phenytoin and other agents such as phenobarbital may produce a syndrome called the fetal hydantoin syndrome, and (3) probably any anticonvulsant increases the risk for birth defects severalfold. Phenytoin also is known to produce gingival hyperplasia, hirsutism, and probably some coarsening of the skin, side effects that are of particular concern for women and children. Thus, in a young woman, carbamazepine might be chosen as a first drug, even though it is more expensive than phenytoin and may be no more effective for seizure control. Pregnant patients taking valproic acid or carbamazepine should have amniotic alpha-fetoprotein levels measured and ultrasonic monitoring at about 16 weeks' gestation. Supplementation with 0.4 mg/d of folic acid is recommended for all potentially pregnant women taking an anticonvulsant, and doses of 5 mg/d for those taking valproate or carbamazepine. A pregnant woman taking phenytoin, phenobarbital, primidone, or carbamazepine should receive 20 mg of vitamin K_1 daily during the last week of pregnancy.

c. **Partial seizures.** Carbamazepine is becoming the first-line drug. The danger of serious hematologic abnormalities is low. The total white blood cell count may drop to around 4000/mm^3 in patients on long-term carbamazepine. Blood counts should be done at intervals, at first monthly, then less frequently. Carbamazepine should be started at a low dosage. For an adult, an appropriate beginning dose is ½ tablet (100 mg) bid. After a week, the dosage is increased by ½ tablet, and increases continue every 3 or 4 days as tolerated, until a dose of 1 tablet (200 mg) tid is reached. At this time, the blood level of the drug should be determined. If the level is in the range of 6 µg/mL, the dosage is maintained at 3/d. If it is significantly below this range, the daily maintenance dose is increased to 4 tablets. Phenytoin is often the first drug used for partial seizures. It is relatively inexpensive. The total daily dose can be given once a day because of a long half-life. At higher doses the plasma levels of phenytoin rise more rapidly (saturation kinetics), and smaller increments and longer intervals should be used for increases. Other drugs such as phenobarbital and primidone (Mysoline) are used less frequently because of sedative side effects. Phenobarbital is one of the major metabolites of primidone; the two drugs should not be used together. Three recently approved anticonvulsants are available to be used as adjunctive therapy: felbamate (Felbatol), gabapentin (Neurontin), and lamotrigine (Lamictal) (Tables 16–2 and 16–3). **Felbamate** must be used with caution because of an increased risk of aplastic anemia and hepatic failure. Written informed consent should be obtained after the risks have been discussed with the patient. **Gabapentin** (Neurontin) has the advantage of not being metabolized. It is excreted unchanged by the kidneys. It does not alter blood levels of other anticonvulsants. In adults, 300-mg capsules are used to initiate therapy, with dosage increases to a maximum of 4800 mg/d in tid or qid divided doses. **Lamotrigine** (Lamictal) also is used as adjunctive treatment of partial seizures. The drug must be started slowly (25 mg qod if on valproate and an enzyme inducer). Increasing the dose very gradually may prevent development of an idiosyncratic rash. Usual maintenance doses are 300–500 mg/d in two divided doses in patients not taking valproate and 100–150 mg/d in those taking valproate.

3. WHEN SHOULD A SECOND DRUG BE USED? Usually, a second drug should be considered when the patient has had another seizure in spite of treatment that has produced therapeutic levels. The serum level of the first drug should be measured, and if it is below the accepted therapeutic range or if the patient has no signs of toxicity, one should first increase the dosage of the initial drug. If seizures continue, a second drug is added. In contrast to past practice, it now is recommended that the first drug be tapered if addition of the second drug achieves seizure control. However, many patients prefer to continue with two drugs if they are seizure free because of concern that stopping the first drug will increase the chances of another seizure.

4. HOW LONG SHOULD AN ANTICONVULSANT BE CONTINUED? Duration of treatment with anticonvulsants has not been established. In approximately 40% of patients who have been seizure free for 2 or more years, seizures recur within 1½ years of discontinuing medication, a risk that should be explained to a patient before discontinuance. Discontinuation should be gradual over a few weeks to minimize the likelihood of withdrawal seizures. **If epileptiform discharges are present on an EEG, stopping the drug is risky.**

5. OTHER MANAGEMENT ISSUES. Poor seizure control can be assessed by in-hospital video-EEG monitoring for several days. Usually, anticonvulsants are withdrawn during the several day hospitalization period.

Nonepileptic pseudoseizures may be documented in some patients. In others, demonstration of a localized epileptic focus at seizure onset may lead to a recommendation for epilepsy surgery.

C. Status Epilepticus

A state of repetitive focal or generalized seizures with incomplete neurologic recovery between seizures is called status epilepticus. Rarely, the only manifestation is altered consciousness (absence or complex partial status). Possible causes include meningitis, cessation of anticonvulsant therapy, withdrawal from ethanol or sedative drugs, electrolyte disturbances, hypoglycemia, subarachnoid hemorrhage, uremia, toxicity from drugs such as high-dose penicillin, meperidine, or theophylline, and recreational drug (cocaine) ingestion. Aggressive anticonvulsant therapy is indicated; there is no single accepted regimen.

Initial management consists of establishing an airway, positioning the patient to avoid aspiration of stomach contents, inserting an IV line, obtaining blood for estimation of glucose, electrolyte, and creatinine levels, and administering 50 mL of 50% glucose. Rapidly acting anticonvulsants are given IV. Commonly, a rapidly acting benzodiazepine (diazepam or lorazepam) is used, followed by a loading dose of a longer-acting agent, such as phenytoin. IV diazepam, in 2-mg increments to a total dose of 10 mg, is often used. Lorazepam, which may have a longer anticonvulsant effect and be less likely to produce respiratory depression, is given in 1–4-mg increments, to a total dosage of 9 mg. With either drug, injections are spaced 5 minutes apart.

The most popular long-acting anticonvulsant for status epilepticus is **phenytoin,** which can be administered IV in a slow push at a rate **no greater than 50 mg/min.** Up to 1 g may be administered over an hour to a patient who has not already been taking this agent. The IV line should contain **normal saline only.** Phenytoin must never be administered intramuscularly because it will precipitate in the muscle and not be reliably absorbed. IV phenytoin can produce cardiac arrhythmias, conduction defects, and hypotension. Blood pressure and pulse are checked frequently, and ECG monitoring is continuous. An alternative long-acting drug, phenobarbital, can also be administered IV in 250-mg doses. Two doses are usually well tolerated. However, respiratory arrest may occur more frequently when phenobarbital is given with a benzodiazepine than when phenobarbital is given alone. Other agents that can be used when seizures continue include lidocaine, propofol, and general anesthetics. Intravenous pentobarbital has been successfully used to stop refractory status epilepticus. The drug is given initially as a bolus of 5 mg/kg. This is followed by 25–50-mg boluses q2–5min until a burst-suppression pattern is seen on EEG. An IV infusion is continued at a rate of 5 mg/kg/h, with gradual decreases after 12 to 24 hours.

Brodie MJ, Dichter MA. Antiepileptic drugs. N Engl J Med 1996;334:168–175.
Brown TR, Mikati M. Status epilepticus. In: Ropper AH, Kennedy SF, eds. Neurological and Neurosurgical Intensive Care, 2nd ed. Rockville, MD: Aspen Publishers; 1988, pp 269–288.
Delgado-Escueta AV, Wasterlain CG, Treiman JDM, et al, eds. Status Epilepticus. Adv Neurol, 1983, vol 34.
Farwell JR, Lee YJ, Hirtz DG, et al. Phenobarbital for febrile seizures—effects on intelligence and on seizure recurrence. N Engl J Med 1990;322:364–369.
Gress D. Stopping seizures. Emergency Med 1980;22:22–29.

Hauser WA, Rich SS, Annegers JF, et al. Seizure recurrence after a first unprovoked seizure: an extended follow-up. Neurology 1990;40:1163–1170.

Johnson LC, DeBolt WL, Long MT, et al. Diagnostic factors in adult males following initial seizures: a 3-year follow-up. Arch Neurol 1972;27:193–197.

Juul-Jensen P. Frequency of recurrence after discontinuance of anticonvulsant therapy in patients with epileptic seizures. Epilepsia 1964;5:352–363.

Levy RJ, Krall RL. Treatment of status epilepticus with lorazepam. Arch Neurol 1984;41:605–611.

Pierelli F, Chatrian GE, Erdly WW, et al. Long-term EEG video-audio monitoring: detection of partial epileptic seizures and psychogenic episodes by 24-hour EEG record review. Epilepsia 1989;30:513–523.

Temkin NR, Dikmen SS, Wilensky AJ, et al. A randomized, double-blind study of phenytoin for the prevention of post-traumatic seizures. N Engl J Med 1990;323:497–502.

II. SLEEP DISORDERS

Daytime sleepiness is a complaint that may require special polysomnography monitoring before a definitive diagnosis is made. It is important **not** to treat patients with stimulant drugs if a precise diagnosis has not been established. The disorders that do require specific management are narcolepsy and sleep apnea. A specialized sleep laboratory is often required to establish the correct diagnosis.

A. Narcolepsy

The narcolepsy syndrome has four components: episodes of irresistible daytime sleepiness (narcolepsy), episodes of sudden loss of postural tone (cataplexy), brief episodes of inability to move on awakening (sleep paralysis), and vivid hallucinations on going to sleep or awakening (hypnagogic hallucinations). Many patients have only one or two of these symptoms. Patients with the narcoleptic syndrome often enter rapid eye movement (REM) sleep almost immediately. **Methylphenidate** (Ritalin) in dosages of 5–10 mg tid is considered to be the most effective drug. An alternative agent is pemoline (Cylert), 18.75 mg each morning, which can be increased as needed up to six tablets per day in divided doses. Drugs should not be prescribed unless the diagnosis is well established. The physician should monitor the number of prescribed pills and use the lowest effective dose. If cataplectic symptoms are bothersome, imipramine (Tofranil) or an analog is often very effective at a dosage of 25 mg bid or tid.

B. Sleep Apnea

This most commonly is due to obstruction to air flow in overweight persons who are snorers. A polysomnogram, with monitoring of air flow and intraesophageal pressure, is used to confirm the diagnosis. Although surgical procedures such as tracheostomy and uvulopalatopharyngoplasty are sometimes necessary, less invasive therapy is often satisfactory. Approaches include weight loss, use of tongue-restraining devices, continuous positive airway pressure, and treatment with agents such as protriptyline and medroxyprogesterone.

C. Restless Legs Syndrome

This is a poorly understood condition characterized by nighttime unpleasant sensations in the limbs relieved by movement. Among medications found to be of limited use, carbidopa/levodopa at doses of one or two 25/100 mg tablets may be the most helpful. Other variably effective drugs are carbamazepine, clonidine hydrochloride (0.2–0.9 mg/d), bromocriptine, clonazepam, and opioids. Amitryptiline is only rarely helpful.

Bliwise DL. Sleep-related respiratory disturbance in elderly persons. Compr Ther 1984;10:8–14.

Kryger M, Roth T, Dement W. Principles and Practice of Sleep Medicine. Philadelphia: WB Saunders, 1989.

O'Keefe ST. Restless legs syndrome. A review. Arch Intern Med 1996;156:243–248.

III. COMA AND ALTERED MENTAL STATUS

Stupor, coma, and delirium are presenting symptoms of cerebral dysfunction due to multiple potential causes. Proper management involves simultaneously establishing a correct diagnosis and instituting measures to prevent complications and to treat rapidly correctable conditions, such as hypoglycemia. Altered mental status implies bilateral cerebral dysfunction or disturbance at the level of the high brainstem, the location of the reticular activating system. Metabolic, toxic, vascular, space-occupying, traumatic, and seizure disorders lead the list of conditions that may manifest in this way. Usually, historical clues are more helpful than physical examination in coming to a rational diagnostic conclusion. Since patients brought to medical attention usually cannot provide accurate information, efforts should be made to seek out relatives, neighbors, or friends who can.

A. Coma

The first measures to be taken when a comatose patient arrives in the emergency room include vital sign assessment, IV line placement, blood withdrawal for determining glucose and electrolyte levels, and IV administration of glucose with thiamine. Taking appropriate measures to maintain blood pressure and respiration then allows time to assess the patient's neurologic and clinical status further. Examination of the head and ear canals for signs of trauma and flexion of the neck to evaluate nuchal rigidity are two quick diagnostic observations to be made. The level of consciousness is assessed by use of verbal commands and, if necessary, noxious stimuli. Assessment of the pupils, visualization of the fundi for papilledema and subhyaloid hemorrhages (the latter common with subarachnoid hemorrhage secondary to rupture of a berry aneurysm), examination of eye movements, and detection of lateralizing motor signs are the most important parts of the neurologic assessment. The most valuable radiologic test is CT scan, but if the patient is febrile and meningitis is strongly suspected, a delay of CSF examination to carry out CT may be unwarranted.

1. COMA DUE TO ENCEPHALITIS. Herpes simplex encephalitis occurs at all ages. Clinical features include fever, convulsions, memory loss, and delirium, followed by stupor and coma. Focal changes on CT or MRI scan usually appear in the frontotemporal areas. Absence of leukocytes in CSF does not exclude the diagnosis. IV acyclovir is recommended if the diagnosis is suspected. If the diagnosis is confirmed by CSF PCR, treatment is continued for up to 3 weeks. (See also Table 3–5.)

2. COMA DUE TO ISCHEMIA, HYPOXIA, OR CARBON MONOXIDE POISONING. Ways to improve survival of cerebral tissues after cardiorespiratory arrest or after exposure to high levels of carbon monoxide are being actively

investigated. Hyperbaric oxygen treatment is indicated for patients in deep coma who have been exposed to high doses of carbon monoxide. For less severely affected persons or for those who have had cerebral ischemia from cardiorespiratory arrest, oxygen is given by endotracheal tube. No drug has been shown to improve outcome in such patients. Use of barbiturates, calcium entry blockers, or blockers of excitatory amino acid (glutamate, aspartate) receptors has been advocated in an attempt to reduce brain damage. Results of animal studies support the use of each of these agents. Thus far, however, only barbiturates have been tested extensively in humans, and results are not encouraging. Studies of calcium entry blockers are in progress, and the search for useful excitatory amino acid blockers is an active area for investigation.

3. COMA DUE TO FAT EMBOLISM. Diffuse encephalopathy from fat embolism occurs in some patients after fracture of a long bone. After a delay of several hours to a few days, the patient becomes stuporous or comatose, often having developed petechiae of skin, conjunctivae, or retina, as well as respiratory distress. Prophylactic use of high-dose methylprednisolone in patients with long-bone fractures has been reported to reduce the incidence of fat embolism (Ann Intern Med 1986; 146:969–973). Once the syndrome has developed, intensive respiratory care is the most important therapy. The use of heparin, steroids, or other agents does not appear to improve the clinical outcome.

B. Delirium

Sudden onset of confusion, often associated with visual hallucinations and impaired consciousness, indicates the presence of delirium. Obtaining a history of previous psychiatric problems, use of medications, substance abuse, and the presence of other medical problems such as diabetes mellitus or thyroid disease is especially important. The presence of fever may suggest the onset of encephalitis or meningitis. In an alcoholic, Wernicke's encephalopathy due to thiamine deficiency is suggested by the presence of nystagmus and ophthalmoplegia. The physician will obtain a blood sample for glucose, electrolytes, CBC, cultures, and drug screen. CT will usually be done to rule out a structural lesion or subarachnoid hemorrhage. Measures similar to those taken with a comatose patient (see above) are carried out. Tremulousness, confusion, hallucinosis, seizures, and delirium tremens usually occur in individuals who have been drinking ethanol heavily for several weeks and who have recently reduced the amount of ethanol consumption. Similar symptoms occur in persons who are withdrawing from barbiturates or other sedative drugs. Withdrawal from narcotics also may be accompanied by similar symptoms, although seizures are unusual. Distinguishing delirium from acute psychosis can be difficult.

Management of the delirious patient requires hospital admission and close observation. The patient should be in a quiet private room with orienting objects, such as a clock and a calendar. The presence of a family member or close friend may be reassuring and should be encouraged. Frequent observation for changes in consciousness and vital signs and monitoring of intake and output is routine. When the patient is in bed, side rails should be raised. Waist and limb restraints may be needed if the patient is combative, is likely to wander, or is being fed parenterally. Medications are used in the lowest doses necessary to keep the patient calm.

Antipsychotic drugs, such as haloperidol (2–5 mg), chlorpromazine (50–100 mg), or thiothixene (20 mg), are used for rapid tranquilization. Lower doses should be used in the elderly. These drugs should be avoided in delirium associated with ethanol or sedative withdrawal because of the danger of precipitating seizures. In this situation, a benzodiazepine is used. Lorazepam 1–2 mg IM can be administered. Chlordiazepoxide hydrochloride 25–100 mg IM can be used. Either drug can be given orally, and repeat doses may be administered every 4 to 6 hours. Diazepam and paraldehyde are also used by some physicians. Propranolol has been used in doses up to 540 mg/d for treating agitated delirium in brain-injured patients. Bradycardia and hypotension are limiting factors. It is important to prevent cumulative effects of whichever drug is chosen. The requirement for sedation will likely diminish within a short time, since the normal course of delirium is improvement within hours to a few days.

Goldberg RJ, Dubin WR, Fogel BS. Behavioral emergencies. Assessment and psychopharmacologic management. Clin Neuropharmacol 1989;12:233–248.

Jacobson DM, Terrence CF, Reinmuth OM. The neurologic manifestations of fat embolism. Neurology 1986;36:847–851.

Plum F, Posner JB. The Diagnosis of Stupor and Coma, 3rd ed. Philadelphia: FA Davis; 1980.

IV. DEMENTIAS

A. Alzheimer's Disease

No medication alters the course of Alzheimer's disease. Mild, transitory symptomatic improvement may occur with some drugs that increase activity in cholinergic systems. However, these agents cannot be recommended with enthusiasm. The list includes lecithin (a source of choline), physostigmine, and tetrahydroaminoacridine **(Tacrine, Cognex).** This agent probably does not improve the dementia significantly, but may improve alertness in the apathetic patient. The recommended dose is 40 mg/d, increasing after 6 weeks to 80 mg/d, with subsequent titration to higher doses if tolerated. Transaminase should be monitored every other week for the first 26 weeks and every 2 to 3 months thereafter. A frequently prescribed ergotamine compound (mixture of equal parts of dihydroergocornine, dihydroergocristine, and dihydrocryptine [Hydergine]) can no longer be recommended. The use of agents that have vasodilating or other rheologic effects is not supported by clinical data.

B. "Treatable" Dementias

Many articles have stressed the importance of diagnosing treatable causes of dementia before assuming a patient has a progressive untreatable disorder. Unfortunately, the proportion of patients with treatable conditions is small among those in whom dementia is the primary complaint. Clinical clues may exist to alert the physician to alternative diagnoses, such as hypothyroidism, normal-pressure hydrocephalus (NPH), or AIDS-related dementia (Table 16–4). Shunting in patients with NPH is most likely to result in improvement in cognitive function when the cause is known and when the

TABLE 16—4. **Differential Diagnosis of Dementia**

CAUSE	CLINICAL CLUES	CONFIRMATORY TESTS*
Alzheimer's disease	No other neurologic signs	
Pick's disease	Symptoms less global than in Alzheimer's disease	CT or MRI may show focal cerebral atrophy
Multiinfarct dementia	Pseudobulbar palsy, episodic worsening	CT may show lacunar infarcts
Depression	Depressed mood	Response to antidepressants
Drugs (tranquilizers, antiparkinsonian agents)	History of drug use, slurred speech, ataxia, lethargy, withdrawal symptoms, or improvement in hospital	Toxicology screen
Chronic subdural hematoma	History of drinking, anticoagulant therapy, lethargy, headache	CT, brain scan
Vitamin B_{12} deficiency	Ataxia, posterior column signs	CBC, B_{12} level, Schilling test
Hydrocephalus	Incontinence, gait disturbance	CT, isotope cisternography
Hypothyroidism	Husky voice, stiff muscles, "hung-up" reflexes	Thyroid studies
Syphilis	Tongue tremor, miotic pupils	VDRL, FTA
Chronic meningitis, (fungus, tumor, tuberculosis)	Other signs of systemic disease	LP for cells, glucose cytology, culture
Huntington's disease	Parent or siblings in mental hospital, fidgety on physical examination	DNA test for expanded trinucleotide repeat
Creutzfeldt-Jakob disease	Progressive over months, myoclonus	EEG: triphasic sharp waves
AIDS-related dementia	History of homosexuality, promiscuity, or IV drug abuse	HIV antibody
Dialysis dementia	Appropriate clinical setting, speech problems, myoclonus, seizures	EEG: slow waves, bursts, spikes

*CT, computed tomography; CBC, complete blood count; VDRL, Venereal Disease Research Laboratory; FTA, fluorescent treponemal antibody; LP, lumbar puncture; EEG, electroencephalogram; HIV, human immunodeficiency virus; MRI, magnetic resonance imaging.
Adapted from Swanson PD. Signs and Symptoms in Neurology. Philadelphia: JB Lippincott; 1984.

duration of symptoms is short (less than 6 months) (Ann Neurol 1986; 20:304–310).

Assuming no specific treatment is available for the dementia, in what areas can the physician assist the patient? In general, it is best to use as few medications as possible. Bothersome hallucinations or nocturnal agitation may respond to a neuroleptic, such as haloperidol. Drugs with anticholinergic actions, such as those used to treat depression and even diphenhydramine for sundowning (nocturnal confusion), can aggravate the dementia or delirium. Urinary retention can also result. Long-term management usually involves assessment of medical, psychologic, and social needs in conjunction with the family and caregivers. Genetic counseling is essential for families of patients with Huntington's disease, which can now be diagnosed with a high degree of certainty using DNA testing for expanded CAG repeats. Caregiver education is valuable. Optimal outcomes in progressive dementias depend on measures designed to preserve caregiver strength and stamina (respite care, recognition of depression) and minimize excess disability due to coexistent illness.

Barry PP, Moskowitz MA. The diagnosis of reversible dementia in the elderly: a critical review. Arch Intern Med 1988;148:1914–1921.

Thompson TL II, Filley CM, Mitchell WD, et al. Lack of efficacy of Hydergine in patients with Alzheimer's disease. N Engl J Med 1990;323:445–448.

V. HEADACHE AND OTHER NEUROLOGIC CAUSES OF PAIN

A. Headache

A patient with **acute** headache should be managed differently from a patient with **chronic** headache.

1. ACUTE HEADACHE. Sudden onset of headache can be an incapacitating and worrisome problem. Perhaps the most important piece of information is whether the headache is of new onset or is one episode of a long-standing pattern. Headache of recent onset should alert the physician to several conditions: acute sinusitis, acute glaucoma, subarachnoid hemorrhage from a leaking berry aneurysm, or bacterial or viral meningitis. The presence of other symptoms or signs, such as tenderness over the frontal or maxillary sinuses, nasal congestion, visual symptoms, fever, and neck stiffness, may make the diagnosis apparent. However, the characteristics of the headache itself may not be specific. Index of suspicion must be high enough so that the appropriate laboratory test (CT, lumbar puncture, or sinus films) is obtained. Approximately 20% of patients with subarachnoid hemorrhage will develop sentinel headaches in the days before aneurysm rupture. A history of sudden agonizing headache, often associated with nausea, vomiting, and neck pain, should arouse suspicion. Assuming that the patient's history and the headache's character support the diagnosis of tension-type or migraine headache, acute pharmacologic treatment may be indicated. Acute muscle contraction headaches should be accompanied by tenderness in the painful areas and resistance to stretch of the painful muscles. Moist heat with a towel soaked in hot water or hot packs may bring relief. Ice packs or gentle massage may also help. Many individuals with tension-type or migraine headache will have relief from aspirin, acetaminophen, or other nonsteroidal anti-inflammatory agents, such as naproxen or ibuprofen. Injections of narcotic analgesics, such as meperidine, should be avoided.

   Ergotamines have been the most widely used agents for aborting migraine headaches. Ergotamines can be given orally, nasally, or per rectum. Usual doses for ergotamine are 2–3 mg PO, 2 mg PR, and 1–2 puffs by inhaler. Sublingual ergotamines are also effective but are not always available. IV or IM dihydroergotamine has been advocated for emergency room treatment of migraine headaches. Up to three doses of

1 mL (1 mg of dihydroergotamine mesylate) can be given at 30-minute or 1-hour intervals. Total weekly dosage should not exceed 6 mL. The drug is contraindicated in pregnancy and in angina, hypertension, or peripheral arterial disease. Other agents used in acute migraine include a phenothiazine such as chlorpromazine 5–10 mg IV, prochlorperazine (Compazine) 2–10 mg IV, or metoclopramide 5–10 mg IV; verapamil 5–10 mg IV; or dexamethasone 20 mg. Propranolol (20 mg PO), used with acetaminophen, can be effective for mild migraine headaches. Ketorolac (Toradol), 60 mg IM, has also been reported to relieve acute headache.

The most recent addition to the armamentarium for migraine abortive therapy is **sumatriptan,** a selective 5-hydroxytryptamine (serotonin) agonist. Initially available for SC injection (6 mg in 0.5 mL), it is now available in 25-mg and 50-mg tablets. A single tablet is taken during the headache and can be followed by a second tablet after 2 hours. The maximum recommended dose in 24 hours is 300 mg. The drug is contraindicated in pregnancy and in patients with risk factors for cardiac disease, as it may cause coronary vasospasm.

2. CHRONIC HEADACHE. Differentiating characteristics of the most common headache types are listed in Table 16–5. A new exhaustive headache classification scheme substitutes the term tension-type for muscle contraction and lists the diagnostic criteria for each headache type and subtype (Cephalalgia 1988;[suppl 7]:1–96). Tension-type or muscle contraction headaches occur frequently, often daily, and may be located in occipital, frontal, or temporal areas. Although usually steady, they may have a throbbing quality or associated nausea. Migraine headaches may be preceded by a visual aura or, rarely, by other symptoms suggesting cerebral ischemia (aphasia or hemisensory or hemiparetic symptoms). The headaches occur episodically, are usually throbbing, and frequently are associated with nausea and other

---

TABLE 16–5. **Classification of Headache**

1. Migraine
   1.1 Migraine without aura
   1.2 Migraine with aura
   1.3 Ophthalmoplegic migraine
2. Tension-type headache
3. Cluster headache and chronic paroxysmal hemicrania
4. Headache associated with head trauma
5. Headache associated with vascular disorders
6. Headache associated with nonvascular intracranial disorders
7. Headache associated with substances or their withdrawal
8. Headache associated with noncephalic infection
9. Headache associated with metabolic abnormality
10. Headache or facial pain associated with disorders of facial or cranial structures
11. Cranial neuralgias, nerve trunk pain, and deafferentiation pain
12. Other types of headache or facial pain
13. Headache, not classifiable

systemic symptoms, such as malaise. Subvarieties of migraine are cluster headaches (daily severe pain, retroorbital location, lacrimation, and nasal stuffiness) and chronic cluster headaches. Temporal arteritis is suspected in older persons with symptoms of malaise, weight loss, and muscle aching. The erythrocyte sedimentation rate is almost always elevated.

a. Chronic tension-type headaches. Understanding that the pain may relate to continued muscle contraction may be helpful to the patient. Demonstrating tenderness and increased muscle tone in painful areas assists in this understanding. Long-term use of narcotic medications should be avoided. Approaches to be encouraged are (1) simple self-administered stretching and relaxation, (2) professional instruction in relaxation, using biofeedback and relaxation-training techniques, and (3) for very severe pain, physical therapy with heat and massage. Low-dose tricyclic antidepressants (amitriptyline 25–50 mg hs) may help patients with a debilitating chronic pain syndrome. Nonsteroidal anti-inflammatory drugs such as naproxen (375–500 mg tid) may be tried for both muscle contraction and migraine prophylaxis.

b. Migraine prophylaxis. Daily medication should be reserved for patients whose headaches occur frequently. The initial drug choice will vary with the physician's experience and will depend on what the patient has tried in the past.

Effective antimigraine drugs have generally been shown to benefit perhaps two thirds of patients when compared with placebos. An agent least likely to produce toxicity should be tried first. If one agent is ineffective, another may be substituted. Aspirin, naproxen, cyproheptadine (Periactin), propranolol, amitriptyline, or a calcium entry blocker may each be tried, with little danger of serious side effects. Recently, divalproex sodium (Depakote) at doses similar to those used for seizure therapy has shown effectiveness in preventing migraine headache. Cyproheptadine has in some instances produced increased appetite and weight gain. Beta-adrenergic blockers are sometimes poorly tolerated because of the occurrence of lassitude, alteration in sleep patterns, or depression. Tricyclic antidepressants often cause sleepiness and dry mouth. Calcium entry blockers are usually well tolerated, but their effectiveness in migraine prophylaxis may be less striking than suggested by early enthusiastic reports. Methysergide (Sansert) is used much less frequently than the others because of the serious side effect of retroperitoneal fibrosis. It is an effective agent for true migraine, and if its use is interrupted every 4 months, there should be little danger of ureteral obstruction. Initially, the dosage should be low (2 mg bid), but if necessary, it can be increased to double this amount. Patients should be warned of side effects, which include angina and intermittent claudication.

B. Face Pain

Pain in the distribution of the face, jaw, or throat must first be diagnosed before a treatment plan can be made. Primary diagnostic considerations are (1) trigeminal and glossopharyngeal neuralgias, (2) disease of teeth, sinuses, or other structures in the head area, (3) pain due to contraction of muscles of mastication, and (4) atypical facial pain.

1. TRIGEMINAL AND GLOSSOPHARYNGEAL NEURALGIAS. These neuralgias share pain characteristics that usually make the clinical diagnosis rather straightforward. The pain occurs suddenly in brief bursts and is usually severe and lancinating. The pain of trigeminal neuralgia (tic douloureux) is almost always in the distribution of the second or third division of the trigeminal nerve; that of glossopharyngeal neuralgia is in the posterior pharynx. The pain is often triggered by stimulation of skin or mucous membrane by such activities as chewing and swallowing. Without such a trigger point the diagnosis should be questioned. The cause is not usually apparent but may be irritation of the affected nerve root by a redundant arterial branch within the posterior intracranial fossa. Although relief may be obtained by surgical intervention, in which a sponge is placed between the nerve root and adjacent artery, or by electrolytic damage to a nerve branch, many patients can be treated with antiseizure medication with good effect. Carbamazepine is begun at a dosage of 100 mg qd or bid, and the amount is gradually increased until a therapeutic level is reached. Blood levels of 6 to 12 μg/mL are usually tolerated without serious side effects. If the pain persists, phenytoin may be used in doses similar to those effective for seizure disorders.

2. ATYPICAL FACE PAIN. Surgical procedures must be avoided in patients whose face pain is not typical of the above neuralgias. The pain is usually more constant, is poorly localized, and is not relieved by anticonvulsant therapy. In some cases, the pain is due to chronic contraction of muscles of mastication, and relief is obtained by measures used by dentists to reduce muscle tension.

C. Drug Withdrawal from Patients with Chronic Pain

Specialty clinics to deal with patients suffering from chronic pain have been established in a number of medical centers. Use of behavioral approaches for managing such patients is emphasized. Many patients with chronic pain have become dependent on narcotic and sedative drugs. A popular method for withdrawal of medications is the use of a "pain cocktail" (Pain 1986; 26:153–165). For patients taking narcotics, methadone is used in doses equivalent to those of the narcotic the patient is taking. Phenobarbital is used to replace sedative drugs. A pain cocktail is prepared in which one or both of these two drugs are added to a taste-masked liquid. The patient is given 10 mL of the pain cocktail every 6 hours. Doses of methadone and phenobarbital are then reduced each day by 15% to 20% and 10%, respectively. Rapid tapering may require inpatient observation.

Buckley FP, Sizemore WA, Charlton JE. Medication management in patients with chronic nonmalignant pain: a review of the use of a drug withdrawal protocol. Pain 1986;26:153–165.

Classification Committee of the International Headache Society. Classification and diagnostic criteria for headache disorders, cranial neuralgias and facial pain. Cephalalgia 1988;8 (Suppl 7):1–96.

Foley KM, Payne R, eds. Current Therapy for Pain. Toronto: BC Decker; 1987.

Goadsby PJ, Oleson J. Diagnosis and management of migraine. Br Med J 1996;312:1279–1283.

Harden RN, Carter TD, Gilman CS, et al. Ketorolac in acute headache management. Headache 1991;31:463–464.

Mathew NT, Saper JR, Silberstein SD, et al. Migraine prophylaxis with divalproex. Arch Neurol 1995;52:281–286.

Meyer JS, Hardenberg J. Clinical effectiveness of calcium entry blockers in prophylactic treatment of migraine and cluster headache. Headache 1983;23:266–277.

Raskin NH, Schwartz RK. Interval therapy of migraine: long-term results. Headache 1980;20: 336–340.

Swanson PD. Signs and Symptoms in Neurology. Philadelphia: JB Lippincott; 1984.

VI. BRAIN TUMORS, INCREASED INTRACRANIAL PRESSURE, AND SPINAL CORD COMPRESSION

Surgical management of space-occupying lesions of the brain or spinal cord is beyond the scope of this chapter. There are, however, certain medical aspects of therapy. The management of increased intracranial pressure is also important for other conditions, such as stroke, generalized cerebral ischemia, and benign intracranial hypertension (pseudotumor cerebri).

A. Brain Tumors

1. **PITUITARY TUMORS.** Adenomas and microadenomas of the pituitary can arise from different cell types. The type most amenable to medical treatment is the **prolactinoma,** which secretes prolactin and produces galactorrhea and hypogonadism as early symptoms. This diagnosis can be confirmed by the serum prolactin levels. Tumor size is determined by radiologic studies. Bromocriptine, a dopamine agonist, causes reduction in the size of prolactin-secreting tumors. Dosages below 10 mg/d are effective and are given for several weeks before transsphenoidal tumor removal. Microadenomas do not require surgery. Alternative dopamine agonists, such as pergolide, have longer half-lives and are taken less frequently than bromocriptine.

2. **GLIOMAS.** Tumor debulking and radiation are mainstays of treatment for primary gliomas of the CNS. The tumor is classified according to probable cellular origin (e.g., oligodendroglioma, astrocytoma) and graded (grade I to IV) according to degree of malignancy. Following surgery, most patients receive radiation therapy, which may include a combination of whole-brain radiation and a boost or radionuclide implant to the tumor site. Adjunctive therapy with chemotherapeutic agents can prolong survival in some cases. Modest success has been achieved with nitrosourea-based protocols.

3. **CEREBRAL METASTASES.** Metastases to the brain or to the leptomeningeal spaces are more common than primary brain tumors. Therapy with whole-brain radiation may produce temporary regression. Meningeal carcinomatosis may respond to intrathecal or intraventricular administration of an appropriate chemotherapeutic agent, such as methotrexate. Patients with a large single metastasis may do better if this is surgically removed before radiation. Cerebral metastases frequently are associated with cerebral edema. Long-term administration of corticosteroids is then recommended.

B. Increased Intracranial Pressure

Increases in intracranial pressure of 200 mm CSF or more can occur in any situation in which the volume of intracranial contents is increased. The success of therapy aimed at reducing intracranial pressure depends on the cause of the pressure increase. Thus, measures to reduce cerebral edema may be effective with brain tumors but much less so in edema associated with cerebral infarction.

1. CORTICOSTEROIDS. **Dexamethasone** is the steroid most often used for reducing cerebral swelling associated with primary or metastatic brain tumors. An initial dose of 10 mg, followed by 4 mg q6h is the usual dosage. However, much higher doses (1 mg/kg) have been recommended by some neurosurgeons. Marked reduction in peritumor edema may occur. H_2-receptor agonists and sucralfate should be used to prevent GI ulceration (see Chapter 8, pp. 336–340). Electrolyte and blood glucose levels need to be determined periodically.

2. HYPEROSMOLAR AGENTS. **Mannitol,** given IV as a 20% to 25% solution, is the most widely used agent for reducing brain swelling by increasing serum osmolality. Doses of 0.25–0.75 g/kg body weight are used, and dramatic reduction in intracranial pressure can occur. However, the reduction is temporary, and the effects of repeated infusions of mannitol become less. Acute renal failure has developed in patients receiving total doses of more than 600 g. An initial dose of 0.75–1 g/kg can be used, followed by lower doses of 0.25–0.5 g/kg every 3 to 5 hours, depending on the level of intracranial pressure and the serum osmolality, which may be raised to about 320 mOsm/L. Foley catheterization and strict monitoring of intake and output are mandatory.

3. HYPERVENTILATION. Reducing the Pa_{CO_2} to 25 to 30 mm Hg can reduce cerebral blood volume and hence the intracranial pressure by 20% to 30%. The effect may not be long lasting. This requires an endotracheal tube and frequent monitoring of blood gases.

4. SURGICAL MEASURES. In some clinical situations (e.g., hydrocephalus associated with subarachnoid hemorrhage), removal of CSF by means of a ventriculostomy is useful. Internal decompression of an intracerebral mass (tumor or hemorrhage) may be needed to prevent transtentorial herniation. Rarely, craniectomy (with preservation of the cranial bone and later replacement at the original site) has been life saving in those with large hemispheral infarcts.

5. BENIGN INTRACRANIAL HYPERTENSION. This condition, also called pseudotumor cerebri, is usually of unknown cause. Often, the patient is young and obese and develops headaches. The only physical sign is papilledema. After known causes of increased intracranial pressure are excluded (tumor, hydrocephalus), the diagnosis is considered. In some instances, thrombosis of a draining venous sinus is implicated (e.g., patients with mastoiditis). Other possible causes (hypervitaminosis A, tetracycline, endocrine abnormalities) are usually not present. The goal of treatment is to prevent headaches and blindness. Treatment with periodic spinal punctures for removal of CSF, best performed with an 18-gauge needle, may suffice to prevent headaches. Enough fluid is removed to reduce the pressure to 150 to 180 mm H_2O. Furosemide or acetazolamide in standard doses is used with success in many persons. A rare patient requires decompression of the optic nerves to prevent progressive visual loss. Formal visual field testing should be carried

out at intervals. Lumboperitoneal shunt is an alternative in refractory cases.

C. Acute Spinal Cord Compression

Rapid onset of leg weakness is often the result of spinal cord compression. Spinal cord compression due to trauma or to epidural tumor should be treated immediately with steroids. Based on a randomized study, a patient with traumatic spinal cord compression is immediately treated with an IV bolus of methylprednisolone 30 mg/kg body weight over 15 minutes. After 45 minutes this is followed by a 23-hour infusion of 5.4 mg/kg/h. Patients treated within 8 hours of injury are most likely to benefit. Spinal cord compression due to epidural metastases should also be treated with corticosteroids, although in this situation, the recommended regimen is a 10-mg IV bolus of dexamethasone followed by 4 mg PO q4h. Higher doses provide no additional benefit. Radiologic assessment (MRI or myelography) should be carried out rapidly. Radiation therapy is then instituted. If the patient's condition deteriorates further, neurosurgical decompression may be necessary.

Barrow DL, Tindall GT, Kovacs K, et al. Clinical and pathological effects of bromocriptine on prolactin-secreting and other pituitary tumors. J Neurosurg 1984;60:1–7.

Bracken MB, Shepard MJ, Collins WF, et al. A randomized, controlled trial of methylprednisolone or naloxone in the treatment of acute spinal-cord injury. N Engl J Med 1990;322:1405–1411.

Burger PC. Malignant astrocytic neoplasms: classification, pathologic anatomy, and response to treatment. Semin Oncol 1986;13:16–26.

Dorman HR, Sondheimer JH, Cadnapaphornchai P. Mannitol-induced acute renal failure. Medicine 1990;69:153–159.

Kleinberg DL, Boyd LAE, Wardlaw S, et al. Pergolide for the treatment of pituitary tumors secreting prolactin or growth hormone. N Engl J Med 1983;309:704–709.

Kornblith PL, Walker M. Chemotherapy for malignant gliomas. J Neurosurg 1988;68:1–17.

Leibel SA, Sheline GE. Radiation therapy for neoplasms of the brain. J Neurosurg 1987;66:1–22.

Patchell RA, Cirrincione C, Thaler HT, et al. Single brain metastases: surgery plus radiation or radiation alone. Neurology 1986;36:447–453.

Ropper AH, Kennedy SF. Neurological and Neurosurgical Intensive Care, 2nd ed. Rockville, MD: Aspen Publishers; 1988.

Vecht CJ, Haaxma-Reiche H, van Putten WLJ. Initial bolus of conventional versus high-dose dexamethasone in metastatic spinal cord compression. Neurology 1989;39:1255–1257.

West CR, Avellanosa AM, Barua NR, et al. Intraarterial 1,3-bis(2-chloroethyl)-1-nitrosourea (BCNU) and systemic chemotherapy for malignant gliomas: a follow-up-study. Neurosurgery 1983;13:420–426.

VII. CEREBROVASCULAR DISEASE

Prevention of hemorrhagic and ischemic stroke is far more effective in reducing morbidity than is treatment after the stroke has occurred. One of the most important accomplishments in disease prevention has been reduction in stroke incidence by better control of hypertension. In contrast, morbidity and mortality figures for completed strokes have improved little if at all. In assessing a patient suspected of having a stroke, the first question is whether the event is **ischemic** or **hemorrhagic.** Treatment decisions are determined by the clinical course and by the presumed cause. Especially important is whether an ischemic event is from an embolic source. With hemorrhagic stroke, distinction between primary intracerebral hemorrhage and hemorrhage from a ruptured berry aneurysm is important in directing management of the case.

A. Ischemic Stroke

1. TRANSIENT ISCHEMIC ATTACKS. By convention, transient ischemic attacks (TIAs) are episodes of transient dysfunction of an area of the CNS in the distribution of a supplying artery that **last less than 24 hours.** The usual duration of an episode is 10 to 15 minutes. TIAs can be mimicked by partial seizures and by migraine accompaniments (symptoms thought to be due to cerebral ischemia that may precede an episode of migraine headache and that occur without headache in some individuals). Presyncopal episodes producing global cerebral ischemia due to decrease in cardiac output or blood pressure should not be labeled TIAs.

   Treatment strategies are designed to accomplish the following: (1) medically reduce the incidence of emboli by interfering with platelet aggregation or by reducing thrombus formation with anticoagulants and (2) surgically reduce sources of emboli, increase flow, and prevent occlusion of a major supplying vessel, usually a severely stenotic internal carotid artery.

   a. **Antiplatelet agents.** These are used for stroke prevention in both men and women with TIAs whether or not endarterectomy is performed. **Aspirin** inhibits the enzyme cyclooxygenase in platelets, thus interfering with the formation of thromboxane A_2. Platelet aggregation and adhesion to vessel walls are thereby lessened. The doses of aspirin used in many clinical studies also inhibit prostacyclin formation in the vessel endothelial cells in vitro and could thereby augment platelet adhesion. Studies suggest that low (300 mg/d) aspirin dosage may be as effective as high dosage (900–1200 mg/d) in preventing stroke in patients with TIAs or small strokes. Other agents, such as dipyridamole (Persantine) or sulfinpyrazone (Anturane), have not potentiated the effects of aspirin when tested in large controlled studies. **Ticlopidine** is an antiplatelet agent that also works for stroke prevention in controlled studies. Side effects include diarrhea, rash, and neutropenia. The effective dose is 250 mg bid.

   b. **Anticoagulants.** The use of anticoagulants for stroke prevention in patients with TIAs is controversial. A patient seen for the first time in the period soon after the onset of a TIA may be a candidate for acute anticoagulation with heparin, the rationale being that onset of TIAs may be a harbinger of an impending stroke. CT without contrast enhancement always should be done before initiation of anticoagulation. Lumbar puncture is usually not recommended because hemorrhagic complications (spinal epidural hemorrhage) are more likely to occur unless anticoagulation is delayed. Heparin is given as a constant infusion, at a dose of 1000 U/h. The goal is to bring the partial thromboplastin time to 1.5 times the control value. Bolus heparinization may increase the risk of hemorrhage. If no further TIA occurs, there are no clear guidelines to duration of anticoagulation treatment. Some recommend switching to coumarin and maintaining anticoagulation (prothrombin levels at 1.5 times control) for 3 months. Others may choose to discontinue heparin during the hospital stay after 1 or 2 weeks.

c. **Carotid endarterectomy.** The NASCET study clearly demonstrated the value of endarterectomy in patients with symptoms on the side ipsilateral to an internal carotid artery with stenosis of 70% or greater.

2. EVOLVING STROKE. It is rare for the physician to encounter a stroke patient in whom signs fluctuate clearly enough to justify the designation **stroke in evolution.** This term should be used for the patient in whom signs are clearly worsening on repeated observation or improve only to worsen again. Generally accepted treatment in such patients is acute anticoagulation with heparin, as outlined in the discussion of TIAs. **Thrombolytic therapy** with IV recombinant tissue plasminogen activator (t-PA) may improve prognosis from an ischemic stroke if it is given within 3 hours of symptom onset. However, the NINDS study, which used 0.9 mg/kg (10% bolus, the remainder infused over 60 minutes), found a 20-fold increase in cerebral hemorrhage and that overall mortality was not reduced even though t-PA recipients were 30% more likely to have a good outcome at 3 months. Intraarterial injection of urokinase by an interventional radiologist is under investigation for patients with occlusion of major vessels, such as the basilar artery.

3. COMPLETED STROKE. Most patients coming to the hospital for treatment belong in this category. If there is no evidence that the stroke resulted from an embolus, anticoagulation is not instituted. Fluid overload should be avoided. Attention must be paid to avoiding aspiration, to initiating range of motion to paralyzed limbs, to preventing bed sores by turning and by using protective boots and an appropriate mattress. If the infarct is large and associated with cerebral swelling, **hyperosmotic therapy** with mannitol (0.25 g/kg IV) may be temporarily beneficial. Most studies suggest that **steroids** are not helpful and may even worsen the prognosis. **Hemicraniectomy** has been shown to be lifesaving in some patients with massive right hemisphere infarcts. Survivors often show marked functional impairment.

4. EMBOLIC STROKE. Many ischemic strokes are due to emboli that usually originate in the heart. Embolic cerebral infarctions often become hemorrhagic, but hemorrhage may not be evident in the hours immediately after onset of symptoms. If the source of emboli is evident, as in a patient with a cardiac mural thrombus or with rheumatic heart disease, mitral stenosis, and an enlarged left atrium, anticoagulation is usually recommended. Anticoagulation is not being used to influence the ischemic area but rather to lessen the likelihood of emboli recurrence. In rheumatic heart disease, the estimated risk of recurrent emboli is 1%/d in the first 2 weeks. Because of the risk that anticoagulants will increase the likelihood of hemorrhage into the cerebral infarct, caution must be used in deciding when to begin anticoagulant therapy. Factors that increase the risk of deterioration, such as stupor or coma, and demonstration of a large infarct with swelling or shift of hemispheral structures should alert the clinician to monitor the

patient's status with repeat CT 24 to 48 hours before anticoagulation is begun. Heparin is usually begun IV, 1000 U/h, and the dosage is subsequently adjusted to achieve a PTT of 1.5 times the control value.

B. Hemorrhagic Stroke

1. PRIMARY SUBARACHNOID HEMORRHAGE. Bleeding from a ruptured berry aneurysm usually is confined to the subarachnoid space, although in some instances the stream of blood is directed into the cerebral substance and may enter a ventricle. The diagnosis is usually confirmed by demonstrating subarachnoid blood by CT. Early neurosurgical intervention should be considered in patients who have not been devastated by the hemorrhage. The patient should be in an ICU, in a darkened room. A stool softener and an analgesic such as codeine should be given as needed. Medical management is directed at controlling hypertension, reducing intracranial pressure, and preventing spasm of intracranial arteries. There is no certain way of preventing vasospasm. However, controlled studies with **nimodipine**, a calcium entry blocker, suggest that the drug is of benefit in reducing the severity of neurologic deficits resulting from vasospasm. Nimodipine is given in a dosage of 60 mg (2 capsules) q4h for 21 consecutive days. If a nasogastric tube is required, the contents of the capsule are extracted into a syringe and washed down the tube with 30 mL of normal saline. After the aneurysm has been clipped, maintaining a mean arterial pressure of 100 to 120 mm Hg may help prevent vasospasm. This is achieved by intravascular volume expansion with normal saline and a plasma substitute to raise the pulmonary wedge pressure above 15 mm Hg. The use of antifibrinolytic agents such as aminocaproic acid (Amicar) is controversial.

2. INTRACEREBRAL HEMORRHAGE. Rupture of small penetrating arterial branches occurs most commonly in patients with chronic hypertension. Common sites of primary intracerebral hemorrhage are deep within a cerebral hemisphere (striatum or thalamus), cerebellum, and pons. There is no specific medical therapy to reduce cerebral damage. Some patients may benefit from clot evacuation. More superficial hemorrhages occur in patients who have developed **congophilic (amyloid) angiopathy** of small cerebral vessels. Surgical evacuation is not recommended because of a high risk of rebleeding.

Cerebral Embolism Study Group. Cardioembolic stroke, early anticoagulation, and brain hemorrhage. Arch Intern Med 1987;147:636–640.

Delashaw JB, Broaddus WC, Kassell NF, et al. Treatment of right hemispheric cerebral infarction by hemicraniectomy. Stroke 1990;21:874–881.

Estol C, Caplan LR. Therapy of acute stroke. Clin Neuropharmacol 1990;2:91–120.

Executive Committee for the Asymptomatic Carotid Atherosclerosis Study. Endarterectomy for asymptomatic carotid stenosis. JAMA 1995;273:1421–1428.

Hacke W, Kaste M, Fieschi C, et al. Intravenous thrombolysis with recombinant tissue plasminogen activator for acute hemispheric stroke. JAMA 1995;274:1017–1025.

Hass WK, Easton JD, Adams HP, et al. A randomized trial comparing ticlopidine hydrochloride with aspirin for the prevention of stroke in high-risk patients. N Engl J Med 1989;321:501–507.

Hirsh J. Therapeutic range for the control of oral anticoagulant therapy. Arch Neurol 1986; 43:1162–1164.

Lip GYH, Lowe GDO. Antithrombotic treatment for atrial fibrillation. Br Med J 1996;312:45–49.

National Institute of Neurological Disorders and Stroke, rt-PA Stroke Study Group. Tissue plasminogen activator for acute ischemic stroke. N Engl J Med 1995;333:1581–1587.

North American Symptomatic Carotid Endarterectomy Trial Collaborators. Beneficial effect of carotid endarterectomy in symptomatic patients with high-grade aortic stenosis. N Engl J Med 1991;325:445–453.

VIII. MOVEMENT DISORDERS

Although one could include seizures in this group of conditions, **movement disorders** are usually restricted to movements not accompanied by alteration in consciousness. Many of these conditions arise from disease in the basal ganglia. However, **tremors** may emanate from structures in cerebellum or midbrain, and **myoclonus** may occur with disease in spinal cord, brainstem, or cerebral cortex. In this section, therapy for spasticity also is discussed (Table 16–6).

A. Myoclonus

Myoclonic movements can be simply termed "jerks." They may be focal or segmental, or they may be generalized, involving many muscles synchronously or asynchronously. They can arise by excitation or by disinhibition of neurons at spinal cord, brainstem, or thalamic level. Myoclonic jerks can be benign, as with nocturnal myoclonus, or they can occur as a sign of more serious pathology, such as CNS hypoxia or encephalitis or during the course of certain degenerative disorders. Medical treatment of myoclonic jerks depends on the mechanism of production of myoclonus and the site of pathophysiology. Generalized myoclonus associated with or preceding generalized seizures may respond to anticonvulsants such as sodium valproate. Postanoxic myoclonus may respond to drugs that affect sero-

TABLE 16–6. Therapy of Nonparkinsonism Movement Disorders

CONDITION	TREATMENT	RESULT
Myoclonus (postanoxic)	Clonazepam, valproic acid	Variable
Spasticity	Baclofen, dantrolene	Variable
Chorea (especially Huntington's disease)	Haloperidol, reserpine	Moderate success
Torticollis, tics	Haloperidol	Variable
Dystonias	Botulinum toxin injections	Good, but temporary for focal dystonias
Neuroleptic-induced movement disorders		
Acute dystonia	Diphenhydramine	Very successful
Parkinsonism	Anticholinergics	Moderate to marked
Tardive dyskinesias	Reserpine	Fair to poor
	Choline percursors	Variable
Benign essential tremor	Beta blockers (propranolol, nadolol), sedatives (primidone)	Moderate success
Gilles de la Tourette syndrome	Haloperidol, pimozide, clonidine, sulpiride	Moderate success

toninergic systems. The drug clonazepam may be effective in this situation in dosages of 4–10 mg/d.

B. Spasticity

Spasticity is the term used to describe increased resistance of muscles to passive stretch that is accompanied by hyperactive tendon reflexes. Patients can be severely disabled by increased muscle tone. Spasticity can also be accompanied by involuntary spasms of extension or flexion of muscles. Spasticity can result from damage to descending suprasegmental motor pathways at spinal cord or higher brainstem or hemispheral levels, presumably by removal of descending inhibitory influences on spinal cord activity. Although unilateral spasticity may result from hemispheral damage due, for example, to cerebral infarction, medical treatment is usually used in patients with spinal cord damage from trauma or diseases such as multiple sclerosis.

Pharmacologic treatment of spasticity is limited by side effects of potentially effective drugs. At this time, **baclofen** is considered the most effective agent. Drug administration is begun at a dosage of 5 mg tid and increased every few days. The maximum recommended dose is 80 mg/d, although some patients have required higher doses to obtain relief. Drowsiness, dizziness, and fatigue are common side effects that limit the dose that can be given. Intrathecal baclofen can be self-administered after placement of a catheter implanted in the subarachnoid space. Most such patients receive 300–800 µg/d. Other drugs used for treating spasticity include **benzodiazepines** such as diazepam and **dantrolene.** These agents are of limited use because of side effects. Dantrolene is thought to act peripherally on the excitation-contraction mechanism of muscle. Frequently, patients receiving enough dantrolene to reduce spasticity will develop accompanying weakness. The drug would be used in a patient with severe spasticity who did not respond to baclofen or a benzodiazepine. Treatment is begun with a dose of 25 mg/d, which is increased in 25-mg increments, as tolerated. Doses as high as 400 mg/d have been tolerated by some persons. Tizanidine, an α_2-adrenergic agonist, has been approved for treatment of spasticity. The drug is administered orally in 3 divided doses, beginning 2 mg tid and increasing as tolerated up to 36 mg/d in divided doses.

C. Chorea

This is an involuntary movement that occurs characteristically in Huntington's disease, inherited as an autosomal dominant trait and due to a defective gene on chromosome 4, and Sydenham's chorea, associated with rheumatic fever. Choreiform movements may also be seen in parkinsonian patients receiving excessive levodopa and in patients with tardive dyskinesias. Medical treatment of choreiform movements is not satisfactory. The movements may be lessened by the neurotransmitter-depleting agent reserpine or by neuroleptic drugs such as haloperidol. It is best not to use these agents, however, unless the choreiform movements are large and are incapacitating. Reserpine may be started at doses of 0.5 mg, which are gradually increased until symptoms are improved or until side effects become a problem. The drug can be used in doses that are higher than those used to treat hypertension.

D. Dystonias

Dystonias currently are classified as **focal** or **generalized.** Focal dystonias include spasmodic torticollis and writer's cramp. Medical treatment is usually unsatisfactory. Occasionally, behavioral modification approaches are successful. An approach that appears to bring about good but temporary (3 to 6 months) improvement is the injection under electromyographic control of small amounts of type A botulinum toxin (Occulinum). This therapy can be used for **blepharospasm, spasmodic torticollis, spasmodic dysphonia,** other focal dystonias, and hemifacial spasm.

Generalized dystonias may occur in a variety of pathologic conditions. The principally encountered ones are (1) **tardive dyskinesias,** resulting from prolonged use of neuroleptic or antinausea medications, (2) dystonias occurring in parkinsonian patients being treated with levodopa, and (3) dystonia occurring during the course of the genetic condition termed **dystonia musculorum deformans** or **torsion dystonia.** Levodopa-related dystonias are improved by reducing the amount of antiparkinsonian medication given with each dose. Dystonias caused by neuroleptic or antinausea medication may or may not improve with removal of the offending drug. Medical treatment of these refractory movement disorders is generally unsatisfactory. Of the many medications that have been tried, anticholinergic therapy may be the most satisfactory. Trihexyphenidyl HCl is usually used. Beginning with 1-mg or 2-mg tablets, the dose may be increased as tolerated. Young patients are able to tolerate much higher doses than are older individuals, who can become confused or delirious with toxic amounts of anticholinergic drugs. Dry mouth is often a problem because of decreased saliva. Doses as high as 75 mg have been tolerated by some. Less success is reported with baclofen or clonazepam. Dopamine agonists, antagonists, and depleters have been relatively unsuccessful. A rare form of generalized dystonia responds to small amounts of levodopa, given in the form of Sinemet.

E. Parkinson's Disease

The cardinal symptoms and signs of Parkinson's disease are bradykinesia (slow movement), resting tremor, rigidity of muscles, and problems with balance and walking. These problems may occur individually or together. The response to therapy may be better for one symptom than for another. Some disagreement remains among specialists about which medication to use initially (Table 16–7).

1. LEVODOPA. Levodopa in the form of carbidopa/levodopa (Sinemet) is the most effective antiparkinsonian drug and may be chosen as the initial drug. Carbidopa/levodopa may be started with one yellow tablet (carbidopa 25 mg, levodopa 100 mg) after a meal, and one tablet may be added at another time every 3 to 4 days to a dosage of two tablets tid. The patient should be assessed after 2 or 3 weeks. If the drug is well tolerated, and if it is necessary to increase the dose, one tablet of carbidopa/levodopa 25/250 tid should be substituted. Half-tablet increments can be continued until significant improvement is noted or until side effects prevent further increase. The lowest dose that produces satisfactory improvement is then continued.

TABLE 16-7. **Some Drugs Used to Treat Parkinsonism**

AGENT	MODE OF ACTION	USUAL DAILY DOSAGE	APPROXIMATE $ COST OF 100 TABLETS OR CAPSULES	SIDE EFFECTS
Levodopa	Converted to dopamine	3–6 g	25 (250 mg)	**Peripheral:** nausea, vomiting, hypotension, glaucoma, cardiac arrhythmia; **Central:** memory loss, confusion, hallucinosis, dyskinesia
Levodopa and carbidopa combinations (Sinemet)	Carbidopa blocks peripheral metabolism of levodopa	0.4–1.5 g levodopa	22 (10/100) 25 (25/100) 30 (25/250) 85 (25/100 CR)* 150 (50/200 CR)	Central side effects of levodopa; on-off reaction more common
Bromocriptine (Parlodel)	Dopamine agonist	25–100 mg	95 (2.5 mg)	Confusion, hallucinosis, dyskinesia, nausea
Pergolide (Permax)	Dopamine agonist	3 mg	60 (0.05 mg) 80 (0.25 mg) 270 (1 mg)	Confusion, hallucinosis, dyskinesia, nausea
Anticholinergics Benztropine (Cogentin) Trihexyphenidyl (Artane) Procyclidine (Kemadrin)	Muscarinic blockers Muscarinic blockers Muscarinic blockers	5–6 mg 6–10 mg 6–20 mg	6 (2 mg) 10 (2 mg) 30 (5 mg)	Confusion, memory loss, hallucinations, dry mouth, urinary retention, constipation
Selegiline (deprenyl, Eldepryl)	Monoamine oxidase B inhibitor	10 mg	200 (5 mg)	Insomnia
Antihistamines Diphenhydramine	Muscarinic blocker	50–200 mg	5 (50 mg)	Somnolence
Amantadine (Symmetrel)	Unknown; mild anticholinergic	200 mg	20 (100 mg)	Confusion, hallucinosis, dry mouth, peripheral edema, livedo reticularis

*CR, controlled release.

Problems may occur in patients who take levodopa: (1) Nausea is common and is best managed by reducing the amount taken at one time. In some patients, up to 200 mg of carbidopa may be necessary to optimally inhibit peripheral dopa decarboxylase. Supplementary carbidopa can be prescribed in patients whose carbidopa/levodopa cannot be increased because of nausea. Antinausea drugs such as metoclopramide (Reglan) or prochlorperazine (Compazine) are centrally acting dopamine receptor blockers and, therefore, contraindicated. **Domperidone** is an antinausea drug that does not block brain dopamine receptors. It is available in Canada in 10-mg tablets. (2) Some patients benefit less when the drug is taken after a meal. Absorption of levodopa in the proximal small bowel and transport from blood to brain take place through facilitated transport mechanisms for neutral amino acids. For patients who respond poorly, a trial of low-protein meals is warranted. (3) Although many patients will remain stable with the same levodopa dose for a number of years, others will notice gradual worsening of bradykinesia, tremor, or balance. If there have been no medication side effects, an increased dose may be effective at that time. (4) Some patients will note that symptoms worsen after 3 hours or so and that improvement is delayed for 30 minutes after a dose of levodopa. In such patients, it may be useful to give the same total daily dosage but in smaller doses at shorter intervals, i.e., 2.5 or 3 hours. (5) The total dose may need to be reduced if choreiform movements or facial grimacing is bothersome. (6) On-off effects occur in a small percentage of patients. These are abrupt fluctuations in the parkinsonian symptoms and in dyskinesia that are not easily correlated with the timing of medication. Reduction in dose and shortening the interval between doses may be helpful.

Sinemet-CR, a controlled-release preparation, produces a slower rise and fall in plasma levodopa levels than does the standard form of the drug. One tablet contains 50 mg of carbidopa and 200 mg of levodopa (the same 1:4 ratio as in the standard Sinemet 25/100 tablet) with a 90% release time of 2 to 2.5 hours. This preparation may help with managing the patient with severe fluctuations in clinical response.

2. **OTHER DRUGS FOR PARKINSON'S DISEASE.** Additional medications that are sometimes beneficial include (1) the dopamine agonists bromocriptine (Parlodel) and pergolide (Permax), (2) selegiline (deprenyl, Eldepryl), (3) the anticholinergics such as trihexyphenidyl (Artane), and (4) amantadine (Symmetrel). Each of these agents can be used in combination with Sinemet. Bromocriptine is available in 2.5-mg and 5-mg tablets. Its plasma half-life is three to four times longer than that of levodopa. In controlled studies, bromocriptine improves parkinsonian symptoms, either alone or as a supplement to levodopa. Unfortunately, the drug is expensive, and side effects are frequent. These include mental changes (confusion, psychosis), erythromelalgia, nausea, and dyskinesias. It is difficult to judge the appropriate dose of this agent. Doses as high as 50–100 mg/d have been given, but current recommendations by the manufacturer are to begin with very low doses of 1.25 mg/d and to increase in increments of 1.25–2.5 mg every 2 to 4 weeks,

to the lowest dosage that produces a therapeutic response. **Pergolide** is a dopamine agonist that may be used as an alternative to bromocriptine. Pergolide is usually started at a dosage of 0.05 mg/d, with gradual increases in 0.1–0.15-mg increments every third day up to 0.75 mg/d. If further increments are necessary, doses are then increased in 0.25-mg increments to a dosage of about 3 mg/d. Newer dopamine agonist drugs being developed include pramipexole and ropinirole.

Selegiline is an irreversible inhibitor of the monoamine oxidase isoenzyme, MAO-B, which is the principal form in brain and blood platelets. The drug may prolong the action of levodopa and thereby benefit the patient with rapid wearing off of levodopa effects before the subsequent dose. Two 5-mg tablets suffice to almost completely inhibit MAO-B activity. The drug is given at breakfast and lunch to avoid nighttime insomnia. Selegiline taken early in the course of Parkinson's disease may lengthen the time before levodopa is required.

Trihexyphenidyl is one of several anticholinergic agents used for adjunctive therapy for parkinsonism (Table 16–7). These agents should be given at low initial doses and gradually increased as tolerated. Dry mouth, visual blurring, mental changes, and urinary retention are common side effects that limit the dosages. The effectiveness of these anticholinergic drugs is similar, although some neurologists prefer **ethopropazine** (Parsidol) for treating tremor. Another agent, **diphenhydramine** hydrochloride (Benadryl), has both anticholinergic and antihistaminic actions and may be useful when taken at bedtime in a dose of 25–50 mg.

Amantadine may have effect on dopamine release and reuptake from nerve endings as well as anticholinergic effects. It may be used as a supplemental drug in a dosage of 100–300 mg/d.

F. Nonparkinsonian Tremor

1. Essential tremor is ordinarily confined to the upper extremities and head and usually increased in amplitude by dorsiflexing the wrists or performing a task such as writing or drinking from a glass. Essential tremor only rarely disappears with medical treatment. Two types of drugs are used: (1) beta-adrenergic blockers such as propranolol and (2) sedative-anticonvulsant drugs such as primidone (Mysoline). Many physicians now choose to use low dosages of primidone (50 mg hs) and gradually increase (to 250 mg/d). Others prefer to use propranolol in dosages beginning at 20–40 mg/d and increasing to 160 mg/d (40 mg qid). Dosages of 160 mg bid of long-acting propranolol have been used, as have alternative beta-adrenergic blockers such as metoprolol. Other agents, such as the anxiolytic benzodiazepines, have also been used. Drug side effects may be more bothersome to the patient than the tremor. Many may prefer not to take medications or to take a pill only at certain times, such as before a meal or when anticipating a stressful situation.

2. Action or intention tremor due to damage to cerebellar pathways is refractory to most medical therapy. An occasional patient will report minimal improvement with a benzodiazepine such as diazepam or lorazepam.

G. Wilson's Disease

Hepatolenticular degeneration is inherited as an autosomal recessive disorder with tremor and dystonia seen in childhood or early adulthood. Elevated copper levels in striatum and liver produce clinical symptoms. Copper chelation with D-penicillamine is the treatment of choice. The drug is given PO, beginning at 250 mg/d. The dose should be increased by 250 mg/d every 4 days to prevent too rapid mobilization of intracellular copper, which can lead to irreversible aggravation of clinical symptoms. The average maintenance dose for an adult is between 750 and 2500 mg/d in divided doses. The drug should be given at least 2 hours after a meal to avoid reduced absorption due to food. A diet low in copper is also recommended, as is administration of 25 mg/d of pyridoxine. If symptoms worsen during the initial phase of treatment, the dosage of D-penicillamine should be reduced and later increased gradually over several weeks to months. For patients who cannot tolerate penicillamine, trientine hydrochloride (Syprine) can be used at doses of 400–600 mg taken tid or qid on an empty stomach. For patients in whom chelating agents cannot be used or for asymptomatic patients, zinc acetate or zinc sulfate is recommended at an average dose of 50–200 mg tid given 30 to 60 minutes before meals. Zinc competes with copper for binding sites on the carrier protein metallothionine and prevents intestinal resorption of copper.

Cedarbaum JM. The promise and limitations of controlled-release oral levodopa administration. Clin Neuropharmacol 1989;12:147–166.

Jankovic J, Schwartz K, Donovan DT. Botulinum toxin treatment of cranial-cervical dystonia, spasmodic dysphonia, other focal dystonias and hemifacial spasm. J Neurol Neurosurg Psychiatry 1990;53:633–639.

Markham CH, Diamond SG. Long-term follow-up of early dopa treatment in Parkinson's disease. Ann Neurol 1986;19:365–372.

Parkinson Study Group. Effect of deprenyl on the progression of disability in early Parkinson's disease. N Engl J Med 1989;321:1364–1371.

Smith C, Birnbaum G, Carter JL, et al. Tizanidine treatment of spasticity caused by multiple sclerosis: results of a double-blind, placebo-controlled trial. US Tizanidine Study Group. Neurology 1994;44(Nov. Suppl 9):S34–S42.

Straube A, Swanson PD. Wilson's disease. In: Brandt T, Caplan LR, Dichgans J, et al., eds. Neurological Disorders: Course and Treatment. San Diego: Academic Press; 1996.

Walshe JM, Yealland M. Chelation treatment of neurological Wilson's disease. Q J Med 1993;86:197–204.

IX. MULTIPLE SCLEROSIS

This disorder of unknown cause is a source of frustration for patient and physician because of the uncertainties of prognosis and the difficulties in assessing treatment results. Its course is unpredictable. Some patients have a classic picture of multiple exacerbations and remissions (relapsing-remitting MS). In others there is slow progression (progressive MS); in still others there is little progression. Other forms (progressive-relapsing, secondary progressive) are also recognized. Since the disease is likely to have a viral or immunologic cause, most suggested treatments alter the immune system in some way. At this time, there is no convincing evidence that any treatment alters the ultimate outcome. Nonetheless, certain treatments are used by respected workers in the field. Others are considered to be of no benefit. In this section we mainly discuss those treatments that are accepted as possibly useful and mention some of the others that are controversial or unaccepted by most neurologists.

1. IMMUNOSUPPRESSANT THERAPY. **Corticosteroid** therapy is the most widely used. Its acceptance followed the report of a cooperative study that used ACTH. Treatment with short courses of prednisone at doses of 60–120 mg/d is less used than previously, following an acute optic neuritis treatment trial that suggested that oral prednisone alone was ineffective. High doses of **IV methylprednisolone** (1000 mg) for 3 to 5 days have been suggested to speed recovery after an acute exacerbation of the disease. It is administered in 500 mL of D_5W over 3 hours and may be followed by prednisone (60 mg PO for 11 days with a subsequent rapid taper). The use of **cyclophosphamide** is advocated by few. Long-term therapy with 100–150 mg/d of **azathioprine** is used in a number of countries, although a large controlled study showed only modest benefit. Encouraging reports have shown lower exacerbation rates in relapsing-remitting disease with **interferon-β1a** or 1b. Attacks are decreased by about 30%. Interferon-β1b (Betaseron) is administered SC at a dose of 0.25 mg qod. Injection site reactions and flu-like symptoms are common. Interferon-β1a is given in doses of 30 μg weekly by intramuscular injection. **Copolymer 1** (COP-1) is a synthetic polypeptide manufactured to resemble myelin basic protein. A recent study with 251 patients showed a reduced number of exacerbations in patients with relapsing-remitting MS who received daily SC injections of 20 mg. This drug has been submitted for FDA approval. For chronic progressive MS, a recent double-blind crossover study of 49 patients suggested benefit from the immunosuppressive drug cladribine, given IV in three or four monthly 7-day courses. At present, certain immunologic treatments are used, but none has been shown to arrest the disease irrevocably.

Beck RW, Cleary BA, Trobe JD, et al. The effect of corticosteroids for acute optic neuritis on the subsequent development of multiple sclerosis. The Optic Neuritis Study Group. N Engl J Med 1993;329:1764–1769.

Beutler E, Sipe JC, Romine JS, et al. The treatment of chronic progressive multiple sclerosis with cladribine. Proc Natl Acad Sci USA 1996;93:1716–1720.

IFNB Multiple Sclerosis Study Group and the University of British Columbia MS/MRI Analysis Group. Interferon beta 1b in the treatment of multiple sclerosis: final outcome of the randomized controlled trial. Neurology 1995;45:1277–1285.

Jacobs LD, Cookfaire DL, Rudick RA, et al. Intramuscular interferon beta-1a for disease progression in relapsing multiple sclerosis. Ann Neurol 1996;39:285–294.

Johnson KP, Brooks BR, Cohen JA, et al. Copolymer 1 reduces relapse rate and improves disability in relapsing-remitting multiple sclerosis: results of a phase III multicenter, double-blind, placebo-controlled trial. Neurology 1995;45:1268–1276.

Noseworthy JH, Seland TP, Ebers GC. Therapeutic trials in multiple sclerosis. Can J Neurol Sci 1984;22:355–362.

Rose AS. Cooperative study in the evaluation of therapy in multiple sclerosis: ACTH vs placebo. Final report. Neurology 1970;20:1–59.

Van den Noort S. Immunosuppressant treatment in multiple sclerosis. Clin Neuropharmacol 1985;8:58–63.

Weiner HL, Hafler DA. Immunotherapy of multiple sclerosis. Ann Neurol 1988;23:211–222.

X. NEUROMUSCULAR DISORDERS

A. Amyotrophic Lateral Sclerosis (ALS)

Until recently, ALS has been considered untreatable. Recent studies have suggested increased survival in some patients given 100 mg/d of the antiglutamate agent **riluzole**. This drug is now approved by the FDA for use in the United States. In the randomized, double-blind clinical trial, no benefit was found in the functional status of treated patients. However, at 18 months, treated patients had a 35% lower risk of death or tracheostomy. Side effects include nausea, vomiting, fatigue, and increases in serum alanine aminotransferase levels.

B. Neuropathies and Radiculopathies

Disorders that involve the peripheral nerves can be broadly classified into (1) polyneuropathies, in which peripheral nerves are affected in general, and (2) mononeuropathies, radiculopathies, and plexopathies, in which individual nerves, roots, or nerve plexuses are affected by a pathologic process. Multiple mononeuropathies (mononeuritis multiplex) also occur, usually in the setting of a disorder such as polyarteritis nodosa in which infarcts of multiple nerves can occur.

1. POLYNEUROPATHIES. Causes of polyneuropathies are multiple and include toxic (e.g., arsenic, vincristine, disulfiram, and hexane), metabolic (e.g., diabetes mellitus, uremia), genetic (e.g., Charcot-Marie-Tooth disease), neoplastic ("remote" effect of malignancies), infectious (leprosy, HIV), and immunologic (e.g., Guillain-Barré syndrome and chronic inflammatory demyelinating neuropathy) factors. When a cause is discernible, its removal may result in improvement of the polyneuropathy. Acute and chronic neuropathies of unknown cause are often assumed to be secondary to an immunologic disorder.

   a. **Acute neuropathies.** The term Guillain-Barré syndrome often is applied to polyneuropathies with a rapid onset over a few days. **Treatment of Guillain-Barré syndrome** is, in great part, concerned with preventing complications associated with severe weakness or respiratory paralysis. Treatment measures depend on the extent of the disability and may require admission to an ICU, institution of respiratory assistance, and physical therapy measures to prevent contractures and pressure sores. The use of more specific measures to prevent worsening of Guillain-Barré is increasing. **Plasma exchange** has gained acceptance on the strength of a multicenter-controlled study suggesting that this treatment speeds recovery. Current recommendations are as follows: patients are considered for plasmapheresis who have developed the rapid onset of ascending paralysis thought to represent polyneuropathy of the Guillain-Barré type. Treatment within 7 days of neurologic symptom onset is encouraged. In the randomized multicenter trial reported in 1985, three to five exchanges were carried out over 1 to 2 weeks. A total of 200 mL of plasma was exchanged per kilogram of body weight, the replacement solution usually consisting of Plasmanate or 5% salt-poor albumin. **High-dose intravenous immunoglobulin** is a treatment for neuropathies that are immune-mediated and has also been used for myasthenia gravis. Rapid symptomatic improvement has been reported with both acute and chronic neuropathies, the latter sometimes associated with a monoclonal gammopathy. Improvement has not always been sustained, however. Patients receive a total of 2 g/kg immunoglobulin (Sandoglobulin). The medication is divided into five doses infused in 1–2 L NS over several hours each day. A recent randomized trial showed that intravenous immunoglobulin and plasma exchange had equivalent efficacy. The costs of the two treatments are comparable, but plasma exchange is simpler and more convenient to administer.

Rapidly progressive weakness, usually with onset in muscles innervated by cranial nerves, may be due to **botulism.** The toxin is produced by strains of the organism *Clostridium botulinum* and is usually ingested by eating tainted home-canned vegetables. For inactivation, the toxin requires heating for 30 minutes at 80°F or boiling for 3 minutes. The toxin binds irreversibly to presynaptic membranes, is taken up into cholinergic nerve endings, and prevents release of acetylcholine at neuromuscular junctions, including those of the heart and intestine. Administration of antibody is of uncertain benefit, as toxin binding has already occurred by the time the diagnosis is made. In very early cases, antibody should probably be given to minimize further toxin binding. Severely affected patients will require ventilatory support, which may be needed for weeks or months until the toxic effects eventually diminish. Anticholinesterases and guanidine hydrochloride (a drug that facilitates release of acetylcholine at synapses) are of little benefit.

b. **Chronic inflammatory demyelinating neuropathy (CIDP) and multifocal motor neuropathy (MMN).** These are progressive neuropathies with presumed autoimmune pathogenesis. No single treatment regimen has been shown clearly to be superior. Plasmapheresis, IV IgG, and immunosuppressive medications are used. Recommended treatments include sequential uses of prednisone (60–100 mg/d initially, followed by a tapering dose), IV IgG (1 g/kg/d for 5 days with maintenance doses every 3 to 8 weeks), plasma exchange (two exchanges per week for 3 weeks followed by single exchanges at 1–4-week intervals), azathioprine (2.5–3 mg/kg), methotrexate (7.5–12.5 mg PO weekly), cyclosporine, and cyclophosphamide.

2. RADICULOPATHIES, PLEXOPATHIES, AND MONONEUROPATHIES

a. **Cervical or lumbar radiculopathy.** Acute radicular compression by herniated nucleus pulposus material is associated with pain and paresthesias in the distribution of the compressed nerve root. Avoidance of spine movement, bed rest, use of analgesics and nonsteroidal anti-inflammatory agents usually provide symptomatic relief. If pain persists and if evidence of nerve root damage occurs, x-ray and electrical diagnostic procedures are instituted and surgical decompression is carried out in selected cases.

b. **Entrapment neuropathies.** Certain peripheral nerves are subject to entrapment as they pass through narrow passages or to compression against hard surfaces. Terms such as **carpal tunnel syndrome** (compression of the median nerve at the wrist) and **meralgia paresthetica** (compression of the lateral femoral cutaneous nerve as it passes through the inguinal ligament) are used to denote entrapment of specific nerves. In many cases, nerve compression can be reduced by identifying and eliminating aggravating factors. For example, with median nerve compression in the carpal tunnel, wearing a wrist splint and avoiding repetitive wrist movement will improve symptoms. The use of a nonsteroidal anti-inflammatory agent such as naproxen (Naprosyn), 375 mg bid, may help. Some physicians inject steroids (20–40 mg of methylprednisolone) into the area to reduce inflammatory swelling. This injection should be done only by those familiar with the technique, and it is probably best to refer patients who do not respond to splinting to a hand surgeon for possible surgical decompression.

c. **Brachial neuritis.** The cause is unknown but is presumed to be immunologic because a similar syndrome has occurred after immunization. The affected individual rapidly develops pain and weakness in muscles of an extremity. Usually, the proximal muscles of an arm are involved unilaterally. The syndrome may resemble poliomyelitis, although CSF pleocytosis is not present. A short course of oral prednisone (e.g., 80 mg/d for 3 days, tapering over the next 9 days) is often used, although efficacy is not proved. Severe pain may require analgesics. Physical therapy may be necessary to prevent frozen shoulder.

d. **Bell's palsy.** The cause of acute facial muscle weakness from dysfunction of the 7th cranial nerve usually is unclear, although recent evidence suggests that herpes simplex virus type 1 is strongly associated with Bell's palsy. Most Bell's palsy patients recover satisfactory function, although if axons are damaged, nerve regrowth may be accompanied by synkinetic movements of facial muscles. Controlled clinical studies have suggested that excellent recovery can occur if steroids are given within a few days of onset. One week of prednisone, 60 mg/d PO, followed by a rapid taper over the next week, is recommended in such instances. A randomized double-blind study suggested that patients treated with acyclovir (400 mg five times per day for 10 days) in addition to prednisone had better outcomes than those treated with prednisone alone. Using an eye patch and artificial tears at night helps protect the globe. Surgical decompression of the facial nerve in its bony canal is not indicated.

C. Diseases of Muscle and the Myoneural Junction

The generic term for a disorder involving muscle primarily is **myopathy.** Myopathies include the genetic muscular dystrophies and acquired conditions, such as polymyositis and endocrine myopathies. The periodic paralyses not associated with definite histologic changes may be included as well. Disorders of the myoneural junction, such as myasthenia gravis and the Lambert-Eaton syndrome, are not usually called myopathies.

1. **THE MUSCULAR DYSTROPHIES.** No cure is available for the genetic disorders known as the muscular dystrophies. Some studies suggest, however,

that chronic prednisone therapy retards progression of weakness in patients with **Duchenne muscular dystrophy** (DMD) (Arch Neurol 1987;44:818–822). Beginning doses were 2 mg/kg/d, shifting to an alternate-day schedule of about two thirds of the original 2-day dose. Studies of this type have not been rigidly controlled, and results must be considered promising but not established. Weakness generally is managed in coordination with rehabilitation specialists. Prevention of contractures, use of appropriate assistive devices for ambulation, and proper nutrition require attention. Treatment of heart failure or arrhythmias may require appropriate cardiologic consultation. In DMD a muscle membrane protein, designated **dystrophin,** is deficient. Treatment trials transferring normal myoblasts into skeletal muscles of DMD patients with the hope of synthesizing the missing dystrophin are being carried out.

2. Disorders associated with myotonia. Myotonia is the phenomenon of delay in relaxation after muscle contraction. Clinically, two disorders, both genetic, are associated with clinical myotonia: **myotonic muscular dystrophy** and **myotonia congenita.** The phenomenon of myotonia is usually less incapacitating than is weakness in the former, whereas in the latter, myotonia dominates the clinical picture. Myotonia can be lessened by drugs that act on excitable membranes: the anticonvulsant phenytoin in conventional doses and quinine (300–600 mg tid or qid). Procainamide (3–4 g/d in divided doses) is also effective but should be used with caution as it may potentiate heart block. These agents do not improve the weakness in myotonic dystrophy.

3. Myasthenia gravis. The etiology and treatment of myasthenia gravis (MG), a condition characterized by fatiguing of skeletal muscle, have been extensively studied. Autoimmune damage to the acetylcholine receptors of the neuromuscular junction results in a decreased response to acetylcholine released by the motor neurons. Several therapeutic approaches are used and are based on the following principles: (1) increasing the concentration of acetylcholine at the neuromuscular junction with anticholinesterase drugs and (2) altering the immunologically mediated interference with the acetylcholine receptor.

   Anticholinesterase treatment is used to relieve symptoms. Pyridostigmine (Mestinon) is given PO at intervals of 3 to 4 hours. The long-acting drug comes in 60-mg tablets and in a sustained-release capsule containing 180 mg. To avoid overmedication, the sustained-release preparation should be used only at night in patients who have difficulty swallowing the morning tablet. The drug is begun at one-half or one tablet every 4 hours. Semiobjective testing of muscle fatiguing should be carried out *before* and ½ to 1 hour *after* the dose of pyridostigmine. Muscles shown to fatigue are tested. Ptosis is probably the most easily tested (the examiner should ask the patient to look up until ptosis occurs and then compare the width of the palpebral fissure). The most important muscles affected by the disease, those of the pharynx and of respiration, are harder to test. Detecting speech slurring or nasality after reading aloud or counting for an extended time is one assessment method. Fatigue of arm muscles can be measured by timing how long the patient can hold the arms outstretched. Pulmonary function testing can be used, as can hand dynamometers, if available. The pyridostigmine dose can then be titrated upward by increments of one-half tablet until the response is optimal. A patient's anticholinesterase requirement may change. Myasthenic patients may appear in the emergency room with increased weakness. It is then critical to determine whether the increased weakness represents a worsening of MG or is due to excessive anticholinesterase medication. Weakness due to excessive anticholinesterase is often accompanied by salivation, hyperactive bowel sounds, and diarrhea, and sometimes fasciculations. Further anticholinesterase medication should be withheld to observe whether the weakness improves or worsens. Short-acting anticholinesterase given parenterally (edrophonium [Tensilon]) can be dangerous, produce marked worsening of the patient's weakness, and even lead to respiratory arrest. Patients on anticholinesterases may develop bothersome muscarinic side effects, such as intestinal hypermotility with cramps and diarrhea. Atropine sulfate, at doses of 0.4 mg q6–8h, often helps. A scopolamine transdermal patch has also been used with success.

Therapies to alter the immune system in myasthenia gravis: Thymectomy may bring about a remission in MG, but it has never been subjected to a rigorous randomized trial. Some neurologists restrict thymectomy to younger patients unless there is evidence of thymoma. Some advocate early thymectomy, even when myasthenic symptoms are relatively mild. The patient must play an important role in deciding when and if the procedure will be done. Postoperatively, the need for anticholinesterase may be less than preoperatively, and the dose should be adjusted.

Prednisone has become standard when an anticholinesterase fails. One approach to initiating therapy is to begin at a low dose with gradual increases until benefit is seen, and the other is to begin at a high dose and, after benefit occurs, reduce the total dose and shift to an alternate-day regimen to lessen the severity of steroid side effects. This approach is used most frequently. Initial hospitalization is recommended because of the risk (48% in one series) of symptom exacerbation during initiation of steroid therapy. The patient is started on prednisone 60–100 mg/d. Improvement may occur in a few days or weeks, and an alternate-day regimen is used. Reduction in dose in 10-mg increments can then be instituted as tolerated. Some neurologists recommend reduction by 10 mg every 2 months, but more rapid tapers are often tolerated well with no worsening in symptoms. If weakness recurs, the dose can be increased again, often with repeated improvement. Other immunosuppressive drugs are used if prednisone is ineffective. Azathioprine, at a dose of 2–2.5 mg/kg/d, and cyclophosphamide have been used successfully. High-dose IV immunoglobulin and plasma exchange are also used for providing dramatic, although usually temporary, relief (see section on Guillain-Barré syndrome, p. 646).

4. **PERIODIC PARALYSES.** These genetically determined conditions, usually inherited as autosomal dominant traits, are classified according to

whether the serum potassium level falls or rises during an acute attack. The most common variety is the hypokalemic form, in which attacks of weakness are often precipitated by a high-carbohydrate meal. **Nonfamilial hypokalemic** periodic paralysis is occasionally the result of thyrotoxicosis. It is most common in Asian males. Attacks usually cease when the patient is euthyroid. **Hyperkalemic** and **normokalemic** forms of periodic paralysis may be associated with myotonia and cardiac arrhythmias.

a. **Acute attacks.** These are usually self-limited. Because respiratory muscles are ordinarily not affected, bed rest and fluid replacement usually suffice. Potassium is given only for clearly identified cases of the hypokalemic type. When the diagnosis has been made previously, an acute attack may be shortened by 15 mL of a sugar-free oral solution of 10% potassium chloride (20 mEq). This dose may be repeated several times at hourly intervals. For the hyperkalemic or normokalemic varieties, ingestion of high-carbonate beverages may help abort an attack. If weakness is severe, glucose plus insulin or other measures to treat hyperkalemia are used.

b. **Prophylactic therapy.** For most patients with hypokalemic periodic paralysis, acetazolamide (Diamox) treatment effectively prevents attacks at doses of 125–1500 mg/d. Other drugs that have been used for prevention are the carbonic anhydrase inhibitor dichlorophenamide (50 mg bid or tid), and the potassium-sparing diuretics amiloride (5 mg up to 20 mg/d), triamterene (50 mg tid or qid), and spironolactone (25 mg bid or tid). Propranolol at a dose of 40–80 mg bid or tid has also been used with some success in patients with refractory disease. Hyperkalemic periodic paralysis attacks may also be prevented with acetazolamide or hydrochlorothiazide.

Adour KK, Ruboyianes JM, Von Doersten PG, et al. Bell's palsy treatment with acyclovir and prednisone compared with prednisone alone: a double-blind, randomized, controlled trial. Ann Otol Rhinol Laryngol 1996;105:371–378.

Bunch TW. Prednisone and azathioprine for polymyositis: long-term follow-up. Arthritis Rheum 1981;24:45–48.

Guillain-Barré Syndrome Study Group. Plasmapheresis and acute Guillain-Barré syndrome. Neurology 1985;35:2096–2104.

Havard CWH, Fonseca V. New treatment approaches to myasthenia gravis. Drugs 1990;39:66–73.

Kleyweg RP, van der Meche FGA, Meulster J. Treatment of Guillain-Barré syndrome with high-dose gammaglobulin. Neurology 1988;38:1639–1641.

Lacomblez L, Bensimon G, Leigh PN, et al. Dose-ranging study of riluzole in amyotrophic lateral sclerosis. Lancet 1996;347:1425–1431.

Munsat TL, Scheifer RT. Myotonia. Clin Neuropharmacol 1979;4:83–107.

Murakami S, Mizobuchi M, Nakashiro Y, et al. Bell palsy and herpes simplex virus: identification of viral DNA in endoneural fluid and muscle. Ann Intern Med 1996;124:63–65.

Pascuzzi RM, Coslett HB, Johns TR. Long-term corticosteroid treatment of myasthenia gravis: report of 116 patients. Ann Neurol 1984;15:291–298.

Plasma Exchange/Sandoglobulin Guillain-Barré Syndrome Trial Group. Randomized trial of plasma exchange, intravenous immunoglobulin, and combined treatments in Guillain-Barré syndrome. Lancet 1997;349:225–230.

Riggs JE. Periodic paralysis. Clin Neuropharmacol 1989;12:249–257.

Van Doorn PA, Brand A, Strengers PFW, et al. High-dose intravenous immunoglobulin treatment in chronic inflammatory demyelinating polyneuropathy. Neurology 1990;40:209–212.

APPENDIX
APPENDIX
APPENDIX

From Bennett JC, Plum F (eds.). Cecil Testbook of Medicine, 20th ed. Philadelphia: W. B. Saunders Co.; 1996, pp. 2230–2233.

Drugs—Therapeutic and Toxic Levels

DRUG	SPECIMEN		REFERENCE INTERVAL (CONVENTIONAL UNITS)	REFERENCE INTERVAL (INTERNATIONAL UNITS)
Acetaminophen	Serum or plasma (hep or EDTA)	Therap:	10–30 µg/mL	66–199 µmol/L
		Toxic:	>200 µg/mL	>1324 µmol/L
Amikacin	Serum or plasma (EDTA)	Therap:		
		Peak	25–35 µg/mL	43–60 µmol/L
		Trough (severe infection)	4–8 µg/mL	6.8–13.7 µmol/L
		Toxic:		
		Peak	>35 µg/mL	>60 µmol/L
		Trough	>10 µg/mL	>17 µmol/L
ε-Aminocaproic acid	Serum or plasma (hep or EDTA); trough	Therap:	100–400 µg/mL	0.76–3.05 mmol/L
Amitriptyline	Serum or plasma (hep or EDTA); trough (>12 h after dose)	Therap:	120–250 ng/mL	433–903 nmol/L
		Toxic:	>500 ng/mL	>1805 nmol/L
Amobarbital	Serum	Therap:	1–5 µg/mL	4–22 µmol/L
		Toxic:	>10 µg/mL	>44 µmol/L
Amphetamine	Serum or plasma (hep or EDTA)	Therap:	20–30 ngmL	148–222 nmol/L
		Toxic:	>200 ng/mL	>1480 nmol/L
Bromide	Serum	Therap:	750–1500 µg/mL	9.4–18.7 mmol/L
		Toxic:	>1250 µg/mL	>15.6 mmol/L
Caffeine	Serum or plasma (hep or EDTA)	Therap:	3–15 µg/mL	15–77 µmol/L
		Toxic:	>50 µg/mL	>258 µmol/L
Carbamazepine	Serum or plasma (hep or EDTA); trough	Therap:	4–12 µg/mL	17–51 µmol/L
		Toxic:	>15 µg/mL	>63 µmol/L
Carbenicillin	Serum or plasma	Therap:	Dependent on minimum inhibitory concentration of specific organism	Same
Chloramphenicol	Serum or plasma (hep or EDTA); trough	Toxic:	>250 µg/mL	>660 µmol/L
		Therap:	10–25 µg/mL	31–77 µmol/L
		Toxic:	>25 µg/mL	>77 µmol/L

Drug	Specimen		Conventional	SI
Chlordiazepoxide	Serum or plasma (hep or EDTA); trough	Therap:	700–1000 ng/mL	2.34–3.34 µmol/L
		Toxic:	>5000 ng/mL	>16.7 µmol/L
Chlorpromazine	Serum or plasma (hep or EDTA); trough	Therap:	50–300 ng/mL	157–942 nmol/L
		Toxic:	>750 ng/mL	>2355 nmol/L
Cimetidine	Serum or plasma (hep or EDTA); trough	Therap:	0.5–1.2 µg/mL	2–5 µmol/L
Clonazepam	Serum or plasma (hep or EDTA); trough	Therap:	15–60 ng/mL	48–190 nmol/L
		Toxic:	>80 ng/mL	>254 nmol/L
Clonidine	Serum or plasma (hep or EDTA)	Therap:	1.0–2.0 ng/mL	4.4–8.7 nmol/L
Clorazepate	Serum or plasma (hep or EDTA)	As desmethyldiazepam: Therap:	0.12–1.0 µg/mL	0.36–3.01 µmol/L
Cocaine	Serum or plasma (hep or EDTA); on ice	Therap:	100–500 ng/mL	330–1650 nmol/L
		Toxic:	>1000 ng/mL	>3300 nmol/L
Codeine	Serum	Therap:	10–100 ng/mL	33–334 nmol/L
		Toxic:	>200 ng/mL	>668 nmol/L
Cyclosporine	Serum (12 h after dose)	Therap:	100–400 ng/mL	83–333 nmol/L
		Toxic:	>400 ng/mL	>333 nmol/L
Desipramine	Serum or plasma (hep or EDTA); trough (≥12 h after dose)	Therap:	75–300 ng/mL	281–1125 nmol/L
		Toxic:	>400 ng/mL	>1500 nmol/L
Diazepam	Serum or plasma (hep or EDTA); trough	Therap:	100–1000 ng/mL	0.35–3.51 µmol/L
		Toxic:	>5000 ng/mL	>17.55 µmol/L
Digitoxin	Serum or plasma (hep or EDTA) ≥6 h after dose	Therap:	20–35 ng/mL	26–46 nmol/L
		Toxic:	>45 ng/mL	>59 nmol/L
Digoxin	Serum or plasma (hep or EDTA) trough (≥ 12 h after dose)	Therap: CHF	0.8–1.5 ng/mL	1.0–1.9 nmol/L
		Arrhythmias:	1.5–2.0 ng/mL	1.9–2.6 nmol/L
		Toxic:	>2.5 ng/mL	>3.2 nmol/L
Diphenylhydantoin (see Phenytoin)				
Disopyramide	Serum or plasma (hep or EDTA); trough	Therap: Arrhythmias: Atrial	2.8–3.2 µg/mL	8.3–9.4 µmol/L
		Ventricular	3.3–7.5 µg/mL	9.7–22 µmol/L
		Toxic:	>7 µg/mL	>20.7 µmol/L

Table continued on following page

Drugs—Therapeutic and Toxic Levels (Continued)

DRUG	SPECIMEN		REFERENCE INTERVAL (CONVENTIONAL UNITS)	REFERENCE INTERVAL (INTERNATIONAL UNITS)
Doxepin	Serum or plasma (hep or EDTA);	Therap:	30–150 ng/mL	107–537 nmol/L
	trough (≥12 h after dose)	Toxic:	>500 ng/mL	>1790 nmol/L
Ephedrine	Serum	Therap:	0.05–0.10 μg/mL	0.30–0.61 μmol/L
		Toxic:	>2 μg/mL	>12.1 μmol/L
Ethchlorvynol	Serum or plasma (hep or EDTA)	Therap:	2–8 μg/mL	14–55 μmol/L
		Toxic:	>20 μg/mL	>138 μmol/L
Ethosuximide	Serum or plasma (hep or EDTA);	Therap:	40–100 μg/mL	283–708 μmol/L
	trough	Toxic:	>150 μg/mL	>1062 μmol/L
Fenoprofen	Plasma (EDTA)	Therap:	20–65 μg/mL	82–268 μmol/L
Flecainide	Serum or plasma (hep or EDTA);	Therap:	0.2–1.0 μg/mL	0.5–2.4 μmol/L
	trough	Toxic:	>1.0 μg/mL	>2.4 μmol/L
Flurazepam	Serum or plasma (EDTA)	Therap:	not well defined	
		Toxic:	>0.2 μg/mL	>0.5 μmol/L
Furosemide	Serum (30 min after dose)	Therap:	1–2 μg/mL	3–6 μmol/L
Gentamicin	Serum or plasma (EDTA)	Therap:		
		Peak (severe infection)	8–10 μg/mL	16.7–20.9 μmol/L
		Trough (severe infection)	<2–4 μg/mL	<4.2–8.4 μmol/L
		Toxic:		
		Peak	>10 μg/mL	>21 μmol/L
		Trough	>4 μg/mL	>8.4 μmol/L
Glutethimide	Serum	Therap:	2–6 μg/mL	9–28 μmol/L
		Toxic:	>5 μg/mL	>23 μmol/L
Haloperidol	Serum or plasma (hep or EDTA)	Therap:	6–245 ng/mL	16–652 nmol/L
		Toxic:	not defined	
Ibuprofen	Serum or plasma (hep or EDTA)	Therap:	10–50 μg/mL	49–243 μmol/L
		Toxic:	100–700 μg/mL	485–3395 μmol/L
Imipramine	Serum or plasma (hep or EDTA);	Therap:	125–250 ng/mL	446–893 nmol/L
	trough (≥12 h after dose)	Toxic:	>500 ng/mL	>1784 nmol/L

Drug	Specimen		Conventional Units	SI Units
Isoniazid	Serum or plasma (hep or EDTA)	Therap:	1–7 µg/mL	7–51 µmol/L
		Toxic:	20–710 µg/mL	146–5176 µmol/L
Kanamycin	Serum or plasma (EDTA)	Therap:		
		Peak	25–35 µg/mL	52–72 µmol/L
		Trough (severe infection)	4–8 µg/mL	8–16 µmol/L
		Toxic:		
		Peak	>35 µg/mL	>72 µmol/L
		Trough	>10 µg/mL	>21 µmol/L
Lidocaine	Serum or plasma (hep or EDTA); ≥45 min following bolus dose	Therap:	1.5–6.0 µg/mL	6.4–26 µmol/L
		Toxic:		
		CNS or cardiovascular depression	6–8 µg/mL	26–34.2 µmol/L
		Seizures, obtundation, decreased cardiac output	>8 µg/mL	>34.2 µmol/L
Lithium	Serum or plasma (hep or EDTA); (>12 h after last dose)	Therap:	0.6–1.2 mEq/L	0.6–1.2 nmol/L
		Toxic:	>2 mEq/L	>2 mmol/L
Lorazepam	Serum or plasma (hep or EDTA)	Therap:	50–240 ng/mL	156–746 nmol/L
Meperidine	Serum or plasma (hep or EDTA)	Therap:	400–700 ng/mL	1620–2830 nmol/L
		Toxic:	>1 µg/mL	>4043 nmol/L
Meprobamate	Serum	Therap:	6–12 µg/mL	28–55 µmol/L
		Toxic:	>60 µg/mL	>275 µmol/L
Methadone	Serum or plasma (hep or EDTA)	Therap:	100–400 ng/mL	0.32–1.29 µmol/L
		Toxic:	>2000 ng/mL	>6.46 µmol/L
Methaqualone	Serum or plasma (hep or EDTA)	Therap:	2–3 µg/mL	8–12 µmol/L
		Toxic:	>10 µg/mL	>40 µmol/L
Methotrexate	Serum or plasma (hep or EDTA)	Therap:	variable	variable
		Toxic:		
		Low-dose therapy (1–2 wk)	>9.1 ng/mL	>20 nmol/L
		High-dose therapy (48 h)	>227 ng/mL	>0.5 µmol/L
Methsuximide (N-desmethyl methsuximide)	Serum	Therap:	10–40 µg/mL	53–212 µmol/L
		Toxic:	>40 µg/mL	>212 µmol/L

Table continued on following page

Drugs—Therapeutic and Toxic Levels *(Continued)*

DRUG	SPECIMEN		REFERENCE INTERVAL (CONVENTIONAL UNITS)	REFERENCE INTERVAL (INTERNATIONAL UNITS)
Methyldopa	Plasma (EDTA)	Therap:	1–5 µg/mL	4.7–23.7 µmol/L
		Toxic:	>7 µg/mL	>33 µmol/L
Methyprylon	Serum	Therap:	8–10 µg/mL	43–55 µmol/L
		Toxic:	>50 µg/mL	>273 µmol/L
Morphine	Serum or plasma (hep or EDTA)	Therap:	10–80 ng/mL	35–280 nmol/L
		Toxic:	>200 ng/mL	>700 nmol/L
N-Acetylprocainamide	Serum or plasma (hep or EDTA); trough	Therap:	5–30 µg/mL	18–108 µmol/L
		Toxic:	>40 µg/mL	>144 µmol/L
Netilmicin	Serum or plasma (EDTA)	Therap:		
		Peak (severe infection)	8–10 µg/mL	17–21 µmol/L
		Trough (severe infection)	<4 µg/mL	<8 µmol/L
		Toxic:		
		Peak	>12 µg/mL	>25 µmol/L
		Trough	>4 µg/mL	>8 µmol/L
Nitroprusside	Serum or plasma (EDTA)	As thiocyanate:		
		Therap:	6–29 µg/mL	103–499 µmol/L
Nortriptyline	Serum or plasma (hep or EDTA); trough (≥12 h after dose)	Therap:	50–150 ng/mL	190–570 nmol/L
		Toxic:	>500 ng/mL	>1900 nmol/L
Oxazepam	Serum or plasma (hep or EDTA)	Therap:	0.2–1.4 µg/mL	0.70–4.9 µmol/L
Oxycodone	Serum	Therap:	10–100 ng/mL	32–317 nmol/L
		Toxic:	>200 ng/mL	>634 nmol/L
Paraquat	Whole blood (EDTA)	Toxic:	0.1–1.6 µg/mL	0.39–6.2 µmol/L
	Urine	Occup exp:	0.3 µg/mL	1.17 µmol/L
		Toxic:	0.9–64 µg/mL	3.50–249 µmol/L

Pentazocine	Serum or plasma (EDTA)	Therap:	0.05–0.2 µg/mL	0.2–0.7 µmol/L
		Toxic:	>1 µg/mL	>3.5 µmol/L
	Urine	Toxic:	>3 µg/mL	>10.5 µmol/L
Pentobarbital	Serum or plasma (hep or EDTA); trough	Therap:	1–5 µg/mL	4–22 µmol/L
		Hypnotic	20–50 µg/mL	88–221 µg/mL
		Therap coma	>10 µg/mL	>44 µmol/L
		Toxic:		
Phenacetin	Plasma (EDTA)	Therap:	1–30 µg/mL	6–167 µmol/L
		Toxic:	50–250 µg/mL	279–1395 µmol/L
Phencyclidine	Serum or plasma (hep or EDTA)	Toxic:	90–800 ng/mL	370–3288 nmol/L
Phenobarbital	Serum or plasma (hep or EDTA); trough	Therap:	15–40 µg/mL	65–170 µmol/L
		Toxic:		
		Slowness, ataxia, nystagmus	35–80 µg/mL	151–345 µmol/L
		Coma with reflexes	65–117 µg/mL	280–504 µmol/L
		Coma without reflexes	>100 µg/mL	>430 µmol/L
Phensuximide (both parent and N-desmethyl metabolites)	Serum or plasma (hep or EDTA)	Therap:	40–60 µg/mL	228–324 µmol/L
Phenytoin	Plasma (EDTA)	Therap: (not well defined)	50–100 µg/mL	162–324 µmol/L
		Toxic:	>100 µg/mL	>324 µmol/L
Phenylpropanolamine	Serum	Therap:	0.05–0.10 µg/mL	0.33–0.66 µmol/L
		Toxic:	>5 µg/mL	>33.07 µmol/L
Phenytoin	Serum or plasma (hep or EDTA); trough	Therap:	10–20 µg/mL	40–79 µmol/L
		Toxic:	>20 µg/mL	>79 µmol/L
Primidone	Serum or plasma (hep or EDTA); trough	Therap:	5–12 µg/mL	23–55 µmol/L
		Toxic:	>15 µg/mL	>69 µmol/L
Procainamide	Serum or plasma (hep or EDTA); trough	Therap:	4–10 µg/mL	17–42 µmol/L
		Toxic:	>10–12 µg/mL	>42–51 µmol/L
	Also consider effect of metabolite, N-acetylprocainamide			
Propoxyphene	Plasma (EDTA)	Therap:	0.1–0.4 µg/mL	0.3–1.2 µmol/L
		Toxic:	>0.5 µg/mL	>1.5 µmol/L

Table continued on following page

Drugs—Therapeutic and Toxic Levels (*Continued*)

DRUG	SPECIMEN		REFERENCE INTERVAL (CONVENTIONAL UNITS)	REFERENCE INTERVAL (INTERNATIONAL UNITS)
Propranolol	Serum or plasma (hep or EDTA); trough	Therap:	50–100 ng/mL	193–386 nmol/L
Protriptyline	Serum or plasma (hep or EDTA); trough (≥12 h after dose)	Therap:	70–250 ng/mL	226–950 nmol/L
		Toxic:	>500 ng/mL	>1900 nmol/L
Quinidine	Serum or plasma (hep or EDTA); trough	Therap:	2–5 µg/mL	6–15 µmol/L
		Toxic:	>6 µg/mL	>18 µmol/L
Salicylates	Serum or plasma (hep or EDTA); trough	Therap:	150–300 µg/mL	1086–2172 µmol/L
		Toxic:	>300 µg/mL	>2172 µmol/L
Secobarbital	Serum	Therap:	1–2 µg/mL	4.2–8.4 µmol/L
		Toxic:	>5 µg/mL	>21.0 µmol/L
Theophylline	Serum or plasma (hep or EDTA)	Therap:	8–20 µg/mL	44–111 µmol/L
		Toxic:	>20 µg/mL	>110 µmol/L
Thiocyanate	Serum or plasma (EDTA)	Nonsmoker:	1–4 µg/mL	17–69 µmol/L
		Smoker:	3–12 µg/mL	52–206 µmol/L
		Therap, after nitroprusside infusion:	6–29 µg/mL	103–499 µmol/L
	Urine	Nonsmoker:	1–4 mg/d	17–69 µmol/L
		Smoker:	7–17 mg/d	120–292 µmol/L
Thiopental	Serum or plasma (hep or EDTA); trough	Hypnotic:	1–5 µg/mL	4.1–20.7 µmol/L
		Coma:	30–100 µg/mL	124–413 µmol/L
		Anesthesia:	7–130 µg/mL	29–536 µmol/L
		Toxic conc:	>10 µg/mL	>41 µmol/L

Drug	Specimen		Therapeutic / Toxic	Conventional	SI units
Thioridazine	Serum or plasma (hep or EDTA)		Therap:	1.0–1.5 µg/mL	2.7–4.1 µmol/L
			Toxic:	>10 µg/mL	>27 µmol/L
Tobramycin	Serum or plasma (hep or EDTA)		Therap:		
			Peak (severe infection)	8–10 µg/mL	17–21 µmol/L
			Trough (severe infection)	<4 µg/mL	<9 µmol/L
			Toxic:		
			Peak	>10 µg/mL	>21 µmol/L
			Trough	>4 µg/mL	>9 µmol/L
Tocainide	Serum or plasma (hep or EDTA)		Therap:	4–10 µg/mL	21–52 µmol/L
Tolbutamide	Serum		Therap:	80–240 µg/mL	299–888 µmol/L
			Toxic:	>640 µg/mL	>2368 µmol/L
Valproic acid	Serum or plasma (hep or EDTA); trough		Therap:	50–100 µg/mL	347–693 µmol/L
			Toxic:	>100 µg/mL	>693 µmol/L
Vancomycin	Serum or plasma (hep or EDTA); trough		Therap:	5–10 µg/mL	3–7 µmol/L
			Toxic:	>80–100 µg/mL	>55–69 µmol/L
			(not well established)		
Verapamil	Serum or plasma (hep or EDTA)		Therap:	100–500 ng/mL	220–1100 nmol/L
Warfarin	Serum or plasma (hep or EDTA)		Therap:	1–10 µg/mL	3–32 µmol/L

INDEX
INDEX

INDEX

Note: Page numbers followed by t refer to tables.

Heart *(Continued)*
  in systemic sclerosis, 589, 591
  transplantation of, 200
Heart block, 194–195
  acute myocardial infarction and, 171t
  complete, 171t
  first degree, 171t, 194
  Mobitz type I, 171t, 194, 195
  Mobitz type II, 171t, 194, 195
  third degree, 194
Heart failure, congestive, 176–185. See
    also *Congestive heart failure.*
Helicobacter pylori, in peptic ulcer disease,
    336–337, 338t
Hematoma, subdural, 627t
Hemochromatosis, liver failure in, 372
Hemodialysis, 241–243
  complications of, 242–243
  contraindications to, 242
  dementia and, 627t
  drug therapy during, 251, 251t
  in acute renal failure, 227, 228
  in antiglomerular basement membrane
      nephritis, 261
  in diabetic nephropathy, 257, 257t
  in drug overdosage, 43
  in hyperkalemia, 65
  in myoglobinuric acute renal failure, 232
  indications for, 242
Hemolysis, transfusion-related, 409–410
Hemolytic anemia, 389–392
Hemolytic uremic syndrome, 264
Hemoperfusion, charcoal, in drug over-
    dosage, 43
Hemophilia, 400–402
Hemophilus influenzae, antimicrobials
    against, 82t–85t
Hemoptysis, 280–281
Hemorrhage, in adult respiratory distress
    syndrome, 316
  intracerebral, 637
  subarachnoid, 637
Hemorrhagic stroke, 637
Hemorrhoids, 354
  bleeding with, 363
Hemostasis, disorders of, 396–404. See
    also specific disorders, e.g.,
    Thrombocytopenia.
Henoch-Schönlein purpura, 569
  renal involvement in, 263

Heparin, during pregnancy, 47t
  in deep venous thrombosis, 309, 310t
  in pulmonary embolism, 310t, 311
  in pulmonary embolism prevention,
      313
  preoperative management of, 53–54, 55
Hepatic encephalopathy, 367–368, 367t,
    377
Hepatitis, 365, 366t
  alcoholic, 369–370
  autoimmune, 370
  chronic, 370–372
    in alpha$_1$-antitrypsin deficiency, 372
    in hemochromatosis, 372
    in Wilson's disease, 371–372
  drug-induced, 365–367, 367t, 371
  viral, 371
Hepatitis A immunization, 107t
Hepatitis B immune globulin, 108t
Hepatitis B immunization, 108t
Hepatitis B virus, in hepatocellular carci-
    noma, 466
Hepatitis C virus, blood transfusion trans-
    mission of, 410
  in hepatocellular carcinoma, 466
  mixed cryoglobulinemia and, 569
Hepatocellular carcinoma, 466–467
Hepatolenticular degeneration, 644
Hepatorenal syndrome, 238–239, 368
Hereditary spherocytosis, 390
Herpes simplex virus, antivirals against,
    100t
  cutaneous infection with, 607–608
  in acquired immunodeficiency syn-
      drome, 142t
  rectal infection with, 355
Herpes simplex virus encephalitis, 624
Herpes zoster virus, 609
Heterocyclic antidepressants, 35t
  antidote for, 44t
Hiccups, 340
Hirsutism, 507–508
Histoplasmosis, in acquired immunodefi-
    ciency syndrome, 142t
HMG-CoA reductase inhibitors, during
    pregnancy, 48t
Hoarseness, in gastroesophageal reflux
    disease, 332
Hodgkin's disease, 446–448, 447t
Home parenteral nutrition, 550–551

Percutaneous transluminal coronary angioplasty, in acute myocardial infarction, 167–168
Perdiem Plus (psyllium), during pregnancy,
49t
in constipation, 16, 17t
in diarrhea, 20t
Pergolide (Permax), in Parkinson's disease,
641t, 643
Pericardial effusion, malignant, 427–429,
428t
Pericardial tamponade, in cancer patient,
427–429, 428t
Pericardiocentesis, in cancer patient, 428
Pericardiotomy, in malignant pericardial
effusion, 428t, 429
Pericarditis, after myocardial infarction,
174
in acute renal failure, 226
in systemic lupus erythematosus, 582,
583
Periodic paralysis, 650–651
Peripheral blood stem cell transplantation,
425–426
Peripheral vascular disease, osteomyelitis
in, 120
Peritoneal carcinomatosis, 490
Peritoneal dialysis, acute, 244–245
ambulatory, continuous, 245–247
in diabetic nephropathy, 257–258
drug therapy during, 250–251, 250t
in myoglobinuric acute renal failure,
232
peritonitis during, 125
Peritonitis, 124–125
bacterial, 376–377
with peritoneal dialysis, 245, 245t, 246
Permax (pergolide), in Parkinson's disease,
641t, 643
Perphenazine (Trilafon), during pregnancy,
49t
in psychosis, 25t
Pertussis immunization, 107t
pH, antimicrobial selection and, 75
Pharyngeal dysphagia, 333
Pharyngitis, 94–95
anaerobic, 94–95
group A streptococcal, 94
viral, 94
Phenacemide (Phenurone), 620t

Phenacetin, reference interval for, 659t
Phencyclidine, reference interval for, 659t
Phenelzine (Nardil), in depression, 35t
Phenergan (promethazine), during pregnancy, 48t
in nausea, 23t
Phenobarbital (Luminal), 619t
during pregnancy, 47t
reference interval for, 659t
Phenothiazines, in psychosis, 25t
Phenoxybenzamine (Dibenzyline), during
pregnancy, 48t
in detrusor-sphincter dyssynergia, 40
Phensuximide, reference interval for, 659t
Phentolamine, in hypertensive crisis, 222t
Phenylalanine mustard (melphalan), 415t,
417
Phenylbutazone, in rheumatoid arthritis,
553–556, 555t
reference interval for, 659t
Phenylpropanolamine, during pregnancy,
48t
reference interval for, 659t
Phenytoin (Dilantin), during pregnancy,
47t
for pain, 14
hepatotoxicity of, 366
in seizures, 619t, 622
in status epilepticus, 622
in ventricular arrhythmias, 196t
in ventricular tachycardia, 192
reference interval for, 659t
side effects of, 199t
Pheochromocytoma, 506–507
hypertension with, 223
Phlebotomy, in polycythemia vera, 394
in pulmonary hypertension, 326
Phosphate balance, in chronic renal failure, 239–240
Phosphate supplements, in hypophosphatemia, 68t
Phosphate therapy, in hypercalcemia, 67,
511
in hypercalcemia of malignancy, 432
Phosphodiesterae inhibitors, in congestive
heart failure, 182t
Phosphorus, daily recommended requirements for, 531t
disturbances of, 67–68, 68t
Phosphorus-32, in polycythemia vera, 394